Evidence-Based Cardiology
Second Edition

Evidence-Based Cardiology
Second Edition

Peter J. Sharis, M.D.
Interventional Cardiologist
Cardiovascular Medicine PC
Genesis Heart Institute
Davenport, Iowa

Christopher P. Cannon, M.D.
Associate Professor of Medicine
Harvard Medical School
Brigham and Women's Hospital
Boston, Massachusetts

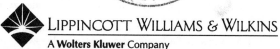

LIPPINCOTT WILLIAMS & WILKINS
A Wolters Kluwer Company

Philadelphia • Baltimore • New York • London
Buenos Aires • Hong Kong • Sydney • Tokyo

Acquisitions Editor : Ruth W. Weinberg
Developmental Editor : Julia Seto
Production Editor : Jeff Somers
Manufacturing Manager : Ben Rivera
Cover Designer : Jeane Norton
Compositor : TechBooks
Printer : RR Donnelley Crawfordsville

Library of Congress Cataloging-in-Publication Data

Sharis, Peter J.
    Evidence-based cardiology / Peter J. Sharis, Christopher P. Cannon.—2nd ed.
      p. ; cm.
    Includes bibliographical references and index.
    ISBN 0-7817-3910-1 (alk. paper)
    1. Heart—Diseases—Handbooks, manuals, etc.   2. Evidence—based
medicine—Handbooks, manuals, etc.   I. Cannon, Christopher P. II. Title.
    [DNLM: 1. Heart Diseases—therapy—Handbooks. 2. Evidence—Based
Medicine—methods—Handbooks. 3. Heart Diseases—diagnosis—Handbooks.
WG 39 S531e 2003]
    RC669.15.S53   2003
    616.1′2—dc21   2003047422

CONTENTS

PREFACE

Perhaps more than any other field of medicine, advances in cardiology are guided by data from large clinical trials. The number of major trials evaluating pharmacologic agents and diagnostic and therapeutic procedures continues to undergo significant growth. Since the publication of the first edition of *Evidence-Based Cardiology,* results of hundreds of trials have been published or presented.

The two primary goals of *Evidence-Based Cardiology* remain the systematic summarization of major trial data and placing the information from these annotated studies in context. The results of major randomized trials in six major topic areas are presented in systematic fashion, including the design, study population, exclusion criteria, treatment regimen, and results; some older trials have been eliminated to limit the book length. Meta-analyses, review articles, nonrandomized and less important trials have abbreviated summaries. Importantly, the chapter overviews preceding the annotated references have been expanded with particular attention to discussing relevant ACC/AHA Practice Guidelines.

Chapter 1 focuses on preventive cardiology, particularly lipid and diet management, but also each of the multiple risk factors for coronary artery disease; in the second edition, the new statin trials and the updated National Cholesterol Education Program (NCEP) Guidelines are reviewed. There is also increased material on other emerging coronary heart disease risk factors and assessment measures, such as high sensitivity C-reactive protein (CRP). Chapter 2 focuses on major revascularization procedures, primarily coronary artery stenting and bypass surgery. New material includes data on drug-eluting stents and distal embolic protection devices. Chapters 3 and 4 cover the wealth of data on acute coronary syndromes. New material includes trial data on invasive management, low molecular heparin therapy and clopidogrel. Chapter 5 focuses on the pharmacologic management of heart failure, with new material on biventricular pacing for CHF. Chapter 6 has been expanded to include both atrial fibrillation with extensive new material on pacemakers and ventricular arrhythmias and implantable cardioverter defibrillators (ICDs).

We wish to acknowledge the co-authors of Chapters 5 and 6 (Duane Pinot and Matt Reynolds), who provided extensive assistance in revising, updating, and expanding these two chapters. We also acknowledge the following cardiologists who provided extremely helpful comments and suggestions on specific chapters: Joe Carrozza and Nicolas Shammas (Chapter 2), C. Michael Gibson (Chapters 3 and 4). And we thank Eugene Braunwald, whose expert mentorship has impressed upon us the importance of well-designed clinical trials to evaluate new therapies, as well as the careful, considerate analysis to incorporate their results into current practice.

1. PREVENTIVE CARDIOLOGY: RISK FACTORS FOR CORONARY ARTERY DISEASE AND PRIMARY AND SECONDARY PREVENTION TRIALS

CHOLESTEROL, LIPIDS, AND DIET

Epidemiology

An estimated 65 million Americans have elevated total cholesterol (TC) levels, and based on the new National Cholesterol Education Cholesterol (NCEP) III Guidelines, 37 million (one in five adults) are eligible for cholesterol-lowering therapy. A 10% decrease in TC is associated with an approximately 10% to 15% lower coronary heart disease (CHD) mortality rate and an approximately 20% decrease in the risk of myocardial infarction (MI) (see *Lancet* 1986;2:933; *JAMA* 1995;274:131). When TC levels are reduced by lifestyle modification (e.g., diet, exercise) and/or pharmacologic intervention, more benefit is derived in younger individuals (*N Engl J Med* 1993;328:313), and the full benefits of a sustained decrease are not achieved for at least 5 years (*BMJ* 1994;308:367). Very low TC levels have been associated with higher mortality rates than those found with normal TC levels (see *Circulation* 1995;92:2396); however, this is likely owing to the higher prevalence of cancer in such individuals. Cardiac risk tables have been created to estimate the risk of CHD death at various cholesterol levels and in combination with other major CRFs. The NCEP III guidelines use modified Framingham risk score tables to estimate the 10-year CHD risk (see **Table 1.2**).

Low-density lipoprotein (LDL) has been shown in several studies, including the Framingham Heart Study, Multiple Risk Factor Intervention Trial (MRFIT), and Lipid Research Clinics (LRC) trial, to be a stronger predictor of CHD than is TC (see *JAMA* 1984;251:351 and 1986;256:2823). As a result, LDL levels are the primary focus of the NCEP III Guidelines. Of note, recent evidence suggests that C-reactive protein, a marker of inflammation, is an even stronger CHD predictor than is LDL (see page 14).

High levels of high-density lipoproteins (HDLs) are associated with a decreased risk of CHD mortality; a 1% lower HDL-C is associated with a 2% to 3% higher CHD risk (8; also see *Am Heart J* 1985;110:1100). The NCEP III guidelines now consider a low HDL level as less than 40 mg/dL (vs. less than 35 mg/dL in NCEP II) an indicator of increased risk, whereas a level of 60 mg/dL or greater is a negative cardiac risk factor (**Table 1.1**). Non-HDL cholesterol levels also have been demonstrated to be predictors of cardiovascular disease (CVD) (10,11) and the new NCEP Guidelines now provide non-HDL goals for various risk categories (see **Table 1.1**).

Growing evidence indicates that high triglyceride (TG) levels are a modest independent predictor of increased CHD mortality (50,52). One analysis of studies with nearly 60,000 participants found that even after adjustment for multiple CRFs, high TG levels are associated with significant 14% and 37% reductions in cardiovascular risk in men and women, respectively (48). Obesity, physical inactivity, glucose intolerance, hypothyroidism, and the use of β-blockers, estrogen, and diuretics are associated with an increased risk of hypertriglyceridemia. The NCEP Guidelines now classify TG levels of less than 150 mg/dL as desirable, 150 to 199 mg/dL as borderline, 200 to 499 mg/dL as high, and 500 mg/dL or greater as very high.

Lipoprotein(a) [Lp(a)], which is structurally similar to LDL except for the addition of a single apolipoprotein(a) molecule, is a weak independent risk factor for CHD. Although individual studies have yielded conflicting results (49,50,52–55), a recent meta-analysis of 27 studies with at least 1 year of follow-up data found a 1.6-fold higher risk among those in top third of Lp(a) levels compared with those in the bottom third (53). Levels are difficult to measure, and various measurement and storage techniques have been used in different studies. Most important, it is difficult to reduce Lp(a) levels significantly with lipid-lowering agents (niacin and estrogen appear best), and the clinical significance of reducing Lp(a) levels is unknown.

TABLE 1.1. NCEP RECOMMENDATIONS FOR THERAPEUTIC LIFESTYLE CHANGES AND DRUG TREATMENT BASED ON LOW-DENSITY LIPOPROTEIN CHOLESTEROL LEVELS

Risk Category	LDL Goal	LDL Level to Initiate TLC	LDL Level at Which to Consider Drug(s)	Non-HDL Goal[a]
CHD or CHD risk equivalents (10-yr risk, >20%)	<100	≥100	>130 (100–129: drug(s) optional)	<130
≥2 Risk factors (10-yr risk, <20%)	<130	≥130	10-yr risk 10–20%, ≥130 10-yr risk <10%, ≥160	<160
0–1 Risk factors	<160	≥160	>190 (160–189: drugs optional)	<190

All LDL levels are in mg/dL. Diabetes is considered a CHD (coronary heart disease) risk equivalent. Positive risk factors include current smoking; hypertension; family history of premature CHD (men =55 yr, women =65 years), HDL <40 mg/dL and age (men =45 years, women =55 years or premature menopause without estrogen replacement therapy). HDL =60 mg/dL is considered a negative risk factor.
HDL, high-density lipoprotein; LDL, low-density lipoprotein; NCEP, National, Cholesterol Education Program.
[a]Non-HDL (total cholesterol − HDL) is a secondary target of therapy in persons with high serum triglycerides (≥200 mg/dL).

National Cholesterol Education Program Guidelines

The NCEP III guidelines recommend that all adults undergo a lipid panel analysis at least once every 5 years, starting at age 20 years (3,6), and now recommend that the initial screening include LDL measurement and TG measurement. Compared with NCEP II, NCEP III has several other changes, including (a) patients with diabetes and other high-risk disorders (peripheral vascular disease, symptomatic carotid disease, abdominal aortic aneurysm) are considered a CHD equivalent; (b) use of a modified Framingham risk table to identify higher-risk patients; (c) non–HDL-C targets for different risk categories; and (d) recognition of the metabolic syndrome.

NCEP LDL goals are listed in **Table 1.1**; of note, a 10-year CHD risk of more than 20% is considered a CHD risk equivalent. **Table 1.2** provides the modified Framingham point scores that should be used to estimate this 10-year risk. Drug therapy is listed as optional for those with CHD/CHD risk equivalents and an LDL of 100 to 129 mg/dL; however, the subsequently published 20,536-patient Heart Protection Study (31) provides persuasive data that drug therapy should be initiated within this range. In elderly patients, the NCEP report recommends considering drug therapy only for primary prevention. Whereas this suggestion was based on limited data, two large recent reports found a significant benefit of drug therapy in older patients, suggesting that such therapy should be routinely used if indicated (32; also see *Arch Intern Med* 2002;162:1395).

Diet and Vitamins

The nutrient composition of the therapeutic lifestyle changes (TLC) diet includes the following: saturated fat, less than 7% of total calories; total fat, 25% to 35% of calories; fiber, 20 to 30 g/day; and cholesterol, less than 200 mg/day. Fiber has minimal impact on cholesterol, and approximately 25% of compliant patients have no response; the average response is a reduction in TC of only 10% to 15%.

Increased vitamin E intake was associated with less CVD in several epidemiologic studies, including the Nurses Health Study (62). In the Cambridge Heart Antioxidant Study (CHAOS) (59), a randomized study of 2,002 CAD patients, vitamin E supplementation was associated with a significantly lower incidence of cardiovascular death and MI. However, in the Alpha-Tocopherol Beta-Carotene Cancer Prevention (ATBC)

TABLE 1.2. ESTIMATE OF 10-YEAR CORONARY HEART DISEASE RISK FOR MEN AND WOMEN (FRAMINGHAM POINT SCORES)

1. Age (yr)

20–34: −9/−7
35–39: −4/−3
40–44: 0/0
45–49: 3/3
50–54: 6/6
55–59: 8/8
60–64: 10/10
65–69: 11/12
70–74: 12/14
75–79: 13/16

2. Total Cholesterol, mg/dL	Age 20–39 yr	Age 40–49 yr	Age 50–59 yr	Age 60–69 yr	Age 70–79 yr
<160	0/0	0/0	0/0	0/0	0/0
160–199	4/4	3/3	2/2	1/1	0/1
200–239	7/8	5/6	3/4	1/2	0/1
240–279	9/11	6/8	4/5	2/3	1/2
≥280	11/13	8/10	5/7	3/4	1/2

3. Smoking Status	Age 20–39 yr	Age 40–49 yr	Age 50–59 yr	Age 60–69 yr	Age 70–79 yr
Nonsmoker	0/0	0/0	0/0	0/0	0/0
Smoker	8/9	5/7	3/4	1/2	1/1

4. HDL (mg/dL)

>60: −1/−1
50–59: 0/0
40–49: 1/1
<40: 2

5. Systolic BP, mm Hg	If Untreated	If Treated
<120	0/0	0/0
120–129	0/1	1/3
130–139	1/2	2/4
140–159	1/3	2/5
≥160	2/4	3/6

Point Total	10-yr Risk (%)	Point Total	10-yr Risk (%)
<0	<1/<1	13	12/2
1	1/<1	14	16/2
2	1/<1	15	20/3
3	1/<1	16	25/4
4	1/<1	17	≥30/5
5	2/<1	18	≥30/6
6	2/<1	19	≥30/8
7	3/<1	20	≥30/11
8	3/<1	21	≥30/14
9	5/1	22	≥30/17
10	6/1	23	≥30/22
11	8/1	24	≥30/27
12	10/1	25	≥30/30

The score for each of the five components should be added together and the total point total used to estimate the 10-year risk of CHD. If the 10-year risk is >20%, this is considered a CHD risk equivalent (see Table 1.1). If the risk is 10–20%, then among those with 2+ CHD risk factors, LDL-lowering drug therapy should be initiated at a LDL level ≥130 (vs. ≥160 if 10-yr risk is <10%) (see Table 1.1).

CHD, coronary heart disease; LDL, low-density lipoprotein; BP, blood pressure; HDL, high-density lipoprotein.

trial (63), GISSI Prevention Study (64), and Heart Outcome Prevention Evaluation (HOPE) study, all found no benefit associated with vitamin E supplementation (65).

No benefit of β-carotene supplementation was observed in the Physicians Health Study (60), whereas the Beta-Carotene and Retinol Efficacy Trial (CARET) was stopped early because of an excess of lung cancer, lung cancer deaths, and all-cause mortality (61), and the ATBC trial found a significant excess of cardiac deaths (63).

Special Diets

1. Fish and omega-3 fatty acid (FA) consumption: In a study of 852 Dutch men, the mortality rate was more than 50% lower among those consuming over 30 g of fish per day (equivalent of one to two dishes per week) (see *N Engl J Med* 1985;312:1305). In the 2,033 patient, randomized Diet and Reinfarction trial, the group advised to increase omega-3 FA intake via fish consumption or fish oil supplementation had a 29% lower mortality compared to no advice group (see *Lancet* 1989;2:757). In a prospective, nested case-control analysis of Physicians' Health Study participants with 17 years of follow-up, men with baseline long-chain n-3 fatty acid (FA) levels in the third and fourth quartiles had significantly reduced risks of sudden death compared with those in first quartile (adjusted RRs, 0.28, 0.19) (73). In the 11,324 patient GISSI Prevenzione trial, supplementation with 850 mg of omega-3 FA decreased sudden death by 45% and all-cause mortality by 20%, even in those receiving standard therapy [e.g., aspirin (ASA), statins]. Evidence also exists that increased fish intake results in a reduced risk of ischemic stroke (see *JAMA* 2002;288:3130).

   Based on these and other data, the American Heart Association (AHA) recently issued recommendations that persons with documented CHD should consume about 1 g of omega-3 FAs per day (74). In those unable to eat sufficient amounts of fish to meet this requirement, it recommends daily supplementation with 1-g fish oil capsules that contain 180 mg of eicosapentaenoic acid and 120 mg of docosahexaenoic acid. In individuals with high TG levels, higher amounts (2 to 4 g/day) should be considered.

2. High fiber: Analysis of 21,930 ABTC patients showed the risk of CHD death to be inversely related to fiber intake [highest quintile (34.8 g/day) vs. lowest quintile (16.1 g/day); RR of CHD death, 0.69] (69). A recent Nurses' Health Study analysis also found a significant association between fiber intake and CHD events. A 10-g/day increase in daily fiber intake was associated with a multivariate RR of 0.81 [95% confidence interval (CI), 0.66 to 0.99; see *JAMA* 1999;281:1998]. Finally, a recent analysis of 39,876 female health professionals found a 21% nonsignificant reduction of cardiovascular events among those in the highest quintile (26.3 g/day) of fiber intake compared with those in lowest quintile (12.5 g/day) (72).

3. Mediterranean (includes more bread, fruit, and margarine, and less meat, butter, and cream): The randomized 605-patient Lyon Heart Study found a 73% reduction in death and MI at 2.3-year follow-up, and a significant 56% all-cause mortality reduction at 3.8-year follow-up (66). The benefits of this diet appear correlated with increased omega-3 FA intake (see *Am J Cardiol* 2000;85:1239).

DRUGS

Bile Resins (e.g., Cholestyramine, Colestipol)

These agents lower lipid levels by binding and blocking the reabsorption of bile acids. These agents typically decrease LDL cholesterol by 15% to 30%, increase HDL by 3% to 5%, and possibly increase TG levels. Compliance is often problematic because of their poor taste and gastrointestinal (GI) side effects, such as abdominal fullness, bloating, flatulence, and constipation. Numerous drug interactions also are found, and use is associated with an increased risk of gallstones. In the Lipid Research Clinic Coronary Primary Prevention Trial (13), cholestyramine use in 3,806 men with a mean TC of 291 mg/dL and LDL of 215 mg/dL resulted in 17% fewer MIs and a 19% reduction in CHD death and MI over the 7.4-year follow-up period. However, the all-cause mortality rate was not significantly different. The Cholesterol Lowering Atherosclerosis Study (CLAS) (34) was a smaller angiographic study that evaluated the combination of colestipol and niacin in 162 men with prior coronary artery bypass graft (CABG) surgery. Drug treatment resulted in lower TC (26%) and LDL levels (43%), higher HDL levels (37%), a higher atherosclerosis regression rate (16.2% vs. 2.4%), and fewer new lesions in bypass grafts. The Familial Atherosclerosis Treatment Study (FATS) (35) and a National Heart, Lung, and Blood Institute study (see *Circulation* 1984;69:313) were angiographic studies that both showed beneficial lipid-lowering effects and better angiographic outcomes in colestipol-treated patients.

Niacin

Niacin is a B vitamin that inhibits the mobilization of free FAs from peripheral tissues, with a resulting decrease in hepatic synthesis of TGs and secretion of very low density lipoproteins (VLDLs). Niacin typically decreases LDL by 10% to 25%, increases HDL by 15% to 35%, decreases TGs by 20% to 50%, and decreases Lp(a). A common side effect is flushing, which is often controllable by daily ASA use. A long-acting formulation of niacin appears to reduce flushing. Other side effects of niacin include hyperglycemia, increased uric acid levels, increased liver function tests, exacerbation of peptic ulcer disease, and rhabdomyolysis (rare). In the Coronary Drug Project (21), a randomized trial enrolling more than 8,000 men with prior MI, the use of niacin, 3 g/day, was associated with a 27% lower nonfatal MI rate at 5-year follow-up and a significant 11% reduction in overall mortality at 15 years. Other trials evaluating the use of niacin in combination with other agents [e.g., CLAS, FATS, HDL-Atherosclerosis Treatment Study (HATS) (34,35,47)] also showed significant favorable changes in lipid levels and reduced rates of CHD mortality.

Fibric Acid Derivatives (e.g., Gemfibrozil, Fenofibrate)

These agents (e.g., gemfibrozil, fenofibrate) typically increase HDL levels by 10% to 15%, decrease triglycerides by 20% to 50%, and have a minimal effect on LDL levels. They are usually well tolerated. The Helsinki Heart Study (14) evaluated the effect of gemfibrozil in 4,081 asymptomatic hypercholesterolemic men. At 5-year follow-up, gemfibrozil use was associated with 34% fewer cardiac events and a 26% lower CHD mortality rate. However, the overall mortality rate was not significantly different because of more deaths due to accidents, violence, and intracranial hemorrhage in the gemfibrozil group. The Veterans Administration HDL Intervention Trial (VA-HIT), which was a secondary prevention trial of 2,531 patients, found that gemfibrozil was associated with a nonsignificant 10% mortality reduction and 20% reduction in the incidence of coronary artery disease (CAD)-related death and MI (27).

The World Health Organization Cooperative Study (12) evaluated clofibrate in 10,627 hypercholesterolemic men. At an average follow-up of 5.3 years, the clofibrate group had 25% fewer nonfatal MIs, but a 47% increase in overall mortality ($p < 0.05$). The Coronary Drug Project found that clofibrate use had no significant effect on all-cause mortality.

Cholesterol Absorption Inhibitors

This new class of agents works by inhibiting the intestinal absorption of dietary and biliary cholesterol by blocking the passage across the intestinal wall. Ezetimibe, now approved by the Food and Drug Administration (FDA), results in moderate LDL reduction when used as monotherapy (18% in one study; see *Clin Ther* 2001;23:1209). More important, its effects appear additive to those provided by the statins (17–19). In one randomized study of 769 patients not at LDL goal at baseline, 72% taking ezetimibe and a statin achieved LDL goal compared with 19% taking statin alone (17). Coadministration is well tolerated (20–22). Therefore ezetimibe should be considered in patients not at LDL goal with statin monotherapy.

3-Hydroxy-3-Methylglutaryl-Coenzyme A Reductase Inhibitors (Statins)

These agents inhibit the rate-limiting step of cholesterol synthesis in the liver and typically decrease LDL by 20% to 60%, increase HDL by 5% to 15%, and decrease TGs by 10% to 20%. Potency (weakest to strongest on milligram-per-milligram basis) may be characterized as follows: fluvastatin, lovastatin, pravastatin, simvastatin, atorvastatin [a sixth agent, rosuvastatin, not yet approved for use in the United States, appears slightly more potent than atorvastatin (see *Am J Cardiol* 2003;91:33 and STELLAR and MERCURY I trial. Results presented at 52nd ACC session, March 2003.)].

All these agents except pravastatin are metabolized by the cytochrome P450 system.

Side effects of the statins are uncommon (approximately 1% to 2%) and include mild GI intolerance, increased liver function test values, myositis (rare and usually with concurrent niacin, cyclosporine, gemfibrozil, or erythromycin). It is important to titrate or increase the dose of a specific agent until the NCEP LDL goal as one analysis of approximately 5,000 CAD patients found that only 25% had met the NCEP LDL goal of less than 100 mg/dL.

Several mechanisms of action ("pleiotropism") are proposed by which these agents achieve significant reductions in CHD and overall mortality:

1. Increased luminal diameter: unlikely because most angiographic trials [e.g., CLAS-I, FATS, MARS, CCAIT, SCRIP, MAAS, PLAC-I, REGRESS, LCAS, SCAT, HATS (34–41,43,45,47,48)] demonstrate minimal or no changes.
2. Restoration of endothelium-dependent vasodilatation: a small study (*Circulation* 1999;99:3227–3233) found that initiation early after acute coronary syndromes (ACSs) (10.4 ± 0.7 days) rapidly improved endothelial function after 6 weeks of therapy (see also *Circulation* 1994;89:2519 and *N Engl J Med* 1995;332:481, 488).
3. Inhibition of thrombus formation (see *JAMA* 1998;279:1643, *J Am Coll Cardiol* 1999;93:1294, and later section on early statin initiation).
4. Antiinflammatory effects: statins significantly reduce C-reactive protein levels (see Pravastatin Inflammation/CRP Evaluation (PRINCE) results (166)].
5. Decreased cholesterol content in lesions, leading to more stable fibrous cap and other plaque-stabilization effects (see *Circulation* 2001;103:926).

A recent meta-analysis of 59 randomized, controlled trials found that several classes of lipid agents lower cholesterol, but only the statins significantly reduced CHD-related and all-cause mortality [34% and 25% RR reductions (RRRs), respectively] (4). In another meta-analysis of only statin trials (3), statin-treated patients had a 22% lower overall mortality rate, a 28% lower cardiovascular mortality rate, and 29% fewer strokes. Another analysis found that the effect of these agents widens with time [7% lower mortality in the first 2 years (25% by 5 years) (see *BMJ* 1994;308: 367–373)].

PRIMARY PREVENTION TRIALS

The West of Scotland Coronary Prevention Study (WOSCOPS) (15) was a randomized, placebo-controlled trial of 6,595 patients with an average TC of 272 mg/dL. At 5 years, the pravastatin group had 29% fewer nonfatal MIs ($p < 0.001$), a 32% lower cardiovascular mortality rate ($p = 0.033$), and a 22% lower overall mortality rate ($p = 0.051$). The Air Force/Texas Coronary Atherosclerosis Prevention Study (AFCAPS/TexCAPS) (16) randomized 9,605 men and postmenopausal women with average TC and LDL levels and below-average HDL levels to lovastatin or placebo. At average follow-up of 5.2 years, the lovastatin group had a 37% reduction ($p < 0.001$) in the risk for acute major coronary events. Only 17% of AFCAPS/TexCAPS patients would be recommended by the NCEP guidelines for drug therapy, suggesting that perhaps the guidelines should be expanded. Finally, the atorvastatin vs. Placebo arm of the Anglo-Scandinavian Cardiac Outcomes Trial (ASCOT) (10,305 patients) was stopped in October 2002 because the atorvastatin group had a significant 36% reduction in nonfatal MI and fatal CHD compared with those with placebo (1.9% vs. 3.0%, $P = 0.0005$) (20).

SECONDARY PREVENTION TRIALS

The Scandinavian Simvastatin Survival Study (4S) (23) was a randomized, placebo-controlled trial enrolling 4,444 patients with an elevated TC ($\geq$213 mg/dL) and a history of CAD. At 5.4-year follow-up, the use of simvastatin, 40 mg/day, was associated with a 25% lower TC, a 35% lower LDL, a 42% lower CHD mortality rate, and a highly significant 30% relative reduction in lower overall mortality rate ($p =$ 0.0003). Simvastatin patients also underwent 34% fewer coronary revascularization procedures and had fewer fatal and nonfatal cerebrovascular events.

The Cholesterol and Recurrent Events (CARE) trial (24) examined the use of pravastatin (40 mg/day) in patients with normal or mildly elevated TC (less than 240 mg/dL). At 5 years, pravastatin was associated with 24% fewer cardiac deaths and nonfatal MIs ($p =$ 0.003). If the baseline LDL level was less than 125 mg/dL, only diabetic patients had a significant benefit.

The Long-term Intervention with Pravastatin in Ischemic Disease (LIPID) trial (25) enrolled more than 9,000 patients with known CAD and average TC levels (155 to 271 mg/dL). Pravastatin (40 mg/day) was associated with a 24% RRR in CHD mortality ($p < 0.001$), 22% RRR in overall mortality rate ($p < 0.001$), 19% RRR in strokes ($p = 0.048$), and 20% RRR in revascularization procedures ($p < 0.001$). Thus both the LIPID and CARE trials provide compelling data to support aggressive lipid lowering with statins in CAD patients with normal TC levels.

The Post-CABG trial (42) was an angiographic trial of 1,351 patients with one patent saphenous venous coronary bypass graft that showed that aggressive LDL-lowering therapy with lovastatin, 40 to 80 mg/day (and cholestyramine added if necessary), to achieve a target LDL of less than 85 mg/dL was associated with less graft atherosclerotic progression and 29% fewer revascularization procedures ($p = 0.03$). These data suggest that achieving very low LDL levels in post-CABG patients is important.

The Atorvastatin versus Revascularization Treatments (AVERT) trial (26) randomized 341 patients with stable one- or two-vessel CAD referred for percutaneous coronary intervention (PCI) to aggressive LDL lowering with atorvastatin 80 mg/day or PCI. At 18-month follow-up, the atorvastatin group had a nonsignificant 36% reduction in cardiovascular events. The results of this study are controversial, with critics pointing out its small size and that enrolled patients were not ideal PCI candidates. In the Lescol Intervention Prevention Study (LIPS), 1,677 patients with stable or unstable angina or silent ischemia after successful first PCI were randomized to fluvastatin, 80 mg/day, or placebo (29). The fluvastatin group had a significantly lower incidence of one or more major events (21.4% vs. 26.7%; RR, 0.78; $p = 0.01$). Subgroup analyses demonstrated even more robust reductions with fluvastatin in diabetics (RR, 0.53; $p = 0.04$) and in those with multivessel disease (RR, 0.66; $p = 0.01$).

The better to determine whether aggressive lipid-lowering therapy with PCI is the optimal care pathway, the Clinical Outcomes Utilizing Revascularization and Aggressive Drug Evaluation (COURAGE) trial is randomizing more than 3,000 patients to PCI, medical therapy, and aggressive lifestyle modification versus medical therapy alone.

Initiation of statin therapy before hospital discharge, in addition to providing probable non–lipid-lowering benefits, results in higher use rates. In the Cardiac Hospitalization Atherosclerosis Management Program (CHAMP) study, statin use increased from 6% to 86% when started in the hospital, and 58% reached their LDL goal (less than 100 mg/dL) versus 6% (see *Am J Cardiol* 2001;87:219).

COMBINED PRIMARY AND SECONDARY PREVENTION TRIALS

In the Heart Protection Study (HPS) (31), which randomized 20,536 patients with CAD, diabetes, or other occlusive arterial disease to simvastatin, 40 mg/day, or placebo, the statin group had a significantly lower all-cause mortality (12.9% vs. 14.7%; $p = 0.003$). Significant benefit also was observed among those with an initial LDL less than 3 mM (116 mg/dL). These results significantly expand the population that should be targeted for lipid-lowering therapy.

In the PROspective Study of Pravastatin i⸺ 'OSPER) study (32), 5,804 patients aged 70 to 82 years wit ⸺ ⸺ sk factors were randomized to pravastatin, 40 mg/day, or pla⸺oo, and the prav⸺ ⸺atin group had a 24% relative reduction in CHD death. This large study provides strong evidence that the benefits associated with statin thera⸺ ⸺ older patients

EARLY STATIN INITIATION TRIA⸺

Several studies have examineds aft ⸺nd n⸺ ⸺ acute coronary events. In the Myocardial Ischeive (⸺ Eve⸺ ⸺olesterol Lowering (MIRACL) study (28), 3,08gina ⸺ ⸺r⸺ ⸺ non–ST elevation MI (STEMI) were enrolleday, ⸺ ⸺iate ⸺ found to have a significant 15% relative redu⸺y ⸺ LDL⸺ ⸺ point compared with placebo, primarily because ven⸺ ⸺fit. ⸺ ⸺ 4.8% vs. 17.4%; $p = 0.048$). This benefit occurrede p⸺ ⸺ P⸺ ⸺ntage by which LDL was lowered, suggesting th⸺ing⸺ ⸺n⸺ ⸺eiotropic effects. The 540-patient Fluvastatin on te N⸺ ⸺mishi⸺ ⸺ ⸺I (FLORIDA) trial was underpowered but found a trend⸺ the fluvastat⸺ ⸺roup toward fewer deaths in patients with severe ischemia at baseline, compared with placeb⸺ ⸺).

In a registry study (RIKS-HIA) of 19,599 post-MI patients, tho⸺ discharged with a statin ($n = 5,528$) had an adjusted 25% lower mortality than did⸺ nonstatin group ($p = 0.001$; see *JAMA* 2001;285:430). A similar analysis of the PURSUIT and GUSTO IIb study populations corroborates these findings: the statin gro⸺p with significantly lower 6-month mortality [1.7% vs. 3.5%; $p < 0.0001$ (p adjusted 0.023); see *Lancet* 2001;357:1063].

Further randomized data on the use of statins after an ACS revascularization will come from the A2Z trial (simvastatin) and Pravastatin or Atorvastatin Evaluation and Infection Therapy (PROVE-IT) TIMI-22 trial.

Triglyceride-Lowering Studies

Agents that are most effective in lowering TG levels are fibric acid derivatives and niacin. A Helsinki Heart Study analysis determined that a subgroup of patients with TG levels of more than 200 mg/dL and an LDL/HDL ratio of more than 5:1 had a 3.8-fold higher risk of cardiac events; furthermore, such patients had their risk reduced by 71% with gemfibrozil treatment (see *Circulation* 1992;85:37). The importance of this ratio has been confirmed in other studies, including a case-control study that found that patients with the higher TG/HDL ratios were 16 times more likely to have an MI (51).

SMOKING

Current smoking is associated with an approximately threefold increased risk of MI and an approximately twofold increased risk of CHD-related death (87–93). Smoking in combination with another major cardiac risk factor [e.g., hypertension (HTN), diabetes, hypercholesterolemia] results in an approximately 20-fold increase in death and MI (88). Among those who quit smoking, the risk gradually returns to baseline after several years (90). Passive or second-hand smoke exposure results in an average 20% to 25% increase in CHD mortality (91,93), whereas frequent or heavy exposure can result in a nearly twofold increased risk (92).

DIABETES

Approximately 15 million individuals in the United States have diabetes mellitus, of whom more than 95% have the non–insulin-dependent variety of diabetes mellitus (NIDDM). The significant decline in CHD mortality seen in the general population in recent decades has not occurred in diabetes (77); 77% of U.S. hospital stays for diabetics are attributable to CVD. NIDDM is associated with approximately two- and threefold increased risks of CHD death in men and women, respectively (see *JAMA* 1991;265:627). The risks of death from MI and CHD are as high in diabetics without prior MIs as in nondiabetics with prior MIs (76,78). As a result, guidelines now consider diabetes a CHD risk equivalent and recommend that all diabetics older than 30 years take ASA ($\geq$81 mg daily). Diabetics also have an approximately twofold increased risk of stroke.

Diabetics frequently have other modifiable risk factors, most often HTN and obesity. Addressing these risk factors [e.g., by exercise, dietary modification, or pharmacologic agent(s)] is essential to reducing an individual's cardiac risk. Tight blood pressure (BP) control significantly reduces the incidence of both macrovascular and microvascular (e.g., retinopathy) complications (82); the Joint National Committee (JNC) VI Guidelines recommend less than 130/85 mm Hg, and the American Diabetes Association and National Kidney Foundation recommend less than 130/80 mm Hg. In particular, angiotensin-converting enzyme (ACE) inhibitors and angiotensin-II–receptor blockers (e.g., losartan, irbesartan) not only lower BP but also protect against the progression of nephropathy [Irbesartan Microalbuminuria Type 2 Diabetes in Hypertensive Patients Study (IRMA II), Reduction of Endpoints in NIDDM with the Angiotensin II Antagonist Losartan Study (RENAAL) Irbesartan in Diabetic Nephropathy Trial (IDNT) (83–85); also see *N Engl J Med* 1993;329:1456].

Intensive glycemic control of individuals with IDDM in the Diabetes Control and Complications Trial (DCCT) resulted in a 34% reduction in LDL levels and a 41% reduction in major cardiovascular and peripheral vascular events (see *N Engl J Med* 1993;329:977). Current American Diabetes Association guidelines (see *Diabetes Care* 1998;21:179) recommend target goals of LDL cholesterol of less than 100 mg/dL; of HDL, more than 45 mg/dL; and of TGs, less than 200 mg/dL.

In the STENO-2 study, intensive therapy, consisting of behavioral modification and drug therapy, which targeted all the previously mentioned areas (hyperglycemia, HTN, dyslipidemia, microalbuminuria), reduced the risk of cardiovascular and microvascular events by about 50% compared with conventional therapy (86).

Metabolic Syndrome

This disorder has received increasing attention and is recognized as a major problem in the NCEP III report. The syndrome is defined as the presence of three or more of the following: (a) abdominal obesity (waist circumference more than 40 in inches men and more than 35 inches in women); (b) triglycerides, 50 mg/dL or more; (c) HDL, less than 40 mg/dL (men) or less than 50 mg/dL (women); (d) BP, 130/85 mm Hg or less; and (e) fasting glucose, 110 mg/dL or less. In the NHANES III survey, the prevalence of the metabolic syndrome was more than 20% (79). A Finnish study found those with the syndrome had a three- to fourfold increased risk of CHD death (80).

HYPERTENSION

Epidemiology

Approximately 50 million Americans have HTN. HTN occurs in the absence of other CRFs in 20%. From ages 30 to 65 years, systolic blood pressure (SBP) and diastolic blood pressure (DBP) increase by approximately 20 and 10 mm Hg, respectively. According to the Joint National Committee (JNC) VI report, only 53% receive treatment, and only 27% have adequate control (less than 140/90 mm Hg); nearly one third are unaware of their HTN, whereas approximately 15% are aware but are receiving no therapy. A Framingham Heart Study analysis (98) showing the age-adjusted prevalence of stage 2 hypertension (SBP $\geq$ 160 mm Hg or DBP $\geq$ 100 mm Hg) declined significantly from 1950 to 1989 (men, 18.5% to 9.2%; women, 28.0% to 7.7%); these findings are likely owing to effective pharmacologic treatment of severe HTN. However, another Framingham analysis found that the lifetime risk of developing HTN is 90% or higher (99). The risks of "mild" HTN are not insignificant; for example, isolated systolic HTN (SBP, 140 to 159 mm Hg) is associated with a 50% to 60% higher incidence of cardiovascular death (95,97); also, the new JNC 7 guidelines stress that

SBP >140 mm Hg is a more important CVD risk factor than diastolic BP in those older than 50 years (94).

Etiology

Approximately 90% to 95% of cases have no known cause (essential HTN). Secondary causes include renal parenchymal disease (2% to 5%), renovascular HTN (approximately 1%), primary aldosteronism (adrenal adenoma, 60%; bilateral hyperplasia, 40%), Cushing syndrome, pheochromocytoma [10% malignancy, 10% bilateral, 10% familial (multiple endocrine neoplasia type 2; MEN II)], coarctation of aorta, numerous drugs [e.g., glucocorticoids, anabolic steroids, nonsteroidal antiinflammatory drugs (NSAIDs) (100), alcohol (see *BMJ* 1994;308:1263), oral contraceptives, cocaine, cyclosporine, sympathomimetics, tricyclic antidepressants, and amphetamines], hyperparathyroidism, and acromegaly.

Diagnosis, Joint National Committee 7 Classification

Unless BP is markedly elevated, it be should measured on three separate occasions before initiating therapy. The new Joint National Committee (JNC 7) classification is as follows (see also **Table 1.3**) (94):

Prehypertension : SBP, 120 to 139 mm Hg; DBP, 80 to 89 mm Hg
Stage I hypertension: SBP, 140 to 159 mm Hg; DBP, 90 to 99 mm Hg
Stage II: SBP, ≥160 mm Hg; DBP, ≥100 mm Hg

Treatment

Nonpharmacologic
Weight loss has been shown to reduce the need for antihypertensive medication(s) (123). The Dietary Approaches to Stop Hypertension (DASH) diet, which consists of a

TABLE 1.3. JNC 7 CLASSIFICATION AND MANAGEMENT OF BLOOD PRESSURE

BP Classification (SBP and DBP, mm HG)	Initial Drug Therapy[a] Without Compelling Indication	With Compelling Indications[b]
Normal (<120 and <80)		
Prehypertension (140–159 or 80–89)	No drug indicated	Drug(s) for compelling indications
Stage 1 hypertension (140–159 or 90–99)	Thiazide-type diuretics for most; may consider ACE inhibitor, ARB, β-blocker, CCB, or combination	Drug(s) for compelling indications: Other antihypertensive drugs (diuretics, ACE inhibitor, ARB, β-blocker, CCB) as needed
Stage 2 hypertension (≥160 or ≥100)	Two-drug combination for most (usually thiazide-type diuretic and ACE inhibitor or ARB or β-blocker or CCB)	Same as above

ARB, angiotensin-receptor blocker; CCB, calcium channel blocker.
[a]Lifestyle modification is recommended for those with prehypertension and stages 1 or 2 hypertension.
[b]See table 6 of JNC 7 Guidelines (examples: post-MI: β-blocker, ACE inhibitor, aldosterone antagonist; heart failure: diuretic, β-blocker, ACE inhibitor, ARB, aldosterone antagonist; diabetes: diuretic, β-blocker, ACE inhibitor, ARB, CCB).
Adapted from Chobanicin AV, et al. (94). Used with permission.

diet rich in fruits, vegetables, and low-fat dairy products, has been shown to reduce BP significantly in hypertensive patients (122). Sodium restriction also appears to have a modest beneficial effect. One meta-analysis of 56 trials showing a 100 mg/day reduction in urinary sodium excretion was associated with a reduction of 3.7 mm Hg in SBP ($p < 0.001$) (102,123). Finally, a recent randomized study (PREMIER) demonstrated the benefit of behavioral modification that included weight loss, Sodium reduction, increased Physical activity, and limited alcohol intake (see *JAMA* 2003;289:2083).

Pharmacologic

The recent JNC 7 guidelines advocate the use of thiazide diuretics for most patients with uncomplicated hypertension, either alone or in combination with drugs from other classes (**Table 1.3**) (94). A meta-analysis of 18 randomized trials enrolling a total of more than 48,000 patients showed that the use of β-blockers and low-dose diuretics was associated with fewer strokes (RRs, 0.71, 0.49, and 0.66) and less congestive heart failure (CHF; RRs, 0.58, 0.17, and 0.58). Low-dose diuretics also were associated with less CAD and lower all-cause mortality rates (RR, 0.90; 95% CI, 0.81 to 0.99) (103).

Several studies have now compared diuretics and β-blockers with newer, more expensive ACE inhibitors and calcium-channel blockers [e.g., CAPP (Cantopril Prevention Project), Nordil (Nordic Diltiazem Study), INVEST (International Verapamil SR-Trandolapril Study), STOP-HTN2 (Swedish Trial in Old Patients with Hypertension-2 Study), CONVINCE (Controlled Onset Verapamil Investigation of Cardiovascular Endpoints Trial)] and found no significant differences in efficacy (111,112,116,119; see *JAMA* 2003;289:2073).

The latest JNC guidelines do provide for the consideration of different agents in specific types of patients or conditions (94). Most important, the use of ACE inhibitors should definitely be considered in individuals with diabetes, CHF with left ventricular (LV) dysfunction, MI complicated by LV dysfunction, chronic kidney disease, prior stroke, and high coronary disease risk. Beta-blockers can be utilized in those with heart failure, MI, diabetes, and high CHD risk. Aldosterone antagonists are indicated in those with heart failure or post-MI Angiotensin-receptor blockers can be utilized in those with diabetes or chronic kidney disease. Elderly patients with isolated systolic HTN may be treated with calcium-channel antagonists (long-acting dihydropyridines) (110). These agents can also be considered in those with high CHD risk or diabetes. In pregnancy, safe agents include labetolol, hydralazine, and methyldopa.

Major Pharmacologic Trials

The Antihypertensive and Lipid-Lowering Treatment to Prevent Heart Attack Trial (ALLHAT) enrolled 33,357 participants aged 55 years or older with HTN and at least one other CHD risk factor (121). Patients received the diuretic chlorthalidone, 12.5 to 25 mg/day; amlodipine, 2.5 to 10 mg/day; or lisinopril, 10 to 40 mg/day [the fourth arm (doxazosin) was stopped early because of increased cardiovascular events and CHF hospitalizations)]. At a mean follow-up of 4.9 years, no significant differences were found between the treatment groups in the incidence of fatal CHD or nonfatal MI (overall rate, 8.9%). Certain secondary outcomes actually occurred less often with the chlorthalidone group compared with the amlodipine group (HF) and lisinopril group (combined CVD, stroke, and HF). Although some criticisms of this important study exist (see comments in annotated summary, page 50), the results suggest that in patients in whom cardiovascular events are the greater risk, a thiazide-type diuretic is the preferred first agent.

The second Australian National Blood Pressure Study (ANBP-2) enrolled 6,083 Caucasian elderly subjects. Patients received any ACE inhibitor or diuretic in an open-label fashion. The ACE inhibitor group had a signicantly lower incidence of death or any cardiovascular event; this benefit was restricted to men (HR 0.83 vs. HR 1.00 in women). This study is methodologically weaker than ALLHAT, but its results suggest Caucasian men may benefit more from ACE inhibitor therapy.

Isolated systolic HTN, which is more common in elderly patients, also warrants treatment (102,107); unfortunately, only one fourth of physicians report routinely starting drug treatment in persons older than 70 years with SBP from 140 to 160 mm Hg.

Target Blood Pressure

The Hypertension Optimal Treatment (HOT) study (118) randomized 18,790 patients to target DBP levels of 90 mm Hg or less, 85 mm Hg or less, or 80 mm Hg or less. The incidence of major events did not differ between the three groups. However, the power to detect such a difference was less than planned for two reasons: (a) actual mean BPs were approximately 2 mm Hg apart instead of 5 mm Hg apart; and (b) only 724 major cardiovascular events occurred over a period of 3.8 years versus the projected 1,100 over a period of 2.5 years. Thus the trial was not adequately powered to determine whether a target DBP of approximately 80 mm Hg results in the fewest major events. Nevertheless, significantly fewer cardiovascular events and deaths were found among diabetic patients assigned to a target DBP of 80 mm Hg or less compared with 90 mm Hg or less ($p = 0.005$; $p = 0.016$). In the African American Study of Kidney (AASK) Disease and Hypertension Study (120), lower BP control (mean, 128/78 mm Hg) was associated with an 18% lower incidence of cardiovascular mortality and hospitalizations compared with higher BP control (mean, 141/85 mm Hg).

OBESITY

Approximately two in three U.S. adults are overweight or obese, compared with one in four in the early 1960s. There are U.S. guidelines for weight for men and women (see *N Engl J Med* 1999;341:427). Another measure, BMI (weight/body surface area), is often used (desirable, 18.0 to 24.9; overweight, 25 to 30; obese, greater than 30).

One analysis of multiple large databases found that obesity reduces life expectancy markedly, especially among younger adults (130). More than 280,000 deaths per year are now attributable to obesity, and it will soon surpass smoking as the primary preventable cause of death in the United States.

Data from the Nurses' Health Study (NHS) show that even modest weight gains over a period of 18 years result in significantly higher risks of CHD death and nonfatal MI; RRs ranged from 1.25 for a 5- to 7.9-kg gain to 2.65 for a 20-kg gain (126). Other studies have shown that a higher waist/hip ratio and greater waist circumference are independent predictors of CHD death and MI (129). In the Framingham Study, variability in weight was associated with increased all-cause and CHD mortality rates (see *N Engl J Med* 1991;324:1839).

SEDENTARY LIFESTYLE AND EXERCISE

Favorable effects associated with exercise include weight loss and favorable alteration of lipoprotein profiles, especially HDL levels (see *N Engl J Med* 2002;347:1483). Observational studies have shown that individuals with low fitness levels have a 25% to 100% increased mortality risk. One meta-analysis showed a nearly twofold risk of CHD death among individuals in sedentary (vs. active) occupations (134).

Studies have shown increasing benefit with increasing intensity and frequency of exercise. An analysis of MRFIT subjects showed a 27% lower CAD mortality rate among subjects with moderate versus less-active physical activity (135). Another study found that running (aerobic) was better than lifting weights (typically more anaerobic) (143).

Although high-intensity, aerobic exercise appears to be best, doing less is better than no activity, as evidenced by two studies of middle-aged women and elderly men that found substantial benefits associated with walking (139,191). An NHS analysis of more than 72,000 women found brisk walking (more than 3 hours a week) associated with a 35% reduction in coronary events (141). Walking also reduces body weight and body fat (see *JAMA* 2003;289:323).

Formal exercise testing can provide a more accurate risk assessment. In the Lipid Research Clinics Mortality Follow-up Study, the least-fit quartile on a standard treadmill test had a greater than eightfold risk of CAD mortality compared with the fittest quartile. In another study of 6,213 men, peak exercise capacity was the strongest predictor of death in those with and without CVD [every 1 metabolic equivalent of the task (MET) increase correlated with a 12% improvement in survival] (142).

Other studies have shown that exertion is a trigger of acute MI, with a markedly increased RR of MI (greater than 100 times) in the 1 hour after heavy exertion in those who exercise infrequently (no more than once per week) (136,137). Thus although exercise is protective, the initiation of any exercise program should generally be preceded by evaluation or consultation with a physician and initiated gradually.

NONMODIFIABLE RISK FACTORS

Family History

A family history of disorders appears most important in those otherwise at low risk. One analysis of 45,317 physicians showed that if a parent had an MI before age 70 years, the RRs of cardiac death, percutaneous transluminal coronary angioplasty (PTCA), and revascularization procedures were approximately twofold higher (144), whereas a study of 21,004 Swedish twins showed that the risk of CHD death was as high as eightfold greater if the other monozygous twin died of CHD before age 55 years (146). A recent cohort analysis of more than 20,000 individuals found that approximately 15% of CHD cases were attributable to family history, independent of other known risk factors (148).

Age

Advancing age is associated with a gradual deterioration in cardiovascular function (e.g., diastolic function, BP regulation) and increasing risks of CHD death (145). The NCEP Guidelines consider age of 45 years or older in men and 55 years or older in women a CAD risk factor (**Table 1.1**).

Gender

CAD–related events are more common in men. This gender disparity is largely owing to a later onset of symptomatic CAD in women (approximately 10 years), which is likely related to the protective effects of estrogen.

ALCOHOL

Several observational studies have shown that moderate alcohol consumption (e.g., one to two drinks per day) is associated with a significantly lower rate of CHD and overall mortality (150,151). A Physicians Health Study analysis reported adjusted relative mortality risks of 0.79 and 0.84 in those consuming one and two drinks per day, respectively (151). Another study of 38,000 male health professionals found consumption of alcohol at least 3 to 4 days per week was associated with a greater than 30% lower rate of MI (153); neither the type of beverage nor the proportion consumed with meals substantially altered this association.

Mechanisms for the benefits of alcohol appear to include increased HDL levels, antiplatelet effects, and improved insulin resistance. Because of the significant health risks associated with more substantial alcohol consumption, many physicians are hesitant to recommend alcohol consumption as a means to reduce cardiovascular risk. AHA Nutrition Committee recommendations include consulting a physician to assess the risks and benefits of alcohol consumption, with contraindications including family history of alcoholism, hypertriglyceridemia, liver disease, uncontrolled HTN, and pregnancy (see *Circulation* 1996;94:3023).

HORMONAL STATUS AND HORMONAL THERAPY

Estrogen replacement therapy in postmenopausal women results in an approximately 15% to 20% reduction in LDL and 15% to 20% elevation in HDL levels. Significant epidemiologic data suggested that estrogen replacement was associated with significantly lower CHD mortality (154,155; also see *N Engl J Med* 1997;336:1769). However, breast cancer rates are 10% to 30% higher, and endometrial cancer occurs up to 6 times more often (see *Lancet* 1998;352:1965).

However, in contrast to the epidemiologic data, the first large prospective, randomized trial [Heart and Estrogen/Progestin Replacement Study (HERS)] showed that a combination of estrogen and progestin in 2,763 women with a CHD event in the preceding 6 months did not result in a significant reduction in cardiovascular death and MI (relative hazard, 0.99) (156,159); the hormone group had more events in year 1 but fewer events in years 4 and 5.

The Women's Health Initiative, which randomized 16,608 postmenopausal women to estrogen and progestin or placebo, was terminated early (at 5.2 years of follow-up) (160). The hormone group had significantly higher rates of CHD (hazard ratio, 1.29), breast cancer (HR, 1.26), and stroke (HR, 1.41), whereas a lower incidence of colorectal cancer (HR, 0.63) and hip fractures (HR, 0.66) was seen. Overall mortality rates were similar. Based on these data, the overall risk–benefit profile for estrogen and progestin therapy does not meet the requirements for a clearly safe and efficacious intervention for primary prevention. The estrogen-only arm of this study is still ongoing.

Raloxifene is a selective estrogen modulator used for treatment of osteoporosis. In the Multiple Outcomes of Raloxifene Evaluation (MORE) trial, 7,705 osteoporotic postmenopausal women were randomized to raloxifene, 60 mg/day; raloxifene, 120 mg/day; or placebo (158). At 4-year follow-up, no significant differences were found between the treatment groups in coronary and cerebrovascular events. However, among the 1,035 women with increased cardiovascular risk at baseline, those assigned to raloxifene (either dose) had a significantly lower risk of cardiovascular events compared with placebo (RR, 0.60; 95% CI, 0.38 to 0.95). Before raloxifene can be advocated for prevention of cardiovascular events, these findings require confirmation in trials with evaluation of cardiovascular outcomes as the primary objective. One such trial is the ongoing Raloxifene Use for The Heart (RUTH) trial, which randomized 10,000 women between June 1998 and August 2000 to raloxifene, 60 mg/day, or placebo; planned median follow-up is 8 years.

C-REACTIVE PROTEIN

C-Reactive protein (CRP) is an acute-phase reactant produced by the liver in response to interleukin 6 (IL-6). A high-sensitivity assay (hsCRP) has allowed accurate measurement at the low levels (less than 10 mg/L) that predict CHD risk. Numerous studies have shown that elevated hsCRP levels are strongly associated with an increased risk of cardiovascular events. CRP also may be more than a marker of CHD risk, as recent research suggests it impairs endothelial vasoreactivity and promotes atherosclerosis (see *Circulation* 2000;102:1000, 2165).

In nested case-control studies of Women's Health Study (WHS) and Women's Health Initiative participants (165,170), the highest hsCRP levels were associated with a more than fourfold higher risk of cardiovascular events and twofold increased risk of CHD, respectively; individuals in the highest quartile of hsCRP had increased rates of stroke (RR, 1.9), MI (RR, 2.9), and peripheral vascular disease (PVD; RR, 4.1). In the Physicians Health Study (PHS), high levels of CRP were associated with increased risk of MI (adjusted RR, 1.5), and those in the highest quartiles of both CRP and total cholesterol had a fivefold higher risk (163). Another study of both PHS and WHS participants found that those in the highest quintiles of CRP *and* TC/HDL had an eight- to ninefold increased risk of major events (see *Circulation* 2001;103: 1813).

CRP also has predictive value in those with known CAD. In the CARE study, those in the highest quintile of CRP levels had nearly a twofold increased risk of recurrent events (166). An analysis of prospective European studies of patients with stable and unstable angina found a 45% increase in nonfatal MI and sudden cardiac death (SCD) in those with increased CRP levels (see *Lancet* 1997;349:962). In patients with ACSs, high CRP levels are predictive of worse prognosis (172). In the initial evaluation of such patients, hsCRP measurement provides additional prognostic information to other markers (see *Circulation* 2002;105:1760) and may prove useful in those with normal troponin levels.

A more impressive finding is that hsCRP appears to be an even stronger predictor of first cardiovascular events than is LDL cholesterol. An analysis of the 27,939 WHS participants found that both baseline LDL and hsCRP levels had a strong linear relation with the incidence of cardiovascular events, although the two were minimally correlated ($r = 0.08$) (171). The adjusted RRs of first cardiovascular events according to increasing quintiles of CRP, as compared with women in the lowest quintile, were 1.4, 1.6, 2.0, and 2.3 ($p < 0.001$), compared with corresponding RRs in increasing quintiles of LDL-C of 0.9, 1.1, 1.3, and 1.5 ($p < 0.001$). Because 46% of major events occurred among those with LDL less than 130 mg/dL, CRP may be particularly helpful in identifying patients at high CHD risk among those with low LDL levels.

CRP levels appear to be effectively lowered by statins. The Pravastatin Inflammation/CRP Evaluation (PRINCE) trial enrolled 2,884 patients (including 1,182 with known CVD off statins for at least 12 weeks) (168). In the primary prevention cohort, pravastatin reduced hsCRP by 16.9% compared with no change with placebo. In the open-labeled CVD cohort (all received statin therapy), a similar 14.3% reduction in hsCRP was found. An analysis of AFCAPS/TexCAPS participants found that lovastatin decreased CRP levels by 14% during the course of the study ($p < 0.001$). If LDL was less than the median (149 mg/dL) and CRP was greater than the median (1.6 mg/L), lovastatin conferred significant benefit (169). In the CARE study, the statin group had a 17% reduction in hsCRP (see *Circulation* 1999;100:230); in those treated with pravastatin, an hsCRP above the 90th percentile was associated with a 54% reduction in recurrent events compared with 25% if hsCRP was less than 9.9 mg/L. Several studies have shown that statins lower hsCRP within weeks of therapy initiation, an effect independent of their effect on LDL cholesterol (see *Circulation* 2001;103:1191; 2002;106:1447). Prospective studies to evaluate whether CRP lowering by statins reduces major events are now ongoing. Finally, it also appears that ezetimibe reduces CRP levels; Preliminary results of 668 patient trial found an 18.2% reduction with simivastatin alone and 34.8% with simivastatin and ezetimibe presented at 52nd ACC Scientific Session, Chicago, IL, March 2003.

In regard to ASA, a PHS analysis found that its use was most beneficial among men in the highest quartile of hsCRP values [56% reduction in MI vs. 14% (lowest quartile)] (163). Studies specifically examining the impact of aspirin on hsCRP are conflicting (see *Circulation* 1999;100:793, *J Thromb Thrombol* 2000;9:37, *J Am Coll Cardiol* 2000;37:2036). Thus further studies are required to determine whether initiation of ASA in patients with high CRP levels results in reduced CHD risk.

Lifestyle modification also lowers hsCRP levels. Several studies have shown that weight loss, exercise, smoking cessation, and modest alcohol consumption reduce hsCRP (see *Circulation* 2002;105:564; 2003;107:443). Because elevated hsCRP levels are seen in those with diabetes and the metabolic syndrome (see *Diabetes Care* 2000;23:1835; *Circulation* 2003;107:391), it is likely that aggressive glycemic control will lower hsCRP levels.

In January 2003, the AHA and Centers for Disease Control (CDC) published a Scientific Statement that identified hsCRP as the most promising inflammatory marker because of the robust data base and its strong ability to predict CHD events (see *Circulation* 2003;107:499). The report does not advocate routine hsCRP screening for primary prevention, but rather selective use in individuals identified as at intermediate risk [10% to 20% risk of CHD at 10 years (with modified Framingham tables)]. It recommends two measurements obtained at least 2 weeks apart. An hsCRP level less than 1.0 mg/L is considered low; 1.0 to 3.0 mg/L is intermediate; and greater than 3.0 mg/L is high. If the level is greater than 10 mg/L, investigations for noncardiac causes should be undertaken. Although no treatment parameters are outlined, an accompanying expert perspective suggests that it is reasonable to consider statin therapy in those with a high hsCRP and an LDL of 130 to 160 mg/dL. Other AHA/CDC recommendations include (a) utility of hsCRP in secondary prevention is limited; (b) hsCRP measurement in ACS patients may be useful as an independent marker of prognosis for recurrent events, including death, MI, and restenosis after PCI, but the benefits of therapy based on this strategy remain uncertain; and (c) little evidence supports serial hsCRP testing to measure disease activity or monitor therapy.

OTHER POTENTIAL RISK FACTORS

Homocysteine

Hyperhomocysteinemia appears to be a modest independent risk factor for coronary heart disease (CHD), cerebrovascular disease, and peripheral vascular disease. Most studies have confirmed that high homocysteine levels are associated with an increased CHD mortality rate (175,179,181); however, other studies have shown no association (156; see also *Stroke* 1994;25:1924). A recent meta-analysis found that in prospective studies, a 25% lower homocysteine level was associated with an 11% lower risk of ischemic heart disease (IHD) and 19% lower stroke risk (174). A recent analysis of 5,569 AFCAPS/TexCAPS participants found that higher baseline homocysteine levels were associated with increased risk of future acute coronary events; however, in contrast to findings in this trial for CRP, homocysteine levels did not help to define low-LDL subgroups with different responses to statin therapy (182).

Two studies reported that folic acid fortification and multivitamin use are associated with lower homocysteine levels (177,178). Randomized trials are ongoing to determine whether lowering homocysteine levels through folate supplementation will result in a reduction in CHD-related events.

Fibrinogen

Several prospective epidemiologic studies have shown fibrinogen to be an independent CAD risk factor (see *N Engl J Med* 1984;311:511 and 1995;332:635, *JAMA* 1987;258:1183, *Circulation* 1991;83:836 and 1997;96:1102). One older meta-analysis of six large studies showed a greater than twofold risk of subsequent MI or stroke in patients with high fibrinogen levels (see *Ann Intern Med* 1993;118:956). A more recent analysis of 18 prospective studies showed a one- to eightfold higher CHD risk among those in the top third of fibrinogen levels (*JAMA* 1998;279:1477). No long-term pharmacologic intervention has been shown to reduce fibrinogen levels significantly.

Infection

Some studies demonstrated an increased risk of CAD in individuals who are seropositive for certain infectious agents. The most robust evidence accumulated to date is for *Chlamydia pneumoniae* (183,184; see also *Circulation* 1998;98:2796). A meta-analysis (performed in 2000) of 15 prospective studies of *C. pneumoniae* immunoglobulin G (IgG) titers, included 3,169 cases, and found a combined OR of CHD of only 1.15 (95% CI, 0.97 to 1.36), suggesting a weak association of *C. pneumoniae* with CHD.

A nested case-control study of PHS subjects and a prospective cohort study of Framingham Heart Study participants found no increased risk of future MI in those with increasing IgG titers to *C. pneumoniae* (see *Circulation* 1999;99:1161, *J Am Coll Cardiol* 2002;40:1408). The Azithromycin in Coronary Artery Disease: Elimination of Myocardial Infection with Chlamydia (ACADEMIC) trial, which treated patients with CAD and elevated *C. pneumoniae* titers with azithromycin, found no difference between the treated and placebo groups in a 3-month composite of four inflammatory markers and clinical outcomes at 6 months (184).

Among unstable angina and non–Q-wave MI patients, The Clarithromycin in Acute Coronary Syndrome Patients in Finland (CLARIFY) study found that clarithromycin reduced the risk of ischemic cardiovascular events compared with placebo (186). In contrast, the AZACS trial found no benefit of azithromycin use in 1,400 unstable angina or acute MI patients (see *Lancet* 2003;361:809), and the larger The Weekly Intervention with Zithromax for Atherosclerosis and its Related Disorders (WIZARD) trial (187), which enrolled more than 7,000 post-MI patients with elevated *C. pneumoniae* titers, showed no significant benefit at 2 years of azithromycin versus placebo. Additional ongoing studies will further examine the use of antibiotics in patients with acute coronary events (e.g., PROVE-IT).

Genetic Markers

The PLA1/PLA2 polymorphism of platelet glycoprotein IIIa and the ACE gene have been most extensively studied. Observational studies of the PLA1/PLA2 polymorphism reported an increased risk of cardiac events among those with the PLA2 allele, whereas larger studies have shown no significant relation (190,191). A meta-analysis performed of 40 studies with a total of 9,095 cases and 12,508 controls found the overall OR of CAD for carriers of the *PLA2* allele was 1.10 (95% CI, 1.03 to 1.18), suggesting a significant but weak association (192). In regard to the ACE gene, a meta-analysis of 15 studies found an approximately 25% increased risk of MI among those homozygous for the deletion allele of the ACE gene (189).

ANTIPLATELET DRUGS FOR PRIMARY AND SECONDARY PREVENTION

Aspirin

Primary Prevention Trials
The PHS found that ASA-treated patients (325 mg every other day) had 44% fewer nonfatal MIs and a nonsignificant 4% reduction in cardiovascular deaths (198). This study was stopped prematurely because of concerns about the high stroke rate (RR, 2.1). A study of 5,139 British physicians found that ASA use (500 mg/day) resulted in a nonsignificant 10% mortality reduction and no effect on the incidence of nonfatal MI (197). In the Swedish Angina Pectoris Aspirin Trial (SAPAT) (198), which randomized 2,035 patients to ASA, 75 mg/day, or placebo, ASA was associated with a 34% reduction in MI and sudden death, but a nonsignificant increase in major bleeds was seen (1.0% vs. 0.7%).

The AHA and the U.S. Preventive Services Task Force have both concluded that currently insufficient evidence exists to recommend for or against routine ASA prophylaxis in primary prevention. Results from the WHS of approximately 40,000 U.S. health professionals will provide the data necessary to assess the balance of benefits and risks of ASA in primary prevention. The American Diabetes Association guidelines recommend that all individuals with diabetes older than 30 years should take ASA because of their increased CHD risk (minimum, 81 mg/day; see *Diabetes Care* 1997;20:1772).

Secondary Prevention Trials
In the second Persantine-Aspirin Reinfarction Study (PARIS II) (1,200), the ASA plus persantine group had a 30% lower 1-year mortality rate. An early meta-analysis that includes the PARIS II results found a similar reduction in mortality with ASA use. In a recent observational study of elderly patients, with no contraindications to ASA, ASA use was associated with a 23% lower mortality rate (192); however, only 76% were given this beneficial therapy at hospital discharge.

The Antithrombotic Trialists' Collaboration recent meta-analysis (published in 2002) examined 287 randomized studies with 135,000 patients in comparisons of antiplatelet therapy versus control and 77,000 in comparisons of different antiplatelet regimens (195). Among high-risk patients [e.g., acute MI, acute stroke, previous stroke or transient ischemic attack (TIA), peripheral arterial disease, atrial fibrillation], antiplatelet therapy reduced the incidence of serious vascular events (nonfatal MI or stroke, vascular death) by approximately one fourth, nonfatal MI by approximately one third, nonfatal stroke by approximately one fourth, and vascular mortality by approximately one sixth (all $p < 0.00001$). In each of the high-risk categories, the absolute benefits outweighed the absolute risks of major extracranial bleeding.

Aspirin resistance is present in 5% to 10% of individuals. In one study, aspirin resistance was associated with a three fold higher risk of death, MI, or stroke compared to aspirin sensitive patients (see *J Am Coll Cardiol* 2003;41:966). Whether aspirin resistant individuals receive adequate or enhanced benefit from Clopidogrel requires futher study.

Clopidogrel

The Clopidogrel versus Aspirin in Patients at Risk of Ischaemic Events (CAPRIE) trial randomized more than 19,000 patients with a recent MI, ischemic stroke, or peripheral arterial disease (PAD) to clopidogrel, 75 mg once daily, or ASA, 325 mg once daily (204) (see page xx). Overall, clopidogrel was associated with a significantly lower incidence in the primary composite end point, consisting of ischemic stroke, MI, or vascular death (5.32% vs. 5.83%/year; $p = 0.043$). Another analysis of all enrolled patients showed a statistically significant 19.2% reduction in the MI event rate ($p = 0.008$) (see *Am J Cardiol* 2002;90:760). Based on these data, the use of clopidogrel in all patients with recent MI or stroke or documented PAD appears to result in a reduced risk of subsequent MI, stroke or CV death. Furthermore, the subsequent results of the CURE and CREDO studies (see Chapters 3 and 2, respectively) confirmed the benefits of clopidogrel for secondary prevention in ACS and PCI patients, respectively. In those with history of stroke or PAD or at high risk for CHD events, the combination of clopidogrel and ASA is being evaluated in large randomized trials [e.g., CHARISMA (target enrollment, approximately 15,000 patients)].

REFERENCES

General Articles

1. **Stampfer MJ,** et al. Primary prevention of coronary heart disease in women through diet and lifestyle. *N Engl J Med* 2000;343:16–22.

   This analysis examined the 84,129 NHS participants who were free of diagnosed CVD, cancer, and diabetes at baseline. During 14 years of follow-up, 296 CHD deaths and 832 nonfatal MIs occurred. Low-risk subjects (only 3% of cohort) were defined as follows: nonsmokers, BMI less than 25, alcohol consumption at least half a drink per day, moderate-to-vigorous physical activity for average of approximately 30 minutes per day, scored in highest 40% of cohort for consumption of a diet high in cereal fiber, marine n-3 fatty acids, and folate, with a high ratio of polyunsaturated to saturated fat, and low in trans fat and glycemic load. After adjustment for age, family history, presence or absence of diagnosed HTN or diagnosed high cholesterol level, and menopausal status, all factors independently and significantly predicted risk. Low-risk women had an 83% RR reduction in CHD death or nonfatal MI compared with all the other women.

2. **Pearson TA,** et al. **AHA Guidelines** for primary prevention of cardiovascular disease and stroke: 2002 update: consensus panel guide to comprehensive risk reduction for adult patients without coronary or other atherosclerotic vascular diseases: American Heart Association Science Advisory and Coordinating Committee. *Circulation* 2002;106:388–391.

Lipids, Cholesterol, and Diet

Review Articles and Meta-Analyses

3. **Hebert PR,** et al. Cholesterol lowering with statin drugs, risk of stroke and total mortality. *JAMA* 1997;278:313–321.

   This meta-analysis of 16 trials included approximately 29,000 patients with an average follow-up of 3.3 years. The use of statins was associated with 22% lower TC and 30% lower LDL levels. Statin-treated patients also had a 22% lower overall mortality rate (95% CI, 12% to 31%), 28% lower cardiovascular mortality (95% CI, 16% to 37%), and 29% fewer strokes (95% CI, 14% to 41%). No increase in deaths was attributable to noncardiovascular causes or cancer.

4. **Bucher HC,** et al. Systematic review of the risk and benefit of different cholesterol-lowering interventions. *Arterioscler Thromb Vasc Biol* 1999;19:187–195.

This analysis of 59 randomized, controlled trials with 85,431 participants included 13 statin trials, 12 fibrate trials, eight bile resin trials, eight hormone trials, two niacin trials, three n-3 fatty acid trials, and 16 dietary intervention studies. Only statins showed a significant reduction in CHD-related mortality (RRR, 0.66; 95% CI, 0.54 to 0.79) and all-cause mortality rates (RRR, 0.75; 95% CI, 0.65 to 0.86). A meta-regression analysis showed that the variability of results across trials was largely explained by the magnitude of cholesterol reduction.

5. **Knopp RH.** Drug treatment of lipid disorders. *N Engl J Med* 1999;341:498–511.

This review discusses the major classes of lipid-lowering agents: statins, bile resins, nicotinic acid, and fibrates. The most extensive section is devoted to the statins; mechanism of action, indications, lipid-lowering effects, comparison of available agents, and adverse effects are concisely described.

6. **NCEP Guidelines.** Expert Panel on Detection, Evaluation, and Treatment of High Blood Cholesterol in Adults: executive summary of the third report of the National Cholesterol Education Program (NCEP) expert panel on detection, evaluation, and treatment of high blood cholesterol in adults (Adult Treatment Panel III). *JAMA* 2001;285:2486–2497.

The guidelines focus on LDL cholesterol goals and cut points for therapeutic lifestyle changes and drug therapy (Table 1.1). High-risk groups are identified by using a modified Framingham point score (Tables 1.2 and 1.3). Attention also is given to TG levels, non-HDL levels, and the metabolic syndrome.

Epidemiology
7. **Martin MJ,** et al. Multiple risk factor intervention trial (**MRFIT**): serum cholesterol, blood pressure and mortality: implications from a cohort of 361,662 men. *Lancet* 1986;2:933–939.

This analysis of 6-year follow-up data showed that cardiovascular mortality correlated with cholesterol levels. Increased cardiovascular mortality risk was seen with TC levels as low as 181 mg/dL. RR was 3.8 for cholesterol levels above the 85th percentile (greater than 253 mg/dL).

8. **Gordon DJ,** et al. High-density lipoprotein cholesterol and cardiovascular disease: four prospective American studies. *Circulation* 1989;79:8–15.

This analysis examined data from the FHS, Lipid Research Clinics Prevalence Mortality Follow-up Study (LRCF) and Coronary Primary Prevention Trial (CPPT), and Multiple Risk Factor Intervention Trial (MRFIT). A 1-mg/dL (0.026 m*M*) increment in HDL-C was associated with a significant CHD risk decrement of 2% in men (FHS, CPPT, and MRFIT) and 3% in women (FHS). In LRCF, in which only fatal outcomes were documented, a 1-mg/dL increment in HDL-C was associated with significant 3.7% (men) and 4.7% (women) decrements in cardiovascular mortality rates.

9. **Pekkanen J,** et al. Ten-year mortality from cardiovascular disease in relation to cholesterol level among men with and without preexisting cardiovascular disease. *N Engl J Med* 1990;322:1700–1707.

The study population was composed of 2,541 white men, 17% with CVD at baseline. At an average follow-up of 10 years, CV mortality was significantly lower in patients with desirable (less than 200 mg/dL) versus high (greater than 240 mg/dL) cholesterol levels: in patients with baseline CVD, 3.8% versus 19.6%; in patients without baseline disease, 1.7% versus 4.9%. Other strong predictors of CV mortality were LDL (more than 160 mg/dL vs. less than 130 mg/dL; RR, 5.9) and HDL levels (more than 45 mg/dL vs. less than 35 mg/dL; RR, 6.0).

10. **Cui Y,** et al. Non-high-density lipoprotein cholesterol level as a predictor of cardiovascular disease mortality. *Arch Intern Med* 2001;161:1413–1419.

This study analyzed data on 2,406 men and 2,056 women aged 40 to 64 years from the Lipid Research Clinics Program Follow-up Study. At follow-up (average, 19 years), baseline levels of HDL-C and non–HDL-C were strong predictors of CVD death in both sexes, whereas LDL-C level was a slightly weaker CVD predictor. Differences of 30 mg/dL in non–HDL-C and LDL-C levels corresponded to increases in CVD risk of 19% and 15%, respectively, in men, and 11% and 8% in women.

11. **Bittner V,** et al. Non-high-density lipoprotein cholesterol levels predict five-year outcome in the Bypass Angioplasty Revascularization Investigation (BARI). *Circulation* 2002;106:2537–2542.

This study analyzed 1,514 BARI study patients with available baseline lipid levels; all had multivessel CAD. At 5 years, non–HDL-C was a strong, independent predictor of nonfatal MI [multivariate RR, 1.049 (95% CI, 1.006 to 1.093) for every 0.26 mM increase] and angina pectoris [multivariate OR, 1.049 (95% CI, 1.004 to 1.096) for every 0.26 mM increase]. No significant association was found with mortality. HDL-C and LDL-C did not predict events during follow-up.

Primary Prevention

12. World Health Organization (**WHO**) Study. Committee of Principal Investigators: a cooperative trial in the primary prevention of ischemic heart disease using clofibrate. *Br Heart J* 1978;40:1069–1118.

Design: Prospective, randomized, placebo-controlled, multicenter study; average follow-up 5.3 years.
Purpose: To evaluate the effects of clofibrate on cholesterol levels and the incidence of major cardiovascular events.
Population: 10,627 men aged 30 to 59 years with high TC levels (upper one third of distribution).
Treatment: Clofibrate, 1.6 g/day, or placebo.
Results: Clofibrate group had 8% lower TC and 20% fewer MIs.

13. Lipid Research Clinics Coronary Primary Prevention Trial. (**LRC-CPPT**) results: reduction in incidence of CHD. *JAMA* 1984;251:351–364.

Design: Prospective, randomized, double-blind, placebo-controlled, multicenter study. Primary end point was CHD-related death and nonfatal MI. The average follow-up was 7.4 years.
Purpose: To evaluate the effects of cholestyramine on cholesterol levels and major cardiac events in hypercholesterolemic men at high risk of CHD events.
Population: 3,806 men aged 35 to 59 years with TC greater than 265 mg/dL and LDL greater than 190 mg/dL.
Treatment: Cholestyramine (24 g/day) or placebo.
Results: Cholestyramine use was associated with 9% lower TC and 13% lower LDL-C. Cholestyramine group had a 19% reduction in CHD-related death and MI (8.1% vs. 9.8%).

14. **Frick MH,** et al. **Helsinki Heart Study**: primary-prevention trial with gemfibrozil in middle-aged men with dyslipidemia. *N Engl J Med* 1987;317:1237–1245.

Design: Prospective, randomized, double-blind, placebo-controlled, multicenter study. Primary end point was cardiac death and MI. The follow-up period was 5 years.
Purpose: To investigate the effect of gemfibrozil on the incidence of CHD in asymptomatic middle-aged men at high risk because of elevated lipid levels.
Population: The 4,081 men aged 40 to 55 years with a non-HDL cholesterol level of ≥200 mg/dL.
Treatment: Gemfibrozil, 600 mg twice daily, or placebo.
Results: Gemfibrozil initially increased HDL levels by more than 10%, followed by a small decline over time. TC and LDL levels were initially decreased by 11% and 10%,

respectively, and remained consistent throughout the trial. The gemfibrozil group had 34% fewer cardiac events (7.3 vs. 41.4/1,000; $p < 0.02$); the decline in incidence became evident in the second year; no significant mortality difference was detected between groups (2.19% vs. 2.07%).

Comments: A subsequent subgroup analysis showed that patients with TG greater than 200 mg/dL and an LDL/HDL ratio of more than 5:1 had a 3.8 times higher risk of cardiac events, and that risk was reduced a substantial 71% with gemfibrozil (see *Circulation* 1992;85:37).

15. **Shepherd J,** et al. West of Scotland Coronary Prevention Study Group (WO-SCOPS): prevention of coronary heart disease with pravastatin in men with hypercholesterolemia. *N Engl J Med* 1995;333:1301–1307.

Design: Prospective, randomized, double-blind, multicenter trial. Primary end point was death from CHD and nonfatal MI. The average follow-up period was 4.9 years.

Purpose: To evaluate the effectiveness of an HMG-CoA reductase inhibitor in preventing events in men with moderate hypercholesterolemia and no history of MI.

Population: 6,544 men aged 45 to 64 years with TC $\geq$252 mg/dL (mean, 272) and no history of MI.

Treatment: Pravastatin, 40 mg once daily, or placebo.

Results: Pravastatin group had 20% lower TC, 26% lower LDL, 31% fewer coronary events (nonfatal MI, death from CHD; $p < 0.001$), 32% lower cardiovascular mortality ($p = 0.033$), and nearly significant 22% overall mortality reduction ($p = 0.051$). The reduction in coronary events was independent of baseline cholesterol level (as in 4S trial).

16. **Downs JR,** et al. for the Air Force/Texas Coronary Atherosclerosis Prevention Study (AFCAPS/TexCAPS) Research Group. Primary prevention of acute coronary events with lovastatin in men and women with average cholesterol levels. *JAMA* 1998;279:1615–1622.

Design: Prospective, randomized, double-blind, multicenter study. Composite primary end point was fatal or nonfatal MI, unstable angina, and SCD. Average follow-up period was 5.2 years.

Purpose: To compare lovastatin with placebo for the prevention of first major coronary events in those without clinically evident atherosclerosis and with average TC and LDL and below-average HDL levels.

Population: 5,608 men aged 45 to 73 years and 997 postmenopausal women aged 55 to 73 years with TC, 180 to 264 mg/dL; LDL, 130 to 190 mg/dL; and HDL, $\geq$45 mg/dL (men) or = 47 mg/dL (women).

Exclusion Criteria: Diabetes managed with insulin or with hemoglobin A_{1c} of 10 or more, and more than 50% ideal weight

Treatment: Lovastatin, 20 to 40 mg once daily, or placebo.

Results: Lovastatin was associated with an RRR of 37% in first acute major coronary events (3.51% vs. 5.54%; $p < 0.001$). Several secondary end points occurred less frequently in the lovastatin group: (a) MI, RRR of 40% ($p = 0.002$); (b) unstable angina, RRR of 32% ($p = 0.02$); (c) coronary revascularization procedures, RRR of 33% ($p = 0.001$); (d) coronary events, RRR of 25% ($p = 0.006$); and (e) cardiovascular events, RRR of 25% ($p = 0.003$). Lovastatin reduced LDL levels by 25% and increased HDL levels by 6%; no significant differences in adverse events were detected.

Comments: Differences between the two groups appeared after 1 year (23 vs. 40 events).

17. **Gagne C,** et al. Ezetimibe Study Group: efficacy and safety of ezetimibe added to ongoing statin therapy for treatment of patients with primary hypercholesterolemia. *Am J Cardiol* 2002;90:1084–1091.

Design: Prospective, randomized, double-blind, placebo-controlled, multicenter trial. Primary end point was percentage change in LDL cholesterol.

Purpose: To evaluate combination therapy with a statin and ezetimibe in patients with primary hypercholesterolemia.

Population: 769 adults with primary hypercholesterolemia who failed to achieve NCEP ATP II goals with dietary alteration and statin monotherapy (stable dose for 6 weeks or more).

Exclusion Criteria: Included MI, CABG surgery, or PTCA in previous 3 months; HF; unstable angina; creatine phosphokinase (CPK) greater than 1.5 times upper limits of normal (ULN); impaired renal function; hepatobiliary disease.

Treatment: Ezetimibe, 10 mg/day, or placebo, in addition to continuation of open-label statin for 8 weeks.

Results: Ezetimibe plus statin therapy reduced LDL levels by 25% (vs. 3.7% reduction with placebo plus statin; $p < 0.001$). HDL-C levels were increased by 2.7% with combination therapy (placebo, 1.0% increase; $p < 0.05$), whereas TGs were decreased by 14.0% (placebo, 2.9% decrease; $p < 0.001$). Among patients not at LDL goal at baseline, 71.5% receiving statin plus ezetimibe versus 18.9% taking statin plus placebo achieved LDL goal ($p < 0.001$). The coadministration of statin and ezetimibe was generally well tolerated.

18. **Dujovne CA,** et al. Ezetimibe Study Group: efficacy and safety of a potent new selective cholesterol absorption inhibitor, ezetimibe, in patients with primary hypercholesterolemia. *Am J Cardiol* 2002;90:1092–1097.

Design: Prospective, randomized, double-blind, placebo-controlled, multicenter trial. Primary end point was the percentage reduction in direct plasma LDL at 12 weeks.

Purpose: To evaluate the safety and efficacy of the new cholesterol-absorption inhibitor ezetimibe.

Population: 892 patients with primary hypercholesterolemia.

Exclusion Criteria: Included MI, CABG surgery, or PTCA in previous 6 months; CHF (NYHA class III or IV); unstable angina; impaired renal function; hepatobiliary disease

Treatment: After 2 weeks or more on an NCEP Step I or stricter diet and a 4- to 8-week single-blind placebo lead-in, those with LDL-C 130 to 250 mg/dL and TGs 350 mg/dL or greater were randomized in 3:1 fashion to ezetimibe, 10 mg, or placebo orally each morning for 12 weeks.

Results: Ezetimibe significantly decreased LDL levels by 17%, compared with a 0.4% increase with placebo ($p < 0.01$). The LDL-lowering effect occurred early (2 weeks) and persisted throughout the 12-week treatment period. Ezetimibe also significantly improved calculated LDL, apolipoprotein B, TC, TGs, HDL, and HDL(3) cholesterol ($p < 0.01$). Ezetimibe was well tolerated: compared with placebo, no differences were seen in laboratory parameters, or GI, liver, or muscle side effects.

19. **Davidson MH,** et al. Ezetimibe coadministered with simvastatin in patients with primary hypercholesterolemia. *J Am Coll Cardiol* 2002;40:2125–2134.

After dietary stabilization, a 2- to 12-week washout period, and a 4-week, single-blind, placebo lead-in period, 591 patients with baseline LDL 145 to 250 mg/dL and TGs 350 mg/dL or more were randomized to one of ten groups administered daily for 12 consecutive weeks: ezetimibe, 10 mg; simvastatin, 10, 20, 40, or 80 mg; ezetimibe, 10 mg plus simvastatin 10, 20, 40, or 80 mg; or placebo. Ezetimibe plus simvastatin resulted in LDL-C reductions of 44% to 57%, TG reductions of 20% to 28%, and HDL increases of 8% to 11%, depending on the simvastatin dose. Compared with simvastatin alone, ezetimibe and simvastatin significantly improved LDL-C (incremental 13.8% reduction; $p < 0.01$), HDL (2.4% increase; $p = 0.03$), and TG (7.5% reduction; $p < 0.01$). Coadministration of ezetimibe with simvastatin was well tolerated and comparable with that of simvastatin alone.

20. **ASCOT-LLA** Sever PS, et al. Prevention of coronary and stroke events with atorvastatin in hypertensive patients who have average or lower-than-average cholesterol concentrations in the Anglo-Scandinavian Cardiac Outcomes Trial-Lipid Lowering Arm (ASCOT-LAA): a multicenter randomized controlled trial. *Lancet* 2003;361:1149–1158

Design: Prospective, randomized, double blind, multicenter trial. Primary end point was nonfatal MI and fatal CHD. Median follow-up: 33 years (trial stopped early).

Purpose: To assess the benefits of cholesterol lowering in primary prevention of CHD in hypertensive patients with normal cholesterol levels.

Population: 10,342 of 19,342 total ASCOT patients with total cholesterol $\leq$250 mg/dL; all were aged 40 to 79 years and with at least three other cardiovascular risk factors in addition to hypertension.

Exclusion Criteria: Included prior MI, currently treated angina, CVA in past 3 months, and heart failure.

Treatment: Atorvastatin 10 mg or placebo.

Results: The atorvastatin group had 36% fewer primary events compared to placebo (1.9% vs. 3.0%, hazard ratio 0.64, $p = 0.0005$). This benefit emerged in the first year of follow-up. There were 13% fewer deaths in the atorvastatin group ($p = 0.16$).

Comments: The rest of the trial, which compares amlodipine $\pm$ perindopril with atenolol $\pm$ bendrofluazide for treating HTN, is ongoing.

Secondary Prevention

21. **Coronary Drug Project.** Coronary Drug Project Research Group: clofibrate and niacin in coronary heart disease. *JAMA* 1975;231:360–381.

Design: Prospective, randomized, multicenter study. Primary end point was all-cause mortality. Mean follow-up was 74 months.

Purpose: To evaluate the effects of clofibrate and niacin on cholesterol levels and major cardiac events.

Population: 8,341 men age 30 to 64 years with ECG-documented prior MI.

Treatment: Clofibrate, 1.8 g/day, or niacin, 3 g/day.

Results: Clofibrate group had a nonsignificant 6% decrease in TC and 7% fewer MIs; niacin group had a 10% decrease in TC, 26% lower TGs, and significant decrease in nonfatal MIs (but not fatal MIs).

Comments: At 15-year follow-up (see *J Am Coll Cardiol* 1986;8:1245), the niacin group had a significant 11% mortality reduction compared with placebo (52.0% vs. 58.2%; $p = 0.0004$).

22. **Buchwald H,** et al. Program on the Surgical Control of Hyperlipidemia (POSCH): changes in sequential coronary arteriograms and subsequent coronary events. *JAMA* 1992;268:1429–1433 (see also *Am J Cardiol* 1990;66:1293).

Design: Prospective, randomized, open-label, multicenter study. Mean follow-up period was 9.7 years.

Purpose: To evaluate whether cholesterol lowering induced by partial ileal bypass surgery would reduce mortality and morbidity due to CHD.

Population: 838 patients with an MI in the prior 6 to 60 months and TC $\geq$ 220 mg/dL or LDL = 140 mg/dL after 6 weeks of dietary therapy.

Exclusion Criteria: Obesity, HTN, and diabetes.

Treatment: Partial ileal bypass of distal 200 cm or one third of small intestine (whichever was greater); all patients were on the AHA phase II diet.

Results: Surgical group had lower TC and LDL cholesterol levels (4.71 vs. 6.14 mM; 2.68 vs. 4.30 mM); surgical group had 35% reduction in incidence of cardiovascular death and MI at 5 years (82 vs. 125 events; $p < 0.001$); surgical group had significantly less angiographic progression ($p < 0.001$ at 5 and 7 years). Fewer surgical patients underwent CABG surgery ($p < 0.0001$) and angioplasty ($p = 0.005$).

23. **Scandinavian Simvastatin Survival Study Group (4S).** Randomised trial of cholesterol lowering in 4444 patients with coronary heart disease: the 4S. *Lancet* 1994;344:1383–1389.

Design: Prospective, randomized, double-blind, placebo-controlled, multicenter study. Primary end point was all-cause mortality. Median follow-up period was 5.4 years.

Purpose: To evaluate whether simvastatin would improve survival of patients with CHD.

Population: 4,444 patients aged 35 to 70 years with angina pectoris or previous MI (≥6 months earlier) and serum cholesterol, 5.5 to 8.0 mM.

Exclusion Criteria: Unstable angina, secondary hypercholesterolemia, planned CABG surgery, or angioplasty.

Treatment: Simvastatin, 20 to 40 mg once daily, or placebo.

Results: Simvastatin group had 25% lower TC, 35% lower LDL, and 8% higher HDL levels; simvastatin patients had significant 30% RRR in overall mortality (8.2% vs. 11.5%; $p = 0.0003$), as well as 39% fewer nonfatal MIs (7.4% vs. 12.1%), 41% fewer IHD deaths (5.0% vs. 8.5%), and 34% fewer myocardial revascularization procedures (11.3% vs. 17.2%). A 35% risk reduction was noted among patients in the lowest quartile of baseline LDL (see *Lancet* 1995;345:1274). Cost analysis showed that simvastatin-treated patients had 34% fewer cardiovascular-related hospital days and that there was \$3,872 savings/patient, reducing the effective drug cost by 88% to 28 cents/day (see *Circulation* 1996;93:1796). A subsequent analysis showed the annual cost of life gained (all costs, including lost wages) ranged from \$3,800 (70-year-old man with a TC level of 309 mg/dL) to \$27,400 (35-year-old woman with a TC level of 213 mg/dL).

24. **Sacks FM,** et al. Cholesterol and Recurrent Events (CARE): the effect of pravastatin on coronary events after MI in patients with average cholesterol levels. *N Engl J Med* 1996;335:1001–1009.

Design: Prospective, randomized, double-blind, placebo-controlled, multicenter study. Primary end point was CHD death and nonfatal MI. Median follow-up period was 5.0 years.

Purpose: To study the effectiveness in a typical population of lowering LDL-C levels to prevent coronary events after MI.

Population: 4,159 patients with MI within the prior 3 to 20 months, TC less than 240 mg/dL (mean, 209) and LDL, 115 to 174 mg/dL (mean, 139).

Exclusion Criteria: EF less than 25%; fasting glucose, 220 mg/dL; symptomatic HF.

Treatment: Pravastatin, 40 mg once daily, or placebo.

Results: Pravastatin group had 24% fewer cardiac deaths and nonfatal MIs (10.2% vs. 13.2%; $p = 0.003$), 26% lower rate of CABG surgery (7.5% vs. 10%; $p = 0.005$), 23% lower rate of balloon angioplasty (8.3% vs. 10.5%), 31% fewer strokes ($p = 0.03$) and nonsignificant 20% mortality reduction ($p = 0.10$). The reduction in primary events was restricted to those with a baseline LDL ≥125 mg/dL (greater than 150 to 175 mg/dL, 35% reduction; 125 to 150 mg/dL, 26% reduction; less than 125 mg/dL, 3% *increase*). Subsequent analysis found pravastatin use associated with a 32% reduction in stroke ($p = 0.03$) and 27% reduction in stroke or TIA ($p = 0.02$) (see *Circulation* 1999;99:216). Another subsequent analysis found that among those with LDL less than 125 mg/dL, only diabetics had a significant reduction in primary events (see *Circulation* 2002;105:1424).

25. **The Long-term Intervention with Pravastatin in Ischaemic Disease (LIPID)** Study Group. Prevention of cardiovascular events and death with pravastatin in patients with coronary heart disease and a broad range of initial cholesterol levels. *N Engl J Med* 1998;339:1349–1357.

Design: Prospective, randomized, double-blind, placebo-controlled, multicenter study. Primary end point was cardiovascular mortality. Mean follow-up period was 6.1 years.

Purpose: To evaluate the effects of lipid-lowering therapy on overall mortality in patients with a history of CAD and average cholesterol levels.

Population: 9,014 patients aged 31 to 75 years with MI or unstable angina within 3 to 36 months before study entry and an initial TC of 155 to 271 mg/dL.

Exclusion Criteria: Renal or hepatic disease, use of cholesterol-lowering medications, and significant medical or surgical event in prior 3 months.

Treatment: Pravastatin, 40 mg daily, or placebo.

Results: Pravastatin group had significant reduction in death from CHD, 6.4% versus 8.3% (RRR, 24%; $p < 0.001$); pravastatin patients also had a lower overall mortality rate (11.0% vs. 14.1%; RRR, 22%; $p < 0.001$), fewer MIs (7.4% vs. 10.3%; RRR,

29%; $p < 0.001$), fewer strokes (3.7% vs. 4.5%; RRR, 19%; $p = 0.048$), and less revascularization (13% vs. 15.7%; RRR, 20%; $p < 0.001$); no significant adverse effects were associated with pravastatin.

26. **Pitt B,** et al. Atorvastatin Versus Revascularization Treatment (**AVERT**) Investigators. Aggressive lipid-lowering therapy compared with angioplasty in stable coronary artery disease. *N Engl J Med* 1999;341:70–76.

Design: Prospective randomized, open-label, multicenter study. Primary end point was 18-month incidence of ischemic events consisting of cardiac death, resuscitation after cardiac arrest, nonfatal MI, cerebrovascular accident, CABG, angioplasty, and worsening angina resulting in hospitalization.

Purpose: To compare percutaneous coronary revascularization with lipid-lowering treatment for reducing ischemic events in patients with IHD and stable angina pectoris.

Population: 341 patients with stable one- or two-vessel CAD, relatively normal LV function, and a LDL $\geq$115 mg/dL who were referred for percutaneous revascularization.

Exclusion Criteria: Included left main or triple-vessel disease, unstable angina, or MI in prior 2 weeks, and LVEF less than 40%.

Treatment: Atorvastatin, 80 mg once daily, or balloon angioplasty, followed by usual care, which could include lipid-lowering treatment.

Results: Atorvastatin group had a 46% reduction in LDL levels (72 mg/dL) compared with an 18% reduction (to 199 mg/dL) in the angioplasty group. Incidence of ischemic events was 36% lower in the atorvastatin group [13% vs. 21%; $p = 0.048$ (but not significant after adjustment for interim analyses)]. In particular, the atorvastatin group had a lower incidence of CABG surgery (1.2% vs. 5.1%) and less frequent hospitalization for worsening angina (6.7% vs. 14.1%).

27. **Rubins HB,** et al. Veterans Affairs HDL Cholesterol Intervention Trial (**VA-HIT**) Study Group. Gemfibrozil for the secondary prevention of coronary heart disease in men with low levels of high-density lipoprotein cholesterol. *N Engl J Med* 1999;341:410–418.

Design: Prospective, randomized, placebo-controlled, double-blind, multicenter study. Primary outcome was a combined incidence of CHD death or nonfatal MI. Mean follow-up was 5.1 years.

Purpose: To evaluate whether increasing HDL cholesterol levels and lowering TG levels would reduce major cardiac events in men with low HDL and LDL cholesterol.

Population: The 2,531 men, aged 74 years, with CHD, HDL $\geq$40 mg/dL, LDL = 140 mg/dL, and triglycerides = 300 mg/dL.

Treatment: Gemfibrozil, 1,200 mg once daily, or placebo.

Results: Gemfibrozil therapy did not significantly reduce LDL levels, but did increase HDL by 6% and decrease TG levels by 31% at 1 year. The gemfibrozil group had a significant reduction in CHD-related death or MI (17.3% vs. 21.7%; RR reduction, 22%; $p = 0.006$). A nonsignificant 10% reduction was noted in all-cause mortality (15.7% vs. 17.4%; $p = 0.23$).

28. **MIRACL** (Myocardial Ischemia Reduction with Aggressive Cholesterol Lowering). Effects of atorvastatin on early recurrent ischemic events in acute coronary syndromes: the MIRACL study: a randomized controlled trial. *JAMA* 2001;285:1711–1718.

Design: Prospective, randomized, double-blind, placebo-controlled, multicenter trial. Primary end point was death, MI, cardiac arrest with resuscitation, or recurrent symptomatic ischemia with objective evidence requiring emergency hospitalization. Follow-up was 4 months.

Purpose: To evaluate the efficacy of early initiation of lipid-lowering therapy with atorvastatin in ACS patients.

Population: 3,086 conservatively managed patients with unstable angina/non-STEMI. Patients had the following: (a) chest pain for longer than 15 minutes at rest or with minimal exertion within 24 hours, and a change from a previous pattern of angina;

(b) new or dynamic ST- or T-wave changes, or new wall-motion abnormality, or positive noninvasive test; (c) troponin or CK-MB greater than 2 times ULN for non-STEMI.

Exclusion Criteria: Serum cholesterol greater than 270 mg/dL, Q-wave MI within 4 weeks, CABG within 3 months, PCI within 6 months, left bundle branch block (LBBB) or paced rhythm, lipid-lowering drugs other than niacin at doses less than 500 mg daily, vitamin E (unless less than 400 IU daily), liver dysfunction [alanine aminotransferase (ALT) greater than twice ULN], insulin-dependent diabetes.

Treatment: Randomization within 24 to 96 hours to high-dose atorvastatin (80 mg/day), or matching placebo.

Results: The atorvastatin group had a significant 15% relative reduction in the composite primary end point compared with placebo (14.8% vs. 17.4%; $p = 0.048$), primarily because of fewer recurrent ischemic events with objective evidence (RR, 0.74; $p = 0.02$). No differences were found between the groups in death, MI, or cardiac arrest. Stroke was significantly decreased in the atorvastatin group (RR, 0.41; $p = 0.02$). Lipid levels were decreased by approximately 40% with atorvastatin, but findings were not coupled to degree of lipid lowering. Only 3% had an increase in liver function tests to more than 3 times normal, and no cases of rhabdomyolysis were observed.

29. **Serruys PW,** et al. for the Lescol Intervention Prevention Study (**LIPS**) Investigators. Fluvastatin for prevention of cardiac events following successful first percutaneous coronary intervention: a randomized controlled trial. *JAMA* 2002;287:3215–3222.

Design: Prospective, randomized, double-blind, placebo-controlled, multicenter trial: primary end point was survival time free of cardiac death, nonfatal MI, or reintervention (major adverse cardiac event; MACE). Median follow-up was 3.9 years.

Purpose: To determine whether fluvastatin reduces MACEs in patients who have undergone PCI.

Population: 1,677 patients aged 18 to 80 years with stable or unstable angina or silent ischemia after successful first PCI with TC levels of 135 to 270 mg/dL, with fasting TG levels less than 400 mg/dL.

Treatment: Fluvastatin, 80 mg/day, or matching placebo; median time between PCI and first dose of study medication was 2.0 days.

Results: MACE-free survival time was significantly longer in the fluvastatin group ($p = 0.01$). Overall, the fluvastatin group had significantly fewer patients who had one or more major events (21.4% vs. 26.7%; RR, 0.78; $p = 0.01$). This result was independent of baseline TC levels. Subgroup analyses demonstrated even more robust MACE reductions with fluvastatin in diabetics (RR, 0.53; $p = 0.04$) and in those with multivessel disease (RR, 0.66; $p = 0.01$). No cases of CPK elevations 10 times or more ULN or rhabdomyolysis were found in the fluvastatin group.

30. **FLORIDA.** Preliminary results presented at the Annual Scientific Session of the American Heart Association, New Orleans, LA, November 2001.

This prospective, randomized, placebo-controlled, multicenter trial enrolled 540 acute MI patients. Patients received fluvastatin, 40 mg twice daily, or placebo, starting within 24 hours of the onset of MI symptoms. At 1 year, fluvastatin therapy was associated with a nonsignificant trend toward less ischemia on 48-hour ambulatory ECG (30% vs. 36%). The reduction in ischemia was slightly more pronounced in patients who had ischemia at baseline (50% vs. 61%; $p = NS$). No difference was noted in clinical event rates between the two groups at 1 year, but the patients with severe ischemia at baseline showed a trend toward a reduction in events with fluvastatin ($p = 0.08$). The lower than expected mortality rate (2% to 4%) made the trial underpowered; therefore the results are not inconsistent with those of the MIRACL trial.

Combined Primary and Secondary Prevention Trials

31. **Heart Protection Study** (HPS) Collaborative Group. MRC/BHF Heart Protection Study of cholesterol lowering with simvastatin in 20,536 high-risk individuals: a randomised placebo-controlled trial. *Lancet* 2002;360:7–22.

Design: Prospective, randomized, double-blind, placebo-controlled, multicenter trial. Primary end point was mortality and fatal or nonfatal vascular events (for subcategory analyses).

Purpose: To determine whether reducing LDL-C may reduce the development of vascular disease, irrespective of initial cholesterol concentrations.

Population: 20,536 U.K. men and women with coronary disease, other occlusive arterial disease, diabetes, or HTN in men older than 65 years.

Exclusion Criteria: Included chronic liver disease, impaired renal function, inflammatory muscle disease, severe HF.

Treatment: Simvastatin, 40 mg daily (average compliance, 85%), or matching placebo (average nonstudy statin use, 17%).

Results: The simvastatin group had a significant reduction in all-cause mortality compared with the placebo group (12.9% vs. 14.7%; $p = 0.0003$), because of a highly significant 18% relative reduction in coronary death rate (5.7% vs. 6.9%; $p = 0.0005$), a marginally significant reduction in other vascular deaths (1.9% vs. 2.2%; $p = 0.07$), and a nonsignificant reduction in nonvascular deaths (5.3% vs. 5.6%; $p = 0.4$). Simvastatin also was associated with lower rates of nonfatal MI or coronary death (8.7% vs. 11.8%; $p < 0.0001$), nonfatal or fatal stroke (4.3% vs. 5.7%; $p < 0.0001$), and coronary or noncoronary revascularization (9.1% vs. 11.7%; $p < 0.0001$). The reductions in major events were not significant in the first year, but were then highly significant for each subsequent year. The proportional reduction in the event rate was similar (and significant) in all subcategories, including those with cerebrovascular disease, PAD, diabetes, those either younger than or older than 70 years at entry, and even those who had an initial LDL-C less than 116 mg/dL (3.0 mM) or TC less than 193 mg/dL (5 mM). The annual excess risk of myopathy with this regimen was only about 0.01%. No significant adverse effects on cancer incidence were found.

Comments: This landmark study demonstrates that adding simvastatin to existing treatments safely provides substantial additional benefits for high-risk patients, irrespective of their initial cholesterol concentrations. After making allowance for noncompliance, actual use of this regimen would likely decrease major event rates by about one third.

32. **Shepherd J,** et al. for the **PROSPER** (PROspective Study of Pravastatin in the Elderly at Risk) Study Group. Pravastatin in elderly individuals at risk of vascular disease (PROSPER): a randomised controlled trial. *Lancet* 2002;360:1623–1630.

Design: Prospective, randomized, double-blind, placebo-controlled, multicenter trial. Primary end point was coronary death, nonfatal MI, and fatal or nonfatal stroke. Average follow-up was 3.2 years.

Purpose: To determine the benefits of pravastatin in an elderly cohort with, or at high risk of developing, CVD and stroke.

Population: 5,804 patients aged 70 to 82 years with a history of, or risk factors for, vascular disease and baseline TC of 4.0 mM to 9.0 mM.

Exclusion Criteria: Included poor cognitive function [Mini Mental State Examination (MMSE) score, less than 24].

Treatment: Pravastatin, 40 mg per day, or placebo.

Results: Pravastatin lowered LDL-C concentrations by 34%. Pravastatin group had a significant reduction in the incidence of the primary composite end point compared with the placebo group (14.1% vs. 16.2%; HR, 0.85; 95% CI, 0.74 to 0.97; $p = 0.014$). The incidence of only CHD death and nonfatal MI also was reduced (HR, 0.81; 95% CI, 0.69 to 0.94; $p = 0.006$), whereas a 24% reduction occurred in death due to coronary disease ($p = 0.043$). Stroke rates were similar (HR, 1.03); the study was underpowered to detect a reduction in stroke due to fewer than expected strokes. A trend toward fewer TIAs was found with pravastatin (HR, 0.75; 95% CI, 0.55 to 1.00;

$p = 0.051$). Pravastatin had no significant effect on cognitive function or disability. New cancer diagnoses were more frequent with pravastatin than with placebo (1.25; 1.04 to 1.51; $p = 0.020$). However, much of this excess occurred early after start of therapy, and inclusion of these data in a meta-analysis of all pravastatin and all statin trials showed no overall increase in risk.

33. **ALLHAT-LLT** (ALLHAT Lipid Lowering Trial): The ALLHAT officers and coordinators for the ALLHAT Collaborative Research Group. Major outcomes in moderately hypercholesterolemic, hypertensive patients randomized to pravastatin versus usual care. *JAMA* 2002;288:2998–3007.

Design: Prospective, randomized, active-controlled, multicenter trial. Primary end point was all-cause mortality. Secondary outcomes included nonfatal MI or fatal CHD (CHD events) combined, cause-specific mortality, and cancer. Mean follow-up was 4.8 years.

Purpose: To determine whether pravastatin compared with usual care reduces all-cause mortality in older, moderately hypercholesterolemic, hypertensive participants with at least one additional CHD risk factor.

Population: 10,355 individuals aged 55 years or older, with LDL-C of 120 to 189 mg/dL (100 to 129 mg/dL if known CHD) and TGs less than 350 mg/dL. During the trial, 32% of usual-care participants with and 29% without CHD started taking lipid-lowering drugs.

Treatment: Pravastatin, 40 mg/day, versus usual care.

Results: At year 4, pravastatin group had 17% lower TC levels compared with an 8% reduction with usual care. Among those who had LDL-C levels assessed, levels were reduced by 28% with pravastatin versus 11% with usual care. All-cause mortality was similar for the two groups [14.9% (pravastatin); 15.3%; $p = 0.88$]. A nonsignificant 9% relative reduction was noted in CHD event rates in the pravastatin group [6-year incidence, 9.3% (pravastatin) vs. 10.4%; RR, 0.91; $p = 0.16$].

Comments: The lack of a significant difference between the usual-care group and those randomized to receive a statin may be explained by the inclusion of statins in the usual-care group for secondary prevention.

Angiographic Analyses

34. **Blankenhorn DH,** et al., Cholesterol-Lowering Atherosclerosis Study (**CLAS-I**). Beneficial effects of combined colestipol-niacin therapy on coronary atherosclerosis and coronary venous bypass grafts. *JAMA* 1987;257:3233–3240.

This prospective, randomized, placebo-controlled, partially blinded, multicenter study enrolled 162 nonsmoking men aged 40 to 59 years who had undergone prior CABG surgery. Patients received colestipol (15 g twice daily) and niacin (3 to 12 g/day), or placebo. At follow-up (2 years), the drug group had 26% lower TC, 43% lower LDL, and 37% higher HDL; as well as higher atherosclerosis regression rate (16.2% vs. 2.4%; $p = 0.002$) and fewer new lesions or adverse changes in bypass grafts ($p < 0.04$ and $p < 0.03$, respectively).

35. **Brown G,** et al., Familial Atherosclerosis Treatment Study (**FATS**). Regression of coronary artery disease as a result of intensive lipid-lowering therapy in men with high levels of apolipoprotein B. *N Engl J Med* 1990;323:1289–1298.

This prospective, randomized, double-blind, placebo-controlled (or colestipol-controlled), multicenter study enrolled 146 men with documented CAD and family history of CAD. Patients were assigned to (a) lovastatin, 20 mg twice daily, and colestipol, 5 mg 3 times daily, for 10 days initially, then increased to 20 g three times daily; (b) niacin, 125 mg twice daily initially, gradually increased to 1 g 4 times daily at 2 months, and colestipol; or (c) placebo, lovastatin, and colestipol (although colestipol was given if LDL was elevated). At follow-up (2.5 years), group c (conventional therapy) had minimal changes in LDL and HDL (−7% and +5%, respectively), whereas the changes were substantial in the treatment groups: colestipol and lovastatin, −46% and +15%; niacin and colestipol, −32% and +43%. Lesion progression in one of nine proximal coronary segments was seen in 46% in the conventional group, compared with 21% and 25% in the two treatment groups, respectively. Lesion regression was more frequently observed in the treatment groups (32% and 39% vs. 11%). Clinical events (death, MI, revascularization for worsening symptoms) occurred significantly less often in the treatment groups (6.5% and 4.2% vs. 19.2%).

36. **Blankenhorn DH,** et al., Monitored Atherosclerosis Regression Study (**MARS**). Coronary angiographic changes with lovastatin therapy. *Ann Intern Med* 1993;119:969–976.

Design: Prospective, randomized, placebo-controlled study. Primary end point was average change from baseline in percentage diameter stenosis of all lesions with ≥20% stenosis baseline. Mean follow-up period was 2.2 years.
Purpose: To evaluate the effects of lovastatin on the progression of atherosclerosis coronary angiographic findings in patients with documented CAD.
Population: 270 patients aged 37 to 67 years with TC of 190 to 295 mg/dL and angiographically documented CAD.
Treatment: Lovastatin, 80 mg/day, or placebo; all patients were put on a cholesterol-lowering diet.
Results: Lovastatin group had 38% lower TC, 38% lower LDL, 8.5% higher HDL, and 0.9% regression of stenoses greater than 50% (vs. +4.1% in the placebo group; $p = 0.005$). Mean percentage diameter of stenosis increased by 2.2% in patients receiving placebo and by 1.6% in lovastatin patients ($p > 0.20$).

37. **Waters D,** et al., Canadian Coronary Atherosclerosis Intervention Trial (**CCAIT**). Effects of monotherapy with an HMG-CoA reductase inhibitor on the progression of coronary atherosclerosis as assessed by serial quantitative angiography: the Canadian Coronary Atherosclerosis Intervention Trial. *Circulation* 1994;89:959–968.

Design: Prospective, randomized, double-blind, placebo-controlled study. Primary end point was a coronary score, defined as per patient mean of minimal luminal diameter (MLD) changes. Follow-up period was 2 years.
Purpose: To evaluate the effect of lovastatin on the progression of atherosclerosis.
Population: 331 patients aged 21 to 50 years with documented atherosclerosis (on angiography in prior 12 weeks) and fasting serum TC of 220 to 300 mg/dL.
Treatment: Lovastatin, 20 mg/day, titrated to 40 to 80 mg/day over a period of 16 weeks to achieve LDL ≥130 mg/dL, or placebo.
Results: Lovastatin reduced TC and LDL levels by 21% and 29%, respectively, and slowed progression of lesions (−0.09 mm vs. +0.05 mm; $p = 0.01$). Lesion progression with no regression at other sites occurred less frequently in the lovastatin group (33% vs. 50%; $p = 0.003$). The lovastatin group also had fewer new coronary lesions ($p = 0.001$). In a subgroup of enrolled women taking lovastatin, TC and LDL decreased by 24% and 32%, respectively; angiographic progression was reduced (28% vs. 59%), and fewer new lesions were observed (4% vs. 45%) (see *Circulation* 1995;92:2404).

38. **Haskell WL,** et al., Stanford Coronary Risk Intervention Project (**SCRIP**). Effects of intensive multiple risk factor reduction on coronary atherosclerosis and clinical events in men and women with coronary artery disease. *Circulation* 1994;89:975–990.

Design: Prospective, randomized, open, multicenter study. Primary end point was angiographic change in minimal artery diameter in segments with visible disease at baseline. Follow-up period was 4 years.
Purpose: To determine the effect of a program of intensive multifactorial risk reduction on the progression of coronary atherosclerosis.
Population: 300 patients (86% men) younger than 75 years with angiographically documented coronary atherosclerosis.
Treatment: Risk reduction composed of low-fat and -cholesterol diet, exercise, no smoking, and antilipid drugs, or usual care.
Results: Risk-reduction group had 22% lower LDL and apolipoprotein B, 20% lower TGs, 12% higher HDL, 20% increase in exercise capacity, and 39% fewer

hospitalizations secondary to cardiac events (17.2% vs. 28.4%; $p = 0.05$). Risk-reduction group showed a 47% reduction in narrowing of diseased segments (change in diameter, -0.024 mm/yr vs. -0.045 mm/yr; $p < 0.02$).

39. **Oliver MF,** et al., Multicentre Anti-Atheroma Study (**MAAS**). Effect of simvastatin on coronary atheroma: the MAAS. *Lancet* 1994;344:633–638.

Design: Prospective, randomized, double-blind, placebo-controlled, multicenter study. Follow-up period was 4 years.
Purpose: To study the effects on coronary atheroma of reducing lipoprotein concentrations with simvastatin in patients with known coronary disease.
Population: The 270 patients with TC of 190 to 295 mg/dL and angiographically documented CAD.
Treatment: Diet and simvastatin, 20 mg once daily, or placebo.
Results: Compared with placebo group, simvastatin patients had 23% lower serum cholesterol, 31% lower LDL, and 9% higher HDL. Simvastatin group had a 2.6% reduction in the mean diameter of stenosis, whereas the placebo group had a 3.6% increase. The simvastatin group also had less disease progression (41 vs. 54 patients) and more frequent lesion regression (33 vs. 20 patients). No significant differences were seen in clinical event rates.

40. **Pitt B,** et al., Pravastatin Limitation of Atherosclerosis in Coronary arteries (**PLAC I**). PLAC I: reduction in atherosclerosis progression and clinical events. *J Am Coll Cardiol* 1995;26:1133–1139.

Design: Prospective, randomized, blinded, placebo-controlled, multicenter study. Follow-up was 3 years.
Purpose: To evaluate the effect of diet and pravastatin on progression of coronary atherosclerosis in patients with mild to moderate hypercholesterolemia and CAD.
Population: 408 patients (mean age, 57 years) with LDL-C of 130 to 190 mg/dL despite diet and at least one stenosis ≥ 50% in a major coronary vessel.
Treatment: Pravastatin, 40 mg once daily, or placebo.
Results: At 3 years, pravastatin patients had 19% lower cholesterol, 28% lower LDL, and 7% higher HDL ($p = 0.001$). Progression of atherosclerosis was reduced by 40% ($p = 0.04$) in the pravastatin group, and they had fewer new lesions and 60% fewer MIs.
Comments: Results were achieved despite only 14% reaching the NCEP goal of LDL ≥ 100 mg/dL.

41. **Jukema JW,** et al., Regression Growth Evaluation Statin Study (**REGRESS**). Effects of lipid lowering by pravastatin on progression and regression of coronary artery disease in symptomatic men with normal to moderately elevated serum cholesterol levels. *Circulation* 1995;91:2528–2540.

Design: Prospective, randomized, double-blind, placebo-controlled, multicenter study. Primary end point was change in average mean segment diameter and change in average minimum obstruction diameter.
Purpose: To determine the effect of 2 years of treatment with an HMG-CoA reductase inhibitor on coronary atherosclerosis.
Population: 885 patients with proven myocardial ischemia and TC of 155 to 310 mg/dL (4 to 8 mM) with angiographically documented coronary disease.
Treatment: Pravastatin, 40 mg once daily, or placebo.
Results: Of patients, 88% had an evaluable angiogram. At 2 years, the pravastatin group had less progression of mean segment diameter and median minimal obstruction (-0.06 vs. -0.10 mm; $p = 0.019$; -0.03 vs. -0.09 mm; $p = 0.001$) and fewer new cardiovascular events (11% vs. 19%; $p = 0.002$). The pravastatin group had lower lipid levels (TC, -20%; LDL, -29%).
Comments: A substudy of 768 patients showed that pravastatin was associated with less transient myocardial ischemia on 48-hour ambulatory monitoring [28% (baseline) to 19% vs. 20% to 23% (placebo); OR, 0.62] (see *Circulation* 1996;94:1503).

42. **Post-CABG** Trial Investigators. The effect of aggressive lowering of LDL choles-terol levels and low-dose anticoagulation on obstructive changes in saphenous venous coronary artery bypass grafts. *N Engl J Med* 1997;336:153–162.

Design: Prospective, randomized, 2 × 2 factorial, multicenter study. Primary end point was substantial progression of graft atherosclerosis (defined as new lesions, progres-sion of lesions present at baseline, new occlusions). Angiography was performed at an average of 4.3 years.

Purpose: To (a) determine whether aggressive lowering of LDL-C in patients with saphenous venous CABGs is more effective than moderate lowering in delayed pro-gression of graft atherosclerosis; and (b) evaluate whether low-dose anticoagulation reduces bypass graft obstruction.

Population: 1,351 patients aged 21 to 74 years with LDL-C of 130 to 175 mg/dL who had undergone CABG surgery in prior 1 to 11 years and had one patent graft.

Exclusion Criteria: Likelihood of revascularization or death within 5 years, EF less than 30%, and unstable angina or MI within prior 6 months.

Treatment: Aggressive lipid-lowering therapy with lovastatin, 40 to 80 mg/day [goal LDL, less than 85 (actual, 93 to 97)] or moderate therapy with lovastatin, 2.5 to 5.0 mg/day [LDL goal, less than 140 (actual, 132 to 136)]. Cholestyramine was added if necessary. Second randomization to low-dose warfarin (mean international normalized ratio, 1.4), or placebo.

Results: Aggressive therapy group had less atherosclerotic progression ($\geq$0.6 mm di-ameter decrease; 27% vs. 39%; $p < 0.001$) and 29% less revascularization (6.5% vs. 9.2%; $p = 0.03$). No difference was detected between warfarin and placebo groups, but at 7.5-year follow-up, low-dose anticoagulation patients had 31% lower incidence of death and MI.

43. **Herd JA,** et al., Lipoprotein and Coronary Atherosclerosis Study (**LCAS**). Ef-fects of fluvastatin on coronary atherosclerosis in patients with mild to moderate cholesterol elevations (LCAS). *Am J Cardiol* 1997;80:278–286.

Design: Prospective, randomized, double-blind, placebo-controlled study. Follow-up period was 2.5 years.

Purpose: To evaluate whether fluvastatin would favorably influence coronary atherosclerosis in patients with mildly to moderately elevated LDL-C.

Population: 429 CAD patients (19% women) aged 35 to 75 years and with LDL choles-terol of 115 to 190 mg/dL.

Treatment: Fluvastatin, 20 mg twice daily, or placebo; 25% with LDL of 160 mg/dL received open-label cholestyramine (maximum, 12 g/day).

Results: Fluvastatin-only subgroup had 22.5% lower LDL (LDL in all fluvastatin pa-tients was reduced by 23.9%). Angiograms at 2.5 years (340 patients) showed that the fluvastatin group had less progression versus placebo (mean lumen diameter, −0.028 vs. −0.100 mm; $p < 0.01$) and a nonsignificant 24% reduction in cardiovascu-lar events (14.5% vs. 19.1%). A subsequent analysis showed that patients with low HDL levels (less than 35 mg/dL) had the greatest angiographic and clinical benefit (see *Circulation* 1999;99:736).

44. **Frick MH,** et al., for Lopid Coronary Angiography Trial (**LOCAT**) Study Group. Prevention of the angiographic progression of coronary and vein-graft atheroscle-rosis by gemfibrozil after coronary bypass surgery in men with low levels of HDL cholesterol. *Circulation* 1997;96:2137–2143.

This prospective, randomized study of 395 post–coronary bypass men with an HDL-cholesterol (HDL-C) of 1.1 mM or less and LDL of 4.5 mM or less. Patients received gemfibrozil, 1,200 mg/day, or placebo. Follow-up angiography was done at an average of 32 months. The gemfibrozil group had a smaller change in average diameter of native coronary segments compared with placebo (−0.01 mm vs. −0.04 mm; $p = 0.009$). The equivalent changes in MLDs of stenoses were −0.04 mm and −0.09 mm, respectively ($p = 0.002$). In aortocoronary bypass grafts, 23 (14%) placebo subjects had new le-sions at follow-up angiography, compared with only four (2%) gemfibrozil subjects ($p < 0.001$).

45. **Teo K,** et al., for the **SCAT** Investigators. Long-term effects of cholesterol lowering and angiotensin-converting enzyme inhibition on coronary atherosclerosis: the Simvastatin/Enalapril Coronary Atherosclerosis Trial (SCAT). *Circulation* 2000;102:1748–1754.

Design: Prospective, randomized, placebo-controlled, 2 × 2 factorial, multicenter trial. Primary end point: death, MI, or CVA. Average follow-up, 4 years.

Purpose: To assess the effects of a statin, an ACE inhibitor, and their combination on the natural history of angiographic coronary disease in patients without hypercholesterolemia.

Population: 460 normocholesterolemic patients; mean baseline TC was 200 mg/dL; TGs, 160 mg/dL; HDL-C, 38 mg/dL; and LDL-C, 129 mg/dL. Of the patients, 90% were taking ASA, and 48% taking β-blockers.

Treatment: Simvastatin, up to 40 mg once daily; enalapril, 10 mg twice daily; their combination; or matching placebos.

Results: The simvastatin group had superior angiographic outcomes with a smaller decrease in mean coronary diameter [0.07 mm vs. 0.14 mm (placebo); $p = 0.004$] as well as mean luminal diameter. Simvastatin group also had a lower incidence of CABG or PCI (6% vs. 12%; $p = 0.02$). Enalapril had no significant effect on angiographic end points, but fewer enalapril patients had death, MI, or CVA (7% vs. 13%; $p = 0.043$). No significant added benefit of combination therapy was noted.

46. **Steiner G, DAIS** (Diabetes Atherosclerosis Intervention Study) Investigators. Effect of fenofibrate on progression of coronary artery disease in type 2 diabetes: the Diabetes Atherosclerosis Intervention Study: a randomised study. *Lancet* 2001;357:905–910.

This prospective, randomized, double-blind, placebo-controlled, multicenter trial enrolled 418 type 2 diabetics with good glycemic control (mean hemoglobin A_{1c}, 7.5%) and at least one visible coronary lesion. Patients received fenofibrate (200 mg/day) or placebo for at least 3 years. The fenofibrate group had a significantly smaller increase in percentage diameter stenosis compared with placebo (mean, 2.1% vs. 3.7%; $p = 0.02$), a significantly smaller decrease in MLD (-0.06 mm vs. -0.10 mm; $p = 0.029$), and a nonsignificantly smaller decrease in mean segment diameter (-0.06 mm vs. -0.08 mm; $p = 0.17$). The trial was not powered to examine clinical end points, but fewer occurred in the fenofibrate group than in the placebo group (38 vs. 50).

47. **Brown BG,** et al. **HATS** (HDL-Atherosclerosis Treatment Study). Simvastatin and niacin, antioxidant vitamins, or the combination for the prevention of coronary disease. *N Engl J Med* 2001;345:1583–1592.

Design: Prospective, randomized, double-blind, placebo-controlled trial. Primary end point was mean change per patient in the most severe coronary stenosis from initial to final arteriogram. Primary clinical end point was the occurrence of a first cardiovascular event (death, MI, stroke, or revascularization). Follow-up was 3 years.

Purpose: To determine whether lipid-lowering and antioxidant therapy provide independent and additive benefits for patients with CAD and low HDL levels.

Population: 160 patients with clinical coronary disease (prior MI, coronary interventions, or confirmed angina), low HDL-C levels (men, less than 35 mg/dL; women, 40 mg/dL or less) and normal LDL-C levels (145 mg/dL or less).

Exclusion Criteria: Included previous CABG surgery, severe HTN, uncontrolled diabetes.

Treatment: Simvastatin plus niacin, vitamins, simvastatin-niacin plus antioxidants, or placebo [niacin placebo was active (only 50 mg), provoked flushing but did not affect lipids].

Results: In the simvastatin-niacin group, LDL decreased by 42% and HDL increased by 26%, whereas the levels were unchanged in antioxidant and placebo groups. The protective increase in HDL with simvastatin plus niacin was attenuated by concurrent therapy with antioxidants. The average stenosis progressed by 3.9% with placebos, 1.8% with antioxidants, and 0.7% with simvastatin-niacin plus antioxidants ($p = 0.004$), and regressed by 0.4% with simvastatin-niacin alone ($p < 0.001$).

Incidence of the composite clinical end point was significantly lower in the simvastatin-niacin–alone group compared with the placebos (3% vs. 24%; $p = 0.003$); the incidence was an intermediate 14% in simvastatin-niacin plus antioxidants group.

Triglycerides
Review Articles and Meta-Analyses
48. **Austin MA,** et al. Hypertriglyceridemia as a cardiovascular risk factor. *Am J Cardiol* 1999;81:7B–12B.

This analysis of 17 studies enrolled 46,413 men and 10,864 women. Average follow-up period was 8.4 years. Elevated TG levels were associated with a 32% increased cardiovascular risk in men and 76% in women. After adjustment for HDL and other risk factors, these increased risks were attenuated but remained statistically significant (men, 14%; women, 37%).

Studies
49. **Criqui MH,** et al. Plasma triglyceride level and mortality from coronary heart disease. *N Engl J Med* 1993;328:1220–1225.

This study analyzed 7,505 patients in the Lipid Research Clinics Follow-up trial. The 12-year incidence of coronary death in both men and women increased with TG levels. However, after adjustment for potential covariates, this association was no longer statistically significant.

50. **Assmann G,** et al. Hypertriglyceridemia and elevated lipoprotein(a) are risk factors for major coronary events in middle-aged men. *Am J Cardiol* 1996;77:1179–1184.

This analysis of 8-year follow-up data of 4,849 Prospective Cardiovascular Munster (PROCAM) study patients, consisting of men aged 40 to 65 years, showed that elevated TG levels were independently associated with an increased risk of major coronary events ($p < 0.001$ in a multivariate analysis). In the small subset (4.3%) of patients with TG greater than 200 mg/dL and LDL/HDL less than 5.0, risk was elevated by sixfold.

51. **Gaziano JM,** et al. Fasting triglycerides, HDL and risk of MI. *Circulation* 1997;96:2520–2525.

This case-control study of 340 MI survivors aged ≥75 years and 340 age-, smoking-, and community-matched controls. After adjustment for age and gender, the risk of MI was 6.8 times higher in those with the highest TG levels, and the risk was even higher (16-fold) in those with the highest TG-to-HDL ratio.

52. **Jeppensen J,** et al. Triglyceride concentration and ischemic heart disease. *Circulation* 1998;97:1029–1036.

This study of 2,906 Copenhagen Male Study participants initially free of CVD found that high fasting TG level is an independent risk factor for IHD. At 8-year follow-up, the risk factor–adjusted RRs of IHD were 1.5 (95% CI, 1.0 to 2.3; $p = 0.05$) and 2.2 (95% CI, 1.4 to 3.4; $p < 0.001$) for middle and higher thirds of TG levels. A clear gradient of risk was found with increasing TG levels within each level of HDL, including high HDL.

Lipoprotein(a)
Review Articles and Meta-Analysis
53. **Danesh J,** et al. Lipoprotein(a) and coronary heart disease: meta-analysis of prospective studies. *Circulation* 2000;102:1082–1085.

This meta-analysis examined 27 prospective studies with at least 1 year of follow-up (mean, 10). Comparison of individuals in the top third of baseline plasma Lp(a) measurements with those in the bottom third resulted in a combined risk ratio of CHD death or nonfatal MI of 1.6 (95% CI, 1.4 to 1.8; $2 p < 0.00001$). The findings were similar when the analyses were restricted to the 18 studies of general populations (combined RR, 1.7; 95% CI, 1.4 to 1.9; 2 p < 0.00001). Despite differences among studies in blood-storage techniques and assay methods, no significant heterogeneity was found among the 18 population-based studies or nine studies of patients with previous disease.

Studies
54. **Ridker PM,** Hennekens CH, et al. A prospective study of lipoprotein(a) and the risk of MI. *JAMA* 1993;270:2195–2199.

This nested case-control study of 296 PHS participants in whom MI subsequently developed and 296 controls, matched for smoking status and age, showed no evidence of an association between Lp(a) levels and the future MI risk. No significant differences were noted between groups in median Lp(a) levels [103.0 mg/L (cases) vs. 102.5 mg/L; p = 0.73]. After adjustment for age and smoking status and even further adjustment for both lipid and nonlipid cardiovascular risk factors, no significant increased MI risk was found with higher Lp(a) levels.

55. **Schaefer EJ,** et al. Lipid Research Clinics Coronary Primary Prevention Trial (**LRC-CPPT**). Lipoprotein(a) levels and risk of coronary heart disease in men. *JAMA* 1994;271:999–1003.

This study enrolled 3,806 men aged 35 to 59 years with TC greater than 265 mg/dL and LDL greater than 190 mg/dL. Patients were randomized to cholestyramine or placebo. Lp(a) was measured in serum obtained (and frozen) before randomization from 233 patients who manifested CHD during the study (7 to 10 years), as well as from 390 CHD-free controls. Lp(a) levels were 21% higher in CHD cases (adjusted p < 0.01).

56. **Bostom AG,** et al. A prospective investigation of elevated lipoprotein(a) detected by electrophoresis and cardiovascular disease in women: the Framingham Heart Study. *Circulation* 1994;90:1688–1695.

A total of 3,103 female Framingham Heart Study participants had Lp(a) indirectly measured at baseline by paper electrophoresis. A positive result was defined as the presence of a detectable sinking pre-β lipoprotein band; band presence was 51% sensitive and 95% specific for detecting plasma lipoprotein levels greater than 30 mg/dL (threshold value associated with increased cardiovascular risk in men). At follow-up (mean, 12 years), multivariate adjusted RR estimates were as follows: MI, 2.37 (1.48 to 3.81), total CHD, 1.61 (1.13 to 2.29), total CVD, 1.44 (1.09 to 1.91).

57. **Bostom AG,** et al. Elevated plasma lipoprotein(a) and coronary heart disease in men <55 years old. *JAMA* 1996;276:544–548.

The study population was composed of 2,191 Framingham Study patients. At follow-up (15 years), an elevated Lp(a) level (greater than 30 mg/dL) was associated with CHD (MI, angina, sudden death): RR, 1.9 (vs. TC greater than 240 mg/dL, 1.8; vs. HDL less than 35 mg/dL, 1.8; vs. smoking, 3.6; vs. glucose intolerance, 2.7).

58. **Nguyen TT,** et al. Predictive value of electrophoretically detected lipoprotein(a) for coronary heart disease and cerebrovascular disease in a community-based cohort of 9936 men and women. *Circulation* 1997;96:1390–1397.

This prospective cohort study was composed of 9,935 people who had undergone lipoprotein analysis between 1968 and 1982. At follow-up (mean, 13.2 years), semi-quantitative levels were measured based on electrophoresis band pattern (0, absent; 1, trace; 2, small increase; 3, increase). A level of 3.0 (by enzyme-linked immunosorbent assay; mean, 55.3 mg/dL) was associated with an increased risk of CAD [adjusted HRs were 1.9 for women (95% CI, 1.3 to 2.9) and 1.6 for men (95% CI, 1.0 to 2.5)].

Antioxidants

Studies

59. **Cambridge Heart Antioxidant Study (CHAOS).** Randomised controlled trial of vitamin E in patients with coronary artery disease: CHAOS. *Lancet* 1996;347:781–786.

Design: Prospective, randomized, double-blind, placebo-controlled, single-center study. Primary end points were nonfatal MI and cardiovascular death plus nonfatal MI. The median follow-up period was 510 days.

Purpose: To evaluate whether high-dose α-tocopherol would reduce subsequent risk of MI and cardiovascular death in patients with known CAD.

Population: 2,002 patients with angiographically proven coronary atherosclerosis.

Exclusion Criteria: Prior use of vitamin supplements containing vitamin E.

Treatment: Vitamin E, 400 IU/day or 800 IU/day, or placebo.

Results: Treatment group had significant reduction in cardiovascular death and nonfatal MI (RR, 0.53; 95% CI, 0.34 to 0.083; $p = 0.005$). The beneficial effects on this composite end point were due to the 66% fewer nonfatal MIs (14 vs. 41 patients; $p = 0.005$); no difference in cardiovascular deaths was detected (27 vs. 23 patients; $p = 0.61$).

60. **Hennekens CH,** et al. **Physicians Health Study.** Lack of effect of long-term supplementation with beta carotene on the incidence of malignant neoplasms and cardiovascular disease. *N Engl J Med* 1996;334:1145–1149.

Design: Prospective, randomized, double-blind, placebo-controlled study. Average follow-up period was 12 years.

Purpose: To evaluate the effect of long-term supplementation of β-carotene on the incidence of CVD and malignant neoplasms.

Population: 22,071 male physicians aged 40 to 84 years (in 1982).

Exclusion Criteria: History of cancer, MI, stroke, or transient cerebral ischemia.

Treatment: Placebo or β-carotene, 50 mg every other day.

Results: A 78% rate of compliance was observed. No significant difference in malignant neoplasms (1,273 vs. 1,293 patients), lung cancer (82 vs. 88 patients), overall mortality (979 vs. 968 patients), cardiovascular-related deaths (338 vs. 313 patients), MIs (468 vs. 489 patients), or strokes (967 vs. 972 strokes) was observed between groups.

61. **Omenn GS,** et al. Beta-Carotene and Retinol Efficacy Trial (**CARET**). Effects of a combination of beta carotene and vitamin A on lung cancer and cardiovascular disease. *N Engl J Med* 1996;334:1150–1155.

Design: Prospective, randomized, double-blind, placebo-controlled, multicenter study. Mean follow-up period was 4 years.

Purpose: To evaluate the effects of a combination of β-carotene and vitamin A on the incidence of lung cancer and cardiovascular-related deaths.

Population: 18,314 smokers, former smokers, and workers exposed to asbestos.

Treatment: β-Carotene, 30 mg, and vitamin A, 25,000 IU, or placebo, once daily.

Results: Trial was stopped 21 months early. Treatment group had increased RRs of lung cancer (1.28; 95% CI, 1.04 to 1.57; $p = 0.02$), lung cancer death (RR, 1.46; 95% CI, 1.47 to 2.0), all-cause mortality (RR, 1.17; 95% CI, 1.03 to 1.33), and cardiovascular death (RR, 1.26; 95% CI, 0.99 to 1.61).

62. **Kushi LH,** et al. Dietary antioxidant vitamins and death from coronary heart disease in postmenopausal women. *N Engl J Med* 1996;334:1156–1162.

Prospective cohort study of 34,486 women without CVD who completed a diet questionnaire in 1986. At follow-up (7 years), increased vitamin E intake correlated with fewer CHD deaths; this association was strongest among nonusers of vitamin: RRs, 0.42 in two highest quintiles of vitamin E intake (vs. lowest quintile). Vitamin E from supplements was not shown to be beneficial, although high doses and duration of use were not definitively addressed. Vitamin A and C intake did not have significant associations with the risk of death from CHD.

63. **Rapola JM,** et al. Alpha-Tocopherol Beta-Carotene Cancer Prevention Study (**ATBC**). Randomised trial of alpha-tocopherol and beta-carotene supplements on incidence of major coronary events in men with previous MI. *Lancet* 1997;349:1715–1720 (editorial, 1710–1711).

Design: Prospective, randomized, double-blind, placebo-controlled study. Primary end point was cardiac death and MI. Follow-up period was 5.3 years.
Purpose: To evaluate the effects of α-tocopherol and β-carotene supplements on the frequency of major coronary events.
Population: 1,862 male smokers aged 50 to 69 years with a history of MI.
Exclusion Criteria: Malignant disease, severe angina, and significant use of vitamins A, E, or β-carotene supplements.
Treatment: α-Tocopherol, 50 mg/day; β-carotene, 20 mg/day; both; or placebo.
Results: No difference was detected between groups in incidence of cardiac death and MI, but the β-carotene and β-carotene plus α-tocopherol groups had more cardiac deaths (RRs, 1.75 and 1.58; $p = 0.007$; $p = 0.03$). α-Tocopherol group had fewer nonfatal MIs [adjusted RR, 0.62 (0.41 to 0.96)]. Authors speculated this to be owing to more fatal MIs.
Comments: β-Carotene serum levels were 19 times normal. Editorial points out that α-tocopherol dose used was one tenth that of CHAOS dose, and a synthetic form was used (CHAOS, natural form).

64. **GISSI-Prevenzione** Investigators. Dietary supplementation with n-3 polyunsaturated fatty acids and vitamin E after myocardial infarction: results of the GISSI-Prevenzione trial. *Lancet* 1999;354:447–455.

Design: Prospective, randomized, open-label, multicenter study. Primary end point was death, nonfatal MI, and stroke. Average follow-up was 3.5 years.
Purpose: To evaluate the independent and combined effects of n-3 polyunsaturated fatty acids (PUFAs) and vitamin E on morbidity and mortality after MI.
Population: 11,324 patients with a MI in the previous 3 months.
Treatment: n-3 PUFA (1 g daily), vitamin E (300 mg/day), both, or none.
Results: The n-3 PUFA group had a significant reduction in death, MI, and stroke [12.3% vs. 14.6% (control); $p = 0.023$]. All-cause mortality was 20% lower in the n-3 PUFA group (8.3% vs. 10.4%). The vitamin E group had a nonsignificant reduction in death, MI, and stroke (13.1% vs. 14.4%). Vitamin E use was associated with a significant 20% reduction in cardiovascular deaths.

65. **HOPE,** The Heart Outcome Prevention Evaluation Study Investigators. Vitamin E supplementation and cardiovascular events in high risk patients. *N Engl J Med* 2000;342:154–160 (see reference 205 for expanded summary/ramipril results).

This prospective, randomized, 2×2 factorial study of 9,541 high-risk patients aged 55 years or older with CAD, stroke, PVD, or diabetes plus one other cardiovascular risk factor included a randomization to vitamin E (400 IU daily) or placebo. Vitamin E supplementation use was not beneficial [incidence of cardiovascular death, MI, and stroke was 16.0% vs. 15.4% (placebo)].

Special Diets

66. **Lyon Diet Heart Study; de Lorgeril M,** et al. A Mediterranean diet reduced mortality after MI. *Lancet* 1994;343:1454–1459.

This prospective, randomized, secondary prevention study enrolled 605 patients with a first MI (91% men). The diet group underwent a 1-hour educational session. At 8 weeks and annually, a diet survey and counseling were administered. At follow-up (average, 27 months), the Mediterranean diet group had a 73% lower incidence of death and nonfatal MI compared with the prudent Western-type diet group (2.7% vs. 11%; $p = 0.001$). A subsequent report with a mean follow-up of 46 months showed persistent benefits (see *Circulation* 1999;99:779).

67. **Ascherio A,** et al. Dietary intake of marine n-3 fatty acids, fish intake and the risk of coronary disease among men. *N Engl J Med* 1995;332:977–982 (editorial, 1024–1025).

This analysis was performed on 44,895 Health Professionals Follow-up Study participants who completed detailed and validated dietary questionnaires. At 6-year follow-up, no significant associations were observed between dietary intake of n-3 fatty acids or fish intake and risk of coronary disease. The multivariate risk of CHD was 1.12 among men in the top quintile of n-3 fatty acid intake compared with men from the bottom quintile (95% CI, 0.96 to 1.31). The risk of CHD death was 0.74 among men who ate any amount of fish compared with those who ate no fish; this finding was significant (95% CI, 0.44 to 1.23), but the risk did not decrease as fish consumption increased. Editorial asserts that a little fish may still do some good, but a greater amount of fish is not necessarily better.

68. **Rimm EB,** et al. Vegetable, fruit and cereal fiber intake and risk of coronary heart disease among men. *JAMA* 1996;275:447–451 (editorial, 486–487).

This observational study included 43,757 male physicians who filled out diet questionnaires. At 6-year follow-up, 41% fewer MIs were found in the highest-fiber quintile. The greatest risk reduction was associated with cereal fiber: RR, 0.71 for each 10-g increase. The editorial points out that the beneficial effect was confined to the highest quintile, probably the result of a healthy lifestyle (only 3.8% smokers, higher vitamin intake, etc.).

69. **Pietinen P,** et al. Intake of dietary fiber and risk of coronary heart disease in a cohort of Finnish men. *Circulation* 1996;94:2720–2727.

This analysis focused on 21,930 ATBC patients (all male smokers aged 50 to 69 years). At follow-up (average, 6.1 years), MI and CHD deaths were found to be inversely associated with fiber intake. The highest quintile (34.8 g/day) versus lowest quintile (16.1 g/day) showed an RR of coronary death of 0.69 ($p < 0.001$ for trend). The same effect was evident after adjustment for CRFs and intake of β-carotene and vitamins C and E. The strongest association was seen with water-soluble and cereal (vs. vegetable or fruit) fibers.

70. **Wolk A,** et al. Long-term intake of dietary fiber and decreased risk of coronary heart disease among women. *JAMA* 1999;281:1998–2004.

This analysis was performed on dietary data collected from NHS participants in 1984, 1986, and 1990 (semiquantitative food-frequency questionnaire). The response rate among the 68,782 women was 80% to 90% during the 10-year follow-up period. Women in the highest quintile of total dietary fiber intake (median, 22.9 g/day) had nearly a 50% lower incidence of major CHD events (age-adjusted RR, 0.53; 95% CI, 0.40 to 0.69) compared with women in the lowest quintile (median, 11.5 g/day). This effect was attenuated after controlling for age, cardiovascular risk factors, dietary factors, and multivitamin supplement use (RR, 0.77; 95% CI, 0.57 to 1.04). The multivariate model found that a 10 g/day increase in total dietary intake resulted in a 19% RRR (95% CI, 1% to 34%).

71. **von Schacky C.** The effect of dietary omega-3 fatty acids on coronary atherosclerosis. *Ann Intern Med* 1999;130:554–562.

This prospective, randomized, double-blind, placebo-controlled trial showed a modest reduction in angiographic progression of CAD with fish oil supplementation. A total of 223 patients with CAD by angiogram was randomized to fish oil concentrate (55% eicosapentaenoic and docosahexaenoic acids), 6 g/day for 3 months, and then 3 g/day, or placebo (fatty acid composition of average European diet), for 21 months. Pairs of angiograms (baseline and 2 years) were evaluated for 80 of 112 placebo recipients and 82 of 111 fish oil recipients. Angiographic analysis showed 48 coronary segments in the placebo group with changes (36 showed mild progression, five showed moderate progression, and seven showed mild regression) and 55 coronary segments in the fish oil group with changes (35 showed mild progression, four showed moderate progression, 14 showed mild regression, and two showed moderate regression;

$p = 0.041$). A trend toward fewer cardiovascular events was found in the fish oil group ($p = 0.10$), although LDL levels tended to be higher in the fish oil group.

72. **Liu S,** et al. A prospective study of dietary fiber intake and risk of cardiovascular disease among women. *J Am Coll Cardiol* 2002;39:49–56.

This prospective cohort study used a semiquantitative food-frequency questionnaire to assess dietary fiber intake among 39,876 female health professionals with no history of CVD or cancer. At 6-year follow-up, 570 incident cases of CVD had occurred, including 177 MIs. Comparing the highest quintile of fiber intake (median, 26.3 g/day) with the lowest quintile (median, 12.5 g/day), the RRs for CVD and MI, adjusted for age and randomized treatment status, were 0.65 (95% CI, 0.51 to 0.84) and 0.46 (95% CI, 0.30 to 0.72), respectively. After further adjustment for CVD risk factors, the RRs were a nonsignificant 0.79 and 0.68.

73. **Albert CM,** et al. Blood levels of long-chain n-3 fatty acids and the risk of sudden death. *N Engl J Med* 2002;346:1113–1118.

Prospective, nested case-control analysis of PHS participants (94 cases, 184 controls matched for age and smoking status). At follow-up (17 years), fatty acid composition in blood was analyzed by gas-liquid chromatography for 94 men in whom sudden death occurred as the first manifestation of CVD and for 184 controls matched for age and smoking status. Baseline blood levels of long-chain n-3 fatty acids were inversely related to the risk of sudden death both before and after adjustment for potential confounders (p values for trend, 0.004, 0.007). Compared with men whose long-chain n-3 fatty acid levels were in the lowest quartile, the RR of sudden death was significantly lower among men with levels in the third quartile (adjusted RR, 0.28; 95% CI, 0.09 to 0.87) and the fourth quartile (adjusted RR, 0.19; 95% CI, 0.05 to 0.71).

74. **Kris-Etherton PM,** et al., for the AHA Nutrition Committee. Fish consumption, fish oil, omega-3 fatty acids, and cardiovascular disease. *Circulation* 2002;106:2747–2757.

The AHA recommends that patients with documented CHD should consume about 1 g of omega-3 fatty acids per day. In those unable to eat sufficient amounts of fish to meet this requirement, it recommends daily supplementation with 1 g fish oil capsules that contain 180 mg of eicosapentaenoic acid and 120 mg of docosahexaenoic acid. In individuals with high TG levels, higher amounts (2 to 4 g/day) can be taken.

Diabetes and Metabolic Syndrome

Epidemiology
75. **Kannel WB.** Lipids, diabetes, and coronary heart disease: insights from the Framingham Heart Study. *Am Heart J* 1985;110:1100–1107.

After risk-factor adjustment, 26-year follow-up data showed that men with diabetes had a 70% increased risk of developing CHD, whereas the risk was 200% higher in women. High HDL levels (approximately 85 mg/dL) were found to be markedly protective, with an RR of CHD at 4 years of only 0.1 to 0.3. The combination of high LDL and low HDL resulted in the greatest risk of CHD: If LDL was 220 mg/dL and HDL was 25 mg/dL, RR was 2.9.

76. **Haffner SM,** et al. Mortality from coronary heart disease in subjects with type 2 diabetes and in nondiabetic subjects with and without prior MI. *N Engl J Med* 1998;339:229–234.

This Finnish-based population study found that diabetic subjects ($n = 1,059$) without a prior MI had a similar risk of subsequent MI compared with nondiabetic subjects ($n = 1,373$) with a prior MI. The 7-year incidence rates of MI among diabetics with and without a prior MI were 45.0% and 22%, compared with 18.8% and 3.5% in nondiabetics. The risk factor–adjusted HR for death from CHD for diabetics without prior MI as compared with nondiabetics with a prior MI was 1.2 (95% CI, 0.6 to 2.4).

77. **Gu K,** et al. Diabetes and decline in heart disease mortality in U.S. adults. *JAMA* 1999;281:1291–1297.

This analysis of data from the First National Health and Nutrition Examination Survey (NHANES I; 1971 to 1975) and NHANES I Epidemiologic Follow-up Survey (1982 to 1984) showed that the declines in heart disease mortality seen in the general population have not occurred in diabetics. The two cohorts were followed up for mortality at an average of 8 to 9 years. Comparing the 1982 to 1984 period with the 1971 to 1975 period, nondiabetic men had a 36.4% decline in age-adjusted heart disease mortality compared with only a 13% decline for men with diabetes. Among women, nondiabetics had a 27% decline, whereas a 23% increase occurred in diabetics. A similar pattern was found for all-cause mortality.

78. **Lotufo PA,** et al. Diabetes and all-cause and coronary heart disease mortality among U.S. male physicians. *Arch Intern Med* 2001;161:242–247.

This prospective cohort study found that the increased mortality risk conferred by diabetes is similar to that conferred by a history of CHD, whereas for CHD mortality, a history of CHD is a more potent predictor than is diabetes. The total cohort of 91,285 U.S. male physicians (aged 40 to 84 years) consisted of four groups: (a) reference group of 82,247 free of both diabetes and CHD (previous MI and/or angina) at baseline; (b) 2,317 with history of diabetes but not CHD; (c) 5,906 with history of CHD but not diabetes; and (d) 815 with a history of both diabetes and CHD. At follow-up (average 5.5 years), compared with men with no diabetes or CHD, the age-adjusted RR of mortality was 2.3 (95% CI, 2.0 to 2.6) among men with diabetes and without CHD, 2.2 (95% CI, 2.0 to 2.4) among men with CHD and without diabetes, and 4.7 (95% CI, 4.0 to 5.4) among men with both diabetes and CHD. The corresponding RRs of CHD death were 3.3, 5.6, and 12.0. Multivariate adjustment for BMI, smoking status, alcohol intake, and activity did not significantly alter these associations.

79. **Ford ES,** et al. Prevalence of the metabolic syndrome among U.S. adults: findings from the third National Health and Nutrition Examination Survey. *JAMA* 2002;287:356–359.

This analysis examined data on 8,814 participants in the Third National Health and Nutrition Examination Survey (1988 to 1994). The ATP III definition of the metabolic syndrome was used: three or more of the following: waist circumference, greater than 102 cm in men and greater than 88 cm in women; triglycerides, 150 mg/dL or greater; HDL, less than 40 mg/dL in men and less than 50 mg/dL in women; BP, greater than 130/85 mm Hg; glucose level, 110 mg/dL or more. Unadjusted and age-adjusted prevalences of metabolic syndrome were 21.8% and 23.7%, respectively. Prevalence increased from 6.7% in those aged 20 through 29 years to 43.5% and 42.0% for those aged 60 to 69 years and 70 years or older, respectively. Age-adjusted prevalences were similar in men (24.0%) and women (23.4%); however, among African Americans, women had a 57% higher prevalence than did men, and among Mexican Americans, women had about a 26% higher prevalence than did men.

80. **Lakka HM,** et al. The metabolic syndrome and total and cardiovascular disease mortality in middle-aged men. *JAMA* 2002;288:2709–2716.

This study analyzed data on 1,209 participants in a population-based, prospective cohort study of Finnish men who were initially free of CVD, cancer, or diabetes. At 11.4 years of follow-up, a total of 109 deaths was found, and the prevalence of the metabolic syndrome ranged from 8.8% to 14.3%, depending on the definition. After adjustment for conventional risk factors, the metabolic syndrome was associated with a significant 2.9- to 4.2-fold increased risk of CHD death (by both NCEP and WHO definitions). With the WHO definition, all-cause mortality was 1.9 times higher in those with the metabolic syndrome. The NCEP definition less consistently predicted CVD and all-cause mortality.

Studies

81. **Lewis EJ,** et al. The effect of angiotensin-converting-enzyme inhibition on diabetic nephropathy: the Collaborative Study Group. *N Engl J Med* 1993;329:1456–1462.

This prospective, randomized, placebo-controlled trial enrolled 409 patients with IDDM in whom urinary protein excretion was 500 mg/day or more and serum creatinine concentration was 2.5 mg/dL or less. Patients received captopril or placebo for a median of 3 years. Doubling of serum creatinine (primary end point) occurred less frequently in the captopril group (25 vs. 43 patients; $p = 0.007$). The reductions in creatinine doubling were 48% in the entire captopril group, 76% in the subgroup with baseline creatinine of 2.0 mg/dL, 55% in the subgroup with creatinine of 1.5 mg/dL, and 17% in the subgroup with creatinine of 1.0 mg/day. Captopril also was associated with a 50% reduction in death, dialysis, or transplantation; this benefit was independent of the small difference in BP between the groups.

82. **UKPDS 38.** Tight blood pressure control and risk of macrovascular and microvascular complications in type 2 diabetes: UK Prospective Diabetes Study Group. *BMJ* 1998;317:703–713.

This prospective, randomized, controlled, multicenter trial enrolled 1,148 type 2 diabetics with HTN (mean entry BP, 160/94 mm Hg). Patients were assigned to tight BP control (goal, 150/85 mm Hg or less) with use of captopril or atenolol as main treatment, or less tight control (goal, 180/105 mm Hg or less). At follow-up (median, 8.4 years), mean BP was significantly reduced in the group assigned tight BP control [144/82 vs. 154/87 mm Hg (looser control); $p < 0.0001$]. Tight-control group had significant relative reductions of 24% in diabetes-related end points, 32% in deaths related to diabetes, 44% in strokes, and 37% in microvascular end points. A nonsignificant reduction was found in all-cause mortality. The tight-control group also had a 34% reduction in risk in the proportion of patients with deterioration of retinopathy by two steps and a 47% reduced risk of deterioration in visual acuity by three lines of the diabetic retinopathy study chart. In a predefined substudy of the tight-control patients (UKPDS 39; see *BMJ* 1998;317:713–720), captopril and atenolol were equally effective in reducing BP, risk of macrovasular end points, and deterioration in retinopathy.

83. **Parving HH,** et al., for the **IRMA II** (Irbesartan in patients with Type 2 Diabetes and Microalbuminuria) Study Group. The effect of irbesartan on the development of diabetic nephropathy in patients with type 2 diabetes. *N Engl J Med* 2001;345:870–878.

This prospective, randomized, double-blind, placebo-controlled, multicenter trial enrolled 590 hypertensive patients with type 2 diabetes and microalbuminuria. Primary end point was time to onset of diabetic nephropathy (urinary albumin excretion rate, more than 200 μg/min and 30% or more higher than baseline level). Patients received irbesartan, 150 mg daily or 300 mg daily, or placebo. At 2-year follow-up, irbesartan groups had a lower incidence of the primary end point compared with the placebo group [5.2% (300 mg) and 9.7% (150 mg) vs. 9.7% (placebo); HRs, 0.30 ($p < 0.001$) and 0.61 ($p = 0.081$)]. Average BPs were 141/83 mm Hg in the 300-mg group, 143/83 mm Hg in the 150-mg group, and 144/83 mm Hg in the placebo group [$p = 0.004$ (SBP placebo compared with SBP of combined irbesartan groups)]. Serious adverse events were less frequent among the patients treated with irbesartan ($p = 0.02$).

84. **Brenner BM,** et al., for the **RENAAL** (Reduction of End points in NIDDM with Angiotensin II Antagonist Losartan) study investigators. Effects of losartan on renal and cardiovascular outcomes in patients with type 2 diabetes and nephropathy. *N Engl J Med* 2001;345:861–869.

This prospective, randomized, double-blind, placebo-controlled, multicenter trial enrolled 1,513 type 2 diabetics with nephropathy (urinary albumin-to-creatinine ratio of 300 or more and serum creatinine, 1.3 to 3.0 mg/dL). Patients received losartan, 50 to 100 mg once daily, or placebo. Both were taken in addition to conventional antihypertensive agents. At a mean follow-up of 3.4 years, the losartan group had a

16% RRR in primary events [doubling of baseline serum creatinine, end-stage renal disease (ESRD), or death] compared with the placebo group (43.5% vs. 47.1%; $p = 0.02$). Losartan reduced serum creatinine doubling by 25% ($p = 0.006$) and ESRD by 28% ($p = 0.002$) but had no significant effect on all-cause mortality. The benefits exceeded those attributable to changes in BP. Losartan also was associated with a lower rate of first hospitalization for HF (RRR, 32%; $p = 0.005$) and a 35% decline in proteinuria ($p < 0.001$ in comparison with placebo).

85. **Lewis EJ,** et al., **IDNT** (Irbesartan Diabetic Nephropathy Trial). Renoprotective effect of the angiotensin-receptor antagonist irbesartan in patients with nephropathy due to type 2 diabetes. *N Engl J Med* 2001;345:851–860.

This prospective, randomized, double-blind, placebo-controlled, multicenter, primary trial enrolled 1,715 hypertensive patients with nephropathy due to type 2 diabetes. Patients received irbesartan (300 mg daily), amlodipine (10 mg daily), or placebo. Target BP was 135/85 mm Hg or less. At mean follow-up of 2.6 years, irbesartan had 20% and 23% fewer primary events (doubling of baseline serum creatinine, ESRD, or death) than did the placebo and amlodipine groups [32.6% vs. 39% ($p = 0.02$) and 41.1%; $p = 0.006$]. Irbesartan was associated with 33% and 37% lower rates of serum creatinine doubling [16.9% vs. 23.7% ($p = 0.003$) and 25.4% ($p < 0.001$)] and 23% lower RR of ESRD than both other groups (14.2% vs. 17.8% and 18.3%; $p = 0.07$ for both comparisons). These differences were not explained by the achieved BP differences. No significant differences were noted between the groups in all-cause mortality or the cardiovascular composite end point.

86. **Gaede P,** et al., **STENO-2.** Multifactorial intervention and cardiovascular disease in patients with type 2 diabetes. *N Engl J Med* 2003;348:383–393.

This prospective, open, parallel trial randomized 160 type 2 diabetics with microalbuminuria to conventional treatment, in accordance with national guidelines, or intensive treatment, with a step-wise implementation of behavior modification and drug therapy that targeted hyperglycemia, HTN, dyslipidemia, and microalbuminuria, as well as secondary prevention of CVD with ASA. At follow-up (mean, 7.8 years), the intensive therapy group had a significantly lower risk of CVD (HR, 0.47; 95% CI, 0.24 to 0.73), nephropathy (HR, 0.39; 95% CI, 0.17 to 0.87), and retinopathy (HR, 0.42; 95% CI, 0.21 to 0.86).

Smoking

87. **Rosenberg L,** et al. The risk of MI after quitting smoking in men under 55 years of age. *N Engl J Med* 1985;313:1511–1514.

This prospective case-control study was composed of 1,873 patients with first MI and 2,775 controls. Among current smokers, defined as smoking within the prior 12 months versus never, the age-adjusted RR of MI was 2.9 (95% CI, 2.4 to 3.4). Among those who had quit smoking 12 to 23 months earlier versus never smokers, the RR of MI was 2.0 (95% CI, 1.1 to 3.8). Those who had quit 2 years earlier had a risk similar to that of never smokers (RR, 1.0).

88. **Willett WC,** et al. Relative and excess risks of coronary heart disease among women who smoke cigarettes. *N Engl J Med* 1987;317:1303–1309.

This analysis focused on 119,404 NHS participants with 6 years of follow-up; 30% were smokers. The number of cigarettes smoked per day was found to be associated with an increased risk of fatal CHD (in multivariate analysis, RR of 5.4 for 25 cigarettes/day), MI (RR, 6.3), and angina pectoris (RR, 2.3). If they smoked one to 14 cigarettes/day, RRs (in multivariate analysis) were 1.8 to 2.5; 15 to 24 cigarettes/day, RRs, 1.5 to 4.7; 45 cigarettes/day, RR of death and MI was 10.8. Overall, smoking was responsible for approximately 50% of events. The greatest absolute risks were seen with smoking in combination with other risk factors: smoking and HTN, RR, 22.2; smoking and hypercholesterolemia, RR, 18.9; smoking and diabetes, RR, 22.3.

89. **Rosenberg L,** et al. Decline in the risk of MI among women who stop smoking. *N Engl J Med* 1990;322:213–217.

This case-control study was composed of 910 patients with a first MI and 2,375 controls (all aged 25 to 64 years). Comparing current smokers with never smokers, the RR of MI was 3.6 (95% CI, 3.0 to 4.4). The difference was less substantial when comparing ex-smokers with never smokers (overall RR, 1.2; 95% CI, 1.0 to 1.7). However, the risk was higher in those who had quit 2 years earlier (RR, 2.6; 95% CI, 1.8 to 3.8), whereas no significant increased risk was seen in those who had quit longer than 3 years earlier.

90. **Kawachi I,** et al. Smoking cessation and time course of decreased risks of coronary heart disease in middle-aged women. *Arch Intern Med* 1994;154:169–175.

This prospective cohort study was composed of 117,006 nurses free of CHD in 1976. The average follow-up period was 11.7 years. In a multivariate analysis, among current smokers versus never smokers, the RR was 4.23 (95% CI, 3.60 to 4.96); among those who started smoking before age 15 years, RR, 9.25; among former smokers, RR, 1.48 (95% CI, 1.22 to 1.79). After quitting, one third of the excess risk was gone at 3 years, and normal risk was attained after 10 to 14 years.

91. **Steenland K,** et al. Environmental tobacco smoke and coronary heart disease in the **ACS CPS-II** cohort. *Circulation* 1996;94:622–628 (editorial, 596–599).

This prospective study was composed of 353,180 women and 126,500 male nonsmokers. A 22% higher CHD mortality rate (95% CI) was observed among men married to current smokers; the corresponding RR for women married to current smokers was 1.1 (95% CI, 0.96 to 1.22). The editorial provides an analysis of data from 14 studies that shows an approximate 20% increased risk of CHD death in nonsmokers married to smokers.

92. **Kawachi I,** et al. A prospective study of passive smoking and coronary heart disease. *Circulation* 1997;95:2374–2379.

This analysis focused on 32,046 NHS participants who did not smoke and were free of CHD in 1982. Exposure was assessed by self-report and only at baseline. At 10-year follow-up, the adjusted CHD risk (nonfatal MI and cardiac death) was significantly higher among those with frequent smoke exposure (RR, 1.91; 95% CI, 1.11 to 3.28), and a trend of increased risk with occasional exposure was noted (RR, 1.58; 95% CI, 0.93 to 2.68). No association was found between duration of living with a smoker and the incidence of CHD.

93. **He J,** et al. Passive smoking and the risk of coronary heart disease: a meta-analysis of epidemiologic studies. *N Engl J Med* 1999;340:920–926.

This analysis of 10 cohort and eight case-control studies showed that nonsmokers exposed to environmental smoke had an RR of CHD of 1.25 (95% CI, 1.17 to 1.32) compared with that of nonsmokers with no such exposure. This association was significant in both men and women and present in those exposed at home or in the workplace. A significant dose-response relation was demonstrated: RR of CHD, 1.23 in those exposed to smoke of 1 to 19 cigarettes/day vs. RR of 1.31 in those exposed to 20 cigarettes/day ($p = 0.006$ for linear trend).

Hypertension

Review Articles/Miscellaneous

94. **JNC 7, Chobanian AV,** et al. The seventh report of the Joint National Committee on prevention, detection, evaluation, and treatment of high blood pressure: the JNC 7 report. *JAMA* 2003;289:2560–2571.

JNC 7 defines HTN as SBP greater than 140 mm Hg and DBP as greater than 90 mm Hg, or taking hypertensive medication(s). JNC 7 introduced a new blood pressure category called, "Prehypertensive," which includes those with SBP 120 to 139 mm Hg or DBP 80 to 89 mm Hg. When pharmacologic intervention is indicated,

JNC 7 advocates the use of diuretics and β-blockers as first-line agents in most patients. As was the case with JNC VI, other therapies (e.g., ACE inhibitors) also are recommended for individuals with specific characteristics (see text for details, pages 10 to 11). If blood pressure is >20 $\neq$ 10 mm Hg above targets (<140 $\neq$ 90 or <130 $\neq$ 80 if diabetic or chronic kidney disease present), initial therapy should be with two agents.

Epidemiology and Risk Factors

95. **Sagie A,** et al. The natural history of borderline isolated systolic hypertension. *N Engl J Med* 1993;329:1912–1917.

This analysis focused on 2,767 of the original participants in the Framingham Heart Study. At 20-year follow-up, 80% with borderline isolated systolic HTN (140 to 159 mm Hg) had progression to definite HTN (SBP, 160 mm Hg, and DBP, 90 mm Hg), compared with 45% of normotensive individuals ($p < 0.001$). After adjustment for multiple risk factors, borderline HTN was associated with an excess long-term risk of CVD (HR, 1.47; 95% CI, 1.24 to 1.74) and cardiovascular death (HR, 1.57; 95% CI, 1.24 to 2.00).

96. **Kannel WB.** Blood pressure as a cardiovascular risk factor. *JAMA* 1996;275: 1571–1576.

This analysis of 36-year follow-data from the Framingham Heart Study shows that from age 30 to 65 years, the average increases in SBP and DBP are 20 and 10 mm Hg, respectively. No evidence of a change was found in the prevalence of HTN over the past four decades. HTN occurs alone in only 20% (i.e., no diabetes, obesity, dyslipidemia). Hypertensive patients had increased RRs (M/F) of CAD (2.0/2.2), stroke (3.8/2.6), PAD (2.0/3.7), and CHF (4.0/3.0). See **Fig. 1.1** of the article for estimated rates of CHD over a 10-year period according to different combinations of risk factors in men and women.

97. **O'Donnell CJ,** et al. Hypertension and borderline isolated systolic hypertension increase risks of cardiovascular disease and mortality in male physicians. *Circulation* 1997;95:1132–1137.

This prospective cohort analysis focused on 18,682 PHS participants, with a mean follow-up of 11.7 years. Isolated SBP (140 to 159 mm Hg) was associated with higher rates of stroke (RR, 1.42) and cardiovascular death (RR, 1.56), as well as a 22% higher all-cause mortality rate and nonsignificant increase in MI rate (RR, 1.26).

98. **Moster d'A,** et al. Trends in the prevalence of hypertension, antihypertensive therapy, and left ventricular hypertrophy from 1950 to 1989. *N Engl J Med* 1999;340:1221–1227.

This analysis focused on 10,333 Framingham Heart Study participants. From 1950 to 1989, the age-adjusted prevalence of SBP, 160 mm Hg, or DBP, 100 mm Hg, declined from 18.5% to 9.2% among men and from 28.0% to 7.7% among women. A decline was noted in ECG evidence of LV hypertrophy: 4.5% to 2.5% and 3.6% to 1.1%.

99. **Vasan RS,** et al. Residual lifetime risk for developing hypertension in middle-aged women and men: the Framingham Heart Study. *JAMA* 2002;287:1003–1010.

Prospective cohort analysis of 1,298 Framingham Heart Study participants who were aged 55 to 65 years and free of HTN at baseline (1976 to 1998). The residual lifetime risks for developing HTN and stage 1 high BP or higher were 90% in both 55- and 65-year-old participants. The lifetime probability of receiving antihypertensive medication was 60%. The risk for HTN remained unchanged for women, but it was approximately 60% higher for men in the 1976 to 1998 period compared with the 1952 to 1975 period. In contrast, the residual lifetime risk for stage 2 high BP or higher (160/100 mm Hg or higher regardless of treatment) was lower in both sexes in the recent period (35% to 57% in 1952 to 1975 vs. 35% to 44% in 1976 to 1998), likely owing to a marked increase in pharmacologic treatment of individuals with substantially elevated BP.

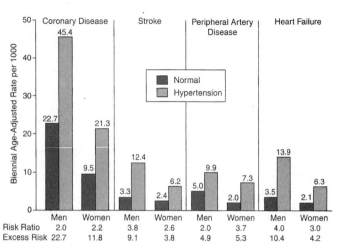

FIG. 1.1. Risk of cardiovascular events by hypertensive status in subjects aged 35 to 64 years, Framingham Study, 36-year follow-up. Coronary disease includes clinical manifestations such as myocardial infarction, angina pectoris, sudden death, other coronary deaths, and coronary insufficiency syndrome; peripheral artery disease is manifested as intermittent claudication. (From Kannel WB. Lipids, diabetes, and coronary heart disease: insights from the Framingham Heart Study. *Am Heart J* 1985;110:1100–1107, with permission.)

Meta-Analyses

100. **Johnson AG,** et al. Do non-steroidal anti-inflammatory drugs affect blood pressure? A meta-analysis. *Ann Intern Med* 1994;121:289–300.

This analysis was performed on data from 38 randomized, placebo-controlled trials and 12 randomized but not placebo-controlled trials (comparing two NSAIDs). NSAID use was associated with a 5.0 mm Hg higher elevated supine mean BP. NSAIDs also antagonized the antihypertensive effect of β-blockers (BP elevation, 6.2 mm Hg). Sulindac and ASA were found to have the least hypertensive effect.

101. **Schmieder RE,** et al. Reversal of left ventricular hypertrophy in essential hypertension: a meta-analysis of randomized double-blind studies. *JAMA* 1996;275:1507–1513.

This meta-analysis of 39 trials showed that a decrease in LV mass correlated significantly with a decrease in SBP ($r = 0.46$; $p < 0.001$) and a longer duration of antihypertensive therapy ($r = 0.38$; $p < 0.01$). ACE inhibitors achieved a greater reduction in LV mass than did β-blockers and diuretics (-13% vs. -6%; $p < 0.05$; -13% vs. -7%; $p = 0.08$).

102. **Midgley JP,** et al. Effect of reduced dietary sodium on blood pressure: a meta-analysis of randomized controlled trials. *JAMA* 1996;275:1590–1597.

This analysis was performed on 56 trials that met inclusion criteria; however, the heterogeneity of these studies was significant, and publication bias was evident. A 100-mg/day reduction in daily urinary sodium excretion was associated with decreases in SBP of 3.7 mm Hg ($p < 0.001$) and DBP of only 0.9 mm Hg ($p = 0.09$). The authors do not recommend universal dietary sodium restriction.

103. **Psaty BM,** et al. Health outcomes associated with antihypertensive therapies used as first-line agents. *JAMA* 1997;277:739–745.

Meta-analysis of 18 randomized, placebo-controlled trials with 48,220 patients. The use of β-blockers and high- and low-dose diuretics was associated with fewer strokes

(RRs of 0.71, 0.49, and 0.66, respectively) and less CHF (RRs of 0.58, 0.17, and 0.58). Low-dose diuretics also were associated with less CAD (RR, 0.72) and lower all-cause mortality (RR, 0.90; 95% CI, 0.81 to 0.99). Calcium-channel blockers and ACE inhibitors are associated with lower BP, but major event and mortality data were limited.

Treatment
Beta Blocker and/or Diuretic Studies
104. Metoprolol Atherosclerosis Prevention in Hypertension (**MAPHY**). Primary prevention with metoprolol in patients with hypertension: mortality results from the MAPHY study. *JAMA* 1988;259:1976–1982.

Design: Prospective, randomized, multicenter, open study. Median follow-up period was 4.2 years.
Purpose: To investigate whether metoprolol lowers cardiovascular complications of high BP to a greater extent than do thiazide diuretics.
Population: 3,234 white men aged 40 to 64 years.
Treatment: Metoprolol (mean dosage, 174 mg/day) or thiazide [hydrochlorothiazide (mean dosage, 46 mg/day) or bendroflumethiazide (mean dosage, 4.4 mg/day)].
Results: Metoprolol group had 48% lower all-cause mortality (4.8 vs. 9.3 deaths/1,000 patient years) and 58% lower CV mortality (2.6 vs. 6.2 deaths/1,000 patient years).

105. Systolic HTN in Elderly Program (**SHEP**). Prevention of stroke by antihypertensive drug therapy in older persons with isolated systolic hypertension. *JAMA* 1991;265:3255–3264.

Design: Prospective, randomized, multicenter, double-blind, placebo-controlled study. Primary outcome was nonfatal and fatal (total) stroke. Average follow-up period was 4.5 years.
Purpose: To assess the ability of antihypertensive drug therapy to decrease the risk of stroke in individuals with isolated systolic HTN.
Population: 4,736 patients aged ≥60 years (14% black, 57% women) with SBP, 160 to 219 mm Hg, and DBP, less than 90 mm Hg; 3,161 patients were taking antihypertensive drug(s).
Treatment: Step 1, chlorthalidone, 12.5 mg/day; dose, 2 25 mg/day; step 2, atenolol, 25 mg/day, and then 50 mg/day.
Results: At 5 years, 36% fewer strokes (5.2 vs. 8.2/1,000; $p = 0.0003$), lower SBP (143 vs. 155 mm Hg), and 27% decrease in nonfatal MI and coronary death were observed.

106. **Dahlof B,** et al., Swedish Trial in Old Patients with Hypertension (**STOP-HTN**). Morbidity and mortality in the STOP-HTN. *Lancet* 1991;338:1281–1285.

Design: Prospective, randomized, double-blind, placebo-controlled, multicenter study. Primary end point was stroke, MI, and other cardiovascular death.
Purpose: To evaluate the effects of several different antihypertensive agents on the incidence of major vascular events in older patients.
Population: 1,627 patients aged 70 to 84 years with SBP, 180 to 230 mm Hg, and DBP, ≥90 mm Hg (or DBP, 105 to 120 mm Hg).
Exclusion Criteria: MI or stroke within prior 12 months, isolated systolic HTN (SBP greater than 180 mm Hg and DBP less than 90 mm Hg).
Treatment: Atenolol (50 mg once daily), hydrochlorothiazide (HCTZ; 25 mg once daily) plus amiloride (2.5 mg once daily), metoprolol (100 mg once daily), pindolol (5 mg once daily), or placebo.
Results: At 25 months, treated patients had a significant 43% RRR in the incidence of all primary outcome measures (3.35%/year vs. 5.55%/year; $p = 0.0031$), 47% RRR in strokes (1.68%/year vs. 3.13%/year), 13% RRR in all MIs (1.44%/year vs. 1.65%/year), 70% RRR in other cardiovascular deaths (0. 25%/year vs. 0.77%/year), 50% RRR in vascular mortality (0.17%/year vs. 0.34%/year), and 43% RRR in total mortality (2.02%/year vs. 3.54%/year; $p = 0.0079$).

107. **Meade TW,** et al. Medical Research Council (**MRC**). MRC trial of treatment of hypertension in older adults: principal results. *BMJ* 1992;304:405–412.

Design: Prospective, randomized, single-blind, placebo-controlled study. Average follow-up period was 5.8 years.

Purpose: To determine whether antihypertensive therapy in men and women aged 65 to 74 years reduces mortality and morbidity due to stroke and CHD.

Population: 4,396 patients not taking any antihypertensive agents and with SBP, 160 to 209 mm Hg, and DBP, less than 115 mm Hg.

Exclusion Criteria: Stroke or MI in prior 3 months, diabetes, and asthma.

Treatment: HCTZ (25 to 50 mg/day), amiloride (2.5 to 5.0 mg/day), atenolol (50 mg/day), or placebo.

Results: Treated patients had 25% fewer strokes ($p = 0.04$) and 19% fewer coronary events ($p = 0.08$). β-Blockers induced nonsignificant reduction; diuretics induced 31% fewer strokes and 44% fewer coronary events.

108. **LaPalio L,** et al. Safety and efficacy of metoprolol in the treatment of hypertension in the elderly. *J Am Geriatr Soc* 1992;40:354–358.

This prospective, open-label, observational study was composed of 21,692 patients aged 50 to 75 years with HTN [SBP $\geq$200 mm Hg and DBP 90 to 104 mm Hg (no prior therapy) or $\geq$95 mm Hg (prior therapy)]. Exclusion criteria included use of β-blockers for angina, CHF, and heart block. Patients received metoprolol, 100 mg/day. If DBP was still less than 90 mm Hg at 4 weeks, HCTZ, 25 mg/day, was added. At 4 weeks, mean BP was reduced from 162/95 to 149/87 mm Hg ($p < 0.001$), and at 8 weeks, to 143/84 mm Hg. At the end of the study, 50% remained taking metoprolol as monotherapy, whereas 27% needed combination therapy.

109. **Neaton JD,** et al. Treatment of mild hypertension study (**TOMHS**): final results. *JAMA* 1993;270:713–724.

Design: Prospective, randomized, multicenter, double-blind, placebo-controlled study. Average follow-up period was 4.4 years.

Purpose: To compare five drug treatments with placebo for long-term management of mild hypertension.

Population: 902 patients aged 45 to 69 years and not taking any antihypertensive medications at initial screening, with DBP, 90 to 99 mm Hg (at two visits).

Treatment: Chlorthalidone, 15 mg/day (diuretic); acebutolol, 400 mg/day (β-blocker); doxazosin, 1 mg/day (α-1 agonist); amlodipine, 5 mg/day; enalapril, 5 mg/day; or placebo (all a.m. dosing). All patients received nutritional and hygienic advice (low weight, low sodium, low alcohol, increased exercise).

Results: Drug therapy reductions were sizable in all six groups (DBP decreased by 8.6 to 12.3 mm Hg). Drug groups had a nonsignificant reduction in death and MACE (5.1% vs. 7.3%; $p = 0.21$). Drug therapy also was associated with better quality of life and decreased resting ECG abnormalities; no differences were seen between the five drug groups in LV mass, lipid levels, and other outcome measures.

Calcium-channel Blocker and/or ACE Inhibitor–focused Studies

110. **Staessen JA,** et al. **Syst-Eur**. Randomised double-blind comparison of placebo and active treatment for older patients with isolated systolic hypertension. *Lancet* 1997;350:757–764.

Design: Prospective, randomized, double-blind, placebo-controlled, multicenter study. Primary end point was fatal and nonfatal stroke. Median follow-up period was 2 years.

Purpose: To investigate whether treatment of isolated systolic HTN could reduce stroke and cardiovascular complications.

Population: 4,695 patients aged $\geq$60 years with average sitting SBP of 160 to 219 mm Hg and DBP of less than 95 mm Hg.

Exclusion Criteria: CHF; creatinine, 180 μM; and MI in prior year.

Treatment: Nitrendipine, 10 to 40 mg/day, with the possible addition of enalapril, 5 to 20 mg/day; and HCTZ, 12.5 to 25 mg/day; or matching placebos.

Results: At 2 years, treated patients had 42% fewer total strokes (7.9 vs. 13.7 per 1,000 patient years; $p = 0.003$) and 31% fewer fatal and nonfatal cardiac end points ($p = 0.03$). Treated patients had significantly lower SBPs and DBPs than did placebo patients (-10.1 mm Hg and -4.5 mm Hg). A trend was seen toward lower CV mortality with active treatment (-27%; $p = 0.07$), but all-cause mortality was not influenced (-14%; $p = 0.22$).

Comments: A subsequent study at mean follow-up of 3.9 years demonstrated a 55% reduction in the risk of dementia with nitrendipine treatment (see *Arch Intern Med* 2002;162:2046).

111. **Captopril Prevention Project (CAPPP).** Effect of angiotensin-converting-enzyme inhibition compared with conventional therapy on cardiovascular morbidity and mortality in hypertension: the Captopril Prevention Project (CAPPP) randomised trial. *Lancet* 1999;353:611–616.

Design: Prospective, randomized, multicenter, open study. Primary composite end points were fatal and nonfatal MI, stroke, and other CV deaths. Mean follow-up period was 6.1 years.
Purpose: To compare the effectiveness of captopril with a conventional antihypertensive regimen of diuretics or β-blockers on cardiovascular morbidity and mortality.
Population: 10,985 patients aged 25 to 66 years with DBP ≥ 100 mm Hg on two occasions.
Exclusion Criteria: Secondary HTN and serum creatinine greater than 150 μM.
Treatment: Captopril, 50 mg once or twice daily; β-blockers (most common: metoprolol and atenolol); or diuretics (most common, HCTZ and bendrofluazide).
Results: Two groups had a similar incidence of composite end point (11.1 and 10.2 events per 1,000 patient years in captopril and conventional therapy groups); captopril group had a trend toward lower CV mortality (RR, 0.77; $p = 0.092$) but a higher incidence of fatal and nonfatal stroke (RR, 1.15; $p = 0.044$); MI rates were similar.
Comments: Lower stroke risk in conventional group probably was owing to lower initial BP (-2 mm Hg).

112. **Hansson L,** et al. Randomised trial of effects of calcium antagonists compared with diuretics and beta-blockers on cardiovascular morbidity and mortality in hypertension: the Nordic Diltiazem (**NORDIL**) study. *Lancet* 2000;356: 359–365.

Design: Prospective, randomized, open, blinded end point, multicenter trial. Primary end point was fatal and nonfatal stroke, MI, and other CV death. Mean follow-up, 4.5 years.
Purpose: To compare the effects of calcium antagonists with those of diuretics and β-blockers on major outcomes in middle-aged hypertensive individuals.
Population: 10,881 patients aged 50 to 74 years with DBP of 100 mm Hg or more.
Treatment: Diltiazem (180 to 360 mg daily) versus diuretics, β-blockers, or both. Additional antihypertensives could be added to achieve DBP less than 90 mm Hg.
Results: SBP and DBP were lowered effectively in the diltiazem and diuretic and β-blocker groups (reduction, 20.3/18.7 vs. 23.3/18.7 mm Hg; difference in systolic reduction, $p < 0.001$). No difference was found between the two groups in the incidence of the primary composite end point [16.6 (diltiazem) vs. 16.2 events per 1,000 patient years]. The diltiazem group had a lower incidence of fatal and nonfatal stroke compared with the diuretic and β-blocker group [6.4 vs. 7.9 events per 1,000 patient years; RR, 0.80 (95% CI, 0.65 to 0.99); $p = 0.04$], whereas the rates of fatal and nonfatal MI were not significantly different [7.4 vs. 6.3 events per 1,000 patient years; RR, 1.16 (0.94 to 1.44); $p = 0.17$].

113. **PROGRESS** (Perindopril pROtection aGainst REcurrent Stroke Study), PROGRESS Collaborative Group. Randomised trial of a perindopril-based blood-pressure-lowering regimen among 6,105 individuals with previous stroke or transient ischaemic attack. *Lancet* 2001;358:1033–1041 (editorial, 1026–1027).

Design: Prospective, randomized, double-blind, placebo-controlled, multicenter trial. Primary end point was total stroke (fatal or nonfatal). Mean follow-up was 3.9 years.
Purpose: To determine the effects of a BP-lowering regimen in hypertensive and non-hypertensive patients with a history of stroke or TIA.

Population: 6,105 individuals with a stroke (hemorrhagic or ischemic) or TIA in the previous 5 years and no major disability.

Treatment: Active treatment [perindopril (4 mg daily) with addition of the diuretic indapamide (2.5 mg daily) at physicians' discretion], or placebo.

Results: At follow-up, active treatment reduced BP by 9/4 mm Hg. In active treatment group, 60% received both drugs, and 40% received perindopril alone. The active treatment group had a significantly lower incidence of stroke compared with the placebo group (10% vs. 14%; 28% RRR; $p < 0.0001$). Active treatment also reduced total major vascular events by 26%. Hypertensive and nonhypertensive subgroups had similar reductions in stroke (all values $p < 0.01$). Combination therapy with perindopril plus indapamide reduced BP by 12/5 mm Hg and stroke risk by 43%, whereas single-drug therapy reduced BP by 5/3 mm Hg and resulted in no significant reduction in stroke incidence.

Comments: Editorialists dispute study's conclusion that treatment with both agents be considered routinely for patients with a history of stroke or TIA, irrespective of BP, and advocate starting treatment with a diuretic, not with combination therapy. They also point out that the 5 mm Hg reduction in systolic BP seen in the perindopril group should translate into an approximate 20% reduction in stroke risk, as seen in many prior studies using diuretics and β-blockers.

114. **Dahlof B,** et al., for the **LIFE** (Losartan Intervention For Endpoint reduction in hypertension) Study Group. Cardiovascular morbidity and mortality in the losartan intervention for endpoint reduction in hypertension study (LIFE): a randomised trial against atenolol. *Lancet* 2002;359:995–1003.

Design: Prospective, randomized, placebo-controlled, blinded, parallel-group, multi-center trial. Primary end point: death, MI, or stroke. Mean follow-up, 4.8 years.

Purpose: Use of losartan compared with atenolol in patients with HTN and left ventricular hypertrophy (LVH).

Population: The 9,193 patients aged 55 to 80 years with previously treated or untreated HTN (SBP, 160 to 200 mm Hg; DBP, 95 to 115 mm Hg; ECG signs of LVH).

Exclusion Criteria: Included secondary HTN; MI or stroke in previous 6 months; angina requiring β-blockers or calcium antagonists; HF or LVEF 40% or less; need for treatment with any angiotensin II–receptor antagonist, any β-blocker, HCTZ, or ACE inhibitor.

Treatment: Losartan-based or atenolol-based regimen after 1 to 2 weeks of placebo. Drugs were dosed to reach a target BP of less than 140/90 mm Hg per titration schedule.

Results: BP was reduced by 30.2/16.6 mm Hg in the losartan group and 29.1/16.8 mm Hg in the atenolol group (treatment difference, $p = 0.017$ for SBP and $p = 0.37$ for DBP). The losartan group had a significantly lower incidence of death, MI, or stroke compared with the atenolol group (11% vs. 13%; HR, 0.87; $p = 0.021$), primarily driven by fewer strokes (5% vs. 7%; HR, 0.75; $p = 0.001$). CV mortality rates were not significantly different (4% vs. 5%; HR, 0.89; $p = 0.21$). Losartan also was associated with a lower incidence of new-onset diabetes (6% vs. 8%; HR, 0.75; $p = 0.001$). A major LIFE substudy examined CV outcomes in 1,195 patients with diabetes, HTN, and ECG signs of LVH (*Lancet* 2002;359:1004). At a mean follow-up of 4.7 years, mean BP decreased to similar levels (losartan, 146/79 mm Hg; atenolol, 148/79 mm Hg). However, the losartan group had a significant 24% RRR in death, MI, or stroke. Losartan also had significant reductions in CV mortality (37% RRR; $p = 0.028$) and all-cause mortality (39% RRR; $p = 0.002$). These substudy results suggest that losartan has benefits beyond BP reduction. In the subgroup of patients with isolated systolic HTN (DBP, less than 90 mm Hg) and LVH (by ECG), the losartan group was associated with 25% fewer primary events compared with atenolol (see *JAMA* 2002;288:1491).

Comments: These results are in contrast to those of the CAPPP, NORDIL, and STOP-HTN2 trials, which compared ACE inhibitors or calcium channel blockers with β-blockers and diuretics for treatment of HTN and found no difference in efficacy. Because this trial examined the efficacy of losartan in high-risk hypertensive patients with signs of LVH, one cannot extrapolate these results to lower-risk patients.

115. **ANBP-2** (Second Australian National Blood Pressure Study). Wing LM, et al. A comparison of outcomes with angiotensin-converting enzyme inhibitors and diuretics for hypertension in the elderly. *N Engl J Med* 2003;348:583–592.

Design: Prospective, randomized, open, multicenter study. Primary end point was death or any cardiovascular event. Median follow-up was 4.1 years.
Purpose: To compare outcomes in older hypertensive subjects receiving ACE inhibitors with those treated with diuretics.
Population: 6,083 subjects aged 65 to 84 years with hypertension.
Treatment: ACE inhibitor or diuretic (enalapril and hydrochlorothiazide recommended, but not mandated).
Results: ACE inhibitor group had a significant reduction in primary events compared to diuretic group (hazard ratio 0.89, 95% CI 0.71 to 1.00, $p = 0.05$). Among men, the HR was 0.83 (95% CI 0.71 to 0.97, $p = 0.02$), while it was 1.00 for women.
Comments: Criticisms of this trial include the open label design, no restrictions on drugs used, and inclusion of "soft" endpoints. Also of note, the study enrolled few or no black patients (% not reported).

116. **INVEST** (International Verapamil SR-Trandolapril Study). Preliminary results presented at 2003 ACC Scientific Session, Chicago, IL.

This prospective, open study randomized 22,576 patients to a verapamil SR or atenololbased approach. At follow-up (range: 2 to 5 years), there was no difference between the arms (RR 0.98) in the incidence of death, nonfatal stroke, or nonfatal MI. The verapamil group did have a lower incidence of new onset diabetes (6.2% vs. 7.3%). This finding appears related to the use of hydrochlorothiazide as the second step in atenolol arm [vs. protective effect of trandolapril (second step in verapamil arm)].

Multiple Agent Studies
117. **Materson BJ,** et al., **VA Cooperative Study**. Single-drug therapy for hypertension in men: a comparison of 6 antihypertensive agents with placebo. *N Engl J Med* 1993;328:914–921.

Design: Prospective, randomized, double-blind, placebo-controlled, multicenter study. Primary end point was DBP less than 95 mm Hg. Follow-up period was 1 year.
Purpose: To compare the effectiveness of several different classes of antihypertensive therapies as monotherapy based on age and race.
Population: The 1,292 men aged ≥21 years with DBP from 95 to 109 mm Hg.
Treatment: HCTZ, 12.5 to 50 mg/day; atenolol, 25 to 100 mg/day; clonidine, 0.2 to 0.6 mg/day; captopril, 25 to 100 mg/day; prazosin, 4 to 20 mg/day; sustained-release diltiazem, 120 to 360 mg/day; or placebo.
Results: Overall success rates (DBP less than 95 mm Hg over a 1-year period) were as follows: diltiazem, 59%; atenolol, 51%; clonidine, 50%; HCTZ, 46%; captopril, 42%; prazosin, 42%; and placebo, 25%. Certain drugs appeared to be more effective in particular subgroups of patients: in blacks (young and old), diltiazem was best; in young whites, captopril was best; and in older whites, atenolol was best. Subsequent 1-year follow-up showed a significant reduction in LVH in those receiving HCTZ, captopril, and atenolol (−42.9, −38.7, and −28.1 g) (see *Circulation* 1997;95: 2007).
Comments: One possible explanation for these findings is that blacks and older patients may be less responsive to ACE inhibition and more responsive to diuretics and calcium-channel blockade because of a higher prevalence of low-renin HTN.

118. **Hansson L,** et al., for the Hypertension Optimal Treatment (**HOT**) study. Effects of intensive blood pressure lowering and low dose aspirin in patients with hypertension: principal results of the Hypertension Optimal Treatment (HOT) randomized trial. *Lancet* 1998;351:1755–1762.

Design: Prospective, randomized, partially open, partially blinded (ASA arm), multicenter study. Mean follow-up period was 3.8 years.

Purpose: To (a) assess the association between major CV events and three different target BPs as well as the actual DBP achieved during treatment; and (b) evaluate whether the addition of low-dose ASA to antihypertensive treatment reduces major CV events.

Population: 18,790 patients aged 50 to 80 years (mean, 61.5 years) with DBP, 100 to 115 mm Hg.

Treatment: Target DBP levels of $\geq$90 mm Hg, =85 mm Hg, or =80 mm Hg. A five-step approach was used: step 1, felodipine, 5 mg/day; step 2, addition of low-dose ACE inhibitor or β-blocker; step 3, felodipine increased to 10 mg/day; step 4, dose of ACE inhibitor or β-blocker increased; and step 5, addition of low-dose alternative agent or HCTZ. All patients were randomized in double-blinded fashion to ASA, 75 mg/day, or placebo.

Results: At 2 years, target DBP was achieved in 85%, 67%, and 75%. Mean DBPs were closely grouped: 85.2, 83.2, and 81.1 mm Hg. Incidence of primary composite end point did not significantly differ between the three groups, but significantly fewer CV events and deaths were noted among diabetic patients assigned to a target DBP of $\geq$80 mm Hg compared with =90 mm Hg ($p = 0.005; p = 0.016$). No differences were found in BP between ASA- and placebo-treated patients. ASA use was associated with 15% fewer major events ($p = 0.03$), 36% reduction in fatal or nonfatal MI ($p = 0.002$), and similar rates of hemorrhagic and ischemic stroke.

Comments: Study was underpowered for two reasons: (a) actual mean DBPs were approximately 2 mm Hg apart instead of 5 mm Hg apart; and (b) only 724 major CV events occurred over a 3.8-year period versus projected 1,100 over a 2.5-year period.

119. **Hansson L,** et al., **STOP-HTN2.** Randomised trial of old and new antihypertensive drugs in elderly patients: cardiovascular mortality and morbidity in the Swedish Trial in Old Patients with Hypertension-2 study. *Lancet* 1999;354:1751–1756.

Design: Prospective, randomized, open (blinded end point evaluation), multicenter study. Primary end point was fatal stroke, fatal MI, or other fatal CV disease.

Purpose: To compare the effects of conventional and newer antihypertensive drugs on CV mortality and morbidity in elderly patients.

Population: 6,614 patients aged 70 to 84 years with HTN (SBP, 180 mm Hg or greater; DBP, 105 mm Hg or greater; or both).

Treatment: Conventional antihypertensive drugs (atenolol, 50 mg; metoprolol, 100 mg; pindolol, 5 mg; or HCTZ, 25 mg plus amiloride, 2.5 mg daily) or newer drugs (enalapril, 10 mg; or lisinopril, 10 mg; or felodipine, 2.5 mg; or isradipine, 2 to 5 mg daily).

Results: BP was decreased similarly in all treatment groups. No difference was found between the treatment groups in the primary combined end point of fatal stroke, fatal myocardial MI, and other fatal CV disease [19.8 events per 1,000 patient years (conventional drugs) vs. 19.8 per 1,000 (newer drugs)]. A similar incidence also was noted in the two treatment groups of fatal and nonfatal stroke, fatal and nonfatal MI, or other CV mortality.

120. **Wright JT Jr,** et al., for the African American Study of Kidney (**AASK**) Disease and Hypertension Study Group. Effect of blood pressure lowering and antihypertensive drug class on progression of hypertensive kidney disease: results from the AASK trial. *JAMA* 2002;288:2421–2431.

Design: Prospective, randomized, 3 × 2 factorial, multicenter trial. Primary end point was rate of change in glomerular filtration rate (GFR; GFR slope). Clinical composite was reduction in GFR by 50% or more (or 25 mL/min or more per 1.73 m^2) from baseline, end-stage renal disease (ESRD), or death. Follow-up was 3.0 to 6.4 years.

Purpose: To compare the effects of two levels of BP control and three antihypertensive drug classes on GFR decline in HTN.

Population: 1,094 African Americans aged 18 to 70 years with hypertensive renal disease (GFR, 20 to 65 mL/min per 1.73 m^2).

Exclusion Criteria: Included DBP less than 95 mm Hg, known diabetes, accelerated or malignant HTN within 6 months, clinical CHF, urinary protein-to-creatinine ratio greater than 2.5.

Treatment: Arterial pressure goals of 102 to 107 mm Hg or 92 mm Hg or less, and to initial treatment with either metoprolol, 50 to 200 mg/day; ramipril, 2.5 to 10 mg/day; or amlodipine, 5 to 10 mg/day. Open-label agents were added to achieve the assigned BP goals.

Results: Achieved BP averaged 128/78 mm Hg in the lower-BP group and 141/85 mm Hg in the higher-BP group. At 4 years, no significant difference was found between the two groups in mean GFR slope from baseline ($p = 0.24$). The lower BP goal did not significantly reduce the rate of the clinical composite outcome (RRR only 2%; 95% CI, −22% to 21%). None of the drug-group comparisons showed consistent significant differences in the GFR slope. However, compared with the metoprolol and amlodipine groups, the ramipril group demonstrated significant risk reductions in the clinical composite outcome of 22% ($p = 0.04$) and 38% ($p = 0.004$), respectively. No significant difference in clinical outcomes was seen between the amlodipine and metoprolol groups.

Comments: Although CV outcomes were not a prespecified outcome measure, CV mortality and hospitalizations were 18% more common in the higher-BP goal group than the lower-BP group.

121. The **ALLHAT** (Antihypertensive and Lipid-Lowering Treatment to Prevent Heart Attack Trial) Officers and Coordinators for the ALLHAT Collaborative Research Group. Major outcomes in high-risk hypertensive patients randomized to angiotensin-converting enzyme inhibitor or calcium channel blocker vs diuretic. *JAMA* 2002;288:2981–2997 (editorials, 3039–3044).

Design: Prospective, randomized, active-controlled, multicenter trial. Primary end point was fatal CHD or nonfatal MI. Secondary outcomes were all-cause mortality, stroke, combined CHD (primary outcome, coronary revascularization, or angina with hospitalization), and combined CVD (combined CHD, stroke, treated angina without hospitalization, HF, and PAD). Mean follow-up was 4.9 years.

Purpose: To determine whether treatment with a calcium channel blocker or an ACE inhibitor lowers the incidence of CHD or other CVD events versus treatment with a diuretic.

Population: 33,357 participants aged 55 years or older with HTN and at least one other CHD risk factor.

Exclusion Criteria: Included history of hospitalized or treated symptomatic HF and/or known LVEF less than 35%.

Treatment: Chlorthalidone, 12.5 to 25 mg/day ($n = 15,255$); amlodipine, 2.5 to 10 mg/day ($n = 9,048$); or lisinopril, 10 to 40 mg/day ($n = 9,054$).

Results: No significant differences were found between the treatment groups in the incidence of fatal CHD or nonfatal MI (overall rate, 8.9%). Compared with chlorthalidone, the RRs for amlodipine and lisinopril were 0.98 (95% CI, 0.90 to 1.07) and 0.99 (95% CI, 0.91 to 1.08), respectively. All-cause mortality rates also were similar. SBP at 5 years was significantly lower with chlorthalidone compared with that in the amlodipine and lisinopril groups (−0.8 mm Hg, −2 mm Hg; $p < 0.001$), whereas DBP was significantly higher with chlorthalidone compared with amlodipine (0.8 mm Hg; $p < 0.001$). For amlodipine versus chlorthalidone, secondary outcomes were similar except for a higher 6-year rate of HF with amlodipine (10.2% vs. 7.7%; RR, 1.38; 95% CI, 1.25 to 1.52). For lisinopril versus chlorthalidone, lisinopril had higher 6-year rates of combined CVD (33.3% vs. 30.9%; RR, 1.10; 95% CI, 1.05 to 1.16); stroke (6.3% vs. 5.6%; RR, 1.15; 95% CI, 1.02 to 1.30); and HF (8.7% vs. 7.7%; RR, 1.19; 95% CI, 1.07 to 1.31). The fourth arm of the trial testing the α-blocker doxazosin was discontinued in January 2000 because of increased CV events and CHF hospitalizations for this agent compared with chlorthalidone (see *JAMA* 2000;283:1967).

Comments: The results from this very large trial suggest that in patients in which CV events are the greater risk, a thiazide-type diuretic is clearly the preferred first agent; however, in patients with kidney disease or with major risk for renal events, ACE inhibitors should be considered. The study results contradict those observed in HOPE, especially the stroke protection that was touted to be independent of BP. Major criticisms of the ALLHAT study include (a) results have limited relevance because most patients require combination therapy for adequate BP control; (b) results appear driven by the experience in black patients → smaller BP reduction in lisinopril group (blacks respond poorly to ACE inhibitors); (c) add-on therapy to ACE inhibitor should have been a diuretic or calcium-channel blocker, not a β-blocker (note: the ongoing ASCOT trial is comparing an ACE inhibitor/calcium-channel blocker combination, amlodipine and perindopril, with a diuretic/β-blocker combination, atenolol and bendrofluazide).

Other Pharmacologic Agent Studies

122. **Levy D,** et al. Hypertension And Lipid Trial (**HALT**). Principal results of the HALT: a multicenter study of doxazosin in patients with hypertension. *Am Heart J* 1996;131:966–973.

Open, noncomparative trial of 851 clinic patients. At 16 weeks, sitting and standing SBP and DBP were significantly lowered by doxazosin (range, 12.5 to 16.1 mm Hg). No significant effect was seen on heart rate. TC was lowered by 2.7% and LDL by 2.4%. The 5-year coronary disease risk was decreased by 14.7% in patients without prior antihypertensive therapy ($p < 0.0001$) and only 1.7% in patients with prior antihypertensive therapy ($p < 0.05$).

123. **OCTAVE** (Omapatrilat Cardiovascular Treatment Assessment Versus Enalapril). Preliminary results were presented at the 51st Annual Scientific Session of the American College of Cardiology, Atlanta, GA, March 2002.

This prospective, randomized, multicenter trial enrolled 25,267 hypertensives. Patients received omapatrilat, a vasopeptidase inhibitor, or enalapril. Omapatrilat showed significantly better reductions in SBP than did enalapril (average, 3 to 4 mm Hg) in all treatment groups, despite the enalapril group's having more frequent increases in dosage and additions of other agents. However, omapatrilat was associated with significantly more cases of angioedema (overall incidence, 2.2% vs. 0.7%). Angioedema rates were even higher in blacks (5.5% vs. 1.6%) and smokers (3.9% vs. 0.8%). Overall mortality rates were similar: 0.18% for enalapril and 0.15% for omapatrilat. Based on the concerns about angioedema, a FDA Advisory Panel voted not to recommend the drug for approval.

Diet Studies

124. **Appel LJ,** et al., for the Dietary Approaches to Stop Hypertension (**DASH**) Research Group. A clinical trial of the effects of dietary patterns on blood pressure. *N Engl J Med* 1997;336:1117–1124.

This prospective, randomized study was composed of 459 adults with SBP less than 160 mm Hg and DBP, 80 to 95 mm Hg. For 3 weeks, all participants were fed a control diet that was low in fruits, vegetables, and dairy products. They were then randomized to the control diet or a diet rich in fruits and vegetables or a combination diet rich in fruits, vegetables, and low-fat dairy products and with reduced saturated fat and total fat. Body weight and sodium intake were not modified. The combination diet resulted in significant reduction in SBP and DBP compared with the control diet (11.4 mm Hg and 5.5 mm Hg, respectively; both $p < 0.001$).

125. **Whelton PK,** et al., Trial of Nonpharmacologic Interventions in the Elderly (**TONE**). Sodium reduction and weight loss in the treatment of hypertension in older persons. *JAMA* 1998;279:839–846.

Prospective, randomized study of 875 individuals aged 60 to 80 years with SBP less than 145 mm Hg and DBP less than 85 mm Hg on a single antihypertensive medication. Obese patients ($n = 585$) were randomized to reduced sodium intake (≥ 1 g/day), weight loss, both, or usual care, whereas nonobese patients ($n = 390$) received reduced sodium or usual care. After 3 months of intervention, discontinuation of the antihypertensive medication was attempted. At a median follow-up of 29 months, reduced sodium intake compared with no reduction in sodium intake was associated with a significant reduction in the incidence of CV events (MI, HF, bypass surgery, angioplasty), recurrent HTN, or reinitiation of antihypertensive therapy (relative HR, 0.69; 95% CI, 0.59 to 0.81; $p < 0.001$), a difference driven by lower rates of the latter two end-point components. Obese patients assigned to weight loss also had a lower incidence of the combined outcome measures compared with those not assigned to weight loss (relative HR, 0.70; 95% CI, 0.57 to 0.87; $p < 0.001$). Overall, weight loss (average, 3.5 kg), and sodium restriction resulted in an approximate 30% decrease in the need for antihypertensive medication.

126. **Sacks FM,** et al., for the **DASH** Sodium Collaborative Research Group. Effects on blood pressure of reduced dietary sodium and the dietary approaches to stop hypertension (DASH) diet. *N Engl J Med* 2001;344:3–10.

This prospective trial randomized 412 participants to a control diet typical of intake in the U.S. or the DASH diet (rich in vegetables, fruits, and low-fat dairy products). Within the assigned diet, participants ate foods with high, intermediate, and low levels of sodium for 30 consecutive days each, in random order. Decreasing sodium intake from the high to intermediate level reduced SBP by 2.1 mm Hg ($p < 0.001$) during the control diet and by 1.3 mm Hg ($p = 0.03$) during the DASH diet. Decreasing intake from the intermediate to low level resulted in further reductions of 4.6 mm Hg during control diet ($p < 0.001$) and 1.7 mm Hg during DASH diet ($p < 0.01$). The effects of sodium were seen in those with and without HTN, blacks, and women and men. The benefits of the DASH diet and low sodium intake were additive, with the largest SBP difference seen between those on the control diet with high sodium intake and DASH diet with low sodium (latter, 7.1 mm Hg lower in those without HTN, 11.5 mm Hg lower in hypertensives). In summary, the reduction of sodium intake to levels below the current recommendation of 100 mmol/day and the DASH diet both reduce BP substantially, with greater effects in combination.

Invasive Therapy
127. **van Jaarsveld BC,** et al., for **DRASTIC** (Dutch Renal Artery Stenosis Intervention Cooperative) Study Group. The effect of balloon angioplasty on hypertension in atherosclerotic renal-artery stenosis. *N Engl J Med* 2000;342:1007–1014.

This prospective, randomized study enrolled 106 hypertensive patients (DBP more than 95 despite at least two drugs) with atherosclerotic renal artery stenosis (50% or more stenosis) and a serum creatinine 2.3 mg/dL or less. Patients underwent percutaneous transluminal renal angioplasty (PTRA) or received drug therapy. BP, doses of antihypertensive drugs, and renal function were assessed at 3 and 12 months, and patency of the renal artery was assessed at 12 months. At 3 months, BPs were similar (169/99 mm Hg [PTRA] and 176/101 mm Hg). PTRA patients were taking fewer daily doses of medication compared with the drug-therapy group (2.1 vs. 3.2; $p < 0.001$). In drug group, 22 patients underwent PTRA after 3 months because of persistent HTN despite treatment with three or more drugs or worsening renal function. At 1 year, no significant differences were found between the groups in SBP and DBP, daily drug doses, or renal function.

Obesity and Weight

128. **Willett WC,** et al. Weight, weight change and coronary heart disease in women: risk within the normal weight range. *JAMA* 1995;273:461–465.

This prospective cohort study was composed of 115,818 nurses aged 30 to 55 years with no history of CAD. Even modest weight gains after 18 years were associated with increased risk (end point was CHD death and nonfatal MI): RR, 1.25 for 5- to 7.9-kg gain; RR, 1.64 for 8- to 10.9-kg gain; 2.65 for 11- to 19-kg gain.

129. **Rextrode KM,** et al. Abdominal adiposity and coronary heart disease in women. *JAMA* 1998;280:1843–1848.

This analysis of 8-year follow-up data of 44,702 NHS participants showed that a higher waist-to-hip ratio and greater waist circumference were associated with an increased risk of CHD. If the waist-to-hip ratio was 0.88, the adjusted RR of CHD death or MI was 3.25 (vs. waist-to-hip ratio less than 0.72). A waist circumference of 38 inches was associated with an adjusted RR of CHD death and MI of 3.06. The independent predictive value of waist-to-hip ratio and waist circumference also was present in a subgroup with a BMI of ≥ 25 kg/m^2.

130. **Bender R,** et al. Effect of age on excess mortality in obesity. *JAMA* 1999; 281:1498–1504.

This prospective cohort study was composed of 6,193 obese patients with a mean BMI of 36.6 kg/m^2 and mean age of 40.4 years. At follow-up (median, 14.8 years), standardized mortality ratios showed that obesity was associated with significantly increased mortality (men, 1.67; women, 1.45). This increased risk associated with obesity decreased with advancing age among both men (18 to 29 years, 2.46; 30 to 39 years, 2.30; 40 to 49 years, 1.99; 50 to 74 years, 1.31) and women (18 to 29 years, 1.81; 30 to 39 years, 2.10; 40 to 49 years, 1.70; 50 to 74 years, 1.26) (trend test, $p < 0.001$).

131. **Wilson PW,** et al. Overweight and obesity as determinants of cardiovascular risk: the Framingham experience. *Arch Intern Med* 2002;162:1867–1872.

This study examined Framingham Heart Study participants aged 35 to 75 years, who were monitored for up to 44 years. The primary outcome was new CVD, which included angina pectoris, MI, CVD, or stroke. Analyses compared overweight (BMI, 25.0 to 29.9) and obese persons (BMI, 30 or more) with a reference group of normal-weight persons (BMI, 18.5 to 24.9). Overweight status was associated with significantly increased risks of HTN (age-adjusted RR: men, 1.46; women, 1.75). New hypercholes-terolemia and diabetes mellitus were less highly associated with excess adiposity. The age-adjusted RR (CI) for CVD was increased among those who were overweight [men, 1.21 (1.05 to 1.40); women, 1.20 (1.03 to 1.41)] and obese [men, 1.46 (1.20 to 1.77); women, 1.64 (1.37 to 1.98)].

132. **Flegal KM,** et al. Prevalence and trends in obesity among U.S. adults, 1999–2000. *JAMA* 2002;288:1723–1727.

Information was obtained from 4,115 adult men and women who participated in the National Health and Nutrition Examination Survey (NHANES). The age-adjusted prevalence of obesity was 30.5% in 1999 to 2000 compared with 22.9% in NHANES III (1988 to 1994; $p < 0.001$). The prevalence of overweight also increased during this period from 55.9% to 64.5% ($p < 0.001$). Extreme obesity (BMI, 40 or more) also increased significantly in the population, from 2.9% to 4.7% ($p = 0.002$). Racial/ethnic groups did not differ significantly in the prevalence of overweight or obesity for men. Among women, overweight and obesity prevalences were highest among non-Hispanic black women (more than 50% over age were obese).

133. **Fontaine KR,** et al. Years of life lost due to obesity. *JAMA* 2003;289:187–193.

This study examined data from U.S. Life Tables (1999), the Third National Health and Nutrition Examination Survey (NHANES III; 1988 to 1994), First National Health and Nutrition Epidemiologic Follow-up Study (NHANES I and II; 1971 to 1992) and NHANES II Mortality Study (1976 to 1992). Among whites, a U-shaped association was found between overweight or obesity and years of life lost (YLL). The optimal BMI (associated with the least YLL or greatest longevity) is 23 to 25 for whites and 23 to 30 for blacks. For any degree of overweight, younger adults typically had greater YLL than did older adults. The maximum YLL for white men aged 20 to 30 years with a severe level of obesity (BMI more than 45) is 13 and is 8 for white women. Among blacks older than 60 years, overweight and moderate obesity were not associated with an increased YLL; only severe obesity resulted in YLL. However, younger blacks with severe levels of obesity had a maximum YLL of 20 for men and 5 for women.

Activity and Exercise

134. **Berlin JA,** Colditz GA. A meta-analysis of physical activity in the prevention of coronary heart disease. *Am J Epidemiol* 1990;132:612–628.

This meta-analysis found a nearly twofold increased risk of death from CHD for individuals with sedentary compared with active occupations (RR, 1.9; 95% CI, 1.6 to 2.2).

135. **Leon AS,** Connett J. Physical activity and 10.5 year mortality in the Multiple Risk Factor Intervention Trial (**MRFIT**). *Int J Epidemiol* 1991;20:690–697.

This analysis focused on 12,138 male MRFIT subjects who had leisure time physical activity (LTPA) assessed by the Minnesota questionnaire. The level of LTPA was inversely related to all-cause mortality, CHD mortality, and CV mortality because those in the lowest LTPA tertile had excess mortality rates of 15%, 27%, and 22%, respectively, compared with men in the middle tertile. No significant further attenuation of risk was seen with additional LTPA (tertile 3).

136. **Mittleman MA,** et al. Triggering of acute MI by heavy physical exertion. *N Engl J Med* 1993;329:1677–1683.

This analysis focused on interviews with 1,228 patients an average of 4 days after MI. Heavy exertion (≥ 6 metabolic equivalents) within 1 hour had occurred in 4.4%. The RR of acute MI in the 1 hour after exertion was 5.9; however, risk correlated with the frequency of exercise (less than once per week: RR, 107; 1 to 2 times: RR, 19.4; 3 to 4 times: RR, 8.6; at least 5 times: RR, 2.4).

137. **Willich SN,** et al. Physical exertion as a trigger of AMI. *N Engl J Med* 1993;329:1684–1690.

This analysis focused on interviews with 1,194 patients at 13 ± 6 days after MI. An increased risk of MI was associated with strenuous activity (≥ 6 metabolic equivalents; 7.1% of patients) at onset of acute MI (RR, 2.1). The RR also was 2.1 for activity within 1 hour; infrequent exercise (less than 4 times per week) was associated with an RR of 6.9 (vs. 1.3).

138. **Blair SN,** et al. Influences of cardiorespiratory fitness and other precursors on cardiovascular disease and all-cause mortality in men and women. *JAMA* 1996;276:205–210.

This observational cohort study of 32,421 patients (78% men) demonstrated independent mortality predictors. Among men, low fitness (RR, 1.52), smoking (1.65), abnormal ECG (1.64), increased TC (1.34), elevated SBP (1.34), and chronic illness (1.63) risks were defined. Among women, low fitness (2.1) and smoking (1.99) risks were defined. It is important to note that a fitness effect occurs with any combination of smoking, TC, and BP.

139. **Kushi LH,** et al. Physical activity and mortality in postmenopausal women. *JAMA* 1997;277:1287–1292.

This prospective cohort study of 40,417 postmenopausal Iowa women, aged 55 to 69 years at baseline (1986), assessed physical activity with a mailed questionnaire. After adjustment for confounders and excluding women with heart disease and those who died in the first 3 years of follow-up, women with regular physical activity had a lower risk of death during follow-up (mean, 7 years), compared with women who did not (RR, 0.77; 95% CI, 0.66 to 0.90). Increasing frequency of moderate activity was associated with reduced risk of death, and a similar pattern was seen for vigorous physical activity. Women with moderate activity but no vigorous activity also benefited; even moderate activity only once per week was associated with lower mortality (RR, 0.78; 95% CI, 0.64 to 0.96).

140. **Hakim AA,** et al. Effects of walking on coronary heart disease in elderly men: the Honolulu Heart Program. *Circulation* 1999;100:9–13.

This study of 2,678 physically capable men aged 71 to 93 years who were observed over a 2- to 4-year follow-up period found that those who walked more than 1.5 miles a day had a lower incidence of developing CHD compared with those who walked less than one-fourth mile a day (2.5% vs. 5.1%; $p < 0.01$) and 0.25 to 1.5 miles/day (4.5%;

$p < 0.01$). These findings were not altered by adjustment for age and other CHD risk factors.

141. **Manson JE,** et al. A prospective study of walking as compared with vigorous exercise in the prevention of coronary heart disease in women. *N Engl J Med* 1999;341:650–658.

This prospective cohort study of 72,488 NHS participants found brisk walking, as assessed by a self-administered questionnaire, was associated with fewer coronary events. In multivariate analyses, women in the highest quintile group [$\geq$3 hours/week at a brisk pace (=3 mph)], had an RR of 0.65 (95% CI, 0.47 to 0.91) compared with those who walked infrequently. Regular vigorous exercise ($\geq$6 METs) was associated with similar risk reductions (30% to 40%).

142. **Myers J,** et al. Exercise capacity and mortality among men referred for exercise testing. *N Engl J Med* 2002;346:793–801.

This analysis examined 6,213 consecutive men referred for exercise treadmill testing (ETT), of whom 3,679 had an abnormal ETT result or a history of CVD, or both. At mean follow-up of 6.2 years, and after adjustment for age, the peak exercise capacity measured in METs was the strongest predictor of the risk of death among both normal subjects and those with CVD. Absolute peak exercise capacity was a stronger predictor of the risk of death than the percentage of the age-predicted value achieved, with each 1-MET increase in exercise capacity conferring a 12% improvement in survival. No interaction was found between the use or nonuse of β-blockade.

143. **Tanasescu M,** et al. Exercise type and intensity in relation to coronary heart disease in men. *JAMA* 2002;288:1994–2000.

This cohort analysis examined the 44,452 U.S. men enrolled in the Health Professionals' Follow-up Study. At follow-up (average, 10.7 years), 1,700 new cases of CHD were found. Total physical activity, running, weight training, and rowing were each inversely associated with risk of CHD. The adjusted RRs of nonfatal MI or fatal CHD corresponding to quintiles of METs for total physical activity were 1.0, 0.90 (95% CI, 0.78 to 1.04), 0.87 (0.75 to 1.00), 0.83 (0.71 to 0.96), and 0.70 (0.59 to 0.82; $p < 0.001$ for trend). Men who ran for an hour or more per week had a 42% RR (RR, 0.58; 95% CI, 0.44 to 0.77) compared with men who did not run ($p < 0.001$ for trend). Weight training for 30 minutes or more per week was associated with a 23% risk reduction (RR, 0.77; 95% CI, 0.61 to 0.98; $p = 0.03$ for trend), whereas rowing for 1 hour or more per week was associated with an 18% risk reduction (RR, 0.82; 05% CI, 0.68 to 0.99). Average exercise intensity was associated with reduced CHD risk, independent of the total volume of physical activity: moderate (4 to 6 METs) and high (6 to 12 METs) activity intensities were associated with 6% and 17% RRRs compared with low activity intensity (less than 4 METs; $p = 0.02$ for trend).

Nonmodifiable Risk Factors

144. **Colditz GA,** et al. A prospective study of parental history of MI and coronary artery disease in men. *Am J Cardiol* 1991;67:933–938.

This prospective study was composed of 45,317 male health professionals aged 40 to 75 years with no diagnosis of CAD. At a mean follow-up of 1.6 years, if a parent had an MI at younger than 70 years, the RRs of cardiac death, MI, PTCA, or CABG were 2.2 (maternal factor) and 1.7 (paternal factor). The risk increased with lower parental age.

145. **Wei JY.** Age and the cardiovascular system. *N Engl J Med* 1992;327:1735–1739.

This review discusses the impact of age on the myocardium, vasculature, cardiac output, diastolic function, BP regulation, and effects of exercise training.

146. **Marenberg ME,** et al. Genetic susceptibility to death from coronary heart disease in a study of twins. *N Engl J Med* 1994;330:1041–1046.

This analysis is composed of data taken from 21,004 Swedish twins in 1961 and 1963; average follow-up was 26 years. Among men, RRs (of death secondary to CHD) if the twin died of CHD at younger than 55 years were 8.1 (monozygous) and 3.8 (dizygous). Among women, RRs were 15.0 and 2.6, respectively; overall, RRs decreased with increased age.

147. **Ciruzzi M,** et al. Frequency of family history in patients with acute MI. *Am J Cardiol* 1997;80:122–127.

This case-control study was composed of 1,060 cases and 1,071 controls. Among cases with a twofold higher incidence of family history (more than one first-degree relative with a history of MI), the incidence of MI was 31% versus 15% for controls. After risk-factor adjustment (age, sex, cholesterol, smoking, diabetes, HTN, BMI, education, social class, exercise), the overall OR was 2.18 (at least one relative, 2.04; two relatives, 3.18). If younger than 55 years with two relatives, the OR was 4.42; $\geq$55 years with two relatives: OR, 3.00; family history plus TC 240 mg/dL: OR, 4.5; family history plus HTN: OR, 4.5; family history plus current smoking: OR, 5.77.

148. **Andresdottir MB,** et al. Fifteen percent of myocardial infarctions and coronary revascularizations explained by family history unrelated to conventional risk factors: the Reykjavik Cohort Study. *Eur Heart J* 2002;23:1655–1663.

This prospective cohort study examined 9,328 men and 10,062 women aged 33 to 81 years in the Reykjavik area, from 1967 to 1996. During follow-up (18 to 19 years), in 2,700 men and 1,070 women, CHD developed. After adjustment for other CRFs, the HR of CHD was highly significant, 1.66 (95% CI, 1.51 to 1.82) and 1.64 (95% CI, 1.43 to 1.89) for men and women, respectively. Family history of MI was attributed to 15.1% of all cases of CHD in men and 16.6% in women, independent of other known risk factors.

Alcohol

149. **Hein HO,** et al. Alcohol consumption, serum LDL cholesterol concentration and risk of ischemic heart disease: 6 year follow-up in the Copenhagen male study. *BMJ* 1996;312:736–741.

This prospective study was composed of 2,826 patients without CAD. At 6 years, 6.1% had experienced a first ischemic event. The association between alcohol and IHD was highly dependent on LDL. With an LDL level of 5.25 mM, among abstainers, the incidence of IHD is 16.4%; among those who have 1 to 21 drinks/week, 8.7%; among those who have $\geq$22 drinks/week, 4.4%. After risk-factor adjustment, RRs were 0.4 ($p < 0.05$) and 0.2 ($p < 0.01$). If LDL level was less than 3.63 mM, no benefit was observed from any level of alcohol consumption.

150. **Camargo CA Jr.** Moderate alcohol consumption and risk for angina pectoris or MI in U.S. male physicians. *Ann Intern Med* 1997;126:372–375.

This prospective cohort study of 22,071 patients confirms the substantial body of data correlating moderate ethanol consumption with decreased CHD risk. One drink/day versus less than one drink/week confers an RR of angina of 0.69 (95% CI, 0.59 to 0.81) and an RR of MI of 0.65 (95% CI, 0.52 to 0.81).

151. **Muntwyler J,** et al. Mortality and light to moderate alcohol consumption after MI. *Lancet* 1998;352:1882–1885.

This analysis is composed of 90,150 men in the PHS, 5,358 with prior MI. At 5-year follow-up, 920 deaths were found. After adjustment for confounders, moderate intake was associated with a significant decrease in total mortality ($p = 0.016$). Mortality RRs were one to four drinks/month, 0.85 (95% CI, 0.69 to 1.05); two to four drinks/week, 0.72 (95% CI, 0.58 to 0.89); one drink/day, 0.79 (95% CI, 0.64 to 9.96); and two drinks/day, 0.84 (95% CI, 0.55 to 1.26).

152. **de Lorgeril M,** et al. Wine drinking and risks of cardiovascular complications after recent acute myocardial infarction. *Circulation* 2002;106:1465–1469.

This analysis examined 437 survivors of a recent MI who had at least two reliable assessments of drinking (and dietary) habits. Average ethanol intake was 7.6% of the total energy intake, of which wine ethanol represented 92%. At 4-year follow-up, 104 CV complications (23.8%) had occurred. In comparison with abstainers, the adjusted risk of complications was significantly reduced by 59% in patients whose average ethanol intake was 7.7% of the total energy intake (about 2 drinks/day), and by 52% in those whose average ethanol intake was of 16% of energy (about 4 drinks/day).

153. **Mukamal KJ,** et al. Roles of drinking pattern and type of alcohol consumed in coronary heart disease in men. *N Engl J Med* 2003;348:109–118.

This study assessed alcohol intake by questionnaires in 38,077 male health professionals free of CVD and cancer at baseline. At 12 years of follow-up, men who consumed alcohol three to four or five to seven days per week had decreased risks of MI compared with those who had less than one drink per week [multivariate RR, 0.68 (95% CI, 0.55 to 0.84) and 0.63 (95% CI, 0.54 to 0.74), respectively]. No single type of beverage conferred additional benefit. A 12.5-g increase in daily alcohol consumption over a 4-year follow-up period was associated with an RR of MI of 0.78.

Hormone Status and Hormonal Replacement

154. **Stampfer MJ,** et al. Postmenopausal estrogen therapy and cardiovascular disease. *N Engl J Med* 1991;325:756–762.

This prospective cohort study was composed of 48,470 postmenopausal women without prior CVD or cancer. After adjustment for risk factors, at an average follow-up of 7 years, estrogen patients had a significant 11% lower total mortality, 28% lower CV mortality, and 44% RRR in the incidence of major coronary disease. No significant difference was found in stroke rates.

155. **Grodstein F,** et al. Postmenopausal estrogen and progestin use and the risk of cardiovascular disease. *N Engl J Med* 1996;335:453–461.

This prospective cohort analysis focused on 59,337 NHS participants who were aged 30 to 55 years and free of known CVD at baseline. At an average follow-up of 11.2 years, combined estrogen and progestin users had a lower incidence of major CHD (MI, death) compared with nonhormone and estrogen-only users (adjusted RRs, 0.39 and 0.60). Thus the addition of progestin does not appear to attenuate the cardioprotective effects of postmenopausal estrogen therapy. No significant differences in stroke rates were found.

156. **Hulley S,** et al. Heart and Estrogen/progestin Replacement Study (**HERS**). Randomized trial of estrogen and progestin for secondary prevention of coronary heart disease in postmenopausal women. *JAMA* 1998;280:605–613.

Design: Prospective, randomized, blinded, placebo-controlled, multicenter study. Average follow-up period was 4.1 years.
Purpose: To determine whether estrogen plus progestin alters the risk for CHD events in postmenopausal women with known coronary disease.
Population: 2,763 women younger than 80 years (mean age, 66.7 years).
Exclusion Criteria: CHD event in previous 6 months, sexual hormone use in previous 3 months, history of pulmonary embolism (PE), deep venous thrombosis (DVT), breast cancer, and endometrial cancer.
Treatment: Conjugated equine estrogens (0.625 mg once daily) and medroxyprogesterone (one tablet once daily) or placebo.
Results: Compliance rates were 82% at 1 year and 75% at 3 years. No difference in primary outcome (MI plus CV death; relative hazard, 0.99) was observed. Lack of effect was observed despite the hormone group having 11% lower LDL and 10% higher HDL (each $p < 0.001$). The hormone group had more events in year 1 and fewer in years 4 and 5. The hormone group had more venous thromboembolism (relative hazard, 2.89; 95% CI, 1.50 to 5.58) and gallbladder disease (relative hazard, 1.38; 95% CI, 1.00 to 1.92).

157. **Tanis BC,** et al. Oral contraceptives and the risk of myocardial infarction. *N Engl J Med* 2001;345:1787–1793.

This population-based, case-control study enrolled 248 women aged 18 to 49 years with a first MI between 1990 and 1995, and 925 control women without a MI who were matched for age, calendar year of index event, and area of residence. An analysis for factor V Leiden and the G20210A mutation in the prothrombin gene was conducted in 217 patients and 763 controls. The risk of MI was twofold higher in those who used any type of combined oral contraceptive compared with nonusers (OR, 2.0; 95% CI, 1.5 to 2.8). The adjusted OR was 2.5 (95% CI, 1.5 to 4.1) among women who used second-generation oral contraceptives (e.g., levonorgestrel) and 1.3 (95% CI, 0.7 to 2.5) among those who used third-generation oral contraceptives (e.g., desogestrel or gestodene). Among women who used oral contraceptives, ORs in those without a prothrombotic mutation compared with those with a mutation were similar (ORs of 2.1 and 1.9, respectively).

158. **Barrett-Connor E,** et al., for the **MORE** Investigators (Multiple Outcomes of Raloxifene Evaluation). Raloxifene and cardiovascular events in osteoporotic postmenopausal women: four-year results from the MORE (Multiple Outcomes of Raloxifene Evaluation) randomized trial. *JAMA* 2002;287:847–857.

Design: Prospective, randomized, double-blind, placebo-controlled, multicenter trial. Primary end point was MI, unstable angina, coronary ischemia, and stroke or TIA.
Purpose: To determine the effect of raloxifene on CV events in osteoporotic post-menopausal women.
Population: 7,705 osteoporotic postmenopausal women (mean age, 67 years); osteo-porosis documented by prior vertebral fracture or bone mineral density score (T score of less than −2.5).
Exclusion Criteria: Stroke or venous thromboembolic disease in prior 10 years.
Treatment: Raloxifene, 60 mg/day; raloxifene, 120 mg/day; or placebo, for 4 years.
Results: No significant differences were noted between the three treatment groups in coronary and cerebrovascular events (raloxifene, 60 mg/day: 3.2%; raloxifene, 120 mg/day: 3.7%; placebo, 3.7%). Among the 1,035 women with increased CV risk at baseline, those assigned to raloxifene (either dose) had a significantly lower risk of CV events compared with placebo (RR, 0.60; 95% CI, 0.38 to 0.95). The number of CV events during the first year was not significantly different in the overall cohort, or among women at increased CV risk ($p = 0.86$) or with evidence of established CHD ($p = 0.60$).

159. **Grady D,** et al. for the HERS Research Group. Cardiovascular disease outcomes during 6.8 years of hormone therapy: Heart and Estrogen/Progestin Replacement Study Follow-up (**HERS II**). *JAMA* 2002;288:49–57.

Design: Prospective, randomized, blinded, placebo-controlled, multicenter trial of 4.1 years' duration (HERS) and subsequent unblinded follow-up for 2.7 years (HERS II). Primary end point was nonfatal MI and CHD death.
Purpose: To determine if the risk reduction observed in the later years of HERS per-sisted and resulted in an overall reduced risk of CHD events with additional years of follow-up.
Population: 2,763 postmenopausal women with CHD and an average age of 67 years at enrollment in HERS; 2,321 women (93% of those surviving) consented to follow-up in HERS II.
Exclusion Criteria: Included age 80 years or older and prior hysterectomy.
Treatment: Conjugated estrogens, 0.625 mg/day, and medroxyprogesterone acetate, 2.5 mg/day, or placebo ($n = 1,383$) during HERS; in HERS II, open-label hormone ther-apy was prescribed at physicians' discretion; at least 80% adherence to hormones declined from 81% (year 1) to 45% (year 6) in the hormone group, and increased from none (year 1) to 8% (year 6) in the placebo group.
Results: No significant differences were found between the groups in primary CHD events or secondary CV events in HERS, HERS II, or overall. The unadjusted rel-ative hazard (RH) for CHD events in HERS was 0.99 (95% CI, 0.81 to 1.22); HERS

II, 1.00 (95% CI, 0.77 to 1.29); and overall, 0.99 (0.84 to 1.17). The overall RHs remained similar after adjustment for potential confounders and differential use of statins between treatment groups (RH, 0.97), and in analyses restricted to women who were adherent to randomized treatment assignment (RH, 0.96). In an accompanying report (*JAMA* 2002;288:58–66), data were presented on thromboembolic events, biliary tract surgery, cancer, fracture, and total mortality. Hormone therapy was associated with an increased risk of venous thromboembolism (unadjusted intention-to-treat RH, 1.40; 95% CI, 0.64 to 3.05; vs. RH of 2.66 in HERS I); the RH was 2.08 overall for the 6.8 years (95% CI, 1.28 to 3.40). The overall RH for biliary tract surgery was 1.48 (95% CI, 1.12 to 1.95); for any cancer, 1.19 (95% CI, 0.95 to 1.50); and for any fracture, 1.04 (95% CI, 0.87 to 1.25). There were 261 deaths among those assigned to hormone therapy and 239 among those assigned to placebo (RH, 1.10; 95% CI, 0.92 to 1.31).

160. Writing Group for the **Women's Health Initiative** Investigators. Risks and benefits of estrogen plus progestin in healthy postmenopausal women: principal results from the Women's Health Initiative randomized controlled trial. *JAMA* 2002;288:321–333 (editorial, 366–368).

Design: Prospective, randomized, controlled, multicenter, primary prevention trial. Primary end point was CHD death and nonfatal MI. Primary adverse outcome was invasive breast cancer. A global index included the two primary outcomes plus stroke, pulmonary embolism (PE), endometrial cancer, colorectal cancer, hip fracture, and death due to all other causes.

Purpose: To assess the major health benefits and risks of the most commonly used combined hormone preparation in the United States.

Population: 16,608 postmenopausal women aged 50 to 79 years with an intact uterus.

Exclusion Criteria: Included prior breast cancer, other prior cancer in previous 10 years, low hematocrit or platelet counts.

Treatment: Equine estrogens, 0.625 mg/day plus medroxyprogesterone acetate, 2.5 mg/day, in one tablet, or placebo.

Results: The estrogen/progestin arm of the trial was terminated early (at 5.2 years follow-up vs. planned 8.5 years) because of excessive risk of global index in hormone group compared with placebo (HR, 1.15; 95% CI, 1.03 to 1.28). The hormone group also had a significantly higher incidence of CHD [HR, 1.29 (1.02 to 1.63)], breast cancer [HR, 1.26 (1.00 to 1.59)], stroke [HR, 1.41 (1.07 to 1.85)], and PE [HR, 2.13 (1.39 to 3.25)], whereas lower rates of colorectal cancer [HR, 0.63 (0.43 to 0.92)] and hip factures [HR, 0.66 (0.45 to 0.98)] occurred, and a trend toward lower rates of endometrial cancer [HR, 0.83 (0.47 to 1.47)]. All-cause mortality rates were similar [HR, 0.98 (0.82 to 1.18)].

Comments: Although mortality rates were similar, the overall risk-benefit profile in this trial is not consistent with the requirements for a clearly safe and efficacious intervention for primary prevention of chronic diseases. The estrogen-only arm was not stopped.

161. **WAVE.** (Women's Angiographic Vitamin and Estrogen Trial). **Waters DD,** et al. Effects of hormone replacement therapy and antioxidant vitamin supplements on coronary atherosclerosis in postmenopausal women: a randomized controlled trial. *JAMA* 2002;288:2432–2440.

Design: Prospective, randomized, placebo-controlled, double-blind, 2 × 2 factorial, multicenter trial. Primary end point was annualized mean (SD) change in MLD of all qualifying coronary lesions.

Purpose: To determine whether hormone replacement therapy (HRT) or antioxidant vitamin supplements, alone or in combination, influence CAD progression in postmenopausal women, as measured by serial quantitative coronary angiography (QCA).

Population: 423 postmenopausal women with at least one 15% to 75% coronary stenosis at baseline coronary angiography.

Treatment: 0.625 mg/d of conjugated equine estrogen (plus 2.5 mg/d of medroxyprogesterone acetate for women if without hysterectomy), or matching placebo, and 400 IU of vitamin E twice daily plus 500 mg of vitamin C twice daily, or placebo.

Results: Mean interval between angiograms was 2.8 years. No differences between groups were found in change in mean MLD: 0.047-mm/yr decrease with HRT, 0.024-mm/yr decrease with HRT placebo, 0.044-mm/yr decrease with antioxidants, and 0.028-mm/yr decrease with vitamin placebo. When patients with intercurrent death or MI were included, the primary outcome showed an increased risk with active HRT ($p = 0.045$), and a trend toward increased risk in the active vitamin group ($p = 0.09$). Death, nonfatal MI, or stroke occurred in 26 HRT patients versus 15 HRT controls (HR, 1.9; 95% CI, 0.97 to 3.6) and in 26 vitamin patients and 18 vitamin controls (HR, 1.5; 95% CI, 0.80 to 2.9).

162. **ESPRIT.** (oEStrogen in the Prevention of ReInfarction Trial). The ESPRIT Team. Oestrogen therapy for prevention of reinfarction in postmenopausal women. *Lancet* 2002;360:2001–2008.

Design: Prospective, randomized, double-blind, placebo-controlled, multicenter, secondary prevention trial. Primary outcomes were reinfarction or cardiac death and all-cause mortality.

Purpose: To ascertain whether unopposed estrogen reduces the risk of further cardiac events in postmenopausal women who survive a first MI.

Population: 1,017 postmenopausal women aged 50 to 69 years who had survived a first MI.

Exclusion Criteria: Included use of HRT or vaginal bleeding in previous year; history of breast, ovarian, or endometrial cancer; history of DVT or pulmonary embolism (PE); severe renal disease; active or chronic liver disease.

Treatment: Estradiol valerate, 2 mg once daily; or placebo, for 2 years. Compliance was poor in both groups [at 2 years, 43% (estradiol) and 63%].

Results: At 2 years, the incidence of cardiac death or reinfarction was similar between the two groups (both 12.1). Similarly, the reduction in all-cause mortality between the estrogen and placebo groups was not significant (rate ratio, 0.79; 95% CI, 0.50 to 1.27; $p = 0.34$).

C-Reactive Protein

163. **Ridker PM,** et al. Inflammation, aspirin, and the risk of cardiovascular disease in apparently healthy men. *N Engl J Med* 1997;336:973–979.

Case-control study of 543 PHS participants who had an MI, stroke, or venous thrombosis, and 543 participants who did not have a vascular event at a long-term follow-up (more than 8 years). Baseline CRP concentrations were significantly higher in men who subsequently had an MI (1.51 vs. 1.13 mg/L; $p < 0.001$) or ischemic stroke (1.38 vs. 1.13 mg/L; $p = 0.02$), but not venous thrombosis (1.26 vs. 1.13 mg/L; $p = 0.34$) than among men without vascular events. Men in the highest quartile of CRP values had, as compared with those in the lowest quartile, an approximately threefold and twofold higher risk of MI and stroke, respectively (RR, 2.9; $p < 0.001$; RR, 1.9; $p = 0.02$). The use of ASA was associated with a substantial (55.7%) reduction ($p = 0.02$) in MI among men in the highest CRP quartile, but only a nonsignificant (13.9%) reduction among those in the lowest quartile.

164. **Ridker PM,** et al. C-reactive protein adds to the predictive value of total and HDL cholesterol in determining risk of first myocardial infarction. *Circulation* 1998;97:2007–2011.

This case-control study of PHS participants analyzed levels of CRP, TC, and HDL in 245 subjects who subsequently developed a first MI and among 372 controls. At follow-up (average period, 9 years), multivariate models incorporating CRP and lipid parameters provided a better method of predicting risk than did models using lipids alone. For example, among those with high levels of both CRP and TC, the risk of MI was increased fivefold ($p = 0.0001$) compared with more modest risk elevations with isolated elevations of CRP (RR, 1.5) or TC (RR, 2.3). CRP levels were predictive of risk for those with low as well as high levels of TC and TC/HDL.

165. **Ridker PM,** et al. Prospective study of C-reactive protein and the risk of future cardiovascular events among apparently healthy women. *Circulation* 1998;98:731–733 (also see *N Engl J Med* 2000;342:836).

This nested case-control study was composed of 122 WHS participants with first cardiovascular event (MI, stroke, coronary angioplasty, coronary bypass surgery, or CV death) and 244 age- and smoking-matched controls free of CVD for 3 years. Elevated CRP levels were strongly associated with increased events ($p = 0.001$); highest levels were associated with an approximately fivefold increase in risk of vascular event (RR, 4.8; 95% CI, 2.3 to 10.1; $p = 0.0004$), and sevenfold increase in MI and stroke (RR, 7.3; 95% CI, 2.7 to 19.9; $p = 0.001$). Risk estimates were independent of other risk factors, and CRP was predictive in both low- and high-risk patients.

166. **Ridker PM,** et al. Inflammation, pravastatin and the risk of coronary events after MI in patients with average cholesterol levels. *Circulation* 1998;98:839–844.

This nested case-control study was composed of 391 CARE patients with MI or cardiovascular death and 391 age- and sex-matched controls. Cases had higher CRP ($p = 0.05$) and serum amyloid A (0.006) levels; the highest quintiles had a significantly higher risk of recurrent events [RRs, 1.77 ($p = 0.02$), 1.74 ($p = 0.02$)]. The greatest risk was seen in placebo patients with elevated CRP and serum amyloid A (RR, 2.81; $p = 0.007$). Overall, the risk association between inflammation and risk was attenuated and nonsignificant in pravastatin patients [RR, 1.29 ($p = 0.5$) vs. RR, 2.11 ($p = 0.048$) in placebo patients].

167. **Koenig W,** et al. C-reactive protein, a sensitive marker of inflammation, predicts future risk of coronary heart disease in initially healthy middle-aged men. *Circulation* 1999;99:237–242.

This analysis focused on 936 men enrolled in MONICA (Monitoring Trends and Determinants in Cardiovascular Disease), a general population cohort study. At 8-year follow-up, the HR ratio of CHD events associated with a one standard deviation increase in the CRP level was 1.67 (95% CI, 1.29 to 2.17), and after adjustment for age and smoking, 1.50 (95% CI, 1.14 to 1.97).

168. **Albert MA,** et al. Effect of statin therapy on C-reactive protein levels: the Pravastatin Inflammation/CRP Evaluation (**PRINCE**): a randomized trial and cohort study. *JAMA* 2001;286:64–70.

Design: Prospective, randomized, placebo-controlled, partially double-blind, partially open, multicenter trial. Primary end point: change in high-sensitivity CRP (hsCRP) at 24 weeks.
Purpose: To determine the antiinflammatory effects of pravastatin as measured by CRP reduction.
Population: 2,884 total patients: 1,702 individuals without CVD and an open-labeled study in 1,182 patients with known CVD off statins for at least 12 weeks.
Treatment: Primary prevention group received pravastatin, 40 mg once daily, or placebo. All patients in secondary prevention received pravastatin.
Results: In the primary prevention cohort, pravastatin reduced hsCRP by 16.9% (decrease of 0.02 mg) compared with no change with placebo. This effect was evident as early as 12 weeks and seen in all subgroups independent of other variables including gender, baseline, or on-treatment lipid levels, diabetes, and use of ASA and HRT. In the open-labeled CVD cohort, a similar 14.3% reduction in hsCRP was seen.

169. **Ridker PM,** et al., for Air Force/Texas Coronary Atherosclerosis Prevention Study Investigators. Measurement of C-reactive protein for the targeting of statin therapy in the primary prevention of acute coronary events. *N Engl J Med* 2001;344:1959–1965.

CRP was measured at baseline and 1 year in 5,742 AFCAPS/TexCAPS participants. At 5 years, higher baseline CRP levels were associated with higher coronary event rates. Lovastatin therapy reduced CRP levels by 14.8% ($p < 0.001$), an effect not explained by lovastatin-induced changes in the lipid profile. In particular, lovastatin was effective among those with a ratio of total-to-HDL cholesterol (TC/HDL) that was lower than the median and a CRP higher than the median ($p = 0.02$). In contrast, lovastatin was ineffective in those with TC/HDL cholesterol and a CRP level that were both lower than the median.

170. **Pradhan AD,** et al. Inflammatory biomarkers, hormone replacement therapy, and incident coronary heart disease: prospective analysis from the Women's Health Initiative observational study. *JAMA* 2002;288:980–987.

This prospective, nested case-control study of postmenopausal women examined the 304 cases in which CHD developed during the Women's Health Initiative; 304 controls were matched by age, smoking status, ethnicity, and follow-up time (median, 2.9 years). Cases had significantly higher median baseline levels of CRP and IL-6 compared with controls (0.33 vs. 0.25 mg/dL; $p < 0.001$; 1.81 vs. 1.47 pg/mL; $p < 0.001$). In matched analyses, the OR for incident CHD in the highest versus lowest quartile was 2.3 for CRP (95% CI, 1.4 to 3.7; p trend = 0.002) and 3.3 for IL-6 (95% CI, 2.0 to 5.5; p trend < 0.001). After additional adjustment for lipid and nonlipid risk factors, both inflammatory markers were significantly associated with a twofold increase in odds for CHD events. Current use of HRT was associated with elevated median CRP levels (no association with IL-6). In analyses comparing individuals with similar baseline levels of either CRP or IL-6, those taking or not taking HRT had similar CHD ORs. Thus use or nonuse of HRT had less importance as a predictor of cardiovascular risk than did baseline levels of either CRP or IL-6.

171. **Ridker PM,** et al. Comparison of C-reactive protein and low-density lipoprotein cholesterol levels in the prediction of first cardiovascular events. *N Engl J Med* 2002;347:1557–1565.

This study measured baseline LDL-C and CRP in 27,939 WHS participants. At a mean follow-up of 8 years, both measures had a strong linear relation with the incidence of CV events, although the two were minimally correlated ($r = 0.08$). After adjustment for age, smoking status, diabetes, BP, use or nonuse of HRT, the RRs of first cardiovascular events (MI, ischemic stroke, coronary revascularization, or cardiovascular death) according to increasing quintiles of CRP, as compared with the women in the lowest quintile, were 1.4, 1.6, 2.0, and 2.3 ($p < 0.001$). Corresponding RRs in increasing quintiles of LDL-C, as compared with the lowest, were 0.9, 1.1, 1.3, and 1.5 ($p < 0.001$). Similar effects were observed in separate analyses of each component of the composite end point. Overall, 46% of major events occurred among those with LDL less than 130 mg/dL. Importantly, because CRP and LDL-C measurements tended to identify different high-risk groups, screening for both biologic markers provided better prognostic information than did screening for either alone.

172. **Mueller C,** et al. Inflammation and long-term mortality after non–ST elevation acute coronary syndrome treated with a very early invasive strategy in 1042 consecutive patients. *Circulation* 2002;105:1412–1415.

Prospective cohort study of 1,042 patients undergoing coronary angiography and subsequent culprit artery stenting within 24 hours. CRP levels were determined on admission. In-hospital mortality was significantly higher in patients with a CRP greater than 10 mg/L (3.7% vs. 1.2% with CRP less than 3 mg/L and vs. 0.8% with CRP of 3 to 10 mg/L; RR, 4.2 for more than 10 mg/L vs. CRP of 10 mg/L or less; $p = 0.004$). At follow-up (mean, 20 months), mortality was 3.4% with CRP less than 3 mg/L, 4.4% with CRP between 3 and 10 mg/L, and 12.7% with CRP more than 10 mg/L (RR, 3.8 for CRP more than 10 mg/L vs. CRP of 10 mg/L or less). In a multivariate analysis, CRP remained an independent predictor of long-term mortality.

173. **Plenge JK,** et al. Simvastatin lowers C-reactive protein within 14 days: an effect independent of low-density lipoprotein cholesterol reduction. *Circulation* 2002;106:1447–1452.

This prospective, randomized, double-blind, crossover study of 40 subjects with elevated LDL-C found that simvastatin lowers hsCRP by 14 days, independent of its effect on LDL-C. Patients received simvastatin, 40 mg/day for 14 days, and then placebo for 14 days, or placebo first, and then simvastatin. Simvastatin reduced LDL-C by 56 mg/dL ($p < 0.0001$) at day 7 and by an additional 8 mg/dL ($p = 0.02$) at day 14. Log(hsCRP) at 14 days was significantly lower in the simvastatin group compared with the placebo group ($p = 0.011$). As noted, no relation was found between the reduction in LDL-C and the decrease in hsCRP.

Other

Homocysteine
Meta-Analysis
174. **Homocysteine Studies Collaboration.** Homocysteine and risk of ischemic heart disease and stroke: a meta-analysis. *JAMA* 2002;288:2015–2022.

This meta-analysis included data from 30 prospective or retrospective studies involving a total of 5,073 IHD events and 1,113 stroke events. Allowances were made for differences between studies, for confounding by known cardiovascular risk factors (CRFs), and for regression dilution bias. Stronger associations were observed in retrospective studies of homocysteine measured in blood collected after the onset of disease than in prospective studies among individuals who had no history of CVD when blood was collected. After adjustment for CRFs in the prospective studies, a 25% lower than usual homocysteine level [about 3 mM (0.41 mg/L)] was associated with an 11% lower IHD risk (OR, 0.89; 95% CI, 0.83 to 0.96) and 19% lower stroke risk (OR, 0.81; 95% CI, 0.69 to 0.95).

Studies
175. **Nygard O,** et al. Total plasma homocysteine and cardiovascular risk profile. *JAMA* 1995;274:1526–1533.

This analysis focused on 16,176 patients aged 40 to 67 years without prior HTN, diabetes, CHD, or CVD. Homocysteine levels were higher in men and increased with age (age 40 to 42 years, 10.8 μM; age 65 to 67 years, 12.2 μM). A strong positive correlation was found, especially among women, with the number of cigarettes smoked per day (0 cigarettes, 1.5; $\geq$20 cigarettes, 11.7), TC (less than 155 mg/dL, 10. 3; $\geq$310 mg/dL, 11.2), DBP (higher than 70 mm Hg, 10.3; higher than 100 mm Hg, 11.2), and heart rate (fewer than 60 beats/min, 10.4; more than 100 beats/min, 11.6). An inverse relation to physical activity was observed (none, 11.1; heavy, 10.4). The precise threshold for increased risk is still unclear.

176. **Morrison HI,** et al. Serum folate and the risk of fatal coronary heart disease. *JAMA* 1996;275:1893–1896.

This retrospective study of 5,056 patients showed that 15-year CHD mortality was correlated with serum folate levels (more than 6 ng/mL vs. less than 3 ng/mL meant a 69% increased risk). An accompanying editorial stresses the need for randomized trials to study whether folate (diet or supplements) would decrease CVD [e.g., three arms, including placebo, folate (dosage 400 to 650 μg/day), and folate plus B_{12}].

177. **Jacques PF,** et al. The effect of folic acid fortification on plasma folate and total homocysteine concentrations. *N Engl J Med* 1999;340:1449–1454.

This study analyzed blood samples of Framingham Offspring Study participants taken from January 1991 to December 1994 and compared them with subsequent samples obtained before fortification of enriched grain with folic acid (January 1995 to September 1996; control group) and after fortification was implemented (September 1997 to March 1998; study group). Among study-group subjects who did not use vitamin supplements, mean folate concentrations more than doubled from the baseline to follow-up visit (4.6 to 10.0 ng/mL; $p < 0.001$), and the prevalence of low folate levels (less than 3 ng/mL) markedly decreased from 22.0% to 1.7% ($p < 0.001$). The mean total homocysteine concentration decreased from 10.1 to 9.4 μM, and the prevalence of high homocysteine levels (more than 13 μM) decreased from 18.7% to 9.8%

($p < 0.001$). No significant changes were noted in folate or homocysteine concentrations in control group subjects.

178. **Ridker PM,** et al. Homocysteine and risk of cardiovascular disease among postmenopausal women. *JAMA* 1999;281:1817–1821.

This prospective, nested case-control study was composed of 122 WHS participants who had CVD and 244 age- and smoking-matched controls. At follow-up (mean, 3 years), case subjects had higher baseline homocysteine levels (14.1 vs. 12.4 μM; $p = 0.02$). The RR of CV events with homocysteine levels in the 95th percentile (≥ 20.7 μM) was 2.6. The increased risk persisted after adjustment for other traditional risk factors. Self-reported vitamin use at study entry was associated with lower homocysteine levels.

179. **Bostom AG,** et al. Nonfasting plasma total homocysteine levels and all-cause and cardiovascular disease mortality in elderly Framingham men and women. *Arch Intern Med* 1999;159:1077–1080.

Nonfasting plasma homocysteine levels were obtained in 1933 Framingham Study participants between 1979 and 1982; mean age was 70 years. At follow-up (median, 10.0 years), proportional hazards modeling showed that homocysteine levels in the upper quartile (≥ 14.26 μM) compared with levels in the lower three quartiles were associated with RRs of all-cause and CV mortality of 2.18 and 2.17, respectively (95% CIs, 1.86 to 2.56 and 1.68 to 2.82). These RR estimates remained significant [1.54 (95% CI, 1.31 to 1.82), 1.52 (1.16 to 1.98)] after adjustment for age, sex, SBP, diabetes, smoking, TC, and HDL.

180. **Folsom AR,** et al. Atherosclerosis Risk in Communities (**ARIC**). Prospective study of coronary heart disease incidence in relation to fasting total homocysteine, related genetic polymorphisms, and B vitamins. *Circulation* 1998;98:204–210.

This prospective analysis focused on 15,792 ARIC participants aged 45 to 64 years (at enrollment); average follow-up period was 3.3 years. Total plasma homocysteine was associated with increased age- and race-adjusted CHD incidence in women ($p < 0.05$) but not men. CHD was associated negatively with plasma pyridoxal 5-phosphate and, in women only, plasma folate and vitamin supplementation. After adjusting for other risk factors, only plasma pyridoxal 5-phosphate was associated with CHD incidence [RR of highest vs. lowest quintile, 0.28 (95% CI, 0.1 to 0.7)]. The C677T mutation of the methylenetetrahydrofolate reductase gene and three mutations of cystathionine B-synthase gene were not associated with CHD incidence.

181. **Nurk E,** et al. Plasma total homocysteine and hospitalizations for cardiovascular disease: the Hordaland Homocysteine Study. *Arch Intern Med* 2002;162:1374–1381.

This prospective cohort study of 17,361 individuals aged 40 to 42 or 65 to 67 years was conducted from April 1992 to May 1998 (mean follow-up, 5.3 years) in western Norway. At baseline, those with preexisting CVD had higher mean total plasma homocysteine (tHcy) values than did individuals without CVD. Risk of CVD hospitalizations increased significantly with increasing baseline tHcy only in the oldest age group. In this group, multiple risk factor–adjusted hospitalization rate ratios in 5-tHcy categories (less than 9, 9 to 11.9, 12 to 14.9, 15 to 19.9, and 20 mM or greater) were as follows: 1.00 (reference level), 1.00, 1.34, 1.67, and 1.94, respectively (p trend <0.001). The relation between tHcy level and CVD hospitalizations was significantly stronger among individuals with preexisting CVD than in those without (hospitalization rate ratio per 5-mM increment, 1.29 vs. 1.10; p for interaction, 0.02).

182. **Ridker PM,** et al., for Air Force/Texas Coronary Atherosclerosis Prevention Study (AFCAPS/TexCAPS) Investigators. Plasma homocysteine concentration, statin therapy, and the risk of first acute coronary events. *Circulation* 2002;105:1776–1779.

A total of 5,569 AFCAPS/TexCAPS participants had homocysteine measured at baseline and 1 year. Median baseline homocysteine levels were significantly higher in those with subsequent acute coronary events [ACEs; 12.1 vs. 10.9 mM (no ACE); $p < 0.001$]. The RRs of future events from lowest to highest quartile of homocysteine were 1.0, 1.6, 1.6, and 2.2 ($p < 0.001$). This increased risk was only modestly attenuated after adjustment for other traditional risk factors. The subgroup of participants with elevated LDL-C and elevated homocysteine levels were at high risk and benefited significantly from lovastatin therapy (RR, 0.46; 95% CI, 0.29 to 0.75). However, in contrast to findings in this trial for CRP, homocysteine levels did *not* help to define low-LDL subgroups with different responses to lovastatin therapy.

Infection

183. **Saikku P,** et al. Chronic *Chlamydia* pneumonia infection as a risk factor for coronary heart disease in the Helsinki Heart Study. *Ann Intern Med* 1992;116:273–278.

This study was composed of 4,071 patients, with 5 years of follow-up. Logistic regression analysis demonstrated that increased IgA and the presence of immune complexes were associated with an increased incidence of CHD [OR, 2.7, 2.1, 2.9 (both)]. After risk-factor adjustment, the ORs were 2.3, 1.8, and 2.6.

184. Azithromycin in Coronary Artery Disease: Elimination of Myocardial Infection with *Chlamydia* (**ACADEMIC**). Randomized secondary prevention trial of azithromycin in patients with coronary artery disease and serological evidence for *Chlamydia pneumoniae* infection. *Circulation* 1999;99:1540–1547.

This prospective, randomized trial was composed of 302 patients with CAD and *C. pneumoniae* titers of 1:16. Patients received azithromycin (500 mg/day for 3 days, and then 500 mg/wk for 3 months) or placebo. No significant difference was found between the two groups in the incidence of the 3-month composite primary end point of four inflammatory markers (CRP, IL-1, IL-6, tumor necrosis factor). At 6 months, the azithromycin group had a lower global rank sum score of these four markers ($p = 0.011$); specifically, change score ranks were significantly lower for CRP ($p = 0.011$) and IL-6 ($p = 0.043$). Antibody titers were unchanged, and no difference was noted in the incidence of CV events at 6 months [nine (azithromycin) vs. seven patients]. These results contradict earlier nonrandomized data.

185. **Danesh J,** et al. *Chlamydia pneumoniae* IgG titres and coronary heart disease: prospective study and meta-analysis. *BMJ* 2000;321:208–213.

This nested case-control analysis (496 cases, 989 controls) found that the OR for CHD among those in the top third of *C. pneumoniae* IgG titers was 1.66 (95% CI, 1.25 to 2.21), but this decreased to 1.22 (0.82 to 1.82) after adjustment for smoking and indicators of socioeconomic status. A meta-analysis of these results with those of 14 other prospective studies of *C. pneumoniae* IgG titers, which included 3,169 cases, yielded a combined OR of 1.15 (95% CI, 0.97 to 1.36), with no significant heterogeneity among the separate studies.

186. **Sinisalo J,** et al., for the Clarithromycin in Acute Coronary Syndrome Patients in Finland (**CLARIFY**) Study Group. Effect of 3 months of antimicrobial treatment with clarithromycin in acute non–Q-wave coronary syndrome. *Circulation* 2002;105:1555–1560.

This prospective, randomized, double-blind trial found that clarithromycin appears to reduce the risk of ischemic CV events in patients with acute non–Q-wave infarction or unstable angina. A total of 148 patients was assigned to either clarithromycin or placebo for 3 months. Primary end point was death, MI, or unstable angina at 3 months. Secondary end point was any CV event during follow-up (average, 1.5 years). At 3 months, a trend was observed toward fewer primary events in the clarithromycin group compared with placebo (11 vs. 19 patients; RR, 0.54; 95% CI, 0.25 to 1.14; $p = 0.10$). At final follow-up, the clarithromycin group had a significant reduction in CV events (RR, 0.49; 95% CI, 0.26 to 0.92; $p = 0.03$).

187. **WIZARD** (Weekly Intervention with Zithromax for Atherosclerosis and its Related Disorders). Preliminary results presented at the ACC 51st Annual Scientific Session Atlanta, GA, March 2002.

This prospective, randomized, placebo-controlled multicenter trial enrolled 7,000 post-MI patients with elevated *C. pneumoniae* titers. Patients received azithromycin (600 mg daily for the first 3 days, and then 600 mg/week for 11 weeks), or placebo. At 2-year follow-up, no significant difference was found between the two groups in the primary composite end point of all-cause mortality, recurrent MI, revascularization, and hospitalization for angina (7% reduction in azithromycin group; HR, 0.93; $p = 0.23$).

Genetics and Miscellaneous

188. **Marenberg ME,** et al. Genetic susceptibility to death from coronary heart disease in a study of twins. *N Engl J Med* 1994;330:1041–1046.

This analysis focused on 21,004 Swedish twins, with 26-year follow-up data. The RRs of death due to CHD if one twin died of CHD at younger than 55 years were 8.1 (monozygous) and 3.8 (dizygous). For women, the RRs were 15.0 and 2.6. Overall, the RRs decreased with increasing age.

189. **Samani NJ,** et al. A meta-analysis of the association of the deletion allele of the ACE gene with MI. *Circulation* 1996;94:708–712.

This analysis focused on 15 studies with 3,394 MI cases and 5,479 controls. The incidence of genotypes was as follows: II, 22.7%; ID, 49%; and DD, 28.3%. The risk of MI was higher in the DD group versus the ID and II groups combined (OR, 1.26; $p < 0.001$). Pairwise ORs were 1.36 for DD and II, 124 for DD and ID, and 1.09 for ID and II ($p = $ NS).

190. **Ridker PM,** et al. PlA1/A2 polymorphism of platelet glycoprotein IIIa and risks of myocardial infarction, stroke, and venous thrombosis. *Lancet* 1997;349:385–388.

This nested case-control study of PHS participants showed no significant association between the PL allele and CVD. The 704 cases consisted of 374 men with a first MI, 209 with strokes, and 121 with venous thrombosis, as well as 704 matched controls. Mean follow-up was 8.6 years. The frequency of the PL allele was similar between cases (MI, 13.5%; stroke, 13.4%; venous thrombosis, 14.5%) and controls (14.8%).

191. **Laule M,** et al. A1/A2 polymorphism of glycoprotein IIIa and association with excess procedural risk for coronary catheter interventions. *Lancet* 1999;353:708–712 (commentary, 687–688).

This study was composed of 1,000 consecutive patients with CAD (by angiography) and 1,000 age- and sex-matched controls; 653 case patients underwent interventions (angioplasty, $n = 271$; stenting, $n = 280$; directional atherectomy, $n = 102$). No evidence was noted that the A2 allele was associated with an excess procedural risk, as assessed by a 30-day composite of death plus MI plus target vessel revascularization (RR, 1.36; $p = 0.37$). No association was found between the allele and the presence of CAD (OR, 0.99). Although these results contrast with the positive results seen in the smaller studies (see *N Engl J Med* 1996;334:1090, *Lancet* 1996;348:485, and *Circulation* 1997;96:1424), they confirm those obtained from the larger PHS and the ECTIM group (see *Thromb Haemost* 1997;77:1170–1181).

192. **Di Castelnuovo A,** et al. Platelet glycoprotein receptor IIIa polymorphism PLA1/PLA2 and coronary risk: a meta-analysis. *Thromb Haemost* 2001;85:626–633.

A total of 34 studies for CAD and six for restenosis after revascularization were identified, with a total of 9,095 cases and 12,508 controls. The overall OR of CAD for carriers of the PLA2 allele was 1.10 (95% CI, 1.03 to 1.18), suggesting a significant but weak association of this polymorphism with CAD.

Antiplatelet Drugs for Primary and Secondary Prevention

Review Articles and Meta-Analyses

193. **Hennekens CH.** Update on aspirin in the treatment and prevention of cardio-vascular disease. *Am Heart J* 1999;137:S9–S13.

This review summarizes the substantial data showing the significant benefits of ASA in secondary prevention, including an approximate 15% reduction in total CV deaths and approximate 25% reduction in major vascular events. The inconclusive data from the only two major primary prevention trials also are discussed.

194. **Weisman SM, Graham DY.** Evaluation of the benefits and risks of low-dose as-pirin in the secondary prevention of cardiovascular and cerebrovascular events. *Arch Intern Med* 2002;162:2197–2202.

This meta-analysis analyzed data from six trials (6,300 patients) that used low-dose ASA (less than 325 mg/day) in approved secondary prevention indications. ASA reduced the incidence of all-cause mortality by 18%, stroke by 20%, MI by 30%, and other "vascular events" by 30%. GI tract bleeding was 2.5 times more common in those taking ASA compared with placebo. Overall, the number needed to treat (NNT) for ASA to prevent one death from any cause was 67, whereas the NNT was 100 for detection of one nonfatal GI bleeding event. In summary, ASA use for the secondary prevention of thromboembolic events has a favorable benefit-to-risk profile and should be encouraged in those at high risk.

195. **Antithrombotic Trialists' Collaboration.** Collaborative meta-analysis of ran-domised trials of antiplatelet therapy for prevention of death, myocardial infarc-tion, and stroke in high risk patients *BMJ* 2002;324:71–86.

This analysis examined 287 randomized studies involving 135,000 patients in com-parisons of antiplatelet therapy versus control and 77,000 in comparisons of different antiplatelet regimens. Among high-risk patients (e.g., acute MI, acute stroke, previous stroke or TIA, PAD, atrial fibrillation), antiplatelet therapy reduced the incidence of serious vascular events (nonfatal MI or stroke, vascular death) by approximately one fourth, non-fatal MI by approximately one third, nonfatal stroke by approximately one fourth, and vascular mortality by approximately one sixth (all p values < 0.00001). No adverse effects were noted on other deaths. In each of the high-risk categories, the absolute benefits outweighed the absolute risks of major extracranial bleeding. Clopidogrel reduced serious vascular events by 10% compared with ASA. Among pa-tients at high risk of immediate coronary occlusion, short-term addition of an intra-venous GP IIb/IIIa antagonist to ASA prevented a further 20 vascular events per 1,000 (p < 0.0001) but caused 23 major (but rarely fatal) extracranial bleeds per 1,000.

196. **Teo KK,** et al., for the ACE Inhibitors Collaborative Group. Effects of long-term treatment with angiotensin-converting-enzyme inhibitors in the presence or absence of aspirin: a systematic review. *Lancet* 2002;360:1037–1043.

This overview examined data on 22,060 patients from six long-term randomized trials evaluating ACE inhibitor (ACEI) therapy. Results from analyses of all trials, except SOLVD, found no significant differences between the risk reductions with ACEI therapy in the presence or absence of ASA in the composite of death, MI, stroke, CHF hospitalization, or revascularization, or in any of its individual components, except MI (interaction $p = 0.01$). Overall, ACEI therapy significantly reduced the risk of major clinical outcomes by 22% (p < 0.0001), with clear reductions in risk both among those receiving ASA at baseline (OR, 0.80; 99% CI, 0.73 to 0.88) and those who were not (OR, 0.71; 99% CI, 0.62 to 0.81; interaction $p = 0.07$).

Studies
Primary Prevention

197. **Peto R,** et al. Randomized trial of prophylactic daily aspirin in British male doctors. *BMJ* 1988;296:313–316.

A total of 5,139 apparently healthy male physicians was randomized in a 2:1 fashion to ASA, 500 mg/day, or no treatment. At follow-up (average, 5.5 years), the ASA group had a nonsignificant 10% mortality reduction, whereas the incidence of confirmed nonfatal MI was similar in both groups (approximately 0.43%/year).

198. **Physicians' Health Study,** Steering Committee of the Physicians Health Study Research Group. Final report on aspirin component of the ongoing Physicians' Health Study. *N Engl J Med* 1989;321:129–135.

Design: Prospective, randomized, double-blind, placebo-controlled study. Average follow-up period was 5 years.
Purpose: To determine whether low-dose ASA decreases CV mortality.
Population: 22,071 male physicians aged 40 to 84 years.
Treatment: ASA, 325 mg every other day, or placebo.
Results: ASA group had a 44% reduction in the risk of MI (0.255%/year vs. 0.44%/year; $p < 0.00001$). This benefit was restricted to those older than 50 years. The ASA group also had a nonsignificant reduction in CV mortality (RR, 0.96), as well as a nonsignificant increase in stroke rate (RR, 2.1; $p = 0.06$). Among 333 patients with chronic stable angina, the risk of MI was reduced an astonishing 87% (see *Ann Intern Med* 1991;114:875).
Comments: This study was stopped early because of the highly significant reduction in nonfatal MIs. However, as a result, the evidence regarding stroke and total CV deaths is inconclusive because of the very low event rates.

199. **Manson JE,** et al. A prospective study of aspirin use and primary prevention of cardiovascular disease in women. *JAMA* 1991;266:521–527.

This analysis of data on approximately 87,000 NHS participants showed that consumption of one to six tablets of ASA per week was associated with a 32% lower incidence of first MI ($p = 0.005$). This benefit was restricted to those older than 50 years and most substantial in smokers and those with HTN and hypercholesterolemia.

200. **Juul-Moller S,** et al., Swedish Angina Pectoris Aspirin Trial (**SAPAT**). Double-blind trial of aspirin in primary prevention of MI in patients with stable chronic angina pectoris. *Lancet* 1992;340:1421–1425.

Design: Prospective, randomized, double-blind, placebo-controlled study. Average follow-up period was 50 months.
Purpose: To compare ASA and placebo in patients with a history of chronic stable angina.
Population: 2,035 chronic stable angina patients aged 30 to 80 years.
Exclusion Criteria: Prior MI, NSAID use, and requirement for anticoagulation.
Treatment: ASA, 75 mg/day, or placebo; all patients received sotalol (40 to 480 mg/day) for symptoms.
Results: ASA group had 34% reduction in MI and sudden death (8.0% vs. 11.8%; $p = 0.003$). A nonsignificant excess of major bleeds was found in the ASA group (20 vs. 13 patients).

201. Collaborative Group of the Primary Prevention Project. Low-dose aspirin and vitamin E in people at cardiovascular risk: a randomised trial. *Lancet* 2001;357:89–95.

Design: Prospective, randomized, open-label, 2 × 2 factorial, multicenter trial. Primary end point was CV death, nonfatal MI, and nonfatal stroke.
Purpose: To determine the benefit of ASA and vitamin E for primary prevention of cardiovascular events (CVDs) in a clinical practice setting.
Population: 4,495 patients aged 50 years or older with one or more CRFs including HTN, hypercholesterolemia, diabetes, obesity, family history of premature MI, or age 65 years or older; approximately 70% had two or more CRFs.
Treatment: Low-dose ASA (100 mg/day) and vitamin E (300 mg/day), either, or neither.
Results: Study was terminated prematurely at a mean follow-up of 3.6 years because the benefit of ASA was demonstrated in similar trials. ASA use was associated with a significantly lower incidence of CV death (0.8% vs. 1.4%; RR, 0.56) and

CV death, MI, or stroke (6.3% vs. 8.2%; RR, 0.77). Bleeding occurred more frequently in the ASA group (1.1% vs. 0.3%). Vitamin E showed no effect on any end points.

Comments: The evidence in support of ASA for primary prevention of CV events has mounted and appears to be independent of dose (100 to 325 mg), age, gender, and CV risk status.

Secondary Prevention

202. **Klimt CR,** et al., Persantine-Aspirin Reinfarction Study (**PARIS II**). PARIS II: secondary coronary prevention with persantine and aspirin. *J Am Coll Cardiol* 1986;7:251–269.

Design: Prospective, randomized, placebo-controlled study. Average follow-up period was 23 months.

Purpose: To evaluate the effectiveness of the combination of ASA and persantine on mortality in patients with a recent MI.

Population: 3,128 patients with an MI 4 weeks to 4 months earlier.

Treatment: Persantine, 75 mg/day, and ASA, 300 mg/day, or placebo.

Results: ASA and persantine group had 30% lower 1-year mortality (24% at end of study).

203. **Krumholz HM,** et al. Aspirin for secondary prevention after acute MI in the elderly: prescribed use and outcomes. *Ann Intern Med* 1996;124:292–298.

Observational study composed of 5,490 consecutive patients without contraindications to ASA. Only 76% were given ASA at hospital discharge. ASA use was associated with a 23% lower 6-month mortality rate. Risk factors for nonprescription were poor EF, diabetes, long stay, low albumin, and discharge to other than home.

204. **Gent M,** et al., Clopidogrel versus Aspirin in Patients at Risk of Ischaemic Events (**CAPRIE**). A randomised, blinded trial of clopidogrel versus aspirin in patients at risk of ischaemic events (CAPRIE). *Lancet* 1996;348:1329–1339.

Design: Prospective, randomized, multicenter study. Primary end point was ischemic stroke, MI, and vascular death. Mean follow-up period was 1.9 years.

Purpose: To compare the effectiveness of clopidogrel with ASA in preventing major vascular events.

Population: 19,185 patients with a history of recent ischemic stroke (1 week to 6 months earlier), MI ($\geq$35 days earlier), or symptomatic PAD.

Treatment: Clopidogrel, 75 mg once daily, or ASA, 325 mg/day.

Exclusion Criteria: Carotid endarterectomy or severe deficit after stroke, uncontrolled HTN, and scheduled major surgery.

Results: Clopidogrel group had a 8.7% reduction in the primary composite end point (5.32 vs. 5.83%/year; $p = 0.043$). The PAD subgroup had a significant 23.8% reduction in the primary end point ($p = 0.003$), whereas the stroke patients had a nonsignificant 7.3% reduction ($p = 0.26$), and MI patients had a nonsignificant 3.7% increase (7.4% reduction if any prior MI). A subsequent analysis of all 8,446 patients with any history of MI showed that clopidogrel was associated with a statistically insignificant 7.4% decrease in the combined end point. No difference was found in incidence of side effects, including neutropenia (clopidogrel, 0.1%; ASA, 0.17).

205. **Mangano DT,** et al., for the Multicenter Study of Perioperative Ischemia Research Group. Aspirin and mortality from coronary bypass surgery. *N Engl J Med* 2002;347:1309–1317.

This prospective, multicenter study of 5,065 patients undergoing CABG surgery found that early use of ASA is associated with a reduced risk of mortality and ischemic complications. During hospitalization, mortality was 3.2%, whereas the incidence of nonfatal cardiac, cerebral, renal, or GI ischemic complications was 16.0%. Among patients who received ASA (up to 650 mg) within 48 hours, mortality was nearly 70% lower [1.3% vs. 4.0% (no ASA); $p < 0.001$]. ASA therapy also was associated with a

48% reduction in the incidence of MI (2.8% vs. 5.4%; $p < 0.001$), a 50% reduction in the incidence of stroke (1.3% vs. 2.6%; $p = 0.01$), a 74% reduction in the incidence of renal failure (0.9% vs. 3.4%; $p < 0.001$), and a 62% reduction in bowel infarction (0.3% vs. 0.8%; $p = 0.01$). Multivariate analysis showed that no other factor or medication was independently associated with reduced rates of these outcomes. Furthermore, the risk of hemorrhage, gastritis, infection, or impaired wound healing was not increased with ASA use (OR, 0.63; 95% CI, 0.54 to 0.74).

Miscellaneous

206. **Gum PA,** et al. Aspirin use and all-cause mortality among patients being evaluated for known or suspected coronary artery disease: a propensity analysis. *JAMA* 2001;286:1187–1194.

This prospective, nonrandomized, observational, single-center cohort study consisted of 6,174 consecutive adults undergoing stress echocardiography for evaluation of known or suspected CAD. ASA was being taken by 2,310 (37%) patients. Patients with contraindications to ASA use (e.g., peptic ulcer disease, renal insufficiency, NSAID use) or significant valvular disease were excluded. At follow-up (median, 3.1 years), 276 (4.5%) patients had died. After adjustment for age, sex, standard CVRFs, use of other medications, CAD history, EF, exercise capacity, heart rate recovery, and echocardiographic ischemia, ASA use was associated with reduced mortality (HR, 0.67; 95% CI, 0.51 to 0.87; $p = 0.002$). After adjusting for the propensity for using ASA and other possible confounders and interactions, ASA remained associated with lower mortality (adjusted HR, 0.56; 95% CI, 0.40 to 0.78; $p < 0.001$). Patient characteristics associated with the largest ASA-related mortality reductions were older age, known CAD, and impaired exercise capacity.

Angiotensin-converting Enzyme Inhibition for Primary and Secondary Prevention

207. **HOPE.** The Heart Outcome Prevention Evaluation Study Investigators. Effects of an ACE inhibitor, ramipril, on cardiovascular events in high risk patients. *N Engl J Med* 2000;342:145–153 (see page xx for Vitamin E results).

Design: Prospective, randomized, double-blind, 2×2 factorial, multicenter study. Primary end point was cardiovascular death, MI, or stroke. Mean follow-up, 4.5 years.
Purpose: To assess the role of an ACEI, ramipril, in patients who at high risk for CV events but without LV dysfunction or HF.
Population: 9,297 high-risk patients aged 55 years or older with CAD, stroke, PVD, or diabetes plus one other CVRF (HTN, elevated TC, low HDL, smoking, documented microalbuminuria).
Exclusion Criteria: Included HF, EF less than 40%, uncontrolled HTN, MI or stroke in previous 4 weeks, overt nephropathy.
Treatment: Ramipril (10 mg once per day orally), vitamin E (400 IU daily), both, or neither (placebo $\times$ 2).
Results: The ramipril group had a 22% relative reduction in CV death, MI, or stroke compared with the placebo group (14.0% vs 17.8%; $p < 0.001$). Ramipril was associated with significantly lower rates of CV death (6.1% vs. 8.1%; RR, 0.74; $p < 0.001$), MI (9.9% vs. 12.3%; RR, 0.80; $p < 0.001$), stroke (3.4% vs. 4.9%; RR, 0.68; $p < 0.001$), all-cause mortality (10.4% vs. 12.2%; RR, 0.84; $p = 0.005$), revascularization procedures (16.3% vs. 18.8%; RR, 0.85; $p < 0.001$), cardiac arrest [0.8% vs. 1.3%; RR, 0.62; $p = 0.02$ (corrected)], HF (9.1% vs. 11.6%; RR, 0.77; $p < 0.001$), and diabetes-related complications (6.4% vs. 7.6%; RR, 0.84; $p = 0.03$). In the MICRO-HOPE substudy of 3,577 diabetics (see *Lancet* 2000;355:253), ramipril reduced primary events by 25%, MI by 22%, stroke by 33%, CV death by 37%, total mortality by 24%, and overt nephropathy by 24% ($p = 0.027$). After adjustment for the changes in SBP (2.4 mm Hg) and DBP (1.0 mm Hg), ramipril still reduced the risk of the combined primary outcome by 25%.

2. INVASIVE PROCEDURES AND REVASCULARIZATION

CORONARY ANGIOGRAPHY

Indications

1. Unstable angina and non–ST-elevation myocardial infarction (NSTEMI; see Chapter 3).
2. Recurrent angina after percutaneous coronary intervention (PCI) or after coronary artery bypass graft (CABG) surgery.
3. Incapacitating angina pectoris despite medical therapy.
4. Complicated myocardial infarction [MI; e.g., recurrent ischemia, heart failure or hypotension, ventricular septal defect, mitral regurgitation, ventricular tachycardia (VT) after 48 hours, history of MI, failed thrombolysis].
5. Preoperative assessment (valve repair/replacement, other high-risk surgery).
6. Positive exercise treadmill test result.
7. Miscellaneous: aortic dissection, unexplained ventricular failure, suspected congenital heart disease, postcardiac transplantation, pericardial tamponade or constriction, persistent precordial chest pain of unclear etiology.

Flow Grade

The Thrombolysis in Myocardial Infarction (TIMI) flow grade system is the most commonly used classification system to assess flow:

Grade 0, no anterograde flow beyond the point of occlusion.
Grade 1, contrast goes beyond occlusion but fails to opacify the entire distal bed.
Grade 2, entire vessel opacified, but the rate of entry to and clearance from the distal bed of the contrast is slower than normal.
Grade 3, normal flow.

The TIMI corrected frame count is a more precise method and allows quantitative assessment of flow as a continuous variable (1). The TIMI myocardial perfusion grade system (grades 0 through 3) provides additional prognostic information to epicardial flow assessment (TIMI grade flow) in acute MI patients receiving thrombolytic therapy (see *Circulation* 2000;101:125, Chapter 4).

Stenosis Morphology

The American College of Cardiology (ACC)/American Heart Association (AHA) Classification (2) is enumerated as follows:

Type A: discrete, concentric, readily accessible, nonangulated segment, smooth contour, little or no calcification, nonstial, no major side branch involved, no thrombus present, less than 10 mm in length.
Type B: tubular, eccentric, moderate tortuosity, moderately angulated segment (45 degrees to 90 degrees), irregular contour, moderate to heavy calcification, total occlusion for ≤3 months, ostial location, bifurcation lesion, thrombus present, longer than 10 mm.
Type B1: one B characteristic.
Type B2: two B characteristics.
Type C: diffuse, excessive tortuosity, extremely angulated segment (greater than 90 degrees), total occlusion for more than 3 months, inability to protect major side branch, degenerated vein graft lesion.

Procedural success rates are typically lower and restenosis rates higher for type B and especially type C lesions.

PERCUTANEOUS CORONARY INTERVENTION

Uses and Indications

1. Stable angina/CAD.
2. Unstable angina/non-ST elevation MI (see Chapter 3).
3. Acute MI (see Chapter 4).

Although stenting is preferable to balloon angioplasty alone for these indications (see later section), stenting is especially effective (or required) for the following:

1. Dissection or abrupt closure.
2. High-risk lesions (e.g., left main disease in patients unable to have CABG).
3. Chronic total occlusions. Restenosis rates also were better than with PTCA [32% vs. 74%, 32% vs. 68%, and 56% vs. 70% in the Stenting in Chronic Coronic Occlusion (SICCO), Gruppo Italiano di Studio sullo Stent nelle Occlusioni Coronariche (GISSOC), and TOSCA trials, respectively (114–116)].
4. Saphenous vein grafts. Lower restenosis rates have been reported in two retrospective analyses (17% vs. 50% with PTCA) (88,89), whereas the randomized Saphenous Vein *de novo* (SAVED) trial found a nonsignificant reduction in restenosis (37% vs. 46%) (119).
5. Diabetic patients. One recent study (131) found that stenting was associated with a 56% relative reduction in restenosis at 6 months compared with PTCA alone (27% vs. 62%, $p < 0.0001$); furthermore, the stent group had lower incidence of cardiac death and nonfatal MI at 4 years (14.8% vs. 26.0%, $p = 0.02$).

The superiority of stenting compared with balloon angioplasty alone is related mostly to a lower incidence of abrupt closure (less than 1% vs. 5%) and lower restenosis rates (15% to 20% for most lesions). Two disadvantages of stenting are difficulty in treating restenosis when it occurs and stent thrombosis [however, incidence is now less than 1% with antiplatelet regimens (see pages 76 to 77)].

Operator and Hospital Volume

Substantial data accumulated in the early and mid 1990s showed better outcomes in patients undergoing PCI performed by high-volume operators and high-volume hospitals (4–8). The best outcomes were achieved by high-volume operators at high-volume facilities (more than 400 cases/year). The recent widespread use of stent technology and glycoprotein (GP) IIb/IIIa inhibitors has reduced overall major adverse event rates but has not attenuated the significant difference between high- and low-volume operators and hospitals (10). Current recommendations of the ACC/AHA Joint Committee and Society for Cardiac Angiography and Intervention (SCAI) suggest a minimum of 75 cases/year to maintain proficiency (*Circulation* 2001;103:3019–3041); of note, the average interventionalist achieves less than 50% of this recommended yearly volume (7). In the treatment of acute MI with primary PCI, outcomes also are better in high-volume centers (recommended level is 36 or more cases/year); some of this benefit is likely related to the shorter door-to-balloon times obtained at such centers (see Chapter 4).

Procedural Details

Access

The right femoral artery is the most common arterial access site. If the patient has severe aortic or femoral vascular disease, radial or brachial artery access is often feasible (see *Am Heart J* 1995;129:1). A 6-French (F) catheter is now most commonly used for diagnostic catheterization. In one study, the use of 6F catheters showed less bleeding and similar procedural success compared with 7F and 8F catheters (14).

Femoral closure devices are being used more frequently. Angioseal and Vasoseal are both collagen-mediated devices. Most studies have found they are associated with a shorter time to hemostasis and ambulation and earlier hospital discharge, but few studies have found significant reductions in major bleeding or vascular complications (see *J Am Coll Cardiol* 1995;25:1685, *Am J Cardiol* 1998;81:1502). One randomized trial directly compared the Angioseal and Vasoseal devices and found no significant differences in times to hemostasis and ambulation or the rates of device failure and vascular complications (see *Cathet Cardiovasc Intervent* 2002;55:421–425). A third approved device is a Perclose, a suture-mediated device. One recent study found that it reduced time to hemostasis and ambulation and was associated with a lower incidence of major complications (*Am J Cardiol* 2000;85:864).

Contrast Agent
Some observational and nonrandomized studies have found low-osmolar ionic contrast agents to result in fewer recurrent ischemic events than nonionic agents, whereas others found no significant reductions in major events with nonionic agents (16). Randomized trials also produced conflicting results (15,17–19); however, the data are consistent in regard to a significant reduction in hypersensitivity and allergic reactions with nonionic agents compared with ionic agents.

Lesion Evaluation
The severity of stenoses is typically first assessed by angiography. Subjective visual assessment and/or quantitative coronary angiography (QCA) are used to grade stenoses from 0 to 100%; the latter is used in clinical trials and usually performed by an independent core laboratory.

Intravascular ultrasound (IVUS) provides three-dimensional imaging, which can better estimate the severity of complex and eccentric lesions; it is more sensitive than fluoroscopy and angiography in detecting coronary calcification. IVUS can assess atheroma within the vessel walls, which often goes undetected by angiography because vascular "remodeling" due to outward displacement of the vessel wall allows early atheroma accumulation without impairing lumen diameter. IVUS also is used after stent deployment and can reveal suboptimal results due to edge dissections [if deep or long (longer than 5 mm), additional stenting is indicated] and malexpansion or malapposition (treated with balloon angioplasty with larger and/or higher pressure balloons).

In the REStenosis after IVUS-guided Stenting (RESIST) study (21), 155 patients who had successful stenting were randomized to no further balloon dilation or additional balloon dilation(s) until IVUS criterion achieved for adequate stent expansion. At 6 months, the lumen cross-sectional area was 20% larger in the IVUS-guided group, but no significant differences were found between the groups in mean luminal diameter or restenosis (4.47 mm^2 vs. 5.36 mm^2; $p = 0.03$). In the Can Routine Ultrasound Influence Stent Expansion (CRUISE) study (22), 522 patients from the Stent Anti-thrombotic Regimen Study (STARS) were enrolled in an IVUS substudy to determine whether IVUS-assisted stenting results in better outcomes when compared with angiography-assisted stenting. At 9 months, the IVUS-guided group had a larger minimal luminal diameter (MLD), a lower residual diameter stenosis, and a significantly lower target vessel revascularization (TVR) rate (8.5% vs. 15.3%; $p < 0.05$), but no significant differences occurred in death or MI rates. In the OPTimization with ICUS to reduce stent restenosis (OPTICUS) study (24), a less selected group of 550 patients with a symptomatic coronary lesion or silent ischemia were assigned to either IVUS-guided or angiography-guided implantation of two or more stents. At 6-month angiography, no significant differences appeared between the two groups in minimal lumen diameter or restenosis rate, and at 1 year, similar incidences were found of major adverse cardiac events (MACEs) and repeated PCI. Given these mixed results and the added expense and time, routine IVUS guidance for stenting is not now recommended.

Measurement of fractional flow reserve (FFR) is an effective method to evaluate stenoses of moderate severity. It can be performed immediately before a potential intervention and requires only the use of a pressure wire and administration of adenosine. FFR is defined as the maximal blood flow to the myocardium in a stenotic segment divided by the theoretic normal maximal flow in the same distribution. The normal value is 1.0, whereas an FFR of 0.75 or less is associated with inducible myocardial ischemia. In one study (20), all patients with an FFR less than 0.75 had reversible myocardial ischemia evident on at least one noninvasive test (bicycle exercise testing, thallium scintigraphy, dobutamine stress echocardiography). After revascularization was performed (PTCA or CABG surgery), all the positive test results reverted to normal. In contrast, 88% of patients with an FFR of 0.75 or more tested negative for reversible ischemia on all the noninvasive tests, and none underwent revascularization (more than 1 year follow-up). In a larger, randomized study of 325 patients (23), 144 patients with an FFR less than 0.75 underwent routine PTCA (reference group), whereas those with an FFR 0.75 or more were randomized to optimal intervention (performance group) or medical therapy (deferral group). At 2 years, the event-free survival was significantly higher in the performance and deferral groups (83% and 89%) compared with the reference group (78%).

Another alternative for noninvasive lesion evaluation is coronary flow velocity reserve (CFVR). A DEBATE II substudy (26) of 379 patients found that a low CFVR (less than 2.5) at the end of PCI was an independent predictor of MACEs at 30 days [odds ratio (OR), 4.71; $p = 0.034$] and at 1 year (OR, 2.06; $p = 0.014$). In another study, a lower CFVR cutoff of less than 2.0 was a more accurate measure of major cardiac events than single-photon emission computed tomography (SPECT) imaging; also, a multivariate analysis found CFVR was the only significant predictor for cardiac events. Discordant results between CFVR and FFR have been observed in 25% to 30% of intermediate lesions. One recent study proposed that an index incorporating CFVR and FFR is a more accurate predictor than either method used alone (see *Circulation* 2002;106:441).

Balloon Angioplasty

Balloon inflations are typically performed at 8 to 12 atmospheres. Higher pressures are often used to perform poststenting dilatations and are often required during treatment of calcified lesions. Prolonged inflation (e.g., 5 minutes) has been shown in randomized studies to result in better procedural success but has no impact on major event rates or restenosis (12,13).

Success rates with balloon angioplasty of approximately 90% to 95% have been achieved in most institutions [vs. 64% success rate in the first major report (11)]. Failures occur when the lesion cannot be crossed, inadequate balloon dilatation is achieved, and abrupt closure occurs. Predictors of failure include chronic occlusion; stenoses that are long, angulated, eccentric, at an ostium or branch point, calcified, and/or associated with intraluminal thrombus; hospital with low volume; low operator volume; saphenous vein grafts (especially if older than 3 years); female gender; and advanced age.

One specific type of balloon deserves mention. The cutting balloon, which consists of several microblades attached to a balloon, permits effective dilation at lower inflation pressures and thus, hypothetically, causes less vessel stretching and trauma. In the CUBA study (53), the cutting balloon was compared with conventional PTCA. Mean luminal diameter at 6 months was larger for the cutting balloon group, but there was no significant difference between groups in the incidence of death, MI, or any target-lesion revascularization. In the randomized CAPAS trial (54), lesions in smaller vessels were examined [less than 3.0 mm (mean, 2.2 mm), compared with 2.5 to 4.0 mm in CUBA]. The cutting-balloon group had a significantly lower 3-month restenosis rate than the PTCA group (25% vs. 42%) and a better 1-year event-free survival rate (72.8% vs. 61.0%). A third, larger randomized trial (1,238 patients) found the cutting balloon associated with a slightly lower TVR rate (11.5% vs. 15.4%; $p = 0.04$) but no difference in the rates of binary restenosis or MACEs (56).

Some operators frequently use the cutting balloon for the treatment of in-stent restenosis (ISR), especially preceding brachytherapy. The cutting balloon does not tend to slip forward or backward ("watermelon seeding"), thus minimizing the chance that areas around the stent will be injured (i.e., fewer dissections), which often necessitates expansion of the radiation field to avoid "geographic miss" [suboptimal radiation to injured area (results in increased restenosis)]. Two recent randomized trials

(RESCUT, REDUCE II) confirmed that the cutting balloon is associated with less slippage and need for lower inflation pressures compared with standard PTCA in treating ISR, but no significant reductions in clinical or angiographic events were found at 6- to 7-month follow-up (57,58).

Stenting

First-generation stents [Palmaz-Schatz (PS) and Gianturco-Roubin] became available in the early 1990s and resulted in lower restenosis rates compared with PTCA in major randomized trials. As a result, subsequent second-generation stents were compared with the earlier stents (vs. PTCA) in trials designed to show "equivalence." A number of these trials were performed [examples: ASCENT (Multilink), BEST (BeStent), EXTRA (XT), GR-II (Gianturco-Roubin II), SCORES (Radius), SMART (Microstent II)] (47–50). The GR-II stent had inferior results compared with the PS stent (48), whereas the others were found to be equivalent but not superior to the PS. However, these trials excluded the most difficult lesion types (e.g., severe calcification and tortuosity) that compose the majority of stent targets. Because these difficult lesions were less amenable to PS stenting, the newer-generation stents were rapidly adopted. Recent randomized stent versus stent trials are similarly designed but have compared newer stents with second-generation stents [examples: TENISS (Tenax coated vs. Nir), MULTILINK-DUET (Multilink vs. Multilink Duet)]; numerous observational and registry studies also compared different stents.

The majority of currently available stents are balloon-expandable, slotted-tube stents, whereas there are a few self-expanding stents (Wallstent, Radius); the latter are very flexible and can be delivered through tortuous vessels, but accurate sizing and placement are challenging. In the past few years, lower profile and smaller stents have become available (2.5 mm, 2.25 mm, 2.0 mm). A *post hoc* analysis of 331 STRESS I-II patients found that stenting resulted in lower restenosis rates than did PTCA in vessels smaller than 3.0 mm (124). Data from several recent randomized trials, however, yielded conflicting results with small-vessel lesions, with three showing similar outcomes between stenting and PTCA (ISAR-SMART, SISA, and COAST studies) (126,128,129), whereas two found lower restenosis rates with stenting [BESMART (127), RAP (presented at 2000 TCT Conference, Washington, D.C.)].

The more robust, significant benefits of stents compared with PTCA have been clearly demonstrated in larger vessels, total occlusions, and saphenous vein graft lesions (see later sections). Drug-coated stents, which received Food and Drug Administration (FDA) approval in 2003, have markedly reduced restenosis rates in several trials (see Restenosis section later).

One covered stent (Jostent) can be used to seal perforations and exclude coronary aneurysms. This covered stent was compared with an uncovered stainless steel stent in the RECOVERS trial for treatment of saphenous vein graft lesions, and resulted in a higher event rate, primarily driven by a higher incidence of non–Q wave MI. Drug-eluting stents are discussed later in the Restenosis section.

Medications
Aspirin
Aspirin, 325 mg before, and continued daily thereafter. Use significantly reduces abrupt closure after balloon angioplasty (157) and significantly reduces stent thrombosis rates. Little is known about lower doses early after PCI.

Heparin
Heparin: initial bolus, 50 to 60 U/kg when used in conjunction with a GP IIb/IIIa inhibitor; higher dosing typically is used when administered alone. The target activated clotting time (ACT) when used alone is 300 to 350 seconds; a low periprocedural ACT is associated with increased complications. One recent study found even less heparin (2,500 U; mean ACT, 185) appears safe in elective cases (67); larger, randomized, blinded studies are needed to examine this issue adequately. Unless PCI is complicated (e.g., residual thrombus), a prolonged heparin infusion is not necessary because it is does not decrease ischemic complications and results in more frequent bleeding (64,65) (see also *J Am Coll Cardiol* 1999;34:461).

Low-molecular-weight Heparin

Low-molecular-weight heparin (LWMH): Several studies have compared unfractionated heparin (UFH) with LWMH during coronary interventions. Conflicting data were found in studies in which LWMH were given for up to 1 month after the procedure. The ENTICES and REDUCE trials found a significant reduction in early ischemic events with enoxaparin or reviparin compared with UFH; these results were not confirmed in the ATLAST or ERA studies. Data regarding bleeding also are conflicting, with two of four studies showing reduced bleeding rates with LWMH. Observations from the NICE-1 and NICE-4 trials in which enoxaparin was used with and without GP IIb/IIIa inhibitors also show that the use of enoxaparin is safe and effective in the interventional setting.

Data from the recently reported INTERACT trial (see Chapter 3) found that enoxaparin was associated with fewer bleeding complications in patients undergoing catheterization, including those requiring subsequent CABG. The A to Z trial found no difference in bleeding with enoxaparin. The larger SYNERGY trial (8,000 patients) will provide additional information on the use of LMWHs in this setting. A quick monitoring method with LWMH has only recently been approved. Anti-Xa levels had been obtained in some studies but take longer to measure than does an ACT. In summary, until more compelling evidence is available demonstrating the superiority of LWMH versus UFH, most operators will likely continue to use UFH in the catheterization laboratory.

Direct Thrombin Inhibitors

In patients with known heparin-induced thrombocytopenia, direct thrombin inhibitors (e.g., lepirudin or bivalirudin) are often administered. Two recent studies examined routine/first-time use of bivalirudin. The Comparison of Abciximab Complications with Hirulog for Ischemic Events Trial (CACHET) study randomized 268 PCI patients and found a significantly lower incidence of death, MI, repeated revascularization, or major bleeding at 7 days in three bivalirudin groups compared with heparin and abciximab (97). The much larger 6,010 patient REPLACE 2 trial compared heparin plus eptifibatide or abciximab with bivalirudin alone (provisional GP IIb/IIIa blocker if needed) (98). Provisional IIb/IIIa-blocker treatment was given to only 7.2% of the bivalirudin group. The bivalirudin group had a nonsignificant reduction in death, MI, urgent revascularization at 30 days, and major in-hospital bleeding (primary end point) compared with heparin plus GP IIb/IIIa blockers (9.2% vs. 10.0%). Bivalirudin was associated with a significantly lower incidence of bleeding (2.4% vs. 4.1%), whereas there was a nonsignificant excess of MI with bivalirudin (7.0% vs. 6.2%). A cost analysis found that use of bivalirudin was associated with a cost savings of $448 per patient. Based on these results, heparin plus IIb/IIIa blockers appears to be the best treatment for high-risk patients, whereas in low-risk patients, bivalirudin may be an alternative anticoagulation strategy in PCI patients.

Thienopyridines

Ticlopidine (250 mg twice daily for 2 to 4 weeks) in conjunction with aspirin and heparin is more effective than an anticoagulant regimen (e.g., intravenous heparin followed by warfarin). In three randomized studies [Intracoronary Stenting and Antithrombotic Regimen (ISAR), Full Anticoagulation versus Aspirin and Ticlopidine (FANTASTIC), and Stent Anticoagulation Restenosis Study (STARS)] (68,72,75), 50% to 80% fewer cardiac end points were reached (**Fig. 2.1**).

Clopidogrel, now commonly is used as an alternative to ticlopidine (58,66,67). Results from one study showed 60% platelet inhibition [measured by using 5 μmol adenosine diphosphate (ADP)] is achieved within 2 to 4 hours of a loading dose of clopidogrel (300 mg) versus 4 to 5 days with regular dosing and 6 to 7 days with ticlopidine, 250 mg twice daily. Results of the Clopidogrel Aspirin Stent International Cooperative Study (CLASSICS) showed clopidogrel (75 mg once daily for 4 weeks $\pm$ 300 mg loading dose) to be as effective as ticlopidine in preventing stent thrombosis and clinical events, but it is much better tolerated (77) (**Fig. 2.1**). More important, as shown in the large Clopidogrel versus Aspirin in Patients at Risk of Ischaemic Events (CAPRIE) trial (see Chapter 1), the risk of neutropenia with clopidogrel is very low (0.1%) and similar to aspirin. Recent data suggest that up to 30% of patients do not respond to clopidogrel

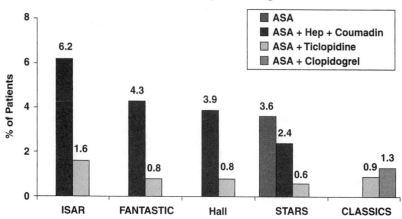

FIG. 2.1. These data from major coronary stent studies show the superiority of a regimen consisting of aspirin and/or ticlopidine or clopidogrel. (Data from refs. 67,71,73, 76.)

primarily due to low levels of enzyme CYP3A4; this drug resistance requires further study.

In the recent PCI-CURE study (78), pretreatment with clopidogrel before PCI was associated with a significantly lower incidence of cardiovascular death, MI, or urgent revascularization at 30 days compared with placebo [4.5% vs. 6.4%; relative risk (RR), 0.70; $p = 0.03$]. Long-term administration of clopidogrel also led to a 31% RR reduction in cardiovascular death or MI (8.8% vs. 12.6%; $p = 0.002$; see **Fig. 2.2**). Only 6% of patients were treated with GP IIb/IIIa inhibitors, but a subanalysis of these data suggests a complementary effect of clopidogrel and GP IIb/IIIa inhibitors; a similar finding also was noted in the ESPRIT trial.

The Clopidogrel in Unstable Angina to Prevent Recurrent Events (CREDO) trial (83) found that a preprocedural loading dose followed by long-term treatment (1 year) with clopidogrel after elective PCI was associated with a 26.9% relative reduction in death, MI, or stroke compared with post-PCI clopidogrel therapy for 1 month [8.5% vs. 11.5% (placebo); $p = 0.02$]. An impressive further 37.4% relative reduction in major events occurred from day 29 to 1 year with clopidogrel ($p = 0.04$; **Fig. 2.3**). As for pretreatment, those given clopidogrel at least 6 hours before PCI had a 38.6% RR reduction in major events at 28 days ($p = 0.05$) compared with no reduction with treatment less than 6 hours before PCI. Among those receiving a GP IIb/IIIa inhibitor (45%) and clopidogrel pretreatment, a 30% reduction in events was found [7.3% vs. 10.3% (no treatment, GP IIb/IIIa); $p = 0.12$]. Finally, a trend toward a higher incidence of major bleeding occurred with clopidogrel (at 1 year, 8.8% vs. 6.7%; $p = 0.07$).

Preliminary results of a recent study found the use of a higher loading dose of clopidogrel (600 mg) may eliminate the need for GPIIb/IIIa inhibition during PCI. A total of 2,159 low-risk patients (excluded if MI within 14 days, ACS or elevated troponins, 100 m) undergoing elective PCI were all given 600 mg $\geq$ 2 hours before PCI and then randomized to abciximab or placebo. At 30 days, there was no difference in death, MI, or urgent TVR between the two groups (4.1% vs. 4.2%; results presented at ACC meeting. Chicago, March 2003).

In summary, the results of PCI-CURE and CREDO support preprocedural loading and long-term therapy with clopidogrel in those scheduled for or expected to undergo PCI. The significant benefits do not appear attenuated by use of GP IIb/IIIa inhibitors.

- PCI-
  CURE

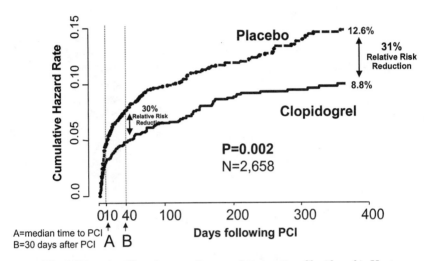

FIG. 2.2. The 2,658-patient Percutaneous Coronary Intervention-Clopidogrel in Unstable angina to prevent Recurrent ischemic Events **(PCI-CURE)** (77) study evaluated pretreatment and extended clopidogrel therapy and found it to be associated with a 31% relative reduction in cardiovascular death or nonfatal myocardial infarction. (Adapted from Mehta SA, et al. *Lancet* 2001;358:527–533, with permission.)

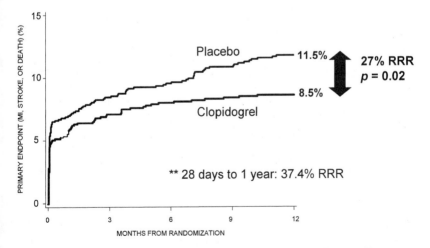

FIG. 2.3. The 2,116-patient Clopidogrel in Unstable angina to Prevent Recurrent Events **(CREDO)** (82) trial demonstrated a substantial 27% reduction in major events (death, myocardial infarction, stroke) at 1 year. Continued clopidogrel therapy from 28 days to 1 year was associated with a further 37% relative reduction in events compared with placebo. (Adapted from Steinbuhl SR, et al. *JAMA* 2002;288:2411–2420, with permission.)

GP IIb/IIIA Antagonists in PCI

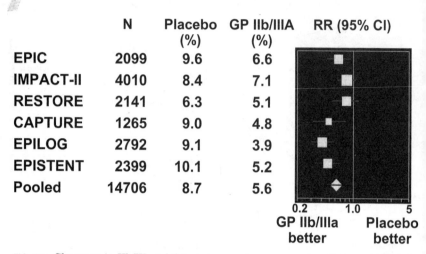

	N	Placebo (%)	GP IIb/IIIA (%)	RR (95% CI)
EPIC	2099	9.6	6.6	
IMPACT-II	4010	8.4	7.1	
RESTORE	2141	6.3	5.1	
CAPTURE	1265	9.0	4.8	
EPILOG	2792	9.1	3.9	
EPISTENT	2399	10.1	5.2	
Pooled	14706	8.7	5.6	

FIG. 2.4. Glycoprotein IIb/IIIa inhibitors in percutaneous coronary intervention and acute coronary syndromes. (Adapted from Topol EJ and Serruys PW. *Circulation* 1998;98:1802–1820, with permission.)

Glycoprotein IIb/IIIa Inhibitor
Over the past several years, GP IIb/IIIa inhibitors have increasingly been used in patients with acute coronary syndromes and those undergoing PCI (**Fig. 2.4**). If used, lower heparin dosage is indicated, with a target ACT of approximately 250 seconds, as the use of a higher ACT target in early trials resulted in increased bleeding. The following three agents are currently available:

Abciximab The monoclonal antibody fragment abciximab binds tightly to the GP IIb/IIIa receptor and has shown impressive results in patients undergoing PCI. In the Evaluation of 7E3 for the Prevention of Ischemic Complications (EPIC) trial (84), composed of 2,099 high-risk patients [acute MI, postinfarct angina with electrocardiographic (ECG) changes, high-risk clinical or angiographic features], the group receiving abciximab, 0.25 mg/kg intravenous bolus, and then 10 μg/min infusion for 12 hours, had 35% fewer end points compared with the placebo group. At 3-year follow-up, this benefit was still present. In the c7E3 Fab Antiplatelet Therapy in Unstable Refractory Refractory Angina (CAPTURE) trial (86), composed of 1,265 unstable angina patients, the abciximab group had a significant 29% reduction in primary composite end point at 30 days but not at 6 months. This loss of benefit is attributed to abciximab infusion being stopped 1 hour after PCI. In the Evaluation in PTCA to Improve Long-term Outcome with Abciximab Glycoprotein IIb/IIIa Blockade (EPILOG) trial (87), composed of 2,792 nonacute coronary syndrome patients, abciximab showed a greater than 50% reduction in primary composite end point at 30 days, and the reduction remained significant at 6 months and 1 year.

In the Evaluation of Platelet IIb/IIIa Inhibitor for Stenting (EPISTENT) trial (89), composed of 2,399 CAD patients randomized to stent plus placebo, stent plus abciximab, or balloon angioplasty plus abciximab, the two abciximab groups had a significantly lower incidence of death, MI, and urgent revascularization at 30 days (5.3% and 6.9% vs. 10.8%). One-year mortality was also lower. A recent meta-analysis of all abciximab trials showed a nearly 30% lower mortality during 6-month to 3-year follow-up ($p = 0.003$; see *J Am Coll Cardiol* 2002;37:2059). Finally, a recent study found intracoronary administration of abciximab in unstable angina or acute MI patients resulted in 50% fewer major cardiac events at 30 days compared to IV administration (see *Circulation* 2003;107:1840); this finding requires verification in additional studies.

Although an antibody response develops in 6% to 7% of patients receiving abciximab after first administration, the Reopro Readministration Registry (R3) reported no significant differences in the incidence of adverse allergic or clinical events or thrombocytopenia in 500 patients receiving repeated abciximab compared with 23,000 patients treated for the first time (92).

Eptifibatide In the Novel Dosing Regimen of Eptifibatide in Planned Coronary Stent Implantation (ESPRIT) study (93), which randomized 2,064 patients undergoing stenting to *double bolus* eptifibatide (two 180-μg/kg boluses 10 minutes apart, and then 2-μg/kg/min for 18 to 24 hours) or placebo, eptifibatide had a significantly lower incidence of death, MI, urgent TVR, and thrombotic bailout GP IIb/IIIa inhibitor therapy within 48 hours (6.4% vs. 10.5%; $p = 0.0015$). This benefit was consistent across different components of the primary end point, including death/MI/TVR [RR, 0.65; 95% confidence interval (CI), 0.47 to 0.87]; death/MI (RR, 0.60; CI, 0.44 to 0.82); and death (RR, 0.5; CI, 0.05 to 5.42). Kaplan–Meier survival curves appeared to separate over time, with most of the difference in mortality occurring between 30 days and 6 months (see *JAMA* 2001;285:2468–2473). A cost-effectiveness analysis found eptifibatide use associated with $1,407 cost per year of life saved (see *JAMA* 2002;287:618).

In the Platelet Glycoprotein IIb/IIIa in Unstable Angina Receptor Suppression Using Integrelin Therapy (PURSUIT) trial (see Chapter 3), a significant reduction in death or MI at 30 days of 31% was observed in patients undergoing PCI.

A recent smaller randomized study (PRICE) (95) of 320 patients examined the costs of eptifibatide compared with abciximab and found the eptifibatide group had both lower in-hospital costs and costs at 30 days, whereas a platelet-inhibition substudy found eptifibatide was associated with earlier and more durable platelet inhibition compared with abciximab ($p < 0.00001$).

Tirofiban The peptidomimetic tirofiban is currently approved by the U.S. FDA for use in acute coronary syndromes with or without PCI, but not in elective PCI. In the Randomized Efficacy Study of Tirofiban for Outcomes and Restenosis (RESTORE) (88), composed of 2,139 patients randomized to tirofiban, 10 μg/kg bolus, and then 0.15 μg/kg/min for 36 hours, or placebo, the tirofiban group had significantly fewer events at 2 days and 7 days but not at 30 days. In the Platelet Receptor Inhibition in Ischemic Syndrome Management in Patients Limited by Unstable Signs and Symptoms (PRISM-PLUS) trial (see Chapter 3), PCI patients showed a reduction in death or MI of approximately 35%. The TARGET trial (94) compared the safety and efficacy of tirofiban with abciximab, randomizing 5,308 patients scheduled for coronary stenting to tirofiban (10 μg/kg bolus, then 0.15 μg/kg/min for 18 to 24 hours) or abciximab. The tirofiban group had a significantly higher incidence of the primary composite end point of death, nonfatal MI, or urgent TVR at 30 days compared with the abciximab group (7.6% vs. 6.0%; $p = 0.038$). This significant difference did not persist at 6-month follow-up. Several investigators suggested that these results were due to underdosing of tirofiban, and recent data documented only 70% platelet inhibition over the first hour, which could explain the poorer outcomes (*Am J Cardiol* 2002;89:647, *Circulation* 2002;106:1470).

Applications of PCI

Stable Angina
Percutaneous Transluminal Coronary Angioplasty versus Medical Therapy
The Angioplasty Compared to Medicine (ACME) study (27) compared PTCA with medical therapy in patients with stable, single-vessel CAD (see pages xxx). The PTCA group had increased exercise time and less use of antianginal medications but had a higher frequency of MI (4%) and emergency coronary artery bypass surgery (2%).

The Veterans Administration Angioplasty Compared to Medicine (VA ACME) study (28) also showed that PTCA in patients with one-vessel coronary artery disease

(CAD) resulted in improved exercise time, less angina, and better quality-of-life score.

The Randomized Intervention Treatment of Angina (RITA-2) trial (29) showed that angioplasty was associated with less angina and longer treadmill time but with an increased incidence of death or MI due to procedure-related MI events. The ongoing Clinical Outcomes Utilizing Revascularization and Aggressive Drug Evaluation (COURAGE) is enrolling more than 2,000 patients with CAD and comparing aggressive medical therapy alone with aggressive medical therapy with added PCI or CABG in all but the highest-risk patients with CAD.

Unstable Angina/Non–ST Elevation Myocardial Infarction

Recent major trials have shown that an early invasive strategy is superior to a conservative approach, especially in high-risk patients (e.g., ST-segment depression, positive cardiac troponin I; see Chapter 3).

Acute ST-Elevation Myocardial Infarction

In experienced centers with short door-to-balloon times, primary PCI has been associated with lower mortality than has thrombolytic therapy (see Chapter 4). However, the availability and institutional volume and experience are limiting factors.

After Thrombolytic Therapy

Studies performed in the 1980s found that routine immediate PTCA was harmful (TAMI I, TIMI IIA, and ECSG trials; see Chapter 4), whereas delayed PTCA (at 18 to 48 hours) was associated with similar outcomes (SWIFT and TIMI IIB; see Chapter 4). PTCA is indicated in patients with high-risk features, such as cardiogenic shock, persistent pain or ischemia, and VT or ventricular fibrillation (VF). Recent data suggest that it can now be performed routinely and safely early after thrombolysis (PACT and TIMI 14; see also *Am J Cardiol* 2001;88:831–836; see Chapter 4).

Stenting versus Percutaneous Transluminal Coronary Angioplasty: Major Trials

All major trials have shown a substantial reduction in restenosis rates with stenting compared with balloon angioplasty alone. Important results include the following:

1. In the Stent Restenosis Study (STRESS) (32), composed of 410 patients, stenting was associated with higher procedural success, less restenosis at 6 months (31% vs. 46%, $p = 0.046$), and a trend toward less revascularization ($p = 0.06$), but there was no significant reduction in clinical events.
2. In the Benestent I study (33), composed of 520 patients, the stent group had lower revascularization but no difference in major clinical events.
3. In the Benestent II study (34), composed of 827 patients, the heparin-coated stent group had a nearly 50% lower restenosis rate versus PTCA (16% vs. 31%).
4. In the EPISTENT study (86,87), composed of 2,399 patients, the rates of TVR at 6 months for stent and stent plus abciximab were significantly lower than those for PTCA and abciximab (10.6% and 8.7% vs. 15.4%; $p = 0.005$, $p < 0.001$).
5. In the START study (36), composed of 452 patients, stenting was associated with a lower 6-month restenosis rate compared with angioplasty (22% vs. 37%; $p < 0.002$) and a greater than 50% reduction in TVR at an extended follow-up of 4 years (12% vs. 25%; $p = 0.0006$).

Primary Stenting versus Percutaneous Transluminal Coronary Angioplasty with Provisional Stenting

In the small Optimal Coronary Balloon Angioplasty with Provisional Stenting versus Primary Stent (OCBAS) study (38), composed of 116 patients, similar angiographic restenosis and TVR rates were observed. In the Optimal PTCA and Provisional Stent versus Primary Stent (OPUS) trial (39), composed of 479 elective PCI patients, the primary stenting group had a significant reduction in the primary composite end point (death, MI, and TVR). The primary stenting group had higher initial costs but lower overall costs by 6 months because of a significantly lower reintervention rate. In the Doppler Endpoints Balloon Angioplasty Trial Europe II (DEBATE II) study (41), 620 elective PCI patients were randomized to primary stenting or balloon angioplasty guided by Doppler flow velocity and angiography. Patients in the latter group were further randomized after optimization (defined as flow reserve greater than 2.5 and diameter stenosis of 35% or less) to either additional stenting or termination of the procedure. *After* the second randomization, stenting was associated with better 1-year event-free survival after both optimal balloon angioplasty (93.5% vs. 84.1%; $p = 0.066$) and suboptimal balloon angioplasty (89.3% vs. 73.3%; $p = 0.005$).

However, in another recent randomized study (42) of 738 elective PCI patients randomized to stenting or PTCA guided by QCA and Doppler CFVR analysis, *optimal* PTCA was associated with a similar incidence of target lesion revascularization (TLR), death, and MI. This also was shown in the FROST trial (French Randomized Optimal Stenting Trial), which randomized 251 patients to systematic stenting or provisional stenting (if postangioplasty CVR less than 2.2 and/or residual stenosis of 35% or more, or as a bailout). At 6 months, no differences were found between the groups in MLD, binary restenosis, or TLR (40).

Although these data from randomized trials are not consistent, it is important to note that most U.S. centers adhere to a primary stenting philosophy, as evidenced by the high stenting rates (greater than 80%) seen in recent national registry data. In particular, routine use of intravascular ultrasound and/or flow reserve to help define an optimal PTCA result is not feasible or even available at many facilities.

Direct Stenting versus Balloon Predilatation

Direct stenting is now performed by many operators and potentially offers numerous advantages, including shorter procedure time, less radiation exposure and contrast use, and overall reduced costs. Possible disadvantages include increased risk of guide trauma and deployment failure. However, with the exclusion criteria used in several trials, such as excessive calcification, severe proximal tortuosity, and occlusion, crossover rates from direct stenting to predilatation have been low (3% to 6%). Most studies comparing direct stenting with predilatation followed by stenting have found no significant difference in major clinical outcomes (44,46; also *Heart* 2002;86:302); one study did find a lower TLR in a direct stenting group (18% vs. 28%; $p = 0.03$) (45). In summary, with careful lesion selection, direct stenting is typically successful, has at least similar clinical outcomes, and provides cost and procedural advantages compared with predilatation.

Coated-stent Studies

Gold-coated stents were developed to provide greater fluoroscopic visualization, but their use was associated with significantly increased restenosis rates in two randomized trials. In one study, the NIR Gold stent had an increased restenosis rate compared with stainless steel stents (46.7% vs. 26.4%; $p < 0.05$) (52). In the other study, the gold-coated Inflow stent was associated with a higher restenosis rate (49.7% vs. 38.1%; $p = 0.003$) and a lower 1-year event-free survival compared with an uncoated stent of similar design (62.9% vs. 73.9%; $p = 0.001$) (51).

Heparin-coated stents were developed to provide better thromboresistance, showing less platelet adhesion and thrombosis in animal models. A heparin-coated stent was compared with PTCA in the Benestent II trial (see earlier) (34) and STENT-PAMI (see Chapter 4). The recent Heparin-Coated Stents in Small Coronary Arteries (COAST) randomized trial compared PTCA with a noncoated stent and heparin-coated stent in 600 patients with lesions in small vessels (2.0 to 2.6 mm) and found no significant differences between the three groups in restenosis rates (129). The ongoing large HEPaNET Registry (target enrollment, 4,000 patients) is examining subacute thrombosis rates in heparin-coated versus uncoated stents. The small ongoing HEAT registry is evaluating the use of the heparin-coated stent and abciximab without heparin during coronary angioplasty.

Numerous drug-eluting stents have been recently developed and are discussed in the restenosis section (see pages 86 to 87).

Repeated Intervention

Repeated PCI is performed only if recurrent symptoms emerge, because up to 50% with angiographic restenosis have no symptoms (see *Circulation* 2001;104:2289). PCI has a high initial success rate (95% to 100%) because restenosis is typically characterized by fibroproliferative tissue as opposed to atherosclerotic plaque. However, recurrent restenosis rates are high, exceeding 50% for diffuse ISR lesions (see *Circulation* 1998;97:318). For treatment of restenosis after prior PTCA, stenting results in better outcomes compared with repeated PTCA; in the randomized REST study (153), the stent group had much lower restenosis and TVR rates compared with PTCA (18% vs. 32% and 10% vs. 27%, respectively).

For treatment of ISR, debulking techniques such as rotational atherectomy (RA) and directional atherectomy appear to be more effective than PTCA alone (see *Am J Cardiol* 1998;82:277, 1345; *J Am Coll Cardiol* 1998;32:1358), but restenosis still occurs in about 30% of cases. Repeated stenting to treat ISR was recently examined in the RIBS (Restenosis Intrastent Balloon versus Stent) study. Preliminary results from this 450-patient study revealed that repeated stenting provided a larger minimal lumen diameter (MLD) immediately after the procedure (2.77 mm vs. 2.26 mm; $p = 0.001$), but this benefit was lost at 6-month follow-up (1.63 mm vs. 1.52 mm; $p = 0.17$). In a prespecified subgroup analysis, it was shown that patients whose target vessel was more than 3 mm in diameter had a lower restenosis rate and a better event-free survival with repeated stenting (27% vs. 48%, $p = 0.007$; 87% vs. 71%, $p < 0.01$).

Complications

In Hospital

1. Death (less than 0.2%).
2. MI (less than 5%). Causes include distal embolization, side-branch occlusion, and obstructive lesion complications such as thrombus, abrupt closure, or severe dissection. Retrospective analyses suggest that even small non–Q-wave MIs [often occurring in the absence of symptoms or electrocardiographic (ECG) changes and detected by routine creatine kinase (CK) and CK-MB measurement] result in increased incidence of ischemic complications and subsequent recurrent MI, revascularization, and death (134). Many of these analyses have problems such as retrospective design, ascertainment bias, high proportion of acute coronary syndrome patients, and inclusion of unsuccessful procedures. One analysis showed that the RR of cardiac mortality increased by 1.05 per 100 U/L increase in CK levels (135). Another study suggests that whereas any elevation of CK-MB is associated with excess mortality risk for 3 to 4 months, a prolonged index hospitalization modifies risk only if there is greater than 5 times elevation (136).
   Post-PCI elevations of the more sensitive troponin assays occur even more frequently. In the TOPSTAR study (137), more than half of patients had an elevated troponin-T level at 24 hours after PCI. In this study, use of a GP IIb/IIIa inhibitor significantly reduced the incidence of troponin elevation. Future, larger studies are needed to confirm these findings, especially whether small troponin elevations with normal CK-MB levels are correlated with worse prognosis.
3. Severe dissection and abrupt closure (less than 1%). Closure results from extensive dissection, thrombosis, or vasospasm. It also may result from stent embolization or misdeployment (see *Am J Cardiol* 2001;88:634) and is more likely to occur if activated clotting time is low (136). Aspirin has been proven to decrease its incidence, whereas GP IIb/IIIa inhibitor use has resulted in a lower incidence of urgent revascularization. Treatment options include (a) conservative medical therapy (reasonable if collateralization is adequate or the amount of jeopardized myocardium is small); (b) stent placement [restores flow in more than 90% of patients, but infarcts occur in up to 20% and reocclusion (over days to weeks) occurs in about 10%]; (c) repeated PTCA (50% success rate; perfusion catheter often is used, which allows balloon inflation for 10 to 30 minutes); or (d) emergency CABG (25% to 50% still have a Q-wave MI).
4. Perforation (less than 0.5%). Small perforations can be sealed with prolonged balloon inflations and/or covered stent(s). Large perforations typically result in pericardial tamponade. One major academic center reported a 0.12% incidence of tamponade in more than 25,000 PCIs (see *Am J Cardiol* 2002;90:1183). Delayed

cardiac tamponade occurred in 45% of cases (mean time from PCI, 4.4 hours); thus tamponade should be considered a cause of late hypotension after PCI.

5. Emergency CABG surgery (less than 0.5%). Data from one large academic center found a decline in incidence from 1.5% in 1992 to 0.14% in 2000 (see *Circulation* 2002;106:2346), usually because of severe dissection, perforation, or recurrent acute closure.

6. Other acute complications: (a) allergic reactions: usually due to contrast agent; if severe, treat with epinephrine; if known, premedication is indicated with prednisone, diphenhydramine (Benadryl), and H_2 blocker; (b) hypotension: multiple causes include hypovolemia (inadequate hydration, blood loss), reduced cardiac output (ischemia, tamponade, arrhythmia), or severe arteriolar vasodilation [vasovagal reaction (especially with femoral sheath placement), excessive nitrates]; (c) arrhythmias: bradycardia (3%), most often due to vasovagal reaction; conduction disturbances (bundle branch block or complete AV block), prophylactic placement of temporary pacemaker is indicated for RA or rheolytic thrombectomy of right coronary; VT and VF (less than 0.5%), occurs most commonly from intracoronary contrast injection (especially right coronary artery).

In Hospital and After Discharge
Stent Thrombosis
Subacute stent thrombosis occurs in 1% to 2% of procedures [used to be more than 5% before high-pressure balloon inflation and antiplatelet regimens were introduced (125)] and typically results in MI or death. Recent evidence suggests clopidogrel nonresponders are at signicantly higher risk of stent thrombosis (see *Thromb Haemost* 2003;89:783); whether such individuals respond to increased doses of clopidogrel and/or alternative agents requires further study. One study showed stent thrombosis had a 90% incidence of MI and a 17% mortality rate (140; see also *J Am Coll Cardiol* 2002;40:1567).

Restenosis
Restenosis usually occurs from 2 to 6 months, and typically results from neointimal hyperplasia and vascular remodeling (not progression of atherosclerosis). The incidence is approximately 30% to 40% for angioplasty alone (up to 50% to 60% for chronic occlusions) and 15% to 20% for stenting. Risk factors can be categorized as clinical (diabetes, unstable angina, smoking, male gender, hypertension, end-stage renal disease, high cholesterol), anatomic [angiographically visible thrombus (152), aortoostial or proximal location, saphenous vein graft, left anterior descending (LAD) artery, chronic occlusion, stenosis longer than 10 mm], or procedural (residual stenosis more than 30%). Recent studies have focused on the effect of stent strut thickness on restenosis rates. The ISAR-STEREO and ISAR-STEREO 2 trials (154,155) were randomized studies that found that thin-strut stents had lower rates of restenosis and TVR compared with thick-strut stents. Critics have asserted that potential confounders occur in these studies, such as stent-deployment pressure and other differences in design and mechanical properties of the tested stents. Drug-coated stents have been shown to reduce restenosis rates markedly (see later section).

Renal Dysfunction
Renal dysfunction: 5% have a transient increase in serum creatinine of 1 mg/dL. Risk is increased with excessive contrast dye load (more than 3 mL/kg. If baseline creatinine is elevated, adequate pre- and posthydration is clearly beneficial (144). The use of *N*-acetylcysteine (Mucomyst) appears to provide protection in those with baseline renal dysfunction [148; also see *N Engl J Med* 2000;343:180; *J Am Coll Cardiol* 2002;40:1383; *Cathet Cardiovasc Intervent* 2002;57:279 (no benefit in latter study)]. Fenoldopam, a selective agonist of the dopamine-1 receptor, showed protective benefit in some early studies (see *Am Heart J* 2002;143:894) but no benefit was observed in the randomized, 315 patient CONTRAST study (148). Finally, cholesterol embolization can cause a late increase in creatinine levels (weeks to months vs. 1 to 2 days with contrast nephropathy), and treatment is supportive, with frank renal failure developing in up to 50%.

Other Postprocedural Complications
Thrombocytopenia can be caused by either heparin (HIT; see *J Am Coll Cardiol* 1998;31:1449) or GP IIb/IIIa inhibitors (incidence ~1%; see *J Am Coll Cardiol* 1998;32:311); if known history of HIT, direct thrombin inhibitors (e.g., hirudin) should be used.

Infection: higher risk with brachial versus femoral approach; some centers administer prophylactic antibiotics when a delayed intervention after sheath exchange is performed.

Vascular complications include femoral or retroperitoneal hematoma, arteriovenous fistula, pseudoaneurysm (140).

Treatment and Prevention of Restenosis

Drug Studies
Numerous therapies have shown no benefit in randomized trials, including aspirin (157), low-molecular-weight heparins (159,167,174,180,184), subcutaneous (s.c.) unfractionated heparin (164), abciximab (181), hirudin (163), 3-hydroxy 3-methyl-glutaryl coenzyme A (HMG-CoA) reductase inhibitors (160,169,182), angiotensin-converting enzyme (ACE) inhibitors (162,186), β-blockers (185), calcium-channel blockers (176,183), n-3 fatty acids (179), platelet-derived growth factor antagonists (161), thromboxane antagonists (158,165), nitric oxide donors (168), antibiotics (187), and antiallergic drugs [e.g., tranilast (190)]. Probucol, an antioxidant agent, showed a modest benefit in the Multivitamins and Probucol (MVP) trial (170) and two smaller trials (171; see *J Am Coll Cardiol* 1997;30:855, 108). MVP patients were elective PTCA patients who were pretreated with probucol for 1 month. Probucol appears to achieve its benefits via a primary effect on remodeling (see *Circulation* 1999;99:30). However, probucol reduces high-density lipoprotein (HDL) levels (by 40% in MVP), and it is unclear if 1 month of pretreatment is needed to achieve the observed benefit and if discontinuation of probucol at 6 months leads to catch-up phenomenon.

Cilostazol, a platelet aggregation inhibitor (currently approved in the United States for treatment of claudication), also has shown promise in several small studies (178; also see *Am J Cardiol* 1997;79:1097, *Int J Cardiol* 2001;78:285–291), but requires further evaluation in a larger randomized trial.

Lowering homocysteine levels with vitamin supplementation to reduce restenosis rates has been examined in recent studies. A prospective, randomized, placebo-controlled trial of 205 patients (188) who underwent successful PTCA found that the folate, vitamin B_{12}, and pyridoxine group had substantially reduced homocysteine levels (from 11.1 μm/L to 7.2 μm/L) and lower rates of restenosis and TVR (19.6% vs. 37.6%; 10.8% vs. 22.3%) compared with placebo. The benefits were observed predominantly in those with PTCA without stenting. However, the 626 patient Folate After Coronary Intervention trial (FACIT) found contradictory results (191). The folate group had smaller minimum luminal diameters than placebo group (1.59 mm vs. 1.74 mm) and higher male incidence (16.8% vs. 10.9%).

Radiation Therapy
Intravascular radiation therapy (IVRT) yielded promising results in initial studies of ISR, with restenosis rates typically less than 20%. Gamma radiation sources were used in the Scripps Coronary Radiation to Inhibit Proliferation Post-Stenting (SCRIPPS) trials, Washington Radiation for In-Stent Restenosis Trial (WRIST), and GAMMA trials (192–194,196,197,200), whereas beta sources were used in the Beta Energy Restenosis Trial (BERT), BETA-WRIST, INHIBIT, START, and BRITE II trials (202,203,207,208). The LONG WRIST study examined lesions 36 to 80 mm in length and found gamma radiation reduced major cardiac events by one-third at 1 year; additional benefit was seen with use of 18 Gy vs. 15 Gy (22% vs. 42%, $p < 0.05$) (201). Data from SVG WRIST demonstrated that the ability of gamma radiation to reduce restenosis also extends to saphenous vein grafts (199); the BRITE SVG trial is evaluating beta radiation in this setting.

Two small studies of beta radiation of *de novo* coronary lesions had positive results (205,206), but the larger (1,455 patients) BETA CATH trial found no benefit associated with radiation (209). Some investigators believe that geographic miss (see later) contributed to the nonsignificant results. No randomized study has directly compared the two types of radiation or the two beta radiation–delivery devices currently approved for use [BetaCath (Novoste), Galileo (Guidant)].

One common problem in many of these trials is geographic miss, a proliferative effect that occurs when subtherapeutic dosing is delivered to injured/treated areas. In the BRIE study, geographic miss occurred in 41% of patients and led to increased rates of restenosis (16.3% vs. 4.3%) (see *J Am Coll Cardiol* 2001;38:415; also see *Circulation* 2001;104:2236). To avoid this issue, the radiation margins should be 5 mm or greater more proximally and distally than the treated areas.

Another issue noted early in the radiation experience was late (more than 1 month) stent thrombosis, which occurred in 6.6% of radiation-treated patients in one study (132). These late events likely occur because radiation delays the healing process. Subsequent studies, such as WRIST and WRIST 12 (195,198) used longer courses of thienopyridine therapy with lower stent thrombosis rates. Current practice is usually 3 to 6 months of clopidogrel for beta radiation without new stent(s), 6 months for gamma radiation without new stent(s), 9 months for beta radiation with new stent(s), and 12 months for gamma radiation with new stent(s).

Concern is expressed that radiation will have long-term sequelae including late development of restenosis and aneursymal dilatation of treated segments. Recent 2-year follow-up data from BERT showed a 15% incidence of restenosis from 6 months to 2 years [four of 30 patients (i.e., small sample size)], whereas no evidence was found of aneurysm or pseudoaneurysm formation (see *Circulation* 2002;106:539).

Drug-Eluting Stents

The most promising approach to the prevention of ISR is the implantation of drug-eluting stents. These stents slowly release drugs that inhibit smooth-muscle cell proliferation, neointimal hyperplasia, or inflammation. Sirolimus (rapamycin) is a naturally occurring macrolide antibiotic which has immunosuppessive properties. It inhibits smooth-muscle cell proliferation and migration by blocking certain aspects of cellular metabolism and thereby preventing mitosis. Sirolimus-coated coronary stents were approved by the U.S. FDA in April 2003.

The earliest study, First-in-Man, treated 45 patients treated with the sirolimus-eluting stent. Three-year follow-up demonstrates event-free survival of 92%; no evidence is found of late events. In the larger, randomized BX VELocity (RAVEL) study, 238 patients with *de novo* lesions received a sirolimus-eluting stent group or an uncoated Bx Velocity stent (210). At 6-month angiographic follow-up, the sirolimus group had a mean late lumen loss of only 0.01 mm compared with 0.80 mm in the control group ($p < 0.0001$). Restenosis occurred in none of the rapamycin patients versus 26% of the controls ($p < 0.0001$). The larger Sirolimus-Eluting Stent in Coronary Lesions (SIRIUS) trial (211) examined the use of this stent in longer lesions (15 mm to 30 mm) and in a more typical patient population (28% with diabetes, 72% with hyperlipidemia, 70% with hypertension, 37% with previous PCI or CABG surgery). In 8-month angiographic data on the first 400 patients, the sirolimus stent group had only a 2% incidence of ISR versus 31.1% of controls; total in-segment restenosis rates were 9.2% and 32.3%, respectively. The proximal margin findings (similar 5.8% restenosis rates in both groups) suggest that balloon injury in this area is associated with pre/post-dilation or stent delivery. A European registry report of 368 patients receiving the sirolimus stent found all 14 stented segments with restenosis were due to *focal* lesions (*Circulation* 2003;107:2178).

This stent is being studied in an even broader array of lesions (SIRIUS excluded ostial lesions, total occlusions, thrombotic lesions) and longer-term follow-up is needed to determine if the restenosis benefit persists, and whether late aneurysmal dilation and/or stent thromboses occur. Other studies must readdress whether the profound reduction in restenosis changes the outcome of PCI versus CABG surgery in patients with multivessel disease. The FREEDOM study will randomize 1,500 patients with multivessel CAD to PCI with sirolimus stents or CABG surgery.

Paclitaxel-eluting stents also show promise but are in earlier stages of testing. Paclitaxel is a taxane derivative that blocks mitosis by interfering with microtubule function; it is cytotoxic at higher doses. Two types of delivery systems are being investigated (polymeric and nonpolymeric). The TAXUS I trial enrolled 61 patients and found no restenosis in the paclitaxel (polymeric) stent group compared with 10% in the control group (see *Circulation* 2003;107:38). However, late loss was less impressive (compared with RAVEL; 0.36 mm vs. 0.71 mm in the control group). The TAXUS II trial (213) enrolled 402 patients and compared a bare stent with two formulations of a paclitaxel-eluting stent (slow or moderate release). At 6 months, MACE was significantly reduced with the drug-eluting stents [slow release, 8.5% vs. 19.5% (control); $p = 0.013$; moderate release, 7.8% vs. 20%; $p = 0.006$]. Binary restenosis rates were much lower with the paclitaxel stents [in-stent, 2.3% (slow release) vs. 17.9%; $p = 0.0002$; 4.7% (moderate release) vs. 20.2%; $p < 0.0001$]. No signs of edge effect were found, with nonsignificant *reductions* seen both in the proximal and distal segments of the segment with the drug-eluting stents versus controls. Researchers will therefore investigate the slow-release formulation in high-risk lesions in TAXUS V, and the moderate-release formulation will be the focus of the international TAXUS VI, also in high-risk lesions.

The TAXUS IV trial enrolled approximately 1,250 patients with *de novo* lesions and will compare the paclitaxel stent with an uncoated stent, whereas TAXUS VII enrolled 528 patients with ISR and is comparing the paclitaxel stent with brachytherapy. The nonpolymer stent delivery system has had promising results in two dose-finding studies [ASPECT (212) and ELUTES]. However, preliminary results of the larger DELIVER study (214), which randomized 1,043 patients to the paclitaxel-coated stent or an uncoated Penta stent, show a nonsignificant reduction in target vessel failure (primary end point) in the paclitaxel group.

DIRECTIONAL ATHERECTOMY

Directional coronary atherectomy (DCA) is an effective debulking technique that uses a cutting device to excise atheromas. DCA requires an 8F or 9F sheath, results in frequent distal embolization, and is a difficult technique with a narrow therapeutic window. Eccentric, noncalcified, short lesions in nontortuous vessel segments are ideal lesions. Current recommendations suggest that more than 20 cases be performed before an operator attempts more difficult lesions.

The Coronary Angioplasty versus Excisional Atherectomy Trial (CAVEAT) I and CAVEAT II (99,101) both showed that DCA achieved better initial success rates compared with balloon angioplasty within native vessel and saphenous vein graft lesions, respectively. However, the atherectomy groups did not have significantly lower higher restenosis rates, and the incidence of death and MI was higher. In the Canadian Coronary Atherectomy Trial (CCAT) (100), the atherectomy group did not have increased complications, but again, the restenosis rate was similar. Two studies that used a more refined/optimal atherectomy technique—the Optimal Atherectomy Restenosis Study (OARS) and Balloon versus Optimal Atherectomy Trial (BOAT) (102,103)—showed lower restenosis rates with atherectomy and similar major complication rates. In the BOAT, directional atherectomy was performed with adjunctive PTCA if indicated.

None of the trials mentioned earlier compared atherectomy with stenting. The recently presented Atherectomy before Multilink Improves Lumen Gain and Clinical Outcomes (AMIGO) trial (108) randomized 753 patients, including those with ostial and bifurcation stenoses and chronic total occlusions, to directional atherectomy and stenting versus stenting alone. No significant differences in restenosis rates were found between groups. However, in the small group of patients (22%) that achieved "optimal" DCA, the restenosis rate was significantly lower. A substantial benefit of DCA and stenting versus stenting alone was seen in bifurcation lesions (restenosis, 9.8% vs. 20.9%). A subsequent randomized trial would be helpful to examine the "optimal" DCA approach before stenting.

ROTATIONAL ATHERECTOMY

RA uses a diamond-coated burr that preferentially ablates atherosclerotic plaque while deflecting away from healthy elastic tissue ("differential cutting"). This technique can facilitate stent delivery and expansion by increasing arterial compliance and lumen diameter in complex, calcified, and diffusely atherosclerotic lesions.

RA was evaluated in the Excimer Laser, Rotational Atherectomy, and Balloon Angioplasty Comparison (ERBAC) trial (111) in patients with type B or C lesions, and the atherectomy group was found to have a better procedural success rate than the balloon angioplasty (PTCA) or excimer laser groups, but the 6-month restenosis rate was higher compared with that observed with PTCA (57% vs. 47%; $p < 0.05$).

After this trial was completed, substantial technical improvements were made, so additional studies were performed. The Study to Determine Rotablator and Transluminal Angioplasty Strategy (STRATAS) (106) randomized 497 patients to aggressive rotablator therapy (70% to 90% burr-to-artery ratio) or standard rotablator (50% to 70% burr-to-artery ratio). At 6 months, no significant differences were observed between the two groups in mean luminal diameter, restenosis, or clinical events. Similar results were seen in the COBRA study (105).

The recent Rotational Atherectomy Does Not Reduce Recurrent In-Stent Restenosis (ARTIST) study (107) examined the use of rotational atherectomy (RA) for the treatment of ISR. The RA and balloon angioplasty (PTCA) group had a higher restenosis at 6 months compared with PTCA alone (65% vs. 51%; $p = 0.039$).

EXCIMER LASER

The Amsterdam-Rotterdam (AMRO) trial (110) found that excimer laser compared with PTCA in patients with long lesions (longer than 10 mm) achieved similar restenosis and clinical event rates. In the ERBAC trial (111), laser therapy was compared with RA and PTCA in patients with type B or C lesions, and PTCA was found to have a lower restenosis rate and less TVR than did laser. Finally, the Laser Angioplasty versus Angioplasty (LAVA) trial (112) showed that laser-facilitated PTCA was associated with more complications and a major event rate similar to that found with PTCA alone. Based on these less than encouraging results, the use of laser treatment has remained limited. It is unclear whether the use of laser therapy by very experienced operators in patients with complex lesions and chronic occlusions (see *J Am Coll Cardiol* 1999;34:25) can achieve better results.

NEWER TECHNIQUES

Thrombectomy

The Possis Angiojet catheter uses high-speed saline jets to generate intense local suction by the Venturi effect, which pulls thrombus into the jets, where it is macerated and then driven down the catheter lumen for external collection. The Vein Graft AngioJet Study randomized 352 patients with angina or MI more than 24 hours before the procedure and thrombus on angiography with intracoronary or graft urokinase (more than 6-hour infusion) or thrombectomy by using the AngioJet system (59). At 30 days, significantly fewer AngioJet patients had experienced MACEs (death, MI, revascularization; 16% vs. 33%; $p < 0.001$). Bradycardia occurred in 24% of those treated with AngioJet and was managed successfully with atropine and temporary pacing. In summary, this technique allows rapid thrombus removal and stenting during the same catheterization session. Many centers are now also using the device for treatment of patients with acute MI who typically have a high thrombus burden.

The EndiCOR X-Sizer thrombectomy device is currently investigational in the United States and approved in Europe. The device uses spinning blades that protrude 0.5 mm from the housing, penetrate the thrombus, entrain the clot, macerate it, and suck it into the catheter. The X-Sizer for Treatment of Thrombus and Atherosclerosis in Coronary Interventions Trial (X-TRACT) randomized 800 high-risk patients with lesion(s) in a saphenous vein graft or a thrombotic native coronary artery to PCI and X-Sizer device or PCI alone (60). Bailout IIb/IIIa inhibitors were required in 0.5% of patients in the thrombectomy device group versus 2.3% of control patients. Among the only 23% of patients who did not receive pre-PCI IIb/IIIa inhibitors, 10% of control patients required bailout IIb/IIIa inhibitor use, compared with 2.1% in the device group. Thirty-day MACE was not different between groups (17.0% vs. 17.4%). However, MI defined as CK-MB more than 8 times normal was reduced by 46% in the X-Sizer group. It is not clear whether this finding translates into long-term mortality benefit. Most important, because this device did not reduce MACE, whereas distal protection reduced MACE by 50% in the SAFER trial (see later), the use of this device would likely be limited to vein graft lesions in which distal protection is not possible [e.g., distal lesions (last 3 cm), poor LV function].

Distal Protection

Distal embolization of friable debris is common during SVG interventions, is a main cause of no reflow, and frequently results in CK release. The Saphenous vein graft Angioplasty Free of Emboli Randomized (SAFER) trial (61) randomized 801 patients with a history of angina, evidence of myocardial ischemia, and more than 50% stenosis in the mid-portion of an SVG with a diameter of 3 to 6 mm, to the GuardWire (Medtronic/PercuSurge) balloon occlusion device or a conventional angioplasty guide wire. The embolic protection group had an impressive 42% relative reduction in MACEs at 30 days (9.6% vs. 16.5%; $p = 0.004$). This reduction was due primarily to fewer MIs (8.6% vs. 14.7%; $p = 0.008$) and "no-reflow" (3% vs. 9%; $p = 0.02$). The benefit of the distal protection device was evident both with and without the use of concomitant GP IIb/IIIa–receptor blockers.

Filter devices provide another method of distal protection that permits TIMI 3 flow during the intervention. In the FilterWireEX During Transluminal Intervention of Saphenous Vein Grafts (FIRE) trial, the FilterWireEx device was compared to the GuardWire; 30-day MACE rates were similar (9.9% vs. 11.6%) (62). Protection devices other filter (e.g., SPIDER) are currently being evaluated in ongoing clinical trials.

CORONARY ARTERY BYPASS SURGERY

Risk factors for operative mortality include advanced age, female gender, smoking, and left ventricular dysfunction (see *J Thorac Cardiovasc Surg* 1994;108:73).

Saphenous Vein Grafts

From 8% to 12% of SVGs occlude in the early postoperative period (most because of technical factors), and 12% to 20% more occlude in the first year (typically because of intimal proliferation and thrombosis), and then 2% to 4% per year (overall 50% at 10 years). Results of the Post-CABG trial (see Chapter 1) showed a 30% to 40% slowing of graft atherosclerosis with very aggressive low-density lipoprotein (LDL)-lowering therapy (average achieved, LDL 90 mg/dL).

Internal Mammary Artery

The patency rate for the internal mammary artery (IMA) is 85% to 95% at 10 years. Use is associated with improved long-term survival. A 27% lower mortality rate was observed in the Coronary Artery Surgery Study (CASS) registry analysis (236). In another analysis, IMA use was associated with a 40% lower 10-year mortality rate among three-vessel disease patients (234).

Coronary Artery Bypass Surgery versus Medical Therapy

Three major clinical trials—the European Coronary Surgery Study (ECSS), CASS, and Veterans Administration (VA) study—helped to define the groups of patients that benefit from bypass surgery. These three studies were performed before the common use of the IMA for revascularization. The ECSS enrolled 768 men aged 65 years or younger and found that surgery resulted in improved survival compared with medical therapy. The majority of the benefit was seen in patients with proximal LAD artery stenoses (220). The CASS enrolled 780 patients aged 65 years or younger and found CABG to be associated with a trend toward lower mortality in patients with three-vessel disease and an ejection fraction of 50% or less (221). Long-term follow-up showed better survival with CABG in patients with left main equivalent disease (severe proximal LAD and left circumflex disease) and left ventricular dysfunction (see *Circulation* 1995;91:2335). The VA study found no significant mortality difference between groups at 11-year follow-up, but CABG was beneficial in certain patients subgroups: (a) three-vessel disease and left ventricular dysfunction, and (b) clinically high-risk patients (at least two of following: resting ST depression, history of MI, or history of hypertension) (20).

An overview of 2,649 patients from these three trials and four smaller studies showed that CABG was associated with a significantly lower mortality rate at 5 years compared with initial medical management (OR, 0.61), 7 years (OR, 0.68), and 10 years (OR, 0.83) (216). The risk reduction was most marked in patients with left main disease and three-vessel disease (Ors, 0.32 and 0.58). High-risk patients (defined as those with two of the following: severe angina, history of hypertension, prior MI, and ST-segment depression at rest) had a 29% mortality reduction with CABG at 10 years compared with a nonsignificant trend toward higher mortality in low-risk patients (no severe angina, hypertension, or prior MI). Overall these results demonstrate that patients with more severe coronary disease, poor LV dysfunction, and high-risk clinical characteristics derive a significant benefit from bypass surgery versus medical therapy.

Coronary Artery Bypass Surgery versus Percutaneous Transluminal Coronary Angioplasty

The RITA-1, German Angioplasty Bypass Surgery Investigation (GABI), Emory Angioplasty versus Surgery Trial (EAST), Coronary Angioplasty versus Bypass Revascularization Investigation (CABRI), and Estudio Randomizado Argentino de Angioplastia versus Cirugia (ERACI) (223–227) all enrolled stable patients with one-to three-vessel CAD. Overall they showed no mortality difference between CABG and PTCA groups. CABG patients did have longer hospitalizations, fewer repeated interventions, and better quality of life (e.g., less angina and better functional status) at follow-up. The Bypass Angioplasty Revascularization Investigation (BARI) study enrolled 1,829 patients (41% with three-vessel CAD); the CABG group had an 85% lower revascularization rate at 5 years, but there was no significant mortality reduction (229). Importantly, a 44% lower rate of mortality ($p = 0.003$) was found among diabetic patients who underwent bypass surgery versus PTCA.

A meta-analysis of eight trials with 3,371 patients published through 1996 (218) showed no significant mortality differences between CABG and PTCA. CABG patients had 90% fewer interventions at 1 year. Only a small proportion of patients screened for these trials (5% to 10%) were actually randomized; thus these findings cannot be readily extrapolated to groups of patients with high-risk characteristics (e.g., left main disease, severe LV dysfunction, chronically occluded vessels).

It also is important to note that these trials were completed before the frequent use of stenting.

The Arterial Revascularization Therapy Study (ARTS) (232), which compared stenting with bypass surgery in 1,200 patients with multivessel CAD, found similar rates of adverse outcomes at 30 days [6.8% (surgery) and 8.7% (stenting)] but a significantly lower incidence of repeated revascularization among bypass patients [0.8% vs. 3.7% (at 1 year: 3.5% vs. 16.8%)]. In the Stent or Surgery (SoS) trial, 988 patients with multivessel CAD were randomized to PCI (78% of lesions stented) or CABG. The CABG group had a lower 1-year revascularization rate (5.8% vs. 20.3%), whereas mortality rates were not significantly different (234). ERACI II was a similarly designed study (215), which enrolled 450 patients and also found a higher revascularization rate in the PCI group [at 18-month follow-up: 16.8% vs. 4.8% (CABG); $p < 0.002$]. However, the PCI group had a significantly lower 30-day and 18-month mortality (0.9% vs. 5.7%; $p < 0.013$; 3.1% vs. 7.5%; $p < 0.017$). A fourth study, the Angina with Extremely Serious Operative Mortality Evaluation (AWESOME) enrolled 554 high-risk VA patients (233). The PCI group had a slightly lower mortality at 30 days and 6 months, but the rates were similar at 3-year follow-up. Once again, the CABG group had a lower revascularization rate (4% vs. 11%).

The use of drug-eluting stents will likely further reduce (or eliminate) the difference in revascularization rates between multivessel PCI and CABG surgery. The FREEDOM trial will address this issue in approximately 1,500 patients (sirolimus-coated stenting vs. CABG).

Transmyocardial Revascularization

Initial studies showed that surgical transmyocardial laser revascularization (TMR) provided symptomatic relief of severe angina (240,241; also see *J Am Coll Cardiol* 1999;33:1021; *Circulation* 1998:II-73). The reduction in anginal symptoms was observed within 48 hours and thought to be due to temporary blood flow through the created channels to the subendocardial area. However, the channels soon close down (necropsy reports show dense fibrous scarring). It was postulated that persistent relief could be the result of angiogenesis, with the creation of new collateral vessels. Studies using a percutaneous approach (PTMR), which creates laser channels from within the heart, found that similar angina relief could be achieved with lower rates of mortality and morbidity (242). Some investigators remained skeptical about these results, attributing the observed benefits to a placebo effect. The DIRECT study (245) was the first double-blind trial conducted and randomized 298 patients to percutaneous laser treatment (with low or high energy) or a placebo procedure. No significant differences were observed between the three groups in exercise tolerance and angina improvement. Another recent randomized trial that also was unblinded found no significant improvement in angina, exercise tolerance, or major events with PTMR compared with maximal medical therapy (244).

REFERENCES

Guidelines and Classification Articles

1. **Gibson CM,** et al. TIMI frame count. *Circulation* 1996;93:879–888.

   This article describes a new method that quantifies coronary artery flow as a continuous variable [vs. assignment to one of four flow grades (i.e., TIMI grade 0, 1, 2, or 3). A total of 393 patients (315 TIMI-4 acute MI patients and 78 subjects without MI) were analyzed. The method was found to be reproducible (difference between two injections, 4.7 ± 3.9). Among normal patients, the LAD artery took 1.7 times longer to fill completely than did the right coronary artery and circumflex arteries (36.2 vs. 20.4, 22.2; both $p < 0.001$). After thrombolysis, mean corrected counts (LAD, divided by 1.7) were 39.2 at 90 minutes and 31.7 by 18 to 36 hours ($p < 0.001$); both were higher than those in patients without acute MI.

2. **Zaacks SM,** et al. Value of the ACC/AHA Stenosis Morphology Classification for coronary interventions in the late 1990s. *Am J Cardiol* 1998;82:43–49.

   This prospective analysis was derived from 957 consecutive interventions in 1,404 lesions from June 1994 to October 1996. The overall procedural success rate was 91.9%. No significant differences in success rates were found between type A, B1, and B2 lesions (96.3%, 95.5%, 95.1%), but all were better than type C (88.2%; $p < 0.003, p < 0.004, p = 0.0001$, respectively). Multiple regression analysis showed that total occlusion and vessel tortuosity were predictive of procedural failure. Lesion type did not predict device use or complications. Actual predictors of complications were bifurcation lesions ($p = 0.0045$), presence of thrombus ($p = 0.0001$), inability to protect a major side branch ($p = 0.0468$), and degenerated vein graft lesions ($p = 0.0283$).

3. **Scanlon PJ,** et al. ACC/AHA guidelines for coronary angiography: a report of the American College of Cardiology/American Heart Association Task Force on Practice Guidelines (Committee on Coronary Angiography). *J Am Coll Cardiol* 1999;33:1756–1824.

   These extensive guidelines begin with a discussion of the utilization, costs, and morbidity and mortality associated with angiography. The majority of the guidelines focus on the use of angiography for specific conditions, including known or suspected CAD (e.g., stable angina, unstable angina, acute MI), and recurrence of symptoms after revascularization, congestive heart failure, valvular disease, and congenital heart disease.

Relation of Operator and Hospital Volume to Outcomes

4. **Jollis JG,** et al. The relation between the volume of coronary angioplasty procedures at hospitals treating Medicare beneficiaries and short-term mortality. *N Engl J Med* 1994;331:1625–1629.

This analysis was conducted on 218,000 Medicare patients who underwent PTCA from 1987 to 1990. A significant mortality difference was found between the 10% treated at the highest- and lowest-volume (fewer than 50 procedures per year) centers (2.5% vs. 3.9%). A difference in the CABG surgery rate was found (2.8% vs. 5.3%).

5. **Kimmel SE,** et al. The relationship between coronary angioplasty procedure volume and major complications. *JAMA* 1995;274:1137–1142.

This cohort study showed an association between low hospital volume and increased complications. The cohort consisted of 19,594 non-MI patients undergoing a first PTCA. Higher volume was associated with lower mortality ($p = 0.04$), emergency bypass surgery ($p < 0.001$), and major complications ($p < 0.001$). Multivariate analysis (adjusted for case mix) showed that the associations persisted, but the mortality difference was not significant. No difference was demonstrated in outcomes when comparing hospitals performing 200 versus more than 200 procedures. However, for hospitals performing 400 to 599 and 600 versus fewer than 200 procedures per year, the adjusted ORs for major complications were 0.66 and 0.54 ($p = 0.03; p = 0.001$).

6. **Ellis SG,** et al. Relation of operator volume and experience to procedural outcome of percutaneous coronary revascularization at hospitals with high interventional volume. *Circulation* 1997;95:2479–2484.

This retrospective analysis focused on 12,985 patients at five centers (1993 through 1994). The data examined were on 38 operators who had 30 cases/year (mean, 163) and who had practiced for 8 ± 5 years. Adverse outcomes (death and death plus Q-wave MI plus emergency CABG were found to be related to the number of cases per year. Fewer (69%) complications existed among patients treated by operators performing more than 270 versus 70 cases/year ($p < 0.001$). This effect was present even among low-risk patients (5.9% vs. 1.7% to 2.4%) and those with only type A and B1 lesions. No effect was seen with years of experience. These difference were not consistent for all operators; hence the controversy surrounding standards applied to all operators.

7. **Jollis JG,** et al. Relationship between physician and hospital coronary angioplasty volume and outcome in elderly patients. *Circulation* 1997;95:2485–2491 (editorial, 2467–2470).

This analysis focused on 97,478 Medicare patients treated by 6,115 physicians at 984 hospitals in 1992. Median procedure volume was only 13 per operator; hospital median was 98. After risk-factor adjustment, low-volume operators were associated with an increased rate of bypass surgery (fewer than 25, 3.8%; 25 to 50, 3.4%; more than 50, 2.6%; $p < 0.001$), and low-volume hospitals were associated with higher bypass surgery and mortality rates (fewer than 100, 3.9%/2.9%; 100 to 200, 3.5%/2.5%; more than 200, 3.0%/2.3%; $p < 0.001$). Improved outcomes were seen with up to 75 and 200 Medicare cases/year, respectively. The accompanying editorial points out that data were acquired in the early stent era and before the use of GP IIb/IIIa inhibition.

8. **Ritchie JL,** et al. Association between percutaneous transluminal coronary angioplasty volumes and outcomes in the Healthcare Cost and Utilization Project 1993–1994. *Am J Cardiol* 1999;83:493–497.

This analysis of 163,527 procedures from 214 centers demonstrated superior outcomes in high-volume institutions (more than 400 cases/year) compared with low-volume centers (fewer than 200 cases/year).

9. **Ritchie JL,** et al. Coronary artery stent outcomes in a Medicare population: less emergency bypass surgery and lower mortality rates in patients with stents. *Am Heart J* 1999;138:437–440.

Analysis of Medicare provider data for fiscal years 1994 and 1996. A total of 74,836 stents was placed during 300,000 coronary interventions. In both the conventional angioplasty and stent groups, a hospital volume of more than 200 cases/year was associated with better short-term outcomes.

10. **McGrath PD,** et al. Relation between operator and hospital volume and outcomes following percutaneous coronary interventions in the era of the coronary stent. *JAMA* 2000;284:3139–3144.

Analysis of Medicare patients aged 65 to 99 years who underwent PCI in 1997. Low-volume operators were defined as those who performed fewer than 30 Medicare interventions/year, whereas high-volume operators performed more than 60/year. Low-volume institutions were defined as those performing fewer than 80 Medicare interventions/year, whereas high volume was considered as more than 160/year. The lowest incidence of 30-day mortality and CABG (4.6%) occurred at high-volume hospitals with a high-volume interventionalist, whereas the highest incidence (6.1%) was seen at low-volume hospitals with low-volume interventionalists.

Technical Aspects

11. **Gruntzig AR,** et al. Nonoperative dilatation of coronary-artery stenosis: percutaneous transluminal coronary angioplasty. *N Engl J Med* 1979;301:61–68.

In this first major report of balloon angioplasty, 50 patients with angina (mean duration, 13 months) underwent angioplasty. All patients received aspirin, 1 g/day for 3 days (starting 1 day before), heparin and dextran during the procedure, and warfarin through follow-up (6 to 9 months). The procedural success rate was 64%. Five patients required CABG surgery, and three had an MI.

12. **Ohman EM,** et al. A randomized comparison of the effects of gradual prolonged vs standard primary balloon inflation on early and late outcome. *Circulation* 1994;89:1118–1125.

This randomized study of 478 patients showed the benefits of prolonged balloon inflation. Patients underwent 15-minute inflation 1 to 2 times or 1-minute inflation 2 to 4 times. The prolonged-inflation group had the higher procedural success ($\leq$50% residual stenosis; 95% vs. 89%; $p = 0.016$) and less dissection (3% vs. 9%; $p = 0.003$). Follow-up angiography performed at an average of 6 months in 77% of patients without in-hospital events showed no significant difference in restenosis rate (44%) or clinical events (death, MI, CABG surgery, or repeated angioplasty); 34% (15-minute group) vs. 26%, $p = 0.15$.

13. **Eltchaninoff H,** et al. Effects of prolonged sequential balloon inflations on results of coronary angioplasty. *Am J Cardiol* 1996;77:1062–1066.

This randomized study showed the short-term favorable results with prolonged balloon inflation. Two hundred eighty-nine patients were randomized to standard balloon inflation (3 to 5 times for $\leq$1 minute) or prolonged inflation (3 to 5 times for 3 to 5 minutes). Prolonged balloon inflation was associated with higher initial success (92% vs. 80%; $p < 0.002$) and decreased dissection rate (14% vs. 30%; $p < 0.001$), but no difference in restenosis at 4 to 6 months (46% vs. 42%).

14. **Metz D,** et al. Comparison of 6F with 7F and 8F guiding catheters for elective coronary angioplasty: results of a prospective, multicenter randomized trial. *Am Heart J* 1997;134:131–137.

This study showed that bleeding and procedural complications decreased with the use of 6F catheters. Four hundred sixty patients with an ejection fraction of 30% and target lesions that could accommodate a 6F catheter were enrolled. No differences were observed in procedural success rates (87%, 6F; 88%, 7F and 8F) or stenting rates (21%, 6F; 25%, 7F and 8F). The 6F group had approximately 40% fewer femoral access site complications (13.8% vs. 23.5%; $p < 0.01$), had shorter procedure and fluoroscopy times, used less contrast, and had shorter post–sheath removal femoral compression times (11.7 vs. 14.1 minutes; $p < 0.01$).

Contrast Agents

15. **Grines CL,** et al. A randomized trial of low osmolar ionic vs nonionic contrast media in patients with MI or unstable angina undergoing percutaneous transluminal coronary angioplasty. *J Am Coll Cardiol* 1996;27:1381–1386 (editorial, 1387–1389).

This randomized study of 211 patients with acute MI or unstable angina showed that the use of ionic low-osmolar contrast media reduced the risk of ischemic complications. Patients received nonionic or ionic low-osmolar contrast media during coronary angiography. The ionic media group had fewer recurrent ischemic events requiring repeated catheterization (3.0% vs. 11.4%; $p = 0.02$) and repeated angioplasty during initial hospitalization (1.0% vs. 5.8%; $p = 0.06$). At 1 month, the ionic contrast group had a reduced need for bypass surgery (none vs. 5.9%; $p = 0.04$) and reported fewer symptoms of any angina or angina at rest (8.5% vs. 20.0%; $p = 0.04$; none vs. 5.9%, $p = 0.04$).

16. **Chevalier B,** et al. Does nonionic contrast medium still modify angioplasty results in the stent era? *J Am Coll Cardiol* 1999;33(suppl A):85A.

This analysis focused on 1,713 consecutive patients (March 1996 to February 1997) undergoing coronary intervention with a low-osmolarity ionic contrast medium (ICM) and 1,826 with a nonionic contrast medium (NICM; March 1997 to February 1998). Clinical and angiographic data were similar in both groups. The incidence of minor and major events, including distal embolization, side-branch occlusion, stent thrombosis, Q-wave MI, and death, were similar in both groups. The authors suggest that the higher use of stenting in the current era (more than 80% in this study) has eliminated the benefits of NICM use.

17. **Schrader R,** et al. A randomized trial comparing the impact of nonionic (iomeprol) versus an ionic (ioxaglate) low osmolar contrast medium on abrupt vessel closure and ischemic complications after coronary angioplasty. *J Am Coll Cardiol* 1999;33:395–402.

This prospective, randomized trial was composed of 2,000 patients undergoing PTCA. The frequency of reocclusions requiring repeated intervention was similar in both groups [in laboratory, 2.9% (iomeprol) and 3.0% (ioxaglate); out of laboratory, 3.1% and 4.1%]. Major ischemic complication rates also were similar (emergency CABG, 0.8% and 0.7%; MI, 1.8% and 2.0%; in-hospital cardiac death, 0.2% and 0.2%). The iomeprol group had higher rates of dissection and stenting (31.6% vs. 25.7%, $p = 0.004$; 31.6% vs. 25.7%, $p = 0.004$), whereas allergic reactions requiring treatment occurred only in the ioxaglate group (0.9%; $p = 0.002$).

18. Contrast Media Utilization in High Risk Percutaneous Transluminal Coronary Angioplasty (**COURT**). Results presented at 71st AHA Scientific Session in Dallas, TX: November 1998.

A total of 853 patients undergoing high-risk interventions was randomized to a nonionic iso-osmolar contrast agent (iodixanol) or an ionic low-osmolar contrast agent (ioxaglate). Angiographic success was significantly better in the nonionic contrast patients (92.2% vs. 85.9%; $p = 0.004$). The nonionic contrast group had a significantly lower incidence of the primary composite end point of in-hospital MI, abrupt closure, recatheterization, or emergency revascularization (5.2% vs. 9.5%).

19. **Bertrand ME,** et al. for the Visipaque in PTCA (**VIP**) Investigators. Influence of a nonionic, isoosmolar contrast medium (iodixanol) versus an ionic, low-osmolar contrast medium (ioxaglate) on major adverse cardiac events in patients undergoing percutaneous transluminal coronary angioplasty: a multicenter, randomized, double-blind study. *Circulation* 2000;101:131–136.

This prospective, randomized, parallel-group, double-blind study enrolled 1,411 patients. Patients received either iodixanol (a nonionic, iso-osmolar contrast medium) or ioxaglate (an ionic, low-osmolar contrast medium) during PTCA. No significant differences were found between the groups in the incidence of the primary composite end point, consisting of death, stroke, MI, CABG surgery, and repeated PTCA at 2 days (iodixanol, 4.7%; ioxaglate, 3.9%; $p = 0.45$) and at 1 month. However, the iodixanol group had a lower incidence of hypersensitivity reactions ($p = 0.007$) and adverse drug reactions ($p = 0.002$) compared with the ioxaglate group.

Lesion Evaluation (Fractional Flow Reserve, Intravascular Ultrasound)

20. **Pijls NHJ,** et al. Measurement of fractional flow reserve to assess the functional severity of coronary-artery stenoses. *N Engl J Med* 1996;334:1703–1708.

A total of 45 consecutive patients with chest pain and a moderate coronary stenosis of approximately 50% underwent bicycle testing, thallium scintigraphy, dobutamine stress echocardiography, and coronary arteriography. In all patients (21) with a fractional flow reserve (FFR) less than 0.75, reversible ischemia was evident on at least one noninvasive test. After revascularization was performed (PTCA or CABG surgery), all positive test results reverted to normal. In contrast, 21 of 24 patients with a FFR 0.75 or more tested negative for reversible ischemia on all the noninvasive tests. None of these patients underwent revascularization through 14 months of follow-up. The sensitivity of FFR in detecting reversible ischemia was 88%, specificity was 100%, positive predictive value was 100%, negative predictive value was 88%, and the accuracy was 93%.

21. **Schiele F,** et al. Impact of intravascular ultrasound guidance in stent deployment on 6-month restenosis rate: a multicenter, randomized study comparing two strategies—with and without intravascular ultrasound guidance. **RESIST** Study Group. REStenosis after IVUS guided STenting. *J Am Coll Cardiol* 1998;32:320–328.

A total of 155 patients who underwent successful stent implantation was randomized into no further balloon dilation or additional balloon dilation(s) until IVUS criterion were achieved for adequate stent expansion. In the latter group, additional dilatation(s) were performed in 39%, with IVUS criterion being achieved in 80%. At 6 months, no significant difference was found between the groups in mean luminal diameter [1.60 mm (no IVUS) vs. 1.70 mm], restenosis rates [28.8% (no IVUS) vs. 22.5%], whereas the lumen cross-sectional area (CSA) was 20% larger in the IVUS-guided group (4.47 mm^2 vs. 5.36 mm^2; $p = 0.03$). Lumen CSA was the only predictor of restenosis by multivariate logistic regression analysis.

22. **Fitzgerald PJ,** et al. Final results of the Can Routine Ultrasound Influence Stent Expansion (**CRUISE**) Study. *Circulation* 2000;102:523–530.

A total of 522 patients from 16 of 45 centers in the Stent Anti-Thrombotic Regimen Study (STARS) was enrolled in this IVUS substudy to determine if IVUS-assisted stenting results in better outcomes when compared with angiography-assisted stenting. At 9 months, the IVUS-guided group had a larger MLD (2.9 mm vs. 2.7 mm; $p < 0.001$), a lower residual diameter stenosis (7.6% vs. 9.8%; $p < 0.001$), and higher final balloon size and inflation pressure (3.88 mm vs. 3.69 mm, and 18.0 atm vs. 16.6 atm; both $p < 0.001$). The IVUS group had a significantly lower TVR rate (8.5% vs. 15.3%; $p < 0.05$), whereas no differences were found in death or MI rates. Additional therapy based on IVUS information was used in 36% of patients (higher pressures in 59%, larger balloons in 33.7%, and an additional stent in 7%). In summary,

IVUS-guided stent deployment results in improved stent expansion and a lower TVR compared with angiographic guidance alone.

23. **Bech GJW,** et al. Fractional flow reserve to determine the appropriateness of angioplasty in moderate coronary stenosis. *Circulation* 2001;103:2928–2934.

This study of 325 scheduled to undergo PTCA of a more than 50% native coronary artery stenosis in a larger than 2.5-mm vessel examined whether deferring PTCA, based on FFR of 0.75 or more, is safe and as least as efficacious as performing PTCA. Patients were excluded if they had evidence of reversible ischemia in the previous 2 months. FFR was less than 0.75 for 144 patients, who underwent routine PTCA (reference group). Another 181 patients had a FFR of 0.75 or more and were randomized to optimal intervention (performance group) or medical therapy (deferral group) in a 1:1 fashion. Primary end point was absence of adverse cardiac events at 2 years, consisting of death, MI, PTCA, and any procedure-related complication requiring major intervention. At 2 years, event-free survival was significantly higher in the performance and deferral groups (83% and 89%) compared with the reference group (78%). The performance and deferral groups had similar rates of freedom from angina (50% vs. 49% at 1 year and 51% vs. 70% at 2 years), whereas the incidence was significantly higher in the reference group (67% at 1 year and 80% at 2 years).

24. **Mudra H,** et al. for the **OPTICUS** (OPTimization with ICUS to reduce stent restenosis) Study Investigators. Randomized comparison of coronary stent implantation under ultrasound or angiographic guidance to reduce stent restenosis (OPTICUS Study). *Circulation* 2001;104:1343–1349.

Prospective, randomized trial of 550 patients with a symptomatic coronary lesion or silent ischemia. Patients were assigned to either IVUS-guided or angiography-guided implantation of two or fewer stents. At 6-month angiography, no significant differences were seen between the two groups in minimal lumen diameter [1.95 mm (IVUS guided) vs. 1.91 mm] or restenosis rate (24.5% vs. 22.8%). At 1 year, the groups also had similar incidences of MACEs and repeated PCI.

25. **Chamuleau SA,** Prognostic value of coronary blood flow velocity and myocardial perfusion in intermediate coronary narrowings and multivessel disease. *J Am Coll Cardiol* 2002;39:852–858.

Prospective, multicenter study of 191 patients with stable angina and multivessel disease scheduled for PTCA. CFVR was measured distal to an intermediate lesion in another artery by using a Doppler guide wire. PTCA of the intermediate lesion was deferred when SPECT was negative or CFVR of 2.0 or more. Reversible perfusion defects were documented in the area of the intermediate lesion in 16%, whereas CFVR was positive in 24%. PTCA of the intermediate lesion was deferred in 182 patients. At 1-year follow-up, CFVR was a more accurate measure of major cardiac events than was SPECT; multivariate analysis showed CFVR as the only significant predictor for cardiac events.

26. **Albertal M,** et al., for the Doppler Endpoints Balloon Angioplasty Trial Europe (**DEBATE) II** Study Group. Coronary flow velocity reserve after percutaneous interventions is predictive of periprocedural outcome. *Circulation* 2002;105:1573–1578.

A total of 379 DEBATE II study patients underwent Doppler flow–guided angioplasty. CFVR measured before PTCA and CFVR in the reference artery were independent predictors of an optimal CFVR (2.5 or more) after balloon angioplasty. A low CFVR (less than 2.5) at the end of the procedure was an independent predictor of MACEs at 30 days (OR, 4.71; $p = 0.034$) and at 1 year (OR, 2.06; $p = 0.014$). After excluding MACE at 30 days, no difference in MACE at 1 year was observed between the patients with and without a CFVR less than 2.5 at the end of the procedure.

Comparison of Angioplasty with Medical Therapy

27. **Parisi AF,** et al. Angioplasty Compared to Medicine (**ACME**): a comparison of angioplasty with medical therapy in the treatment of single-vessel coronary artery disease. *N Engl J Med* 1992;326:10–16.

Design: Prospective, randomized, multicenter study. Primary end point was change in exercise tolerance, frequency of angina attacks, and nitroglycerin use.

Purpose: To compare medical therapy with balloon angioplasty in patients with one significant coronary artery stenosis.

Population: 212 patients with a single 70% to 99% stenosis.

Treatment: The drug therapy group included oral isosorbide dinitrate with sublingual glyceryl trinitrate and/or β-blockers and/or calcium antagonists. The balloon angioplasty group was given calcium antagonists before and for 1 month after the procedure, and heparin and glyceryl trinitrate during and until 12 hours after the procedure. All patients received aspirin, 325 mg orally daily.

Results: Balloon angioplasty (PTCA) was successful in 80% and reduced stenoses from 76% to 36%. The PTCA group had less angina (64% vs. 46%; $p < 0.01$), better exercise performance [+2.1 minutes (6 months vs. baseline exercise test) vs. +0.5 minutes; $p < 0.0001$], and more improvement in quality-of-life score (+8.6 units vs. +2.4 units; $p = 0.03$). However, the PTCA group did have more complications [emergency bypass surgery in two patients, MIs in five (vs. three), and repeated PTCA in 16].

28. **Folland ED,** et al. VA Angioplasty Compared to Medicine (**VA ACME**). Percutaneous transluminal coronary angioplasty vs medical therapy for stable angina pectoris. *J Am Coll Cardiol* 1997;29:1505–1511.

Design: Prospective, randomized, double-blind, multicenter study.

Purpose: To compare balloon angioplasty with medical therapy in patients with documented coronary disease and chronic stable angina.

Population: 328 patients with stable angina and positive exercise treadmill test; 101 patients had two-vessel disease ($\geq$70% stenosis in proximal two thirds), and 227 had one-vessel disease.

Exclusion Criteria: Medically refractory unstable angina, prior coronary revascularization, ejection fraction $\leq$30%.

Treatment: Medical therapy or balloon angioplasty.

Results: Among two-vessel patients, no significant changes were found between treatment groups in exercise treadmill test duration (performed at 2 to 3 years), or freedom from angina and quality of life. However, fewer angioplasty patients had improved perfusion imaging results (59% vs. 75%) and higher average stenosis of worst lesions (74% vs. 56%). Among one-vessel disease patients, the angioplasty group had more improvement in exercise time (+2.1 vs. +0.6 minutes; $p < 0.001$) and quality-of-life score (+7.1 vs. +1.5; $p = 0.01$), and were more angina free (63% vs. 48%; $p = 0.02$).

29. Randomized Intervention Treatment of Angina (**RITA-2**) Trial participants. Coronary angioplasty vs medical therapy for angina: the RITA-2 trial. *Lancet* 1997;350:461–468.

Design: Prospective, randomized, double-blind, multicenter study. Primary end point was death and nonfatal MI. Follow-up period was 2.7 years.

Purpose: To compare the effects of coronary angioplasty and conservative medical care in patients considered suitable for either treatment.

Population: 1,018 patients, 53% with grade 2 angina, 47% with prior MI, only 7% with three-vessel disease.

Exclusion Criteria: Unstable angina in prior 7 days, left main CAD, early revascularization necessary or planned.

Treatment: Medical therapy or balloon angioplasty (in the latter group, the procedure was performed in 93% at a median of 5 weeks).

Results: Angioplasty group had increased rates of death and MI (6.3% vs. 3.3%; $p = 0.02$). Benefit was attributable mostly to procedure-related events. However, the

PTCA group had 7% less grade 2 angina at 2 years and longer exercise treadmill test time at 3 months (+35 seconds; $p < 0.001$).

Stent Studies

Review Articles, Miscellaneous

30. **Goy J-J,** Eeckhout E. Intracoronary stenting. *Lancet* 1998;351:1943–1949.

The focus of this review is on the indications for stenting, including elective stenting for primary and secondary prevention of restenosis, bail-out, SVG disease, chronic total occlusion, and acute MI. Future directions are discussed, including randomized trials to compare stenting and bypass surgery, different types of stents, coated stents, and radiation therapy.

31. **Sigwart U,** et al. Intravascular stenting to prevent occlusion and restenosis after transluminal angioplasty. *N Engl J Med* 1987;316:701–706.

In this first major report of coronary stenting, 24 stents were placed in 19 patients with restenosis ($n = 17$) or abrupt closure ($n = 4$) after PTCA or SVG disease ($n = 3$). Three patients had stent thrombosis (one death), and 0 of 12 had restenosis at 3- to 6-month angiography.

Stenting Compared with PTCA

32. **Fischman DL,** et al. Stent Restenosis Study (**STRESS**). A randomized comparison of coronary-stent placement and balloon angioplasty in the treatment of coronary artery disease. *N Engl J Med* 1994;331:496–501.

Design: Prospective, randomized, open-label, multicenter study. Primary end point was angiographic restenosis.
Purpose: To compare the results of elective balloon angioplasty with PS stent implantation on clinical outcomes and restenosis in patients with *de novo* coronary lesions.
Population: 410 patients with *de novo* 70% stenotic lesions ≤15 mm long and in vessels with a diameter of ≥3 mm.
Exclusion Criteria: MI in previous 7 days, EF less than 40%, diffuse coronary or left main artery disease, and angiographic evidence of thrombus.
Treatment: Balloon angioplasty or PS stent. All patients received aspirin, 325 mg daily. Stented patients received dextran (started 2 hours before the procedure); heparin, 10,000 to 15,000 U before the procedure and infusion for 4–6 hours after sheath removal; dipyridamole, 75 mg 3 times daily for 1 month; and warfarin for 1 month.
Results: Stent group had better procedural success (96.1% vs. 89.6%; $p = 0.011$), greater increase in lumen diameter (1.7 mm vs. 1.2 mm; $p < 0.001$; at 6 months, 1.56 mm vs. 1.24 mm; $p < 0.01$), and a lower rate of restenosis at 6 months (31% vs. 42%; $p = 0.046$). No significant difference in early clinical events (days 0 to 14) was observed between the two groups (19.5% vs. 23.8%). The stent group had a nonsignificant reduction in revascularization rate (10% vs. 15%; $p = 0.06$). At 1-year follow-up (see *Am J Cardiol* 1998;81:860–865), 154 (75%) patients assigned to stent implantation and 141 (70%) to PTCA were free of all clinical events (death, MI, or any revascularization procedure).
Comments: The 1-year cost analysis showed the cost of stenting to be $800 more per patient despite lower costs during follow-up (see *Circulation* 1995;92:2480).

33. **Benestent I,** Serruys PW, et al. A comparison of balloon-expandable stent implantation with balloon angioplasty in patients with coronary artery disease. *N Engl J Med* 1994;331:489–495.

Design: Prospective, randomized, multicenter study. Primary end point was death, stroke, MI, CABG, or need for repeated percutaneous intervention during hospitalization.

Purpose: To compare elective balloon angioplasty with PS stenting in patients with stable angina and *de novo* coronary lesions.

Population: 520 patients aged 30 to 75 years with stable angina and one *de novo* coronary lesion shorter than 15 mm and in vessel larger than 3 mm in diameter.

Treatment: Balloon angioplasty or PS stenting. All patients received aspirin, 250 to 500 mg/day, and dipyridamole, 75 mg 3 times daily (started 1 day before procedure and continued for more than 6 months); heparin, 10,000 U was given before the procedure. Stented patients received dextran, 1,000 mL over 6 to 8 hours, and then warfarin for 3 months (target international normalized ratio, 2.5 to 3.5).

Results: No differences were observed between groups in incidence of death, stroke, MI, or subsequent revascularization during index hospitalization, and no differences were observed in composite end point of in-hospital clinical events (6.2% and 6.9%). At 7 months, the stent group had a significant reduction in primary composite end point (20.1% vs. 29.6%; $p = 0.02$), with the majority of this difference attributed to fewer second angioplasties (10% vs. 20.6%; $p = 0.001$). The stent group had more vascular complications (13.5% vs. 3.1%; $p < 0.001$) and longer hospital stays (8.5 vs. 3.1 days; $p = 0.001$). The 1-year follow-up data showed similar rates of death, stroke, MI, and CABG, but the stent group had 26% fewer primary end points (23% vs. 31%; $p = 0.04$), primarily because of approximately 50% fewer repeated PTCAs (10% vs. 21%; $p = 0.001$) (see *J Am Coll Cardiol* 1996;27:255). At 5-year follow-up, the stent group still had an approximate 10% absolute lower incidence of TVR (17.2% vs. 27.3%; $p = 0.008$; see *J Am Coll Cardiol* 2001;37:1598–1600).

Comments: Results suggest that stenting reduces repeated interventions but not major clinical events. Longer hospital stay with stenting was attributable to the aggressive antithrombotic regimen.

34. **Benestent II,** Serruys PW, et al. for the Benestent Study Group. Randomised comparison of heparin-coated stents with balloon angioplasty in selected patients with coronary artery disease (Benestent II). *Lancet* 1998;352:673–681.

Design: Prospective, randomized, double-blind, multicenter study. Primary end point was death, MI, and need for revascularization at 6 months.

Purpose: To compare elective balloon angioplasty with heparin-coated PS stents in patients with *de novo* coronary artery lesions.

Population: 827 patients with stable angina or stabilized unstable angina with one or more *de novo* lesions longer than 18 mm and in vessels ≥3 mm in diameter.

Exclusion Criteria: Left main disease, lesion at bifurcation with side-branch diameter greater than 2.0 mm, ejection fraction less than 30%, and MI in prior 7 days.

Treatment: Heparin-coated stents (10, 15, or 20 mm) or balloon angioplasty, and 1:1 subrandomization to clinical or angiographic follow-up. Stent patients received ticlopidine, 250 mg twice daily for 1 month.

Results: Stent group had an approximately one-third lower incidence of primary end point (12.8% vs. 19.3%; $p = 0.013$). The 30-day stent thrombosis rate was only 0.2%. In the subgroup undergoing angiographic follow-up, stented patients had a larger mean lumen diameter (1.89 mm vs. 1.66 mm; $p = 0.0002$) and less restenosis (16% vs. 31%; $p = 0.0008$). In the group assigned to clinical follow-up, the stent group had superior 1-year event-free survival [89% vs. 79%; $p = 0.004$ (RRs: cardiac events, 0.66; TVR, 0.60)]. The stent group patients with angiographic follow-up underwent 2.5 times more interventions (13.5% vs. 5.4%) than did clinical follow-up patients, whereas this ratio was only 1.5 among balloon angioplasty patients (18.7% vs. 12.4%).

35. **Versaci F,** et al. A comparison of coronary artery stenting with angioplasty for isolated stenosis of the proximal left anterior descending coronary artery. *N Engl J Med* 1997;336:817–822.

This randomized trial was composed of 120 patients with an ejection fraction ≥40%, no MI within the previous month, and isolated stenoses of the LAD artery. Patients underwent stenting (using high-pressure inflation and warfarin for 3 months) or balloon angioplasty (PTCA). All patients received aspirin and diltiazem (first doses given 1 day before the procedure) and intravenous heparin during the procedure. Procedural success rates were similar (stent, 95%; PTCA, 93%). The stent group had superior outcomes: lower 1-year event-free survival (no recurrent angina, MI, death; 87% vs. 70%; $p = 0.04$) and more than 50% reduction in restenosis (19% vs. 40%; $p = 0.02$). Stented patients had a longer hospital stay (6.5 vs. 5.0 days; $p = 0.04$), but this was likely owing to warfarin use, which has now been supplanted by aggressive antiplatelet regimens. The authors emphasize the need for a study comparing CABG with stenting.

36. **Betriu A,** et al. Randomized comparison of coronary stent implantation and balloon angioplasty in the treatment of de novo coronary artery lesions (**START**): a four-year follow-up. *J Am Coll Cardiol* 1999;34:1498–1506.

Design: Prospective, randomized, multicenter study. Primary end points were the rate of restenosis at 6 months and a composite of death, MI, and TVR at 4 years of clinical follow-up.

Purpose: To evaluate whether stent implantation in *de novo* coronary artery lesions would result in lower restenosis rates and better long-term clinical outcomes than balloon angioplasty.

Population: 452 patients with either stable or unstable angina.

Treatment: Stent implantation (229 patients) or standard balloon angioplasty (223 patients). Stent patients received aspirin, dipyridamole, dextran, calcium channel blocker, heparin, and warfarin; after the first 100 stents, oral ticlopidine replaced dextran, dipyridamole, and warfarin.

Results: Procedural success rate was achieved in 84% and 95% of angioplasty and stent patients, respectively. At 6 months, the stent group had a lower restenosis compared with the angioplasty group (22% vs. 37%; $p < 0.002$). At 4 years, no differences were found in mortality or nonfatal MI between the two groups. However, the stent group had a lower TVR rate (12% vs. 25% in the angioplasty group; $p = 0.0006$). Most of the repeated procedures (84%) were performed within 6 months.

37. **Witkowski A,** et al., on behalf of **AS** (Angioplasty or Stent) trial investigators. A randomized comparison of elective high-pressure stenting with balloon angioplasty: six-month angiographic and two-year clinical follow-up. *Am Heart J* 2000;140:264–271.

Design: Prospective, randomized, single-blind, multicenter study. Primary end points were restenosis at 6 months and event-free survival at 2 years.

Purpose: To determine whether routine high-pressure stenting with an antiplatelet regimen can show similar results.

Population: 400 patients with CCS class I to IV angina, single *de novo* lesion more than 50% and less than 15-mm length, and vessel diameter 2.5 mm or more.

Exclusion Criteria: Acute or recent MI, contraindication(s) to heparin, aspirin, or ticlopidine; left main lesions, bifurcation lesion, total occlusion.

Treatment: Balloon angioplasty or PS 153 stent using 14 atm or more after predilatation of target lesion. All received aspirin, 300 mg/day, and ticlopidine, 250 mg twice daily, started 2 or more days before the procedure and continued for 1 month.

Results: At 6 months, a trend toward a lower incidence of restenosis was found in the stent group (18.2% vs. 24.0%; $p = 0.055$). At 2 years, the stent group had a higher event-free survival rate compared with the angioplasty group (83.1% vs. 73.5%; $p = 0.017$). This difference was driven by a lower TVR rate in the stent group (17.2% vs. 25.5% in the angioplasty group; $p = 0.02$), whereas no significant differences were seen in the incidence of death or MI between the groups.

Provisional Stenting

38. **Rodriguez R,** et al., on behalf of the OCBAS Investigators. Optimal coronary balloon angioplasty with provisional stenting versus primary stent (**OCBAS**). *J Am Coll Cardiol* 1998;32:1351–1357.

Design: Prospective, randomized, multicenter study. Primary end point was angiographic restenosis and TVR at 6 months.

Purpose: To determine any significant difference in restenosis rates between lesions treated with primary elective stenting versus those treated with optimal balloon angioplasty.

Population: 116 patients with symptomatic CAD undergoing successful balloon angioplasty (as determined by angiography at 30 minutes) of *de novo* lesions in native coronary arteries.

Exclusion Criteria: Lesions longer than 20 mm and in vessels less than 2.5 mm diameter, diffuse disease, or severe tortuosity.

Treatment: Balloon angioplasty (PTCA) alone or PTCA followed by elective coronary stenting.

Results: Of the patients, 13.5% crossed over to stenting. Angiographic restenosis and TVR rates were similar [19.2% (stent) vs. 16.4% (PTCA); 17.5% vs. 13.5%]. Immediate and follow-up angiography showed that short-term gain was significantly higher in the stent than in the PTCA group (1.95 mm vs. 1.50 mm; $p < 0.03$), but this was offset by a higher late loss (0.63 vs. 0.26 mm; $p = 0.01$). Overall costs (hospital and follow-up) were lower in the PTCA group ($398,480 vs. $591,740; $p < 0.02$).

39. **Weaver WD,** et al. Optimum percutaneous transluminal coronary angioplasty compared with routine stent strategy trial (**OPUS-1**): a randomised trial. *Lancet* 2000;355:2199–2203.

Design: Prospective, randomized, open, multicenter study. Primary end point was death, MI, and TVR at 6 months.

Purpose: Whether routine implantation of coronary stents is the best strategy to treat flow-limiting coronary stenoses is unclear. An alternative approach is to do balloon angioplasty and provisionally use stents only to treat suboptimal results. The multicenter trial compared the outcomes of patients treated with these strategies.

Population: 479 patients aged 21 to 81 years with stable or unstable angina or MI more than 24 hours earlier and 70% coronary artery stenosis (≤ 2 mm length, vessel diameter ≥ 3 mm).

Treatment: Systematic stenting or provisional stenting (undertaken if residual stenosis greater than 20%, impending abrupt closure, stenosis was ≥ 2 mm, or flow-limiting dissection). IVUS was used at the physician's discretion. Abciximab was used in fewer than 15% of patients. All patients received aspirin and ticlopidine.

Results: Stents were implanted in 98.7% of the routine stenting group, whereas 37% of patients assigned to initial PTCA had more than one stent placed because of suboptimal angioplasty results. At 6 months, the primary stenting group had a significantly lower incidence of death, MI, or TVR (6.1% vs. 14.9%; $p = 0.003$). The majority of this benefit was owing to a lower TVR rate (4% vs. 10%; $p = 0.007$). The provisional stent group had higher initial costs, but the overall costs at 6 months were similar in both groups.

40. **Lafont A,** et al. The French Randomized Optimal Stenting Trial (**FROST**): a prospective evaluation of provisional stenting guided by coronary velocity reserve and quantitative coronary angiography. *J Am Coll Cardiol* 2000;36:404–409.

Design: Prospective, randomized, open, multicenter study. Primary end point was the 6-month angiographic minimal lumen diameter (MLD).

Purpose: To compare systematic stenting with provisional stenting guided by Doppler measurements of coronary velocity reserve and quantitative coronary angiography.

Population: 251 patients undergoing elective PTCA.

Treatment: Provisional stenting (stenting performed if post-PTCA coronary velocity reserve was less than 2.2 and/or residual stenosis 35% or more or as bailout) or to systematic stenting.

Results: Stenting was performed in 48.4% of the provisional stenting group and all systematic stenting patients. At 6 months, no significant differences were found between the groups in MLD [1.90 mm (provisional) vs. 1.99 mm; $p = 0.39$] or binary restenosis rate (27.1% vs. 21.4%; $p = 0.37$). The rates of TLR and MACEs (death, acute MI, and TLR) were similar in both groups (15.1% vs. 14.4%; 15.1% vs. 16.0%).

41. **Serruys PW,** on behalf of Doppler Endpoints Balloon Angioplasty Trial Europe (**DEBATE**) **II** Study Group. Randomized comparison of primary stenting and provisional balloon angioplasty guided by flow velocity measurement. *Circulation* 2000;102:2930–2937.

Design: Prospective, randomized, double-blind, multicenter study. Primary end point was death, nonfatal MI, and TLR.

Purpose: To determine if provisional stenting is as effective as and less expensive than primary stenting.

Population: 620 patients scheduled to undergo angioplasty for stable or unstable angina pectoris and with documented myocardial ischemia due to a single *de novo* lesion shorter than 25 mm.

Exclusion Criteria: MI in prior week, total occlusion, ostial or bifurcation lesions, vessel with target lesion previously bypassed, vessel tortuous or containing thrombus.

Treatment: Primary stenting or balloon angioplasty guided by Doppler flow velocity and angiography. Patients in latter group were further randomized after optimization to either additional stenting or termination of the procedure. Optimal result defined as flow reserve greater than 2.5 and diameter stenosis 35% or greater.

Results: Bailout stenting occurred in 25% of patients in the balloon angioplasty group. No differences were found between the two groups in event-free survival at 1 year (primary stenting, 86.6%; provisional angioplasty, 85.6%). Costs at 1 year were higher in the provisional angioplasty group (EUR 6573 vs. EUR 5885; $p = 0.014$), primarily because of longer hospitalizations and higher rate of surgical revascularization. After the second randomization, stenting was associated with better 1-year event-free survival after both optimal balloon angioplasty (93.5% vs. 84.1%; $p = 0.066$) and suboptimal balloon angioplasty (89.3% vs. 73.3%; $p = 0.005$).

Comments: An unexpected observation was a further reduction in MACEs in patients stented after optimal balloon angioplasty.

42. **Di Mario C,** et al. Randomized comparison of elective stent implantation and coronary balloon angioplasty and intracoronary Doppler. *Circulation* 2000;102:2938–2944.

Design: Prospective, randomized, double-blind, multicenter study. Primary end point was a composite of death, MI, and TLR at 1 year.

Purpose: To compare the outcomes of balloon angioplasty with provisional stenting with primary stenting.

Population: 738 patients with lesions suitable for stent implantation.

Exclusion Criteria: Recent MI (24 hours or less), prior MI with akinesis or dyskinesis in target vessel territory, chronic total occlusion, graft and ostial stenoses, second restenosis after PTCA, stent restenosis, planned rotational or directional atherectomy.

Treatment: Elective stent implantations (370 patients, 386 lesions) or PTCA guided by quantitative coronary angiography (QCA) and Doppler CFR analysis (368 patients, 384 lesions). Balloon angioplasty result was considered "optimal" if the final lesion diameter by QCA less than 35%; no type C through F dissections were found, and CFR distal to the stenosis was greater than 2.0.

Results: Optimal PTCA was achieved in 166 (43%) lesions. The main reasons for suboptimal PTCA were CFR 2.0 or less (62% cases) and significant residual stenosis (44% of cases). At 1 year, no significant difference was found in the primary composite end point of death, MI, and TLR (17.8% in elective stent group and 18.9% in guided PTCA group). When compared with provisional stenting, *optimal* PTCA was associated with a similar incidence of TLR (17.6% vs. 14.1% for provisional stenting; $p = $ NS) and death, MI, and TLR (20.1% and 18.0%, respectively; $p = $ NS).

Comments: Optimal PTCA achieved only in 43% of cases. Capacity to measure CFR is not available in every interventional laboratory, and it requires both operator and laboratory experience.

43. **Frey AW,** et al. Ultrasound-guided stratification for provisional stenting with focal balloon combination catheter: results from the randomized Strategy for Intracoronary ultrasound-guided PTCA and Stenting (**SIPS**) trial. *Circulation* 2000;102:2497–2502.

Design: Prospective, randomized, multicenter study. Clinical end points included procedure success (less than 50% residual stenosis in the absence of repeated revascularization, MI, or death before discharge), angiographic restenosis, TLR, and a composite of death, MI, and repeated revascularization (MACE).

Purpose: To determine whether routine intracoronary ultrasound guidance (ICUS) can improve outcomes of provisional stenting when compared with standard angiography.

Population: 269 patients undergoing elective coronary intervention.

Exclusion Criteria: Emergency intervention, planned atherectomy, chronic total occlusion.

Treatment: ICUS or angiography-guided provisional stenting. Stenting was discouraged unless a significant dissection was present or angiographic results were unacceptable. In the ICUS group, inflations were performed until the minimal lumen area was more than 65% of the mean reference area.

Results: The ICUS group had a significantly higher procedural success rate than the angiography group (94.7% vs. 87.4%; $p = 0.033$), a larger short-term gain (1.85 mm vs. 1.67 mm; $p = 0.02$), and a similar minimal lumen diameter (2.49 mm vs. 2.38 mm; $p = 0.12$). Stenting rates were similar (50.3% and 50.5%, respectively; $p = 0.96$), but a trend toward a lower short-term TLR rate was seen in the ICUS group (2.3% vs. 5.7%; $p = 0.15$). At 6-month follow-up, no significant differences were found in restenosis rates (29% vs. 35%; $p = 0.42$). At 2-year follow-up, the ICUS group had a lower incidence of clinically driven TLR compared with the angiographic group (17% vs. 29%; $p = 0.02$), whereas no significant differences were seen in overall MACE rates (30% vs. 37%; $p = 0.2$).

Direct Stenting

44. **Brito FS Jr,** et al., for The **DIRECT** Study Investigators. Comparison of direct stenting versus stenting with predilation for the treatment of selected coronary narrowings. *Am J Cardiol* 2002;89:115–120.

This prospective, multicenter trial randomized 411 patients to direct stenting or balloon predilatation followed by stent implantation. Lesions with severe calcification were excluded. Angiographic success rates were 100% with direct stenting (2.8% requiring balloon predilation) and 98.6% with routine predilation ($p = 0.12$). Direct stenting was associated with decreased use of balloons and a trend toward reduced procedure time (22.7 vs. 25.6 minutes; $p = 0.07$). Fluoroscopy time and contrast volume were not different between groups. At 6 months, mortality, MI, and TVR rates were similar in both groups. MACE-free survival rates were 87.5% for direct stenting and 85.5% for the predilation group ($p = 0.0002$ for equivalence).

45. **Brueck M,** et al. Direct coronary stenting versus predilatation followed by stent placement. *Am J Cardiol* 2002;90:1187–1192.

This prospective, randomized study enrolled 335 symptomatic patients with single or multiple coronary lesions (severity, 60% to 95%; length, 30 mm or shorter; diameter, 2.5 to 4.0 mm). Lesion exclusion criteria: excessive calcification, severe proximal tortuosity, occlusion. Patients were assigned to direct stenting or stenting after predilation. In the direct stent group, there was a 5% crossover rate to predilation. Direct stenting was associated with shorter procedural time (42.1 vs. 51.5 minutes; $p = 0.004$), less radiation exposure time (10.3 vs. 12.5 minutes; $p = 0.002$), less contrast dye used (163 vs. 197 mL; $p < 0.0001$), and lower procedural costs. In-hospital complication rate were similar. At 6 months, direct stenting was associated with a lower rate of angiographic binary restenosis (20% vs. 31%; $p = 0.048$) and target lesion revascularization (18% vs. 28%; $p = 0.03$).

46. **TRENDS** (Tetra Randomized European Direct Stenting). Preliminary results presented at the Transcatheter Cardiovascular Therapeutics meeting, Washington, DC: September 2002.

This prospective, randomized, multicenter trial of 941 patients showed that direct stenting and stenting with predilatation yield comparable angiographic and clinical results. Both treatment groups had similar characteristics, with eccentric and type B lesions predominating. Exclusion criteria included chronic occlusions and unprotected left main stenoses. Only 5.7% of patients in the direct-stenting group crossed over to predilatation; this was because of failure to cross the target lesion in 25 of 31 cases. At 6-month angiography, no difference was found between the groups in MLD [2.91 mm (direct stenting) vs. 2.95 mm] or binary restenosis (11.6% vs. 11.4%). Resource use was less with the direct-stent approach, including shorter procedure time (34.3 minutes vs. 37.5 minutes; $p = 0.01$) and less contrast use (175 mL vs. 186 mL; $p = 0.05$). No significant difference was found between the groups in death, MI, and TLR (7.1% vs. 8.8%).

Stent versus Stent Studies

47. **Carrozza JP,** et al. Final acute, 30-day, and 6-month clinical and angiographic outcome from the multicenter randomized EXTRA trial comparing the operator-mounted XT and Palmaz-Schatz coronary stents. *Circulation* 1998;98:I–661.

A total of 649 patients with 70% or more stenosis and lesion length of 25 mm or less in native coronary was randomized to XT or PS stent. No significant differences were found between the groups in major adverse events, restenosis [28% (XT) vs. 35%] or TLR [8.2% (XT) vs. 9.0%].

48. **Lansky AJ,** et al. Randomized comparison of GR-II stent and Palmaz-Schatz stent for elective treatment of coronary stenoses. *Circulation* 2000;102:1364–1368.

This prospective study randomized 755 patients to either Gianturco-Robin (GR)-II or PS stent implantation. At 30 days, the composite MACE rate was significantly higher in the GR-II group compared with the PS group (4.2% vs. 1.3%; $p < 0.01$). This difference was mostly owing to more frequent subacute stent thrombosis in the GR-II group (3.9% vs. 0.3%; $p = 0.001$). At 1 year, the TLR rate (primary end point) also was significantly higher in the GR-II group (27.4% vs. 15.3%; $p < 0.001$).

49. **Baim DS,** et al., for the **NIRVANA** (NIR Vascular Advanced North American Trial) Investigators. Final results of a randomized trial comparing the NIR stent to the Palmaz-Schatz stent for narrowings in native coronary arteries. *Am J Cardiol* 2001;87:152–156.

This prospective study randomized 849 patients with single coronary lesions to the NIR stent or the PS. At 30 days, the two groups had a similar incidence of MACEs (death, MI, repeated TLR; 4.3% vs. 4.4%). The primary end point of target vessel failure at 9 months occurred in 16.0% of NIR patients compared with 17.2% of PS patients, with the NIR proving to be equal or superior to the PS stent ($p < 0.001$ by test for equivalency). Angiographic restudy in 71% found no significant difference in restenosis rates [19.3% (NIR) vs. 22.4%].

50. **Baim DS,** et al., for the **ASCENT** Investigators (ACS MultLink Stent Clinical Equivalence in De Novo Lesions Trial). Final results of a randomized trial comparing the MULTI-LINK stent with the Palmaz-Schatz stent for narrowings in native coronary arteries. *Am J Cardiol* 2001;87:157–162.

This prospective, randomized, multicenter trial enrolled 1,040 patients with single, *de novo* native vessel lesions. Patients received ACS Multilink (ML) stent or PS stent. At 30 days, no significant differences were found between the groups in MACEs [5.0% (ML) vs. 6.5%]. The primary end point of target vessel failure at 9 months occurred in 15.1% of ML-treated patients compared with 16.7% of PS-treated patients, with the ML proving to be equal or superior to the PS stent ($p < 0.001$ by test for equivalency).

Angiographic restudy in a prespecified subgroup showed a nonsignificant trend toward reduced restenosis with the ML stent (16.0% vs. 22.1%).

Coated-Stent Studies

51. **Kastrati A,** et al. Increased risk of restenosis after placement of gold-coated stents: results of a randomized trial comparing gold-coated with uncoated steel stents in patients with coronary artery disease. *Circulation* 2001;101:2478–2483.

This prospective, randomized, multicenter study enrolled 731 patients with symptomatic CAD. Patients received either a gold-coated Inflow stent or an uncoated Inflow stainless steel stent. All received ticlopidine for 4 weeks. At 30 days, no difference was found between the two groups in the incidence of death, MI, or TVR [7.9% (gold) vs. 5.8%; $p = 0.25$]. At 6 months, the gold-stent group had a significantly higher incidence of restenosis compared with the uncoated-stent group (49.7% vs. 38.1%; $p = 0.003$). At 1 year, the gold-stent group had a significantly lower event-free survival (62.9% vs. 73.9%; $p = 0.001$).

52. **Park SJ,** et al. Comparison of gold-coated NIR stents with uncoated NIR stents in patients with coronary artery disease. *Am J Cardiol* 2002;89:872–875.

This prospective, randomized, multicenter (6) trial enrolled 216 patients with stenoses greater than 50% and shorter than 20 mm in vessels with 2.5 mm diameter or larger. Patients received either an uncoated NIR stent or a gold-coated NIR stent. All received ticlopidine (or cilostazol) starting 48 hours before the procedure and for 4 weeks. At angiographic follow-up, the gold-stent group had a significantly higher restenosis rate compared with the uncoated-stent group (46.7% vs. 26.4%; $p < 0.05$). At 9 months, the gold-stent group had a 22.7% TLR rate compared with 15.1% in the uncoated-stent group ($p = 0.15$).

Newer Devices/Techniques

Cutting Balloon
53. **CUBA** (Cutting Balloon versus Conventional Angioplasty Study). *Eur Heart J* 1998;19(abstr suppl):48.

A total of 306 patients with a *de novo* lesion shorter than 15 mm in native vessel with a diameter of 2.5 to 4.0 mm were randomized to cutting balloon or conventional PTCA. Exclusion criteria were bifurcation lesions, calcified lesions, thrombus, and severe tortuosity or angulation, with a 6-month angiographic follow-up and a 7-month clinical follow-up. Stent implantation was required in 12% in the conventional balloon group compared with 8% in the cutting balloon group. Postprocedure MLD was 2.0 ± 0.4 mm for both groups, whereas MLD at 6 months was 1.7 ± 0.8 mm for the cutting balloon group and 1.5 ± 0.7 mm for the balloon group. At 7 months, the incidence of death, MI, or any TLR was 20% for the cutting balloon group and 26% for the conventional balloon group ($p = $ NS).

54. **Izumi M,** et al. Final results of the **CAPAS** trial. *Am Heart J* 2001;142:782–789.

A total of 248 type B/C lesions in small vessels (smaller than 3 mm diameter) were randomly assigned to cutting balloon angioplasty (CBA) or conventional balloon angioplasty (PTCA). At follow-up angiography (3 months), restenosis was significantly lower in the CBA group compared with the PTCA group (25.2% vs. 41.5%; $p = 0.009$). At 1 year, the event-free survival rate was 72.8% in the cutting balloon group and 61.0% in the PTCA group ($p = 0.047$).

55. **Adamian M,** et al. Cutting balloon angioplasty for the treatment of in-stent restenosis: a matched comparison with rotational atherectomy, additional stent implantation and balloon angioplasty. *J Am Coll Cardiol* 2001;38:672–679.

A total of 648 lesions with ISR was divided into four groups according to treatment strategy: CBA, RA, additional stenting, and PTCA. After the matching process, 258 lesions were entered into the analysis. Acute lumen gain was significantly higher in the stent group (2.12 mm) compared with the CBA, RA, and PTCA groups (1.70 mm, 1.79 mm, and 1.56 mm, respectively). However, the lumen loss at follow-up was lower for the CBA versus RA and stent groups (0.63 mm vs. 1.30 mm and 1.36 mm, respectively; $p < 0.0001$), resulting in a lower recurrent restenosis rate in CBA group (20% vs. 35.9% and 41.4%, respectively; $p < 0.05$). By multivariate analysis, predictors of TLR were CBA (OR, 0.17; $p = 0.001$) and diffuse restenosis at baseline (OR, 2.07; $p = 0.02$).

56. **Mauri L,** et al. Cutting balloon angioplasty for the prevention of restenosis: results of the Cutting Balloon Global Randomized Trial. *Am J Cardiol* 2002;90:1079–1083.

This prospective, multicenter center randomized 1,238 patients to CB treatment or standard PTCA. At 6 months, binary angiographic restenosis rates (primary end point) were 31.4% for CB and 30.4% for PTCA. Freedom from TVR was slightly higher in the CB group (88.5% vs. 84.6%; log-rank $p = 0.04$). Coronary perforations occurred only in CB arm (0.8% vs. none; $p = 0.03$). At 270 days, the rates of MI, death, and total MACEs for CB and PTCA were 4.7% versus 2.4% ($p = 0.03$), 1.3% versus 0.3% ($p = 0.06$), and 13.6% versus 15.1% ($p = 0.34$), respectively.

57. **RESCUT** (Restenosis Cutting Balloon Evaluation). Preliminary results presented at Transcatheter Cardiovascular Therapeutics meeting, Washington, DC: September 2002.

This prospective, randomized trial was conducted at 23 European centers and enrolled 382 patients with ISR. Patients were assigned to CB or standard balloon angioplasty (PTCA). The CB did dilate the target lesion wider at significantly lower inflation pressures compared with PTCA (3.18 mm vs. 3.07 mm; $p < 0.01$; 9.9 atm vs. 12.6 atm; $p < 0.01$). Balloon slippage also occurred much less often with the CB (6.5% vs. 25.1%; $p < 0.01$), and there was a trend toward less stenting in the CB group (3.9% vs. 8.0%; $p = 0.07$). However, at 7 months, no significant differences were found between the CB and PTCA groups in the rates of binary restenosis by QCA (29.3% vs. 31.3%) or a clinical-event composite of death, MI, or TLR (18% vs. 19%).

58. **REDUCE II** (Restenosis Reduction by Cutting Balloon Evaluation). Preliminary results presented at Transcatheter Cardiovascular Therapeutics meeting, Washington, DC: September 2002.

This prospective, randomized, multicenter trial enrolled 466 patients with ISR. Patients were treated with the CB or a standard balloon. Procedural results were similar with both balloons, with no significant differences in QCA parameters. The CB group had a lower incidence of in-hospital death, MI, or TLR (4.0% vs. 8.2% for the standard balloon; $p = 0.049$). However, at 6-month angiographic follow-up, no significant differences were found between the groups in the rates of binary restenosis, percentage stenosis, and MLD.

Thrombectomy

59. **Kuntz RE,** et al. Atrial comparing rheolytic thrombectomy with intracoronary urokinase for coronary and vein graft thrombus (the Vein Graft AngioJet Study [VeGAS 2]). *Am J Cardiol* 2002;89:326–330.

Design: Prospective, randomized, open, multicenter study. Primary end point was death, Q-wave MI, emergency coronary bypass surgery, TLR, stroke, or stent thrombosis at 30 days.

Purpose: To evaluate the safety and efficacy of rheolytic thrombectomy in CAD. Comparison of safety and efficacy of rheolytic thrombectomy (AngioJet) versus thrombolytic therapy (intracoronary urokinase).

Population: 352 patients with angina or MI more than 24 hours before the procedure and thrombus on angiography with discrete, mobile, intraluminal defect or a total occlusion with thrombus confirmed by multi-sidehole infusion catheter.

Exclusion Criteria: MI or thrombolytic therapy in previous 24 hours, more than two vessels requiring treatment, target vessel smaller than 2.0 mm diameter.

Treatment: Standard intracoronary or graft urokinase (more than 6-hour continuous infusion) or thrombectomy using the AngioJet system. Adjunctive thrombolytics and abciximab were discouraged, and crossover to AngioJet was prohibited. Short-term 30-day success was defined as more than 20% improvement in MLD, a final diameter stenosis of ≤50%, TIMI grade III flow, and freedom from major coronary events.

Results: Procedural success was significantly higher in the AngioJet group than in the urokinase group (86% vs. 72%; $p = 0.002$). Both treatments were equally effective with respect to the 30-day primary end point (AngioJet, 29%; urokinase, 30%). However, AngioJet patients had fewer MACEs (death, MI, revascularization; 16% vs. 33%; $p < 0.001$). Bradycardia occurred in 24% of those treated with AngioJet and was managed successfully with atropine and temporary pacing.

Comments: Trial was terminated early because of the growing safety difference between the two groups as well as reservations of investigators about using urokinase. Furthermore, mechanical thrombectomy allowed rapid thrombus removal and stenting during the same catheterization session.

60. **X-TRACT** (X-Sizer for Treatment of Thrombus and Atherosclerosis in Coronary Interventions Trial). Preliminary results presented at Transcatheter Cardiovascular Therapeutics, Washington, DC: September 2002.

This prospective, randomized, open, multicenter trial enrolled 800 high-risk patients with lesion(s) in an SVG or a thrombotic native coronary artery. Most patients had unstable angina and three-vessel disease. Patients were stratified according to preinterventional GP IIb/IIIa inhibitor use, and then randomized to either PCI with use of the X-Sizer device or PCI alone. Bailout GP IIb/IIIa inhibitors were required in 0.5% of patients in the thrombectomy device group versus 2.3% of control patients. However, GP IIb/IIIa inhibitors were used in 77% of patients, so this primary end point of bailout GP IIb/IIIa–inhibitor therapy applied to only a minority of patients. Among patients who did not receive preintervention GP IIb/IIIa inhibitors, 10% of control patients required bailout use, compared with 2.1% in the device group. The overall incidence of bailout use of a IIb/IIIa inhibitor or a thrombectomy device was reduced in the device group by more than 50%, from 4.8% to 1.8% ($p = 0.02$). Thirty-day MACE was not different between groups (17.0% vs. 17.4%). However, MI defined as CK-MB more than 8 times normal was reduced by 46% in the X-Sizer group. It is not clear whether this effect translates into mortality benefit downstream. When the analysis was limited only to vessels containing thrombus, large MI was reduced by 50%, and death or large MI by 54%. In no-thrombus lesions, a trend occurred to increased overall MACE and only a weak trend for reduction in death and large MI; thus the device has no role in fibrotic calcified lesions. Most important, because this device did not reduce MACE, whereas distal protection reduced MACE by 50% in the SAFER trial, the use of this device would likely be limited to vein graft lesions where distal protection is not possible [e.g., distal lesions (last 3 cm), poor LV function].

Distal Protection

61. **Baim DS,** et al. on behalf of Saphenous vein graft Angioplasty Free of Emboli Randomized (**SAFER**) Trial Investigators. Randomized trial of a distal embolic protection device during percutaneous intervention of saphenous vein aorto-coronary bypass grafts. *Circulation* 2002;105:1285–1290.

Design: Prospective, randomized, controlled, multicenter study. Primary end point was death, MI, emergency bypass surgery, or TVR (MACE) at 30 days.

Purpose: To compare clinical outcomes after SVG stenting plus GuardWire distal protection versus that performed over a conventional guide wire (control arm).

Population: 801 patients with a history of angina, evidence of myocardial ischemia, and greater than 50% stenosis in the mid-portion of an SVG with a diameter of 3 to 6 mm. In the first 142 patients, the lesion could not occupy more than one third of graft length.

Exclusion Criteria: Recent MI, ejection fraction less than 25%, creatinine greater than 2.5 mg/dL (unless receiving long-term hemodialysis), planned use of an atherectomy device.

Treatment: The 0.014-inch PercuSurge GuardWire balloon occlusion device or conventional 0.014-inch angioplasty guide wire. GP IIb/IIIa–receptor blocker could be used at the discretion of the operator.

Results: The embolic protection group had a 42% relative reduction in MACE at 30 days (9.6% vs. 16.5%; $p = 0.004$). This reduction was due primarily to fewer MIs (8.6% vs. 14.7%; $p = 0.008$) and "no-reflow" (3% vs. 9%; $p = 0.02$). The benefit of the distal protection device was evident both with and without the use of concomitant GP IIb/IIIa–receptor blockers.

Comments: The use of distal embolization protection devices in other territories, such as native coronary, carotid, and renal arteries, has yet to be fully examined.

62. **FIRE** (FilterWireEx During Transluminal Intervention of Saphenous Vein Grafts) trial. Preliminary results presented at the 52nd ACC Scientific Sessions, Chicago, IL: March 2003.

This prospective, randomized, open, multicenter trial enrolled 651 patients with SVG lesion(s). Patients were treated using the GuardWire of FilterWireEx (Boston Scientific). At 30 days, male rates were similar [9.9% (FilterWireEx) vs. 11.6%].

Adjunctive Pharmacologic Therapy

Aspirin

63. **Schwartz L,** et al. Aspirin and dipyridamole in the prevention of restenosis after percutaneous transluminal coronary angioplasty. *N Engl J Med* 1988;318:1714–1719.

This prospective, randomized, double-blind, placebo-controlled study enrolled 376 patients undergoing planned PTCA. Patients received an aspirin-dipyridamole combination (330 mg to 75 mg t.i.d.), beginning 24 hours before PTCA and until follow-up angiography, or placebo. At follow-up angiography (249 patients), no differences were observed between the two groups in binary restenosis rates [37.7% vs. 38.6% (placebo)]. However, the aspirin-dipyridamole group had significantly fewer periprocedural Q-wave MIs compared with the placebo group (6.9% vs. 1.6%; $p = 0.0113$).

Heparin

64. **Friedman HZ,** et al. Randomized prospective evaluation of prolonged vs abbreviated intravenous heparin treatment after PTCA. *J Am Coll Cardiol* 1994;24:1214–1219.

Design: Prospective, randomized, open, single-center study.

Purpose: To compare continuous prolonged heparin therapy with abbreviated heparin therapy with early sheath removal after uncomplicated coronary angioplasty.

Population: 238 patients who underwent successful elective coronary angioplasty (46 were excluded because of unfavorable procedural results).

Exclusion Criteria: Recent MI, unstable angina, and uncompensated LV dysfunction.

Treatment: All patients received an initial bolus of 10,000 to 15,000 U of heparin and then an infusion at 10 U/kg/h (titrated to ACT, 160 to 190 seconds) for 24 hours or no additional heparin with sheath removal 3 to 4 hours later.

Results: Abbreviated heparin group had fewer bleeding complications [zero vs. eight patients (one blood transfusion, seven inguinal hematomas); $p < 0.001$]. Abbreviated infusion patients also were discharged earlier (after 23 vs. 42 hours; $p < 0.001$), resulting in a cost savings of $1,370/patient.

65. **Garachemani AR,** et al. Prolonged heparin after uncomplicated coronary interventions: a prospective, randomized trial. *Am Heart J* 1998;136:352–356 (editorial 183–185).

This prospective randomized trial was composed of 191 consecutive patients who underwent successful coronary angioplasty. Patients received prolonged intravenous heparin (12 to 20 hours) or no postprocedural heparin. Stents were used in 33% and 36% of patients. MIs occurred in 3% and 4%, whereas vascular complications were seen in 3% and 1%. Accompanying editorial contains results from a meta-analysis of six studies comprising 2,186 patients. Postprocedural heparin was associated with a nonsignificant OR of 0.91 (0.45 to 1.84) for ischemic complications and an OR of 2.54 (1.44 to 4.47) for bleeding complications (27 additional episodes/1,000 patients treated).

66. **Lincoff AM,** et al. Precursor to EPILOG (**PROLOG**) Investigators. Standard versus low-dose, weight-adjusted heparin in patients treated with the platelet glycoprotein IIb/IIIa receptor antibody fragment abciximab (c7E3 Fab) during percutaneous coronary revascularization. *Am J Cardiol* 1997;79:286–291.

This randomized 2 × 2 factorial pilot study was composed of a total of 103 patients undergoing PCI with concomitant abciximab (0.25 mg/kg intravenous bolus, and then 10 μg/min for 12 hours) were randomized to standard or high-dose heparin (100 U/kg bolus before PCI and then hourly boluses to keep ACT 300 to 350 seconds, or continuous infusion at 10 U/kg/hr without further ACT measurements), or low-dose heparin (70 U/kg and then 30 U/kg boluses during the procedure, or continuous infusion at 7 U/kg/hr without further ACT measurements). There was a separate randomization to early or late sheath removal. The early sheath-removal group had heparin discontinued immediately after PCI and sheaths removed at 6 hours, whereas the late group had heparin continued for 12 hours and sheaths removed 4 to 6 hours later. No difference was found between the groups in the incidence of ischemic events at 7 days. The early sheath-removal group had a smaller decrease in mean hemoglobin from baseline ($p = 0.03$), and nonsignificant trends occurred toward less minor non-CABG bleeding with low-dose heparin and early sheath removal.

67. **Kaluski E,** et al. Minimal heparinization in coronary angioplasty: how much heparin is really warranted? *Am J Cardiol* 2000;85:953–956.

Prospective, randomized, open study of 341 consecutive patients undergoing non-emergency PTCA. Patients received 2,500 U of unfractionated heparin before PTCA with the intention of no additional boluses. Mean ACT at 5 minutes was 185 seconds. Two in-hospital deaths and one Q-wave MI occurred. Six (2%) patients had abrupt coronary occlusion within 14 days after PTCA, requiring repeated TVR. Six-month clinical follow-up in 184 patients revealed three cardiac deaths (one arrhythmic, two after cardiac surgery), one Q-wave MI, and 9.7% repeated TVR. These results warrant larger, randomized, double-blind heparin dose-optimization studies.

Antithrombotic Regimens to Prevent Stent Thrombosis
68. **Schomig A,** et al. Intracoronary Stenting and Antithrombotic Regimen (**ISAR**). A randomized comparison of antiplatelet and anticoagulant therapy after the placement of coronary artery stents. *N Engl J Med* 1996;334:1084–1089.

Design: Prospective, randomized, open, multicenter study. Primary cardiac end points were cardiovascular death, MI, bypass surgery, and repeated target vessel intervention. Additional noncardiac end point was death from noncardiac causes, cerebrovascular accidents, severe hemorrhage, and peripheral vascular events.
Purpose: To compare the early outcome of patients given a combined antiplatelet regimen or conventional anticoagulation after coronary stent placement.
Population: 517 patients who underwent successful stenting.
Exclusion Criteria: Cardiogenic shock and stenting intended as a bridge to CABG surgery.
Treatment: Intravenous heparin for 12 hours; ticlopidine, 250 mg twice daily, and aspirin; or intravenous heparin for 5 to 10 days, phenprocoumon, and aspirin.
Results: At 30 days, the antiplatelet group had 75% fewer cardiac end points (1.6% vs. 6.2%), including a significant reduction in MI (0.8% vs. 4.2%; $p = 0.02$). The antiplatelet group had a 90% reduction in the primary noncardiac end point (1.2% vs. 12.3%; $p < 0.001$), including an 87% reduction in peripheral vascular events (0.8% vs. 6.2%; $p = 0.001$) and no bleeding complications (vs. 6.5%; $p < 0.001$). Antiplatelet therapy also was associated with 86% fewer stent reocclusions (0.8% vs. 5.4%; $p = 0.004$).

69. **Karrillon GJ,** et al. **French Multicenter Registry.** Intracoronary stent implantation without ultrasound guidance and with replacement of conventional anticoagulation by antiplatelet therapy. *Circulation* 1996;94:1519–1527.

The results of this large registry study of 2,900 patients confirm that the benefits of an antiplatelet regimen can be achieved without ultrasonographic guidance. Patients were treated with aspirin, 100 mg/day, and ticlopidine, 250 mg/day, for 1 month. Low-molecular-weight heparin use was reduced in four stages (1 month to none). At 1 month, the subacute closure rate was 1.8% (peak incidence at 5 to 8 days; 12 of 51 died), and the acute MI rate was 0.6%; CABG surgery was performed in 0.3%. A higher stent thrombosis rate was seen with balloons smaller than 3 mm ($\leq$2.5 mm, 10%; 3 mm, 2.3%; 3.5 mm, 1%), in bailout situations (6.7% vs. 1.4%), and in patients with unstable angina or acute MI (2.2% vs. 1.1%; $p = 0.02$).

70. **Goods CM,** et al. Comparison of aspirin alone versus aspirin and ticlopidine after coronary artery angioplasty stenting. *Am J Cardiol* 1996;78:1042–1044.

The results of this prospective, nonrandomized study show that aspirin alone is not an adequate antithrombotic regimen after stenting. Aspirin and ticlopidine were used in 338 patients, and aspirin alone, in only 46 patients. Inclusion criteria included adequate coverage of intimal dissections, absence of residual filling defects, and normal flow in the stented vessel at the end of the procedure. The aspirin and ticlopidine group had a significantly lower stent thrombosis rate (0.9% vs. 6.5%; $p = 0.02$), fewer deaths (0.3% vs. 4.4%; $p = 0.04$), and fewer Q-wave MIs (none vs. 6.5%; $p = 0.002$).

71. **Albiero M,** et al. Results of a consecutive series of patients receiving only antiplatelet therapy after optimized stent implantation: comparison of aspirin alone vs combined ticlopidine and aspirin therapy. *Circulation* 1997;95:1145–1156 (editorial, 1098–1100).

This analysis focused on 801 patients treated with antiplatelet therapy only (aspirin, $n = 264$; aspirin plus ticlopidine, $n = 537$). The first 575 patients were not randomized. At 1 month, no difference in subacute stent thrombosis (1.9% vs. 1.3%; $p = 0.5$) or major clinical events (1.9%, 2.0%) was observed. The combination therapy group had a higher discontinuation rate [1.9% (0.6% with neutropenia) vs. none; $p = 0.04$]. The accompanying editorial points out some weaknesses of this primarily observational study: six different stent types were used; the aspirin arm was smaller; and the use of antiplatelets for abrupt closure, acute MI, or with suboptimal results was not addressed.

72. **Bertrand ME,** et al. Full Anticoagulation versus Aspirin and Ticlopidine (**FANTASTIC**). Randomized multicenter comparison of conventional anticoagulation versus antiplatelet therapy in unplanned and elective coronary stenting. *Circulation* 1998;98:1597–1603.

Design: Prospective, randomized, multicenter study. Primary end point was bleeding and peripheral vascular complications. Secondary end points were death, MI, and stent occlusion.

Purpose: To compare the effects of aggressive antiplatelet treatment with anticoagulation after implantation of a Wiktor stent on bleeding rates and stent thrombosis rates.

Population: 485 patients undergoing elective (58%) or unplanned (42%) coronary stenting.

Exclusion Criteria: Platelet count less than 150,000, bleeding disorders, recent (less than 6 months) gastrointestinal bleeding, recent stroke, angiographic evidence of thrombus at target site, and allergy to aspirin or ticlopidine.

Treatment: Antiplatelet therapy with aspirin, 100 to 325 mg/day, and ticlopidine, 250 mg twice daily for 6 weeks [first dose (500 mg) given in catheterization laboratory], or anticoagulation with heparin (target activated partial thromboplastin time, 2.0 to 2.5 times control), and then warfarin for 6 weeks (target international normalized ratio, 2.5 to 3.0). The anticoagulation group also received aspirin. All patients received heparin, 10,000-U bolus before the procedure.

Results: Successful stent implantation was achieved in 99%. The antiplatelet group had fewer bleeding and peripheral vascular complications (13.5% vs. 21%; OR, 0.6; $p = 0.03$). Major cardiac events in electively stented patients were less common in the antiplatelet group (2.4% vs. 9.9%; OR, 0.23; $p = 0.01$). Antiplatelet patients had a shorter average hospital stay (4.3 vs. 6.4 days; $p = 0.0001$).

73. **Urban P,** et al. for the Multicenter Aspirin and Ticlopidine Trial after Intracoronary Stenting (**MATTIS**) investigators. Randomized evaluation of anticoagulation versus antiplatelet therapy after coronary stent implantation in high-risk patients. *Circulation* 1998;98:2126–2132.

Design: Prospective, randomized, multicenter study. Primary composite end point was cardiovascular death, MI, and repeated revascularization at 30 days.
Purpose: To compare antiplatelet therapy with anticoagulation in high-risk patients undergoing coronary stent implantation.
Population: 350 patients randomized within 6 hours of stent implantation who met the eligibility criteria: (a) stent(s) was placed to treat abrupt closure after balloon angioplasty; (b) suboptimal angiographic result was achieved; (c) the stented segment measured more than 45 mm (or was composed of three stents); (d) the vessel in question was small (i.e., largest balloon used was ≤2.5 mm). Eight different stent types were used by investigators.
Exclusion Criteria: Recent MI, persistent ischemia, administration of GP IIb/IIIa inhibitors before or during procedure, and intervention planned within 30-day follow-up period.
Treatment: Aspirin, 250 mg once daily, and ticlopidine, 250 mg twice daily for 30 days, or aspirin, 250 mg once daily, and oral anticoagulation (target international normalized ratio, 2.5 to 3.0).
Results: Antiplatelet group demonstrated a trend toward fewer cardiac end points (5.6% vs. 11%; $p = 0.07$) and significant reduction in major vascular and bleeding complications (1.7% vs. 6.9%; $p = 0.02$). The incidence of subacute stent thrombosis was not precisely known (no angiographic end point). In three patients (1.7%) treated with ticlopidine, asymptomatic agranulocytopenia developed.

74. **Leon MB,** et al. for the Stent Anticoagulation Restenosis Study (**STARS**) investigators. A clinical trial comparing three antithrombotic-drug regimens after coronary-artery stenting. *N Engl J Med* 1998;339:1665–1671.

Design: Prospective, randomized, open, multicenter study (50). The 30-day primary composite end point was death, MI, TLR, and angiographically evident thrombosis.
Purpose: To compare clinical outcomes for three antithrombotic regimens after elective coronary stenting.
Population: 1,653 patients who underwent successful stenting of a more than 60% stenosis in a native coronary artery with a diameter of 3 to 4 mm.
Exclusion Criteria: MI in prior 7 days, abciximab administration, and planned revascularization within 30 days.
Treatment: Aspirin, 325 mg daily; aspirin, 325 mg daily, and intravenous heparin followed by warfarin (target international normalized ratio, 2.0 to 2.5); or aspirin, 325 mg daily, and ticlopidine, 250 mg twice daily.
Results: Aspirin plus ticlopidine group had a significant reduction in the incidence of primary composite end points for aspirin and warfarin (0.5% vs. 2.7%) and for aspirin alone (3.6%; $p < 0.001$ for comparison of all three groups). Hemorrhagic and vascular surgical complications occurred less frequently with aspirin alone: 1.8% vs. 5.5% (aspirin plus ticlopidine), and 6.2% (aspirin and warfarin) and 0.4% versus 2.0% and 2.0%. No significant differences were observed in the incidences of neutropenia or thrombocytopenia (overall incidence, 0.3%).

75. **Steinbuhl SR,** et al. The duration of pretreatment with ticlopidine prior to stenting is associated with the risk of procedure-related non-Q-wave MIs. *J Am Coll Cardiol* 1998;32:1366–1380.

This retrospective study showed the benefits of beginning ticlopidine several days before stenting. Outcomes were analyzed in 175 consecutive patients treated with ticlopidine before stenting. Non–Q-wave MI was defined as CK greater than the upper limit of normal and the CK-MB fraction $\geq 4\%$. Longer duration of ticlopidine pretreatment was strongly associated with a lower incidence of procedure-related non–Q-wave MI: more than 1 day, 29%; 1 to 2 days, 14%; ≥ 3 days, 5% (χ^2 for trend 9.6; $p = 0.002$).

76. **Moussa I,** et al. Effectiveness of clopidogrel and aspirin versus ticlopidine and aspirin in preventing stent thrombosis after coronary stent implantation. *Circulation* 1999;99:2364–2366.

This observational study was composed of 1,689 patients undergoing coronary stent implantation; 1,406 received ticlopidine (500 mg loading dose, and then 250 mg twice daily) and aspirin (325 mg once daily), and 283 received clopidogrel (300 mg loading dose and then 75 mg once daily) and aspirin. Exclusion criteria included requirement for oral anticoagulation, abciximab administration, and procedural failure. At 1-month follow-up, the two groups had a similar incidence of stent thrombosis [1.5% (ticlopidine plus aspirin) vs. 1.4%] and MACEs (3.1% vs. 2.4%). The clopidogrel plus aspirin group had a significantly lower incidence of side effects, consisting of neutropenia, diarrhea, or rash (5.3% vs. 10.6%; RR 0.53; $p = 0.006$).

77. **Bertrand ME,** et al. Double-blind study of the safety of clopidogrel with and without a loading dose in combination with aspirin, compared with ticlopidine in combination with aspirin after coronary stenting: the Clopidogrel Aspirin Stent International Cooperative Study (**CLASSICS**). *Circulation* 2000;102:624–629.

Design: Prospective, randomized, double-blind, placebo-controlled, multicenter study. The primary end point was a composite of major peripheral or bleeding complications, neutropenia, thrombocytopenia, or early discontinuation of the drug because of a noncardiac event. Secondary end point was cardiac events, consisting of cardiovascular death, MI, or TVR.

Purpose: To demonstrate that clopidogrel has an efficacy similar to and better tolerability than ticlopidine.

Population: 1,020 patients who had undergone successful planned or unplanned coronary stenting (one or two stents) in a single-vessel (reference vessel diameter, more than 2.8 mm) with the use of any non–heparin-coated stent(s).

Exclusion Criteria: Included acute ST-elevation MI; CK $2 \times$ normal or greater; stent(s) in left main coronary artery, vein grafts, or at a major bifurcation; oral anticoagulants, GP IIb/IIIa–receptor antagonists or other antiplatelet agents, except for aspirin, in previous month (or required after the procedure); percutaneous or surgical revascularization (PTCA, CABG) in the previous 2 months.

Treatment: Ticlopidine, 250 mg twice daily for 4 weeks; clopidogrel, 75 mg once daily for 4 weeks; or clopidogrel, 300 mg loading dose followed by 75 mg once daily (days 2 to 28). All patients received aspirin, 325 mg once daily.

Results: The clopidogrel groups had a significantly lower incidence of the primary composite end point, which consisted of major bleeding, neutropenia, thrombocytopenia, and early discontinuation of therapy: 2.9% (loading dose group) and 6.4% [clopidogrel, 75 mg/day (all clopidogrel patients, 4.6%) vs. 9.1% for ticlopidine ($p = 0.005$)]. No significant differences were seen among the three groups in the incidence of the secondary end point (0.9%, 1.5%, and 1.2% of patients, respectively).

Comments: Clopidogrel appears to have superior safety and tolerability compared with ticlopidine and acceptable efficacy in the prevention of MACEs after coronary stenting. Although this study was not developed to determine efficacy, the results support the use of clopidogrel as an alternative to ticlopidine after coronary stenting.

78. **PCI-CURE** (Clopidogrel in Unstable angina to prevent Recurrent ischemic Events), Mehta SR, et al. Effects of pretreatment with clopidogrel and aspirin followed by long-term therapy in patients undergoing percutaneous coronary intervention: the PCI-CURE study. *Lancet* 2001;358:527–533.

Design: Prospective, randomized, placebo-controlled, double-blinded, multicenter trial. Primary end point was 30-day composite of cardiovascular death, MI, or urgent TVR and cardiovascular death or MI to end of trial. Mean follow-up was 8 months.

Purpose: To determine if pretreatment with clopidogrel before PCI would be superior to placebo in preventing major ischemic events after PCI and if long-term treatment with clopidogrel for up to 1 year after PCI would result in additional benefit.

Population: 2,658 patients with mean age 61 years and acute coronary syndromes who were hospitalized within 24 hours of onset of symptoms. ECG evidence of new ischemia (but less than 1-mm ST elevation) or elevated concentrations of cardiac enzymes ($2\times$ normal or more) was required.

Exclusion Criteria: Contraindications to antithrombotic or antiplatelet therapy, high bleeding risk, NYHA class IV heart failure, need for oral anticoagulation, coronary revascularization in previous 3 months, GP IIb/IIIa–receptor inhibitors in previous 3 days.

Treatment: Clopidogrel, 300 mg loading dose, or matching placebo followed by 75 mg clopidogrel, or matching placebo once daily for 3 to 12 months (mean, 9 months). Patients underwent PCI at a mean 10 days after randomization. All received aspirin, 75 to 325 mg once daily. The use of GP IIb/IIIa–receptor antagonists was discouraged but allowed during PCI.

Results: Before PCI, the clopidogrel group had a lower incidence of MI or refractory ischemia compared with placebo (12.% vs. 15.3%; RR, 0.76; $p = 0.008$). At 30 days after PCI, the clopidogrel group had a lower incidence in the primary composite outcome of cardiovascular death, MI, or urgent revascularization (4.5% vs. 6.4%; RR, 0.70; $p = 0.03$). Long-term administration of clopidogrel after PCI was associated with a lower rate of the composite end point ($p = 0.03$) and cardiovascular death or MI ($p = 0.047$). Including events before and after PCI, the clopidogrel group was associated with a 31% lower incidence of cardiovascular death or MI (8.8% vs. 12.6%; $p = 0.002$; see Fig. 2.3). Clopidogrel use was associated with similar rate of major bleeding compared with placebo.

79. **Steinbuhl R,** et al. Ticlopidine pretreatment before coronary stenting is associated with sustained decrease in adverse cardiac events: data from the evaluation of platelet IIb/IIIa Inhibitor for Stenting (**EPISTENT**) Trial. *Circulation* 2001;103:1403–1409.

Design: Nonrandomized, multicenter study. Primary composite end points were all-cause mortality, nonfatal MI, or urgent revascularization at 30 days, and at 1 year, all-cause mortality, MI, and TVR.

Purpose: To determine whether pretreatment with ticlopidine before coronary stenting results in a sustained reduction in adverse cardiac events.

Population: Included 1,603 patients enrolled in the EPISTENT trial who were randomized to either placebo or abciximab. Of these, 932 patients received pretreatment with ticlopidine before stenting, at the discretion of the investigator.

Exclusion Criteria: see EPISTENT trial.

Treatment: Abciximab (bolus and 12-hour infusion) and stenting, placebo and stenting, or abciximab and balloon angioplasty. Investigators were encouraged to treat all patients with ticlopidine according to their usual practice before stenting. All were pretreated with aspirin.

Results: Among patients randomized to placebo, ticlopidine pretreatment was associated with a significant decrease in death, MI, or TVR at 1 year (adjusted HR, 0.73; 95% CI, 0.54 to 0.98; $p = 0.036$). At 30-day follow-up, the primary end point had occurred in 13.4% of patients in the no-abciximab or ticlopidine group, 8.9% of patients in the placebo + ticlopidine group, 5.5% of patients in the abciximab/no-ticlopidine group ($p = 0.028$ vs. placebo and plus ticlopidine) and 5.2% of patients in the abciximab + ticlopidine group. The benefit of pretreatment with ticlopidine in the placebo group was primarily attributable to a lower incidence of MI (8.4% vs. 12.5%; $p = 0.048$). At 1 year, fewer primary events occurred in the placebo group in patients pretreated with ticlopidine compared with patients not pretreated with ticlopidine (20.7% vs. 28.5%; $p = 0.008$), whereas no difference was related to pretreatment with ticlopidine in the abciximab group (19.5% for abciximab + ticlopidine vs. 20.9% for abciximab/no ticlopidine). Controlling for patient characteristics and for the propensity to use ticlopidine, Cox regression model identified ticlopidine pretreatment as an independent predictor of the need for TVR at 1 year (hazard ratio, 0.62; 95% CI, 0.43 to 0.89; $p = 0.01$) in both placebo-treated and abciximab-treated patients. By multivariate modeling, however, the beneficial effect of ticlopidine on TVR was diminished by treatment with abciximab.

Comments: Duration of pretreatment with ticlopidine was uncertain. Beneficial effect of ticlopidine in placebo-treated group may have been due to an antiplatelet effect in aspirin-resistant patients.

80. **Taniuchi M,** et al. Randomized comparison of ticlopidine and clopidogrel after intracoronary stent implantation in a broad patient population. *Circulation* 2001;104:539–543.

Design: Prospective, randomized, double-blind, placebo-controlled, parallel-group study. Primary end point was failure to complete the 2-week therapy.

Purpose: To determine the relative safety of a 2-week treatment with clopidogrel plus aspirin compared with ticlopidine plus aspirin in patients undergoing coronary stenting.

Population: 1,067 patients who had undergone successful stent implantation

Exclusion Criteria: Known intolerance to aspirin, ticlopidine, or clopidogrel.

Treatment: Loading dose of ticlopidine, 500 mg, followed by ticlopidine, 250 mg b.i.d., plus aspirin, 325 mg/day, for 14 days (522 patients), or a loading dose of clopidogrel, 300 mg, followed by clopidogrel, 75 mg/day, plus aspirin, 325 mg/day, for 14 days (494 patients).

Results: The primary end point occurred in 3.64% of patients in the ticlopidine group and in 1.62% of patients in the clopidogrel loading-dose group ($p = 0.04$). The most common adverse event requiring ticlopidine discontinuation was rash (0.96% in the ticlopidine group and 0.2% in the clopidogrel group). No significant differences were noted in rates of thrombocytopenia (0.57% in the ticlopidine group and 1.01% in the clopidogrel group) and neutropenia (0.38% and none, respectively). A trend toward a higher incidence of cardiac death was found in the ticlopidine group (1.53% vs. 0.61%), whereas the incidence of stent thrombosis was similar among the two groups (2.02% vs. 1.92%). The majority of stent thrombosis occurred during the first 8 days of treatment, whereas only one event per group occurred after the 2-week treatment period. At 30-day follow-up, the incidence of MACE was 4.6% in the ticlopidine group and 3.85% in the clopidogrel group.

81. **Bhatt DL,** et al. Meta-analysis of randomized and registry comparisons of ticlopidine with clopidogrel after stenting. *J Am Coll Cardiol* 2002;39:9–14.

Data were pooled and analyzed from published trials and registries comparing clopidogrel with ticlopidine in a total of 13,955 patients undergoing stenting. The pooled rate of MACEs was 2.10% in the clopidogrel group and 4.04% in the ticlopidine group. After adjustment for trial heterogeneity, the OR for ischemic events was lower with clopidogrel compared with ticlopidine (95% CI, 0.59 to 0.89; $p = 0.002$). The clopidogrel group also had a significantly lower mortality compared with the ticlopidine group (0.48% vs. 1.09%; OR, 0.55; 95% CI, 0.37 to 0.82; $p = 0.003$). The authors note that these findings may be due to the more rapid onset of an antiplatelet effect with the loading dose of clopidogrel, which was used in most of these studies, or to better patient compliance with clopidogrel therapy.

82. **Hongo RH,** et al. The effect of clopidogrel in combination with aspirin when given before coronary artery bypass grafting. *J Am Coll Cardiol* 2002;40:231–237.

This nonrandomized observational study of 224 consecutive patients undergoing nonemergency first-time CABG compared those with preoperative clopidogrel exposure within 7 days ($n = 59$) with those without exposure ($n = 165$). Groups had comparable baseline characteristics. The clopidogrel group had higher 24-hour mean chest tube output (1.2 L vs. 0.84 L; $p = 0.001$) and more transfusions of red blood cells (2.51 U vs. 1.74 U; $p = 0.036$), platelets (0.86 U vs. 0.24 U; $p = 0.001$), and fresh frozen plasma (0.68 U vs. 0.24 U; $p = 0.015$). Reoperation for bleeding was tenfold higher in clopidogrel group (6.8% vs. 0.6%; $p = 0.018$). The clopidogrel group also had a trend toward less hospital discharge within 5 days (33.9% vs. 46.7%; $p = 0.094$).

83. **Steinhubl SR,** et al. for the Clopidogrel in Unstable angina to Prevent Recurrent Events **CREDO** Investigators. Early and sustained dual oral antiplatelet therapy following percutaneous coronary intervention. *JAMA* 2002;288:2411–2420.

Design: Prospective, randomized, double-blind, placebo-controlled, multicenter study. Primary end points were death, MI, or stroke at 1 year, and death, MI, or urgent TVR at 28 days in the per-protocol population.
Purpose: To evaluate long-term treatment (1 year) with clopidogrel after elective PCI and initiation of clopidogrel with a preprocedure loading dose, both in addition to aspirin therapy.
Population: 2,116 patients scheduled to undergo elective PCI or deemed at high likelihood of undergoing PCI.
Exclusion Criteria: Included contraindications to antithrombotic/antiplatelet therapy; failed PCI in previous 2 weeks; coronary anatomy not amenable to stenting or greater than 50% left main stenosis; planned staged procedure; administration of the following medications before randomization: GP IIb/IIIa inhibitors (within 7 days), clopidogrel (10 days), thrombolytics (24 hours).
Treatment: Clopidogrel loading dose (300 mg), or placebo, 3 to 24 hours before PCI. All patients then received clopidogrel, 75 mg/day, through day 28. From day 29 through 12 months, loading-dose patients received clopidogrel, 75 mg/day, and control patients received placebo. Both groups received aspirin throughout the study. GP IIb/IIIa inhibitors were administered in 45% of the per-protocol population. PCI was performed in 86%.
Results: At 1 year, long-term clopidogrel therapy was associated with a 26.9% relative reduction in death, MI, or stroke [8.5% vs. 11.5% (placebo); $p = 0.02$]. Although not a prespecified analysis, a further 37.4% relative reduction in major events occurred from day 29 to 1 year with clopidogrel ($p = 0.04$). At 28 days, clopidogrel pretreatment was associated with a nonsignificant 18.5% relative reduction in death, MI, or urgent TVR (6.8% vs. 8.3%; $p = 0.23$). However, in a prespecified subgroup analysis, those given clopidogrel at least 6 hours before PCI had a significant 38.6% RR reduction ($p = 0.05$) compared with no reduction with treatment less than 6 hours before PCI. Among those receiving a GP IIb/IIIa inhibitor and clopidogrel pretreatment, a 30% reduction in events was found [7.3% vs. 10.3% (no pretreatment, GP IIb/IIIa); $p = 0.12$]. A trend toward a higher incidence of major bleeding was found with clopidogrel (at 1 year, 8.8% vs. 6.7%; $p = 0.07$).
Comments: This trial, together with CURE and PCI-CURE, support long-term use of clopidogrel plus aspirin post PCI.

Glycoprotein IIb/IIIa Inhibitors

84. Evaluation of 7E3 for the Prevention of Ischemic Complications (**EPIC**). Use of a monoclonal antibody directed vs platelet glycoprotein IIb/IIIa receptor in high-risk percutaneous transluminal coronary angioplasty. *N Engl J Med* 1994;330:956–961.

Design: Prospective, randomized, double-blind, multicenter study. The 30-day primary composite end point was death, MI, CABG surgery, repeated PCI for acute ischemia, and stenting due to procedural failure, or placement of an intraaortic balloon pump.
Purpose: To determine whether the monoclonal antibody c7E3 Fab provides clinical benefit in patients undergoing coronary angioplasty or atherectomy.
Population: 2,099 high-risk patients, defined as having experienced acute MI with onset of symptoms within previous 12 hours, two episodes of postinfarct angina within previous 24 hours with ECG changes, or high-risk clinical or angiographic features, who underwent percutaneous intervention (PTCA, 90%; directional atherectomy, 5%; both, 5%).
Exclusion Criteria: Included bleeding diathesis, major surgery in prior 6 weeks, and stroke in prior 2 years.

Treatment: Abciximab, 0.25 mg/kg intravenous bolus (started 10 minutes before procedure), and then 10 μg/min infusion for 12 hours, abciximab or placebo. All patients received heparin (10,000- to 12,000-U bolus; target ACT, 300 to 350 seconds).

Results: Abciximab bolus plus infusion group had 35% fewer end points (death, MI, unplanned surgical revascularization, repeated percutaneous procedure, need for intraaortic balloon pump): 12.8% versus 11.4% (bolus only; $p = 0.43$) and 8.3% (placebo; $p = 0.008$). A significant reduction was observed in the MI rate only: 5.2% versus 8.6% for placebo ($p = 0.013$). Abciximab was associated with more bleeding episodes: 14% versus 7% ($p = 0.001$). Follow-up studies have shown abciximab to be associated with persistent significant reductions at 6 months (27% vs. 35.1%; $p = 0.001$; see *Lancet* 1994;343:881) and 3 years [41.1% vs. 47.4% (bolus only) and 47.2% (placebo), $p = 0.009$; see *JAMA* 1997;278:479]. Three-year follow-up also showed that the subgroup of patients with an evolving MI or refractory unstable angina (28% of patients) had a significant 60% reduction in mortality rate (5.1% vs. 12.7%; $p = 0.01$).

Comments: Significant bleeding likely was due to high heparin dosing.

85. Integrelin to Minimise Platelet Aggregation and Coronary Thrombosis II (**IMPACT II**). Randomised placebo-controlled trial of effect of eptifibatide on complications of percutaneous coronary intervention: IMPACT-II. *Lancet* 1997;349:1422–1428 (editorial, 1409–1410).

Design: Prospective, randomized, double-blind, multicenter study. The 30-day primary composite end point was death, MI, unplanned surgical or repeated percutaneous revascularization, or stenting for abrupt closure.

Purpose: To determine the effectiveness of eptifibatide in reducing ischemic complications in patients undergoing nonsurgical coronary revascularization.

Population: 4,010 patients who underwent elective, urgent, or emergency percutaneous intervention (PTCA, 91% to 93%).

Exclusion Criteria: Bleeding diathesis, major surgery in prior 6 weeks, and any history of stroke.

Treatment: Eptifibatide, 135 μg/kg intravenous bolus (10 to 60 minutes before procedure), and then 0.5 or 0.75 μg/kg/min for 20 to 24 hours; or placebo.

Results: At 30 days, a nonsignificant reduction in the primary composite end point was observed: 9.2% (135/0.5 group) and 9.9% (135/0.75 group) versus 11.4% (placebo) ($p = 0.063, 0.22$). On-treatment analysis showed that the 135/0.5 group had a significant 22% reduction in composite primary end point (9.1% vs. 11.6%; $p = 0.035$). No significant differences in bleeding or transfusion rates were observed.

86. c7E3 Fab Antiplatelet Therapy in Unstable Refractory Angina (**CAPTURE**). Randomized, placebo-controlled trial of abciximab before and during coronary intervention in refractory unstable angina: the CAPTURE study. *Lancet* 1997;349:1429–1435 (editorial 1409–1410).

Design: Prospective, randomized, placebo-controlled, multicenter study. The 30-day primary end point was death, MI, or urgent intervention for recurrent ischemia.

Purpose: To assess whether abciximab given before and until briefly after PCI improves outcome in patients with refractory unstable angina.

Population: 1,265 patients with chest pain at rest with ST-segment depression or elevation or abnormal T waves, with one or more episodes (rest pain and/or ECG changes) occurring more than 2 hours after the start of intravenous heparin and nitrate therapy.

Exclusion Criteria: Recent MI, persisting ischemia that required immediate intervention, and left main stenosis as shown by angiography.

Treatment: After angiography, patients were randomized to abciximab (0.25 mg/kg bolus, and then 10 μg/min) or placebo for 18 to 24 hours before and 1 hour after PCI (balloon angioplasty with stenting only if necessary to maintain vessel patency). Goal ACT was 300 seconds.

Results: Trial was stopped early because of significant treatment effect (1,400 patients planned). The abciximab group had a 29% reduction in 30-day primary end points of death, MI, and ischemia requiring intervention (11.3% vs. 15.9%; $p = 0.012$). Most of this difference was due to fewer MIs (defined as CK or CK-MB 3 times the upper limit of normal in two samples): 4.1% vs. 8.2% ($p = 0.002$). MIs occurred less frequently before and after PTCA in abciximab patients (0.6% vs. 2.1%; $p = 0.029$; 2.6% vs. 5.5%, $p = 0.043$). Importantly, no difference in event rates was seen at 6 months (31% vs. 30.8%). A twofold higher major bleeding rate was observed in the abciximab group (3.8% vs. 1.9%; $p = 0.043$). An ECG ischemia substudy (332 patients monitored from start of treatment to 6 hours after intervention) showed that the abciximab group had a lower incidence of two episodes of significant ($\geq$1 mm) ST segment deviation (5% vs. 14%; $p < 0.01$) (see *Circulation* 1998;98:1358).

Comments: In contrast to other studies, patients given abciximab for a substantial period before intervention and only briefly afterward had a reduction in events during the 18- to 24-hour interval before intervention. Lack of long-term benefits is likely owing to lack of 12-hour postintervention infusion.

87. Evaluation in PTCA to Improve Long-term Outcome with Abciximab Glycoprotein IIb/IIIa Blockade (**EPILOG**) investigators. Platelet glycoprotein IIb/IIIa receptor blockade and low-dose heparin during percutaneous coronary revascularization. *N Engl J Med* 1997;336:1689–1696 (editorial 1748–1749).

Design: Prospective, randomized, double-blind, multicenter study. Thirty-day composite primary end point was death, MI, ischemia requiring urgent coronary bypass surgery, or repeated percutaneous coronary revascularization.

Purpose: To determine whether the clinical benefits of abciximab extend to all patients undergoing coronary intervention and to evaluate whether hemorrhagic complications are reduced by adjusting heparin dosing.

Population: 2,792 patients undergoing urgent or elective revascularization.

Exclusion Criteria: Acute MI or unstable angina with ECG changes in prior 24 hours, planned stenting or atherectomy, PCI in prior 3 months, anticoagulant therapy, major surgery or bleeding in prior 6 weeks.

Treatment: Abciximab [0.25 mg/kg intravenous bolus (10 to 60 minutes before procedure), and then 0.125 μg/kg/min for 12 hours] plus heparin (100 U/kg bolus), abciximab plus heparin, 70 U/kg, or placebo plus heparin, 100 U/kg.

Results: Abciximab groups had lower 30-day incidences of death, MI, and urgent revascularization: 5.4% and 5.2% versus 11.7% (OR, 0.45, 0.43; both $p < 0.001$). Fewer large non–Q-wave MIs also were observed (CK 5 times normal): 2.5% and 2% versus 5.6% ($p < 0.001$). Similar major bleeding rates were observed, but abciximab plus standard heparin was associated with more minor bleeds [7.4% vs. 4% (low heparin); $p < 0.001$]. At 6 months, similar rates of repeated revascularization and a smaller reduction in composite end points were observed (death, MI, and any revascularization): 22.3% and 22.8% versus 25.8% ($p = 0.04$). One-year follow-up showed persistent benefit in abciximab groups (incidences of primary end points were 9.6% and 9.5% in abciximab plus low-dose heparin and abciximab plus standard heparin groups, respectively, vs. 16.1% in placebo group; see *Circulation* 1999; 99:1951).

Comments: In an effort to reduce bleeding rates, sheaths were removed as soon as possible, and no routine postprocedural heparin was administered.

88. Randomized Efficacy Study of Tirofiban for Outcomes and Restenosis (**RE-STORE**) Investigators. Effects of platelet GP IIb/IIIa blockade with tirofiban on adverse cardiac events in patients with unstable angina or acute MI undergoing coronary angioplasty. *Circulation* 1997;96:1445–1453.

Design: Prospective, randomized, double-blind, placebo-controlled, multicenter study. Primary composite end point was death, MI, CABG due to failed PTCA or recurrent ischemia, repeated PTCA of target vessel due to ischemia or stenting for actual or threatened abrupt closure.

Purpose: To evaluate the effectiveness of tirofiban in patients undergoing high-risk coronary interventions.

Population: 2,139 patients seen within 72 hours of onset of symptoms with a 60% stenosis.

Exclusion Criteria: Included scheduled stenting or adjunctive rotablation.

Treatment: Tirofiban (10 μg/kg intravenous bolus over 3 minutes and then 0.15 μg/kg/min for 36 hours) or placebo. All patients were taking aspirin and heparin.

Results: For the initial procedure, PTCA was performed in 92% to 93%, and atherectomy in 7% to 8% of patients. At 30 days, a similar incidence of primary composite end points was observed (10.3% vs. 12.2%; $p = 0.16$). If only urgent/emergency CABG and PTCA are included, the rates are 8% versus 10.5% ($p = 0.052$). However, the tirofiban group had significantly fewer events at 2 days and 7 days (RR, 0.62; $p = 0.005$; RR, 0.73, $p = 0.022$), mostly because of less reinfarction and repeated PTCA [at 2 days, 2.7% vs. 4.4% ($p = 0.039$) and 1.1% vs. 3.2% ($p = 0.001$); at 7 days, 3.6% vs. 5.3% ($p = 0.055$) and 2.7% vs. 4.4% ($p = 0.034$)]. Similar rates of major bleeding and thrombocytopenia were observed [5.3% vs. 3.7% ($p = 0.096$) and 1.1% vs. 0.9%].

89. Evaluation of Platelet IIb/IIIa Inhibitor for Stenting (**EPISTENT**) Investigators. Randomized placebo-controlled and balloon-angioplasty-controlled trial to assess safety of coronary stenting with use of platelet glycoprotein IIb/IIIa blockade. *Lancet* 1998;352:87–92.

Design: Prospective, randomized, double-blind, placebo-controlled multicenter study. Primary composite end point was death, MI, and urgent revascularization at 30 days.

Purpose: To evaluate the effects of platelet GP IIb/IIIa blockade with abciximab in conjunction with elective coronary stenting in patients with 60% coronary lesions.

Population: 2,399 patients with ischemic heart disease and suitable coronary artery lesions (e.g., stenosis $\geq$60%).

Exclusion Criteria: Unprotected left main stenosis, stroke within prior 2 years, PCI in past 3 months, systolic blood pressure (SBP) greater than 180 mm Hg, and diastolic blood pressure (DBP) greater than 100 mm Hg.

Treatment: Stent plus placebo, stent plus abciximab [0.25 mg/kg bolus up to 60 minutes before intervention, and then 0.125 μg/kg/min (maximum, 10 μg/min) for 12 hours], or balloon angioplasty plus abciximab. All patients were given aspirin and heparin (70 U/kg and 100 U/kg boluses in abciximab and placebo groups, respectively). Ticlopidine administration before enrollment was encouraged.

Results: Stent plus abciximab group had more than 50% reduction in 30-day composite end points compared with the stent plus placebo group (5.3% vs. 10.8%; $p < 0.01$), whereas the balloon angioplasty plus abciximab group had a 36% reduction (6.9%; $p = 0.007$). Death and large MIs (defined as CK greater than 5 times normal) occurred less frequently in the abciximab groups [3.0% and 4.7% vs. 7.8% (placebo)]. However, the rates of Q-wave MI were similar (0.9% to 1.5%). No significant differences were seen in major bleeding complications (1.4% to 2.2%).

90. **Lincoff AM,** et al. Complementary clinical benefits of coronary-artery stenting and blockade of platelet glycoprotein IIb/IIa receptors. *N Engl J Med* 1999;341:319–327.

This report of the 6-month EPISTENT results demonstrates persistent benefits of stenting in combination with abciximab. The incidence of composite end points was 6.4% in the stent plus abciximab group, 9.2% in the angioplasty plus abciximab group, and 12.1% in the stent-alone group. The mortality rate with stent plus abciximab also was significantly lower than that with angioplasty plus abciximab [0.5% vs 1.8%; $p = 0.02$ (stent alone: 1.2%, $p = 0.12$)]. This mortality benefit persisted at 1 year.

91. Evaluation of Oral Xemilofiban in Controlling Thrombotic Events (**EXCITE**). Results presented at the 48th ACC Scientific Session in New Orleans, LA: March 1999.

This prospective, randomized, double-blind, multicenter trial was composed of 7,232 patients with stable angina (43%), unstable angina (45%) or MI more than 24 hours earlier who had undergone successful PTC revascularization (PTCR) of a more than 70% stenosis. Patients received xemilofiban, 20 mg, 20 to 90 minutes before PTCR (stents placed in 70%), and then 10 or 20 mg 3 times daily for 6 months, or placebo. At 6-month follow-up, the treatment groups had a similar incidence of the primary composite end point, consisting of death, MI, and urgent revascularization: 9.1% for placebo; 9.3% for xemilofiban, 10 mg; and 8.2% for xemilofiban, 20 mg [$p = 0.238$ (placebo vs. xemilofiban, 20 mg)].

92. ReoPro Readministration Registry (**R3**). *Circulation* 1998;98:(abstr suppl):I-17.

This multicenter registry (22 U.S. sites) was designed to evaluate the repeated use of abciximab as an adjunct to coronary intervention. Approximately 2% of the screened patients (500 of 23,454 angioplasty cases) were included in the analysis.

No significant differences were observed in the incidence of adverse allergic and clinical events at baseline and 2 months and the incidence of thrombocytopenia.

93. The **ESPRIT** Investigators. Novel dosing regimen of eptifibatide in planned coronary stent implantation (ESPRIT): a randomised, placebo-controlled trial. *Lancet* 2000;356:2037–2044.

Design: Prospective, randomized, double-blind, placebo-controlled, multicenter study. Primary end point was death, MI, urgent TVR, and thrombotic bailout GP IIb/IIIa inhibitor therapy within 48 hours. Secondary end point was a composite of death, MI, and urgent TVR at 30 days.
Purpose: To determine whether double-bolus dosing of eptifibatide can improve outcomes of patients undergoing coronary stenting.
Population: 2,064 patients scheduled to undergo stent implantation.
Exclusion Criteria: These included ongoing chest pain necessitating urgent PCI, MI in prior 24 hours, PCI in prior 90 days, or planned staged PCI within 30 days, stroke or transient ischemic attack (TIA) in prior month, bleeding diathesis, major surgery in prior 6 weeks, SBP greater than 200 mm Hg or DBP greater than 110 mm Hg, platelet count less than 100,000, Cr greater than 350 μM.
Treatment: Placebo or eptifibatide (two 180 μg/kg boluses 10 minutes apart, and then 2 μg/kg/min for 18 to 24 hours). Bailout blinded GP IIb/IIIa receptor was available.
Results: The eptifibatide group had a significantly lower incidence of the primary composite end point (6.4% vs. 10.5%; $p = 0.0015$). This benefit was consistent across different components of the primary end point, including death/MI/TVR (RR, 0.65; 95% CI, 0.47 to 0.87), death/MI (RR, 0.60; CI, 0.44 to 0.82), and death (RR, 0.5; CI, 0.05 to 5.42). At 30 days, the eptifibatide group also had a reduction in the secondary end point of death, MI, and urgent TVR (6.8% vs. 10.5%; $p = 0.0034$). Eptifibatide group did have a higher incidence of major bleeding compared with placebo (1.3% vs. 0.4%; $p = 0.027$). No significant differences in major bleeding were found in the lowest tercile of ACT (ACT less than 244 seconds; 0.6% in both groups). At 6-month follow-up, the composite end point of death or MI had occurred in 7.5% of eptifibatide-treated patients and 11.5% of placebo-treated patients (RR, 0.63; 95% CI, 0.47 to 0.84; $p = 0.002$), whereas the composite of death, MI, or TVR had occurred in 14.2% and 18.2% of patients, respectively (RR, 0.75; 95% CI, 0.60 to 0.93). The 6-month mortality rate was 0.8% in the eptifibatide group and 1.4% in the placebo group (RR, 0.56; 95% CI, 0.24 to 1.34; $p = 0.19$). Kaplan-Meier survival curves appeared to separate over time, with most of the difference in mortality occurring between 30 days and 6 months (see *JAMA* 2001;285:2468–2473). At 1-year follow-up, the significant difference continued to persist (6.6% vs. 10.5%; $p = 0.015$), and a cost analysis found eptifibatide use associated with $1,407 per year of life saved (see *JAMA* 2002;287:618).
Comments: The persistent benefit observed at 6 and 12 months further supports the use of GP IIb/IIIa–receptor blockers as standard of care for patients undergoing stent implantation.

94. **Topol EJ**, et al. for the **TARGET** Investigators. Comparison of two platelet glycoprotein IIb/IIIa inhibitors, tirofiban and abciximab, for the prevention of

ischemic events with percutaneous coronary revascularization. *N Engl J Med* 2001;344:1888–1894.

Design: Prospective, randomized, double-blind, double-dummy, multicenter study. Primary end points: death, nonfatal MI, or urgent TVR at 30 days.

Purpose: To compare the safety and efficacy of the two GP IIb/IIIa inhibitors, tirofiban and abciximab.

Population: 5,308 patients scheduled for coronary stenting with greater than 70% stenoses in either *de novo* or restenotic lesions in native coronary arteries or bypass grafts.

Exclusion Criteria: Cardiogenic shock, acute STEMI, serum creatinine 2.5 mg/dL or greater, high risk for bleeding or ongoing bleeding, platelet count less than 120,000.

Treatment: Tirofiban (10 μg/kg bolus, and then 0.15 μg/kg/min for 18 to 24 hours) or abciximab [0.25 mg/kg bolus and then 0.125 μg/kg/min (maximum, 10 μg/min) for 12 hours]. All received preprocedure aspirin (250 to 500 mg). Clopidogrel loading dose (300 mg) was given, when possible, 2 to 6 hours before PCI and then continued for 30 days (75 mg once daily). All were given initial heparin bolus of 70 U/kg, with a target ACT of 250 seconds.

Results: In both groups, 95% underwent stenting. The abciximab group had a significantly lower incidence of the primary composite end point of death, nonfatal MI, or urgent TVR compared with the tirofiban group (6.0% vs. 7.6%; $p = 0.038$). The abciximab group had fewer MIs (CK-MB, 3 times or more upper limit of normal or new Q waves; 5.4% vs. 6.9%; $p = 0.04$), whereas no significant differences were found between the two groups in 30-day mortality (0.4% vs. 0.5%; $p = 0.66$) or urgent TVR (0.7% vs. 0.8%; $p = 0.49$). Subgroup analysis showed superiority of abciximab in all subgroups, including age (younger than 65 or 65 years or older), gender, diabetes, and clopidogrel pretreatment. No significant differences were seen between the two groups in major bleeding complications or transfusions [0.7% (abciximab) vs. 0.9%; $p = $ NS], but tirofiban was associated with lower rates of minor bleeding episodes (2.8% vs. 4.3%; $p < 0.001$) and thrombocytopenia (less than 100,000/mm^3; 0.1% vs. 0.9%; $p < 0.001$). At 6 months, however, no significant difference were found between the groups in the incidence of the primary composite end point (14.8% vs. 14.3%; $p = 0.59$) (see *Lancet* 2002;360:355–360).

Comments: Two studies found the TARGET tirofiban dosing results in lower platelet inhibition levels compared those with abciximab, especially from 15 to 60 minutes after drug administration, which typically coincides with iatrogenic vessel injury (see *Am J Cardiol* 2002;89:647, 1293).

95. **PRICE** Investigators. Comparative 30-day economic and clinical outcomes of platelet glycoprotein IIb/IIIa inhibitor use during elective percutaneous coronary intervention: Prairie ReoPro versus Integrilin Cost Evaluation (PRICE) Trial. *Am Heart J* 2001;141:402–409.

Prospective, randomized, double-blind study of 320 consecutive patients undergoing elective PTCA or stenting. Patients received adjunctive abciximab or eptifibatide therapy. The eptifibatide group had lower total in-hospital costs (primary end point) compared with the abciximab group (median, $7,207 vs. $8,268; $p = 0.009$). The eptifibatide group also had lower median costs at 30 days ($7,207 vs. $8,336; $p = 0.009$). No significant differences were found between the groups in incidence of death, nonfatal MI, and urgent revascularization [4.9% vs. 5.1% (hospital discharge), 5.6% vs. 6.3% (30 days)]. In a platelet-inhibition substudy (155 patients; Ultegra Rapid Platelet Function Assay), eptifibatide was associated with earlier and more durable platelet inhibition compared with abciximab ($p < 0.00001$).

Thrombin Inhibitors

96. **Bittl A,** et al. Hirulog Angioplasty Study investigators (**HAS**). Treatment with bivalirudin (hirulog) as compared with heparin during coronary angioplasty for unstable or postinfarction angina. *N Engl J Med* 1995;333:764–769 (also see *Am Heart J* 2001;142:952–959).

Design: Prospective, randomized, double-blind, multicenter study. Primary composite end point was death in hospital, MI, abrupt vessel closure, or rapid clinical deterioration of cardiac origin. Follow-up period was 6 months.

Purpose: To evaluate whether bivalirudin is more effective than heparin in reducing mortality and ischemic events in unstable or postinfarction angina patients undergoing angioplasty.

Population: 4,098 patients undergoing coronary angioplasty (PTCA) for unstable angina or postinfarct angina.

Treatment: Bivalirudin, 1.0 mg/kg bolus, and then 2.5 mg/kg/hr for 4 hours and 1.0 mg/kg/hr for 14 to 20 hours, or heparin, 175 U/kg bolus, and then 15 U/kg/hr for 18 to 24 hours. Agents were started immediately before angioplasty, and doses were adjusted according to ACTs. All patients received aspirin (300 to 325 mg daily).

Results: Overall, no significant difference occurred between the groups in the incidence of the primary composite end point at 6 months (11.4% vs. 12.2%). At 7 days, however, fewer events were found in the bivalirudin group (6.2% vs. 7.9%; $p = 0.039$). Among postinfarction angina patients, bivalirudin was associated with a significant reduction in composite end points (9.1% vs. 14.2%; $p = 0.04$), although at 6 months, the cumulative rates of death, MI, and repeated revascularization were similar (20.5% vs. 25.1%; $p = 0.1$). Bivalirudin was associated with decreased bleeding (3.8% vs. 9.8%; $p < 0.001$).

97. **Lincoff AM,** et al. Bivalirudin with planned or provisional abciximab versus low-dose heparin and abciximab during percutaneous coronary revascularization: results of the Comparison of Abciximab Complications with Hirulog for Ischemic Events Trial (**CACHET**). *Am Heart J* 2002;143:847–853.

This pilot study evaluated bivalirudin for the first time with stenting or in combination with GP IIb/IIIa antagonists. A total of 268 PCI patients who were randomized in three sequential phases to bivalirudin [1.0 mg/kg bolus, and then 2.5 mg/kg/hr for 4 hours plus abciximab (phase A), 0.5-mg/kg bolus, and then infusion of 1.75 mg/kg/hr for procedure duration plus provisional ("rescue") abciximab (phase B), or 0.75-mg/kg bolus, and then 1.75 mg/kg/hr for procedure duration plus provisional abciximab (phase C)] OR to control regimen of low-dose weight-adjusted heparin with abciximab. Provisional abciximab was used in 24% of phase B and C patients. The composite end point of death, MI, repeated revascularization, or major bleeding at 7 days occurred in 3.3%, 5.9%, none, and 10.6% of the patients in the bivalirudin phases A through C and heparin plus abciximab groups, respectively ($p = 0.018$ for the pooled bivalirudin groups vs. the heparin group).

98. **REPLACE-2.** Lincoff AM, et al. Bilvalirudin and provisional glycoprotein IIb/IIIa blockade compared with heparin and planned glycoprotein IIb/IIIa. blockade during percutaneous coronary intervention: the REPLACE-2 randomized trial. *JAMA* 2003;289:853–863.

This prospective, randomized, double-blind, triple-dummy, multicenter trial randomized 6,010 PCI patients to heparin plus a GP IIb/IIIa blocker (eptifibatide or abciximab) or to bivalirudin alone (0.75 mg/kg bolus plus 1.75 mg/kg/hr for duration of PCI) with the provisional addition of a GP IIb/IIIa blocker if needed in a double-blind, triple-dummy design. Provisional GP IIb/IIIa–blocker treatment was given to 7.2% of the bivalirudin group and 5.2% of the heparin and GP IIb/IIIa–blocker group. A nonsignificant reduction in death, MI, urgent revascularization at 30 days and major in-hospital bleeding (primary end point) with bivalirudin was found compared with heparin plus GP IIb/IIIa blockers (9.2% vs. 10.0%; $p = 0.32$). Among the four components, the only significant difference between the groups was a significantly lower incidence of bleeding with bivalirudin (2.4% vs. 4.1%). The secondary triple end point (death, MI, urgent revascularization) showed a trend toward fewer events in the heparin-plus-IIb/IIIa-blocker group [7.1% vs. 7.6% (bivalirudin)]; the difference was driven by a nonsignificant excess of MI with bivalirudin (7.0% vs. 6.2%). A cost analysis found that use of bivalirudin was associated with a cost savings of $448 per patient.

Directional Atherectomy Studies

99. **Topol EJ,** et al., Coronary Angioplasty versus Excisional Atherectomy Trial (**CAVEAT**). A comparison of directional atherectomy with coronary angioplasty in patients with coronary artery disease. *N Engl J Med* 1993;329:221–227.

Design: Prospective, randomized, controlled, multicenter study. Primary end point was angiographic restenosis at 6 months.
Purpose: To compare outcomes in patients undergoing balloon angioplasty (PTCA) with those having DCA.
Population: 1,012 patients with symptomatic CAD and no prior intracoronary interventions.
Treatment: PTCA or DCA.
Results: The atherectomy group had a higher initial success rate ($\leq$50% stenosis; 89% vs. 80%) but was associated with a higher rate of early complications (11% vs. 5%) and higher hospital costs. At 6-month angiography, the atherectomy group showed a trend toward lower restenosis (50% vs. 57%; $p = 0.06$) and a higher probability of death or MI (8.6% vs. 4.6%; $p = 0$).

100. **Adelman AG,** et al. Canadian Coronary Atherectomy Trial (**CCAT**). A comparison of directional atherectomy with balloon angioplasty for lesions of the left anterior descending coronary artery. *N Engl J Med* 1993;329:228–233.

Design: Prospective, randomized, open-label, multicenter study. Primary end point was restenosis at follow-up angiography (median, 5.9 months).
Purpose: To compare restenosis rates for balloon angioplasty and directional atherectomy in lesions of the proximal LAD artery.
Population: 274 patients with *de novo* 60% stenosis of the LAD artery.
Treatment: Balloon angioplasty or directional atherectomy.
Results: Atherectomy group had a nonsignificantly higher success rate (94% vs. 88%; $p = 0.06$); no difference in complication rates was observed (5% vs. 6%). At follow-up angiography, restenosis rates and MLDs were similar [43% (angioplasty) vs. 46% (atherectomy); 1.61 vs. 1.55 mm].

101. **CAVEAT-II.** Holmes DR Jr, et al. A multicenter, randomized trial of coronary angioplasty vs directional atherectomy for patients with saphenous vein bypass graft lesions. *Circulation* 1995;91:1966–1974.

Design: Prospective, randomized, open label, multicenter study.
Purpose: To compare outcomes after directional atherectomy versus balloon angioplasty in patients with *de novo* venous bypass graft stenosis.
Population: 305 patients with *de novo,* nonocclusive SVG stenoses ($\geq$60%) who were suitable candidates for atherectomy or angioplasty.
Treatment: Balloon angioplasty or directional atherectomy.
Results: Higher initial angiographic success was observed with atherectomy (89.2% vs. 79.0%; $p = 0.019$). No significant differences in either angiographic restenosis [45.6% (atherectomy) vs. 50.5% (angioplasty)] or target vessel reintervention [18.6% (atherectomy) vs. 26.2% (PTCA); $p = 0.09$] were observed. No difference in death or Q-wave MI rates were observed. However, the atherectomy group did have more frequent distal embolization (13.4% vs. 5.1%; $p = 0.012$) and a trend toward increased incidence of non–Q-wave MI (16.1% vs. 9.6%; $p = 0.09$).

102. **Simonton CA,** et al. Optimal directional atherectomy: final results of the Optimal Atherectomy Restenosis Study (**OARS.**) *Circulation* 1998;97:332–339.

Design: Prospective, multicenter registry study. Primary end point was angiographic restenosis at 6 months.
Purpose: To determine if use of an optimal atherectomy technique would translate into a lower rate of late clinical and angiographic restenosis.
Population: 199 patients aged 18 to 80 years with angina or a positive functional study and after angiographic criteria: (a) target vessel reference diameter, 3.0 to 4.5 mm;

(b) culprit lesion(s) with 60% stenosis; and (c) mild to moderate tortuosity and mild or no target lesion calcification. DCA and adjunctive angioplasty were performed if necessary to achieve less than 15% residual stenosis; 213 lesions met the criteria.
Treatment: DCA (7F device).
Results: Frequent (87%) postatherectomy angioplasty was performed. The short-term procedural success rate was 97.5%. The mean rate of residual stenosis was only 7%. The major complication rate was 2.5% (death, emergency bypass surgery, Q-wave MI). Non–Q-wave MI (CK-MB more than 3 times normal) occurred in 14%. At 1-year follow-up, the TLR rate was 17.8%. The 6-month restenosis rate was 28.9% (major predictor: smaller postprocedural lumen diameter).
Comments: A lower restenosis rate was observed than in prior directional atherectomy trials.

103. **Baim DS,** et al. for the Balloon vs Optimal Atherectomy Trial (**BOAT**) Investigators. Final results of the Balloon vs Optimal Atherectomy Trial (BOAT). *Circulation* 1998;97:322–331.

Design: Prospective, randomized, double-blind, multicenter study. Primary end point was restenosis rate at follow-up angiography (median, 6.9 months).
Purpose: To compare the optimal DCA technique with conventional balloon angioplasty on restenosis.
Population: 1,000 patients with single *de novo,* native vessel lesions in vessels larger than 3 mm in diameter.
Treatment: DCA (large device used) with aggressive tissue removal and use of adjunctive PTCA if indicated, or PTCA alone.
Results: DCA group had a higher procedural success rate (99% vs. 97%; $p = 0.02$) and a lower rate of residual stenosis (15% vs. 28%; $p < 0.0001$). Similar rates of major complication were observed (2.8% vs. 3.3%). However, DCA was associated with more frequent CK-MB elevations (more than 3 times normal; 16% vs. 6%; $p < 0.0001$). At follow-up angiography, the DCA group had a lower restenosis rate (primary end point): 31.4% vs. 39.8% ($p = 0.016$). At 1-year follow-up, the DCA group had nonsignificant reductions in mortality (0.6% vs. 1.6%; $p = 0.14$), TVR (17.1% vs. 19.7%; $p = 0.33$), target-site revascularization (15.3% vs. 18.3%; $p = 0.23$), and target vessel failure (death, Q-wave MI, or TVR; 21.1% vs. 24.8%; $p = 0.17$).

104. **Suzuki T,** et al. Effects of adjunctive balloon angioplasty after intravascular ultrasound-guided optimal directional coronary atherectomy: the result of Adjunctive Balloon Angioplasty After Coronary Atherectomy Study (**ABACAS**). *J Am Coll Cardiol* 1999;34:1028–1035.

Design: Prospective, randomized, open, multicenter, study. Primary end point was angiographic restenosis at 6 months.
Purpose: To evaluate balloon angioplasty (PTCA) after DCA compared with DCA alone and the outcome of IVUS-guided aggressive DCA.
Population: 214 patients (of 225) who underwent IVUS-guided DCA and had optimal debulking were randomized.
Exclusion Criteria: MI in prior month, left main or ostial RCA lesion, diffuse disease, lesion with thrombus, lesion with marked calcification, angulated lesion (greater than 60 degrees), significant vessel tortuosity.
Treatment: Adjunctive PTCA or no further therapy. DCA was performed with the Simpson Coronary AteroCath and IVUS guidance to achieve angiographic criteria of less than 30% or adequate debulking (estimated plaque area, less than 50%).
Results: The adjunctive PTCA group had a higher MLD [2.88 mm vs. 2.6 mm (DCA alone); $p = 0.006$] and lower residual stenosis (10.8% vs. 15%; $p = 0.009$) by postprocedural QCA. Ultrasound analysis also demonstrated a larger MLD in the PTCA group (3.26 mm vs. 3.04 mm; $p < 0.001$) as well as a lower residual plaque mass (42.6% vs. 45.6%; $p < 0.001$). At 6 months, however, the restenosis and TLR rates were similar [23.6% vs. 19.6% (DCA alone); 20.6% vs. 15.2%].

Rotational Atherectomy Studies

105. **Dill T,** et al. A randomized comparison of balloon angioplasty versus rotational atherectomy in complex coronary lesions (**COBRA** study). *Eur Heart J* 2000;21:1759–1766.

Design: Prospective, randomized, open-label, multicenter study. Primary end points were procedural success, 6-month restenosis rates in the treated segments, and major cardiac events during follow-up.
Purpose: To compare outcomes between RA and balloon angioplasty for the treatment of complex coronary artery lesions.
Population: 502 patients aged 20 to 80 years with angina and angiographic CAD with target lesion stenosis of 70% to 99% and mean lumen diameter of 1 mm or less for a length of 5 mm or more. Lesions were required to be complex (calcified, ostial or bifurcational, eccentric, diffuse, or within angulated segment).
Exclusion Criteria: Unstable angina, MI in previous 4 weeks, prior PCI of target vessel within 2 months, left ventricular ejection fraction (LVEF) less than 30%.
Treatment: Rotablation (burr sizes, 1.25 to 2.5) or balloon angioplasty. All received ASA, nitroglycerin, nifedipine, and heparin (15 to 20 KU with target ACT, 350 seconds or more). Stenting allowed bailout for unsatisfactory outcomes.
Results: Procedural success was achieved more frequently with rotablation compared with angioplasty (85% vs. 78%; $p = 0.038$). No difference was found between PTCA and rotablation with respect to procedure-related complications such as Q-wave infarctions (both groups, 2.4%), emergency bypass surgery (1.2% vs. 2.4%), and death (1.6% vs. 0.4%). A higher incidence of stenting occurred after PTCA (14.9% vs. 6.4%; $p < 0.002$), mostly because of bailout or unsatisfactory results. If bailout stenting is included as an end point, procedural success rates were 84% for rotablation and were 73% for angioplasty ($p = 0.006$). At 6 months, the restenosis rates were similar in both groups (rotablation, 49%; PTCA, 51%).

106. **Whitlow PL,** et al. Results of the study to determine rotablator and transluminal angioplasty strategy (**STRATAS**). *Am J Cardiol* 2001;87:699–705.

Design: Prospective, randomized, open, multicenter study. Primary end point was major cardiac adverse events at 6 months.
Purpose: To compare outcomes of an aggressive rotablator strategy and a conventional rotablator strategy.
Population: 497 patients with stenoses in native coronary arteries with lesion length less than 20 mm and vessel size less than 3.25 mm. A restenotic lesion was treated in 15% of routine and 16% of aggressive strategy patients.
Treatment: Aggressive rotablator therapy (70% to 90% burr/artery ratio) with no or low pressure (1 atm) adjunctive balloon inflation or standard rotablation (burr/artery ratio, 0.6 to 0.8) with adjunctive balloon dilatation (balloon/artery ratio, 1.1 to 1.3).
Results: Final MLD and residual stenosis were similar in both groups [1.97 mm (routine), 1.95 mm; 26%, 27%]. The aggressive group had a higher maximum burr size (2.1 vs. 1.8 mm), burr/artery ratio (0.82 vs. 0.71), and number of burrs used (2.7 vs. 1.9; all p values <0.0001). The aggressive group had a higher incidence of elevated CK-MB (more than 5 times normal; 11% vs. 7%). CK-MB elevation was associated with a decrease in rpm of more than 5,000 from baseline for a cumulative time longer than 5 seconds ($p = 0.002$). At 6 months, no significant differences were found between the two groups in binary restenosis [52% (routine) vs. 58% (aggressive)], whereas a trend toward fewer routine patients undergoing target lesion revascularization was noted (22% vs. 31%). Multivariable analysis indicated that LAD location (OR, 1.67; $p = 0.02$) and operator-reported excessive speed decrease more than 5,000 rpm (OR, 1.74; $p = 0.01$) were significantly associated with restenosis.

107. **vom Dahl J,** et al. Rotational Atherectomy Does Not Reduce Recurrent In-Stent Restenosis: results of the Angioplasty Versus Rotational Atherectomy for Treatment of Diffuse In-Stent Restenosis Trial (**ARTIST**). *Circulation* 2002;105:583–588.

Design: Prospective, randomized, multicenter (24 European sites). Primary end point was MLD assessed by QCA at 6 months.

Purpose: To determine the safety and efficacy of RA with balloon angioplasty (PTCA) compared with PTCA alone for the treatment of diffuse ISR.

Population: 298 patients with angina and/or objective evidence of target vessel–related ischemia and all of following: documented ISR more than 70% within a stent ±5 mm of stent edges, stent diameter 2.5 mm or more, ISR as only lesion for treatment, length of ISR of 10 to 50 mm, lesion accessible for rotablation.

Exclusion Criteria: Included MI within 30 days, LVEF less than 30%, intraluminal thrombus or dissection, unprotected ostial stenoses, stents obviously not fully expanded, stents at or directly distal to a bend of greater than 45 degrees, stents implanted within previous 3 months.

Treatment: RA with PTCA or PTCA alone. Rotablation was performed by using a stepped-burr approach followed by adjunctive PTCA with low (6 atm) inflation pressure. Use of GP IIb/IIIa inhibitors was discouraged.

Results: Initial procedural success rates (residual stenosis less than 30%) were similar in both groups (89% PTCA, 88% RA). However, at 6-month angiography, the PTCA group had superior results with a mean net gain in MLD of 0.67 mm versus 0.45 mm for RA ($p = 0.0019$). The mean gain in diameter of stenosis was 25% and 17% ($p = 0.002$), resulting in binary restenosis rates of 51% (PTCA) and 65% (RA; $p = 0.039$). Six-month event-free survival also was significantly higher after PTCA (91.3%) compared with RA (79.6%; $p = 0.0052$). A subset of 86 patients underwent IVUS, which showed that the main difference between the two groups was the absence of stent overexpansion during PTCA after rotablation.

108. **AMIGO.** Atherectomy and Multilink stenting Improves Gain in Outcome trial. Preliminary results presented at the 51th ACC Annual Scientific Session, Atlanta, GA: March 2002.

This prospective, multicenter (six European sites) study randomized 753 patients to DCA plus stenting or stenting alone. The average lesion length was 14.6 mm in the DCA/stent group and 14.3 mm in the stent-only group. At 8 months, no significant overall difference was found in binary restenosis rates (24.1% in DCA/stent group vs. 19.7% in the stent-only group; $p = NS$). Restenosis rates were 21.8% for the stent-only patients and 31.8% for those having suboptimal DCA. However, in the small group of patients (21.5%) that achieved optimal DCA, the restenosis rate was only 16.2%. Restenosis rates among bifurcated lesions were 9.8% for DCA/stent and 20.9% for stent-only treatment. The "optimal" DCA approach before stenting should undergo further study in a subsequent randomized trial.

Excimer Laser

109. **Deckelbaum LI,** et al. Percutaneous Excimer Laser Coronary Angioplasty (**PELCA**) Trial: effect of intracoronary saline infusion on dissection during excimer coronary angioplasty: a randomized trial. *J Am Coll Cardiol* 1995;26:1264–1269.

This small randomized study was composed of 63 patients who received 1 to 2 mL/sec of normal saline or a blood medium during excimer laser angioplasty. Saline-treated patients had a lower mean dissection grade [0. 43 vs. 0.91 (scale, 0 to 5)] and 71% fewer significant dissections (grade 2, 7% vs. 24%; $p < 0.05$). The proposed mechanism of benefit was minimization of blood irradiation leading to less arterial wall damage.

110. **Appelman YEA,** et al., Amsterdam-Rotterdam (**AMRO**) Trial. Randomised trial of excimer angioplasty vs balloon angioplasty for treatment of obstructive coronary artery disease. *Lancet* 1996;347:79–84.

This prospective, randomized, double-blind, multicenter study enrolled 308 patients with stable angina and coronary lesions longer than 10 mm. Patients were assigned to excimer laser or balloon angioplasty. The primary clinical end point was cardiac death, MI, bypass surgery, and repeated angioplasty. Primary angiographic end point was

MLD at 6 months. The similar angiographic success rates were similar in both groups [80% (laser) vs. 79%]. No significant differences in lumen gain [0.4 mm (laser) vs. 0.48 mm (angioplasty); $p = 0.34$] or restenosis rate (51.6% vs. 41.2%; $p = 0.13$) were observed. The clinical event rates were similar (MI, 4.6% vs. 5.7%; bypass surgery, 10.6% vs. 10.8%; repeated angioplasty, 21.2% vs. 18.5%).

111. **Reifart N,** et al. Excimer Laser, Rotational Atherectomy and Balloon Angioplasty Comparison Study (**ERBAC**). Randomized comparison of angioplasty of complex lesions at a single center. *Circulation* 1997;96:91–98.

This prospective, randomized, single-center study enrolled 685 patients with type B or C lesions. Patients were assigned to balloon angioplasty (PTCA), laser, or RA. The primary end point was procedural success rate (defined as less than 50% stenosis without in-hospital death, MI, or coronary bypass surgery). The RA group had best procedural success rate [89% vs. 80% (PTCA) and 77% (laser); $p = 0.0019$]. No difference in the incidence of in-hospital complications was observed. At 6-month follow-up, the PTCA group had undergone less revascularization of target lesions [31.9% vs. 42.4% (atherectomy) and 46% (laser); $p = 0.013$] and had a lower restenosis rate [47% vs. 57% ($p = $ NS) and 59% ($p < 0.05$)].

112. **Stone GW,** et al. for the Laser Angioplasty vs Angioplasty (**LAVA**) Trial Investigators. Prospective, randomized, multicenter comparison of laser-facilitated balloon angioplasty vs stand-alone balloon angioplasty in patients with obstructive coronary artery disease. *J Am Coll Cardiol* 1997;30:1714–1721.

This prospective, randomized, multicenter study enrolled 215 patients with 244 lesions in vessels ≥ 2 mm in diameter that were successfully crossed with a guide wire. Patients were assigned to holmium laser–facilitated balloon angioplasty or balloon angioplasty. Similar in-hospital clinical success rates were observed [89.7% (laser) vs. 93.9% (angioplasty alone); $p = 0.27$]. No significant difference was observed in postprocedural diameter stenosis (18.3% vs. 19.5%). However, the laser group had significantly more major and minor procedural complications (18.0% vs. 3.1%; $p = 0.0004$), MIs (4.3% vs. none; $p = 0.04$), and total in-hospital major adverse events (10.3% vs. 4.1%; $p = 0.08$). At mean follow-up of 11 months, no significant differences in late or event-free survival between the two groups were observed.

113. **Koster R,** et al. Laser angioplasty of restenosed coronary stents: results of a multicenter surveillance trial: the Laser Angioplasty of Restenosed Stents (**LARS**) Investigators. *J Am Coll Cardiol* 1999;34:25–32.

Prospective, nonrandomized, multicenter, surveillance trial of 440 patients with restenoses or occlusions in 527 stents. Patient underwent debulking with a xenon chloride excimer laser unit followed by adjunctive balloon angioplasty. Abciximab was used at the discretion of the investigator. Laser angioplasty success, defined as 50% diameter stenosis or less after laser treatment or successful passage with a 1.7-mm or 2.0-mm eccentric laser catheter, was achieved in 92% of patients. Procedural success, defined as laser angioplasty success followed by 30% or less stenosis with or without balloon angioplasty, occurred in 91%. Use of large or eccentric catheters was associated with a higher success rate and lower residual stenosis. Perforations after laser treatment occurred in 0.9% of patients, and after balloon angioplasty, in 0.2%. Dissections were visible in 4.8% of patients after laser treatment and in 9.3% after balloon angioplasty. Repeated interventions during hospitalization were required in 0.9% of patients.

Special Situations

Chronic Total Occlusions
Angioplasty
114. **Violaris AG,** et al. Long-term luminal renarrowing after successful elective coronary angioplasty of total occlusion. *Circulation* 1995;91:2140–2150 (editorial 2113–2114).

This analysis focused on 2,930 patients from four prospective restenosis trials, 7% with chronic occlusions. The occluded group had a higher restenosis rate (44.7% vs. 34.0%; RR, 1.58; $p < 0.001$), mostly due to more reocclusions (19.2% vs. 5.0%). The occluded group also had more absolute mean LD loss (0.43 vs. 0.31 mm; $p < 0.001$). The accompanying editorial points out that the occluded group had more prior MIs. Subsequent decreased distal bed flow could lead to slower flow, especially after angioplasty, causing increased reocclusion.

Stenting

115. **Sirnes PA,** et al. Stenting in Chronic Coronary Occlusion (**SICCO**): a randomized, controlled trial of adding stent implantation after successful angioplasty. *J Am Coll Cardiol* 1996;28:1444–1451.

Design: Prospective, randomized, multicenter study. Primary end point was restenosis rate at 6 months.
Purpose: To assess the potential benefit of additional stent implantation after successful angioplasty of a chronic coronary occlusion.
Population: 119 patients undergoing balloon angioplasty of an occluded native coronary artery.
Exclusion Criteria: Indications for stenting (e.g., major dissection), occlusions more than 2 weeks old, vessel diameter less than 2.5 mm, and visible thrombus.
Treatment: Stenting (or not) after successful balloon angioplasty.
Results: Stent group had less restenosis at 6 months (32% vs. 74%; $p < 0.001$). At long-term follow-up (33 $\pm$ 6 months), the stent group had fewer cardiac events (cardiovascular death, lesion-related acute MI, repeated lesion-related revascularization, or angiographic documentation of reocclusion): 24.1%; vs. 59.3%; OR, 0.22 ($p = 0.002$; see *J Am Coll Cardiol* 1998;22:305).

116. **Rubatelli P,** et al. Gruppo Italiano di Studio sullo Stent nelle Occlusioni Coronariche (**GISSOC**). Stent implantation vs balloon angioplasty in chronic coronary occlusions: results from the GISSOC trial. *J Am Coll Cardiol* 1998;32:90–96.

This randomized study was composed of 110 patients who underwent successful PTCA of a chronically occluded vessel 3 mm in diameter. Patients were randomized to PS stenting and warfarin for 1 month, or to no other therapy. Repeated angiography (at mean 9 months) revealed that the stent group had a larger mean LD (1.74 mm vs. 0.85 mm; $p < 0.001$), lower restenosis rate (32% vs. 68%; $p < 0.001$), and less reocclusion (8% vs. 34%; $p = 0.003$). The stent group also had less recurrent ischemia (14% vs. 46%; $p = 0.002$) and TLR (5.3% vs. 22%; $p = 0.038$), although hospitalization was prolonged.

117. **Buller CE,** et al. Total Occlusion Study of Canada (**TOSCA**) Investigators. Primary stenting versus balloon angioplasty in occluded coronary arteries. *Circulation* 1999;100:236–242.

This prospective, multicenter, randomized trial of primary stenting (with heparin-coated PS stent) versus balloon angioplasty was composed of 410 patients with symptomatic nonacute total occlusion (TIMI grade 0/1 flow) of native coronary arteries. Randomization occurred after successful placement of a guide wire across the occlusion and was stratified by duration of occlusion ($\leq$6 weeks vs. more than 6 weeks/unknown). The crossover rate to the stent arm was 10%. The overall incidence of the primary end point, failure of sustained TIMI grade 3 flow at 6 months (confirmed by angiography), was significantly lower in the stent group (10.9% vs. 19.5%; $p = 0.024$). The stent group also had a lower restenosis rate (less than 50% diameter stenosis; 55% vs. 70%; $p < 0.01$) and less TVR at 6 months (8.4% vs. 15.4%; $p = 0.03$).

Saphenous Vein Graft Lesions
Angioplasty

118. **Feyter PJ,** et al. Balloon angioplasty for the treatment of lesions in saphenous vein grafts. *J Am Coll Cardiol* 1993;21:1539–1549.

This review estimates an initial success rate of 90% and restenosis rate of 42%. The poorest outcomes were seen in patients with chronic total occlusions, diffuse SVG disease, and presence of chronic graft thrombus.

Stenting
119. **Wong SC,** et al. Immediate results and late outcomes after stent implantation in saphenous vein graft lesions: the multicenter U.S. Palmaz-Schatz stent experience. *J Am Coll Cardiol* 1995;26:704–712.

This analysis focused on 589 stented patients; a 97% procedural success rate was achieved. The anticoagulant regimen used consisted of ASA, 325 mg 4 times daily, and dipyridamole, 75 mg 3 times daily, started 24 to 48 hours before the procedure, dextran and heparin during the procedure, and then warfarin [target prothrombin time (PT), 16 to 18 seconds] and dipyridamole for 1 month, and ASA indefinitely. Stent thrombosis occurred in 1.4%, and major vascular or bleeding complications in 14%. The 6-month restenosis rate was 29.7%. Independent predictors included (a) restenotic lesions (46% vs. 18%); (b) small reference size (less than 3 mm; 47% vs. 26%); (c) history of diabetes; and (d) higher poststent residual stenosis. These results compare favorably with those observed in similar patients with PTCA. In CAVEAT II, a 51% restenosis rate was seen with PTCA.

120. **Savage MP,** et al. Saphenous Vein *de novo* (**SAVED**). Stent placement compared with balloon angioplasty for obstructed coronary bypass grafts. *N Engl J Med* 1997;338:740–747.

Design: Prospective, randomized, multicenter study. Primary end point was restenosis.
Purpose: To compare stent implantation with balloon angioplasty for the treatment of obstructive disease of venous bypass grafts.
Population: 220 patients with obstructed coronary bypass grafts.
Exclusion Criteria: MI in prior 7 days, ejection fraction less than 25%, diffuse disease that would require more than stents, and presence of thrombus.
Treatment: PS stent or balloon angioplasty.
Results: Stent group had higher procedural efficacy, defined as residual stenosis less than 50% without cardiac complications (92% vs. 69%; $p < 0.001$). However, the stent group had more hemorrhagic complications (17% vs. 5%; $p < 0.01$). Restenosis rates were not significantly different [37% (stent group) vs. 46%; $p = 0.24$], but the stent group had a lower incidence in the composite end points of freedom from death, MI, repeated bypass surgery, and TLR (73% vs. 58%; $p = 0.03$).

Other
121. **Braden GA,** et al. Transluminal extraction catheter atherectomy followed by immediate stenting in treatment of saphenous vein grafts. *J Am Coll Cardiol* 1997;30:657–663.

This observational study evaluated transluminal extraction catheter atherectomy followed by PS stenting in 49 consecutive patients with 53 vein grafts more than 9 years old. The procedural success rate was 98%, with MLD increasing from 1.3 mm at baseline to 3.9 mm after the transluminal extraction catheter-stent procedure. The event-free survival rate to hospital discharge was 90%. At follow-up (mean, 13 months), only 26% had experienced one adverse outcome (revascularization rate was 11%; nonfatal MI rate, 9%; death rate, 11%).

Small Vessels
122. **Elezi S,** et al. Vessel size and long-term outcome after coronary stent placement. *Circulation* 1998;98:1875–1880.

This retrospective analysis of 2,602 patients who underwent successful stenting showed that small vessel size predisposes to restenosis. Patients were divided into three groups: less than 2.8-mm, 2.8-mm to 3.2-mm, and more than 3.2-mm vessels. The less than 2.8-mm group had the lowest 1-year event-free survival (69.5% vs. 77.5% and 81%; $p < 0.001$). Late lumen loss was similar between the three groups, but the less than 2.8-mm group had a higher angiographic restenosis rate (38.6% vs. 28.4%

and 20.4%). The highest restenosis rate (53.5%) was seen in the less than 2.8-mm patients with diabetes and complex lesions.

123. **Akiyama T,** et al. Angiographic and clinical outcome following coronary stenting of small vessels. *J Am Coll Cardiol* 1998;32:1610–1618.

This analysis showed that stenting of small vessels is associated with poorer outcomes. A total of 1,298 consecutive patients with 1,673 lesions was identified; angiographic follow-up was done in 75%. Patients with smaller than 3-mm vessels versus 3 mm showed no difference in procedural success or subacute stent thrombosis rates (95.9% vs. 95.4%; 1.4% vs. 1.5%) but had a higher restenosis rate (32.6% vs. 19.9%; $p < 0.0001$) and a lower rate of event-free survival (63% vs. 71.3%; $p = 0.007$).

124. **Savage MP,** et al. Efficacy of coronary stenting versus balloon angioplasty in small coronary arteries: Stent Restenosis Study (STRESS) Investigators. *J Am Coll Cardiol* 1998;31:307–311.

Angiographic substudy of 331 STRESS I-II patients who had symptomatic CAD, *de novo* greater than 70% stenosis in native coronary vessel, lesion length less than 15 mm, and reference vessel diameter less than 3.0 mm by QCA. Patients underwent PS stenting (163) or balloon angioplasty (168). Compared with angioplasty, stenting was associated with a larger postprocedural lumen diameter (2.26 mm vs. 1.80 mm; $p < 0.001$), and this advantage persisted at 6 months (1.54 mm vs. 1.27 mm; $p < 0.001$). The binary restenosis rates at 6 months were 34% for stenting and 55% for angioplasty ($p < 0.001$). At 1 year, the event-free (death, MI, or revascularization) survival rate was better with stenting (78% vs. 67%; $p = 0.019$), primarily because of a lower TLR rate with stenting (16.1% vs. 26.6%; $p = 0.015$).

125. **Suwaidi JA,** et al. Immediate and one-year outcome of intracoronary stent implantation in small coronary arteries with 2.5-mm stents. *Am Heart J* 2000;140:898–905.

This single-center registry study examined 651 patients with stenoses in coronary arteries treated with 2.5-mm stents ($n = 108$) or 2.5-mm conventional balloon angioplasty. Patients who received treatment with both 2.5-mm and 3.0-mm or greater stent placement or balloons were excluded. Angiographic success rate was higher in the stent group (97.2% vs. 90.2%; $p = 0.02$). In-hospital complication rates were similar. At 1-year follow-up, no significant differences were found between the groups in survival [96.2% (stent) vs. 95.2% (balloon)], Q-wave MI (none vs. 0.4%), or CABG surgery (8.4% vs. 6.8%), but the stent group had more adverse cardiac events (35.4% vs. 22.1%; $p = 0.05$). However, after excluding GR II stent use, stenting was not independently associated with reduced cardiac events.

126. **Kastrati A,** et al. A randomized trial comparing stenting with balloon angioplasty in small vessels in patients with symptomatic coronary artery disease. **ISAR-SMART** Study Investigators. Intracoronary Stenting or Angioplasty for Restenosis Reduction in Small Arteries. *Circulation* 2000;102:2593–2598.

Design: Prospective, randomized, multicenter study. Primary end point was the incidence of angiographic restenosis at 6 months.
Purpose: To assess whether, compared with PTCA, stenting of small coronary vessels is associated with a reduction of restenosis.
Population: 404 patients with symptomatic CAD with lesions in vessels with 2.0-mm to 2.8-mm diameter.
Exclusion Criteria: Included acute MI in previous 3 days, left main stenoses, ISR.
Treatment: Stenting or PTCA. Adjunct therapy consisted of abciximab, ticlopidine, and ASA.
Results: In the PTCA group, 16.5% received at least one stent. Six-month angiographic restenosis rates were similar between the two groups [35.7% (stent) vs. 37.4% (PTCA); $p = 0.74$]. At 7 months, similar rates were found of death or MI (3.4% vs. 3.0%) and TVR (20.1% vs. 16.5%; $p = 0.35$).
Comments: In a prespecified subgroup analysis of the 98 (24%) patients with long lesions (15 mm), stenting was associated with a significant 41% relative reduction

in restenosis compared with PTCA (35.6% vs. 60.6%; $p = 0.028$); however, 1-year TVR rates were not significantly different (see *Am J Cardiol* 2002;89:58).

127. **Koning R,** et al. for the **BESMART** (BeStent in Small Arteries) Trial Investigators. Stent placement compared with balloon angioplasty for small coronary arteries: in-hospital and 6-month clinical and angiographic results. *Circulation* 2001;104:1604–1608.

Design: Prospective, randomized, double-blind, multicenter study. Primary end point was angiographic restenosis rate at 6 months.
Purpose: To compare the results of balloon angioplasty with stenting in small arteries.
Population: 381 symptomatic patients with *de novo* focal lesions in small coronary vessels (less than 3.0 mm).
Exclusion Criteria: Ostial and/or bifurcation lesion, LVEF 30%, MI in previous 3 days, contraindication to ASA or ticlopidine.
Treatment: Stent implantation or standard balloon angioplasty.
Results: Angiographic success rates were similar [97.6% (stent), 93.9% (PTCA)]. At follow-up angiography (obtained in 91%), the stent group had a significant 55% relative reduction in restenosis (21% vs. 47%; $p = 0.0001$). Repeated TLR was less frequent in the stent group (13% vs. 25%; $p = 0.0006$).

128. **Doucet S,** et al. for the Stent In Small Arteries (**SISA**) Trial Investigators. Stent placement to prevent restenosis after angioplasty in small coronary arteries. *Circulation* 2001;104:2029–2033.

- *Design:* Prospective, randomized, multicenter study. Primary end point was angiographic restenosis at 6 months (repeated angiography performed in 85.3%).
- *Purpose:* To compare the effects of stenting and angioplasty in small vessels on restenosis rates and other major outcomes.
- *Population:* 351 patients with stable angina, stabilized unstable angina, or documented silent ischemia with a *de novo* lesion and with reference vessel diameter between 2.3 mm and 2.9 mm.
- *Treatment:* Balloon angioplasty (PTCA) alone or stent implantation.
- *Results:* Angiographic success was achieved in 98.2% of stent patients versus 93.9% of PTCA patients ($p = 0.0065$). In the angioplasty group, 37 (20.3%) patients crossed over to stent implantation. Clinical success was higher in the stent group (95.3% vs. 87.9%; $p = 0.007$). No differences were found in major in-hospital cardiac complications including death (none), Q-wave MI (none), non–Q-wave MI (4.9% in the PTCA group vs. 1.8% in the stent group), CABG surgery (0.5% vs. 0.6%), and repeated angioplasty (2.7% vs. 0.6%). A trend toward fewer in-hospital events was seen in the stent group (3.0% vs. 7.1% in angioplasty group; $p = 0.076$), driven primarily by a lower incidence of non–Q-wave MI in the stent group. At 6 months, no significant differences were seen in the rates of angiographic restenosis [28% (stenting) vs. 32.9%] or TVR (17.8% vs. 20.3%).

129. **COAST** (Heparin-Coated Stents in Small Coronary Arteries). Havde M, et al. Heparin-coated stent placement for the treatment of stenoses in small coronary arteries of symptomatic patients. *Circulation* 2003;107:1265–1270.

Prospective, randomized, multicenter study of 588 patients from 21 European centers with coronary stenoses in 2.0-mm to 2.6-mm diameter vessels. Patients underwent PTCA, placement of a noncoated stent, or placement of a heparin-coated stent. All patients were pretreated with ASA and 10,000 U of heparin. At the 6-month follow-up (80% had angiogrphy), there were, no significant differences between the three treatment groups in the primary end point of restenosis (PTCA, 32%; noncoated stent, 25%; heparin-coated stent, 30%). No differences existed between groups in adverse events, death, or event-free survival.

Diabetes
130. **Kip KE,** et al. Coronary angioplasty in diabetic patients: the NHLBI PTCA Registry. *Circulation* 1996;94:1818–1825.

In this analysis of the 1985 to 1986 NHLBI Registry, 281 diabetic and 1,833 nondiabetic patients were studied. The diabetic group was older and had more three-vessel coronary disease, atherosclerotic lesions, and comorbidities. At 9-year follow-up, diabetic patients had a twofold higher mortality rate (35.9% vs. 17.9%) and increased incidence of nonfatal MI (29% vs. 18.5%), CABG surgery (36.7% vs. 27.4%), and repeated PTCA (43.7% vs. 36.5%).

131. **Elezi S,** et al. Diabetes mellitus and the clinical and angiographic outcomes after coronary stent placement. *J Am Coll Cardiol* 1998;32:1866–1873.

This analysis of 715 patients with diabetes and 2,839 patients without diabetes showed less-favorable outcomes in the diabetic group. At 6 months, the incidence of angiographic restenosis and stent vessel occlusion was higher among diabetics (37.5% vs. 28.3%; $p < 0.001$; 5.3% vs. 3.4%; $p = 0.037$). At 1 year, the diabetic group had lower rates of event-free survival and survival free of MI (73.1% vs. 78.5%; $p < 0.001$; 89.9% vs. 94.4%; $p < 0.001$). Multivariate analyses found that diabetes was an independent predictor of adverse clinical events and restenosis.

132. **Van Belle E,** et al. Effects of coronary stenting on vessel patency and long-term clinical outcome after percutaneous coronary revascularization in diabetic patients. *J Am Coll Cardiol* 2002;40:410–417.

A total of 314 diabetics undergoing stenting ($n = 157$) or balloon angioplasty ($n = 157$) was matched for gender, diabetes treatment regimen, stenosis location, reference diameter, and MLD. Other baseline characteristics were similar between groups. At 6 months, the stent group had a significantly lower restenosis rate (27% vs. 62%; $p < 0.0001$) and occlusion rate (4% vs. 13%; $p < 0.005$) than the angioplasty group. The ejection fraction in the stent group remained unchanged at 6 months, whereas the angioplasty group had a significant decrease ($p = 0.02$). At 4-year follow-up, the stent group had lower rates of cardiac death and nonfatal MI (14.8% vs. 26.0%; $p = 0.02$) and revascularization (35.4% vs. 52.1%).

Complications

Review Article

133. **O'Meara JJ,** Dehmer GJ. Care of the patient and management of complications after percutaneous coronary artery interventions. *Ann Intern Med* 1998;127:458–471.

This review focused on common postintervention complications, including acute closure and thrombosis, vascular access problems, chest pain, elevated CK levels, contrast-induced nephropathy, and radiation-induced skin injury. The middle section covers management considerations after 48 hours, such as restenosis and functional studies. The concluding section covers issues specific to atherectomy, excimer laser angioplasty, and stents.

Postintervention CK/CK-MB and Troponin Studies

134. **Abdelmeguid AE,** et al. Significance of mild transient release of CK-MB fraction after percutaneous coronary interventions. *Circulation* 1996;94:1528–1536.

This retrospective analysis focused on 4,484 patients after PTCA or directional atherectomy. No elevations were detected in 3,776 patients; the CK level was 100 to 180 IU/L, and MB, greater than 4% in 450 patients, and CK, 181 to 360 IU/L, and MB, more than 4% in 258 patients. CK-MB elevation predictors included atherectomy (OR, 4.1) and catheterization laboratory complications (OR, 2.6). At 3 years, the group with elevated CK and CK-MB had more MIs (RR, 1.3), cardiac deaths (RR, 1.3), and ischemic complications (death, MI, revascularization; 48.9% vs. 43.3% vs. 37.3%).

135. **Kong TQ Jr,** et al. Prognostic implication of CK elevation following elective coronary artery interventions. *JAMA* 1997;277:461–466.

This retrospective cohort study was composed of 253 consecutive patients with CK and CK-MB elevations and 120 patients without CK elevations. The CK elevation group had increased cardiac mortality ($p = 0.02$), highest if more than 3 times normal (RR, 1.05 per 100 U/L CK increase). The effect was independent of procedure type and outcome. Top mortality predictors were peak CK and ejection fraction (both $p < 0.001$).

136. **Tardiff BE,** et al. Clinical outcomes after detection of elevated cardiac enzymes in patients undergoing percutaneous intervention. *J Am Coll Cardiol* 1999;33:88–96.

This analysis of the IMPACT-II database showed that even small elevations in cardiac enzymes are associated with an increased short-term risk of adverse outcomes. No CK-MB elevation was seen in 1,779 (76%) patients, whereas levels were elevated to 1 to 3 times the upper limit of normal (ULN) in 323 patients (13.8%), 3 to 5 times ULN in 3.6%, 5 to 10 times ULN in 3.7%, and more than 10 times ULN in 2.9%. For all devices, including stents, CK-MB elevations of any magnitude were associated with an increased incidence of the composite end point at 30 days and 6 months (at 6 months, normal CK-MB level was 20.2% to 27.3%; CK-MB, 1 to 3 times ULN was 29.6% to 40.0%). The degree of risk correlated with the increase in enzymes, even for patients who had undergone successful procedures without abrupt closure. As seen in other studies, atherectomy performed in conjunction with angioplasty was associated with a greater incidence of postprocedural CK-MB elevations than was angioplasty alone ($p < 0.0001$).

137. **Bonz AW,** et al. Effect of additional temporary glycoprotein IIb/IIIa receptor inhibition on troponin release in elective percutaneous coronary interventions after pretreatment with aspirin and clopidogrel (**TOPSTAR** Trial). *J Am Coll Cardiol* 2002;40:662–668.

This prospective, randomized, double-blind, placebo-controlled, single-center study enrolled 109 patients with stable angina undergoing PCI. All were pretreated with a loading dose of clopidogrel (375 mg) and ASA (500 mg) 1 day before PCI. Patients were randomized to received tirofiban (10-μg/kg bolus and then 0.15 μg/kg/min for 18 hours) or placebo. At 12, 24, and 48 hours after PCI, the tirofiban-treated patients had a lower incidence of troponin T release (12 hours, 40% vs. 63%; $p < 0.05$; 24 hours, 48% vs. 69%; $p < 0.05$; 48 hours, 58% vs. 74%; $p < 0.08$). At 9 months, the tirofiban group had a lower incidence of death, MI, and TVR (2.3% vs. 13.0%; $p < 0.05$). Future, larger studies are needed to confirm these findings, especially whether small troponin elevations with normal CK-MB levels are correlated with worse prognosis.

Also see *Ann Clin Biochem* 2002;39:392–397: troponin I 2.0 or more seen in 27% and correlated with an increased incidence of recurrent angina, repeated PCI, coronary bypass surgery, and cardiac death at 2 years.

138. **Ellis SG,** et al. Death following CK-MB elevation after coronary intervention: identification of an early risk period: importance of CK-MB level, completeness of revascularization, ventricular function, and probable benefit of statin therapy. *Circulation* 2002;106:1205–1210.

This analysis examined 8,409 consecutive nonacute MI patients with successful PCI and no emergency surgery or Q-wave MI; average follow-up was 3.2 years. Post-PCI CK-MB was above normal on routine ascertainment in 17.2%. Patients were prospectively stratified into those with CK-MB 1 to 5 times or CK-MB more than 5 times normal. No patient with CK-MB 1 to 5 times normal died during the first week after PCI, and excess risk of early death for patients with CK-MB elevation occurred mostly in the first 3 to 4 months. The actuarial 4-month risk of death was 8.9%, 1.9%, and 1.2% for patients with CK-MB greater than 5 times, CK-MB 1 to 5 times, and CK-MB more than 1 time normal ($p < 0.001$). Incomplete revascularization ($p < 0.001$), CHF class ($p = 0.005$), and no statin treatment at hospital discharge ($p = 0.009$) were associated with death at 4 months.

Stent Thrombosis
139. **Mak KH,** et al. Subacute stent thrombosis: evolving issues and current concepts. *J Am Coll Cardiol* 1996;27:494–503.

This excellent review discusses the advances in stenting technique and antithrombotic regimens that have led to a significant reduction in incidence of subacute stent thrombosis. The importance of antiplatelet therapy is emphasized.

140. **Hasdai D,** et al. Coronary angioplasty and intracoronary thrombolysis are of limited efficacy in resolving early intracoronary stent thrombosis. *J Am Coll Cardiol* 1996;28:361–367 (editorial, 368–370).

This retrospective analysis focused on 29 of 1,761 consecutive patients with early ($\leq$30 days) stent thrombosis occurring in 44 stents. Acute MI occurred in 90% of patients, and five (17%) patients died. Fourteen patients were treated with balloon angioplasty (PTCA), seven with PTCA and urokinase, and two with urokinase only. Among these treated patients, flow was restored in 48% (six of 14, four of seven, and one of two). Editorial points out that risk factors for stent thrombosis include emergency use and preexisting thrombus (see *Circulation* 1994;89:1126).

141. **Moussa I,** et al. Subacute stent thrombosis in the era of intravascular ultrasound-guided coronary stenting without anticoagulation: frequency, predictors and outcome. *J Am Coll Cardiol* 1997;29:6–12.

This retrospective analysis focused on 1,001 patients with 1,334 lesions. Subacute stent thrombosis occurred in 1.9%. Predictors of subacute stent thrombosis included low ejection fraction ($p = 0.019$), combination of different stents ($p = 0.013$) and postprocedural dissection ($p = 0.014$), and slow flow ($p = 0.0001$).

142. **Costa MA,** et al. Late coronary occlusion after intracoronary brachytherapy. *Circulation* 1999;100:789–792.

This analysis of 108 patients who underwent PCI followed by intracoronary β-radiation to treat ISR. Of 91 patients with more than 2 months' follow-up, six patients (6.6%) experienced sudden thrombotic events confirmed by angiography at 2 to 15 months after intervention. Two patients had been treated with PTCA only, and four received new stents.

Other

143. **Baumbach A,** et al. Acute complications of excimer laser coronary angioplasty: a detailed analysis of multicenter results. *J Am Coll Cardiol* 1994;23:1305–1313.

In this retrospective analysis of 1,469 patients, 7% had major complications (death, emergency or urgent bypass surgery). ACTs were obtained before, after a 10,000-U bolus of heparin, and at the end of the procedure. The group with complications had lower ACTs during and after the procedure: less than 250 seconds in 61% versus 27%. Complications were seen in all patients with a final ACT less than 250 seconds, but only in 0.3% with ACT longer than 300 seconds.

144. **Solomon R,** et al. Effects of saline, mannitol, and furosemide on acute decreases in renal function induced by radiocontrast agents. *N Engl J Med* 1994;331:1416–1420.

Prospective, randomized study of 78 patients with chronic renal insufficiency (mean creatinine, 2.1 mg/dL) who underwent coronary angiography. Patients received 0.45% saline alone for 12 hours before and 12 hours after angiography, saline plus mannitol, or saline plus furosemide. Mannitol and furosemide were given just before angiography. An increase in the creatinine of 0.5 mg/dL or more after angiography was seen in 26%. The saline group had a lower incidence of elevated creatinine compared with the mannitol and furosemide groups (11% vs. 28% and 40%; $p = 0.05$). The mean increase in serum creatinine 48 hours after angiography was significantly greater in the furosemide group ($p = 0.01$) than in the saline group.

145. **Narins CR,** et al. Relation between activated clotting time during angioplasty and abrupt closure. *Circulation* 1996;93:667–671.

This study correlated low ACTs with adverse outcomes. The analysis focused on 62 of 1,290 consecutive nonemergency angioplasty patients with in- or out-of-catheterization laboratory closure and 124 matched controls. Abrupt closure patients had a lower initial and minimum ACT (350 vs. 380 seconds; 345 vs. 370 seconds). High ACTs were not associated with more major bleeding complications.

146. **Schaub F,** et al. Management of 219 consecutive cases of postcatheterization pseudoaneurysm. *J Am Coll Cardiol* 1997;30:670–675.

This analysis focused on 219 patients with postcatheterization pseudoaneurysm. A compression bandage was reapplied in 132 patients with 32% success [more likely if small pseudoaneurysm (10 mm; 71% vs. 95%) and patient not anticoagulated (72% vs. 93%)]. Ultrasound-guided compression repair was undertaken in 124 patients (primary treatment modality in 49). The success rate was 84%, higher if preceded by reapplied bandage (89% vs. 76%; $p = 0.04$). Overall, surgical repair was necessary in only 7% of patients.

147. **Piana RN,** et al. Effect of transient abrupt vessel closure during otherwise successful angioplasty for unstable angina on clinical outcome at six months. *J Am Coll Cardiol* 1999;33:73–78.

A multivariate analysis of 4,098 Hirulog Angioplasty Study (HAS) patients found uncomplicated abrupt vessel closure to be the strongest independent predictor of MACEs at 6 months (OR, 3.6; 95% CI, 2.5 to 5.1; $p < 0.001$). Other predictors included multivessel angioplasty, target lesion in the LAD artery, and diabetes (all values of $p = 0.02$).

148. **Kay J,** et al. Acetylcysteine for prevention of acute deterioration of renal function following elective coronary angiography and intervention: a randomized controlled trial. *JAMA* 2003;289:553–558.

Prospective, randomized, double-blind, placebo-controlled trial of 200 patients with stable moderate renal insufficiency (creatinine clearance, less than 60 mL/min) who underwent elective coronary angiography. Patients received oral acetylcysteine, 600 mg twice daily, or placebo, on the day before and the day of angiography. The acetylcysteine group had a significantly lower incidence of a greater than 25% increase in serum creatinine level within 48 hours compared with placebo (4% vs. 12%; relative $p = 0.03$). Average serum creatinine also was lower in the acetylcysteine group (1.22 mg/dL vs. 1.38 mg/dL; $p = 0.006$). The benefit of acetylcysteine was present in all patient subgroups and persisted for at least 7 days.

149. **CONTRAST.** Preliminary results presented at 52nd ACC Scientific Sessions, Chicago, IL: March 2003.

This prospective, randomized, multicenter study enrolled 315 patients with baseline creatinine clearance (CvCl) of <60 cm³/min. Patients received fenoldopam (0.05 to 0.10 μg/kg/min or placebo, starting 1 hour before angiography and continuing for 12 hours thereafter. There was no significant difference between the groups in primary end point of $\geq 2.5\%$. Serum creatinine increase in first 96 hours [36.6% (fenoldopam) vs. 30.1%, $p = 0.54$].

Restenosis

Review Articles and Miscellaneous

150. **Frishman WH,** et al. Medical therapies for the prevention of restenosis after coronary interventions. *Curr Probl Cardiol* 1998;23:538–635.

This extensive review covers the definition and pathophysiologic characteristics of restenosis. The largest section discusses the pharmacologic approaches to restenosis, including antiplatelet and antithrombotic agents, antiinflammatory drugs, lipid-lowering agents, and radiotherapy.

151. **Violaris AG,** et al. Role of angiographically identifiable thrombus on long-term renarrowing after PTCA. *Circulation* 1996;93:889–897.

This analysis focused on 2,950 patients with 3,583 lesions, 160 with thrombus. Thrombotic lesions were associated with a 45% higher restenosis rate (at 6 months,

43% vs. 34%; $p = 0.01$), mostly due to increased total occlusion rate (13.8% vs. 5.7%; $p < 0.001$).

152. **Belle EV,** et al. Restenosis rates in diabetic patients. *Circulation* 1997;96:1454–1460 (editorial, 1374–1377).

This retrospective analysis showed an increased risk of restenosis among diabetic patients undergoing balloon angioplasty but not stenting. A total of 300 stented patients (single-native-vessel procedure, no high-pressure balloon inflation; 19% diabetics) and 300 balloon angioplasty (PTCA) patients was analyzed. The PTCA group had a nearly twofold higher restenosis rate (63% vs. 36%; $p = 0.0002$), whereas among stented patients, diabetics and nondiabetics had a similar rate of restenosis (25% vs. 27%). Editorial points out that these findings suggest that vascular remodeling (vs. neointimal proliferation) drives the excess in post-PTCA restenosis in diabetics. However, these findings contradict those of other studies that have shown no special benefit with stenting in diabetics: [see *Ann Intern Med* 1993;118:344: restenosis in 55% (diabetics) vs. 20%; *J Am Coll Cardiol* 1997;29:188A: 40% vs. 24%; *J Am Coll Cardiol* 1997;29:455A: 29% vs. 23%]. One possible explanation for the differences in results is that the lack of high-pressure balloon inflation in this stented population led to less vessel damage and subsequently less intimal proliferation (the latter may be especially important in the restenotic process in diabetics).

Repeated Percutaneous Coronary Intervention for Restenosis after Percutaneous Transluminal Coronary Angiography

153. **Erbel R,** et al., **REST** (Restenosis Stent Study). Coronary-artery stenting compared with balloon angioplasty for restenosis after initial balloon angioplasty. *N Engl J Med* 1998;339:1672–1678.

Design: Prospective, randomized, multicenter study. Primary end point was angiographic evidence of restenosis at 6 months.
Purpose: To determine whether coronary stenting, as compared with balloon angioplasty, reduces restenosis after prior successful balloon angioplasty.
Population: 383 patients with clinical and angiographic evidence of restenosis after successful balloon angioplasty.
Treatment: Standard balloon angioplasty or PS stent implantation; crossover to stenting was allowed if symptomatic dissection occurred that could not be managed with repeated balloon inflations.
Results: Stent group had a significantly lower restenosis rate (18% vs. 32%; $p = 0.03$) and less TVR (10% vs. 27%; $p = 0.001$). The difference resulted from smaller MLD in angioplasty (1.85 vs. 2.04 mm; $p = 0.01$). The stent group had better event-free survival at 250 days (84% vs. 72%; $p = 0.04$), but a nonsignificant increase was found in death and MI (at 6 months, 5.6% vs. 2.3%). Subacute thrombosis occurred more frequently in the stent group (3.9% vs. 0.6%).
Comments: These results are consistent with prior studies (26–29) that have shown a reduction in TVR but an excess of the hard end points of death and MI.

Effect of Stent Design (Strut Thickness)

154. **Kastrati A,** et al. Intracoronary stenting and angiographic results: Strut Thickness Effect on Restenosis Outcomes (**ISAR-STEREO**) Trial. *Circulation* 2001;103:2816–2821.

This prospective, randomized study of 651 patients examined whether stents with different strut thickness result in similar restenosis rates and clinical outcomes. Patients receive either a thin-strut stent (ACS MultiLink stent) or thick-strut stent (ACS MultiLink Duett stent). At 30 days, urgent TVR was the same in the two groups (both 1.5%); mortality and MI rates also were similar. At 6 months' follow-up angiography [obtained in 79% (thin strut) and 82%], the primary end point of restenosis was significantly lower in the thin-strut group compared with the thick-strut group (15% vs. 25.8%; $p = 0.003$). At 1-year follow-up, 8.6% of the thin-strut stent patients and 13.8% of the thick-strut stent patients required TVR because of restenosis-related ischemia

($p = 0.03$). This study shows that even small changes in stent design can result in different angiographic and clinical outcomes.

155. **ISAR-STEREO 2.** Intracoronary Stenting and Angiographic results: Strut Thickness Effect on Restenosis Outcome Trial –2: preliminary results presented at American College of Cardiology, 51st Annual Scientific Session, Atlanta, GA, March 2001.

This prospective, randomized study also evaluated the effect of stent strut thickness on restenosis rates in 611 patients with stenoses in native coronary arteries 2.8 mm or more in diameter. Patients received a thin-strut stent (50 mm thickness) or thick-strut stent (140 mm thickness). Vessel size, lesion length, MLD, and GP IIb/IIIa platelet inhibitor use were similar in both groups. At 6 months, QCA showed that the thin-strut group had a greater MLD and less late lumen loss compared with the thick-strut group, as well as a significantly lower binary restenosis rate (17.9% vs. 31.4%; $p < 0.001$). Clinical restenosis (TVR) also was significantly lower in the thin-strut group (12.3% vs. 20.9%; $p = 0.002$). A careful examination of potential confounders such as stent-deployment pressure is needed.

156. **Briguori C,** et al. In-stent restenosis in small coronary arteries: impact of strut thickness. *J Am Coll Cardiol* 2002;40:403–409.

Retrospective analysis of 821 patients who had successful stenting in small native vessels (3.0 mm reference diameter) and had angiographic follow-up available. The thin-strut group (less than 0.10 mm) included 400 patients with 505 lesions, whereas the thick-strut group had 421 patients with 436 lesions. The thin-strut group had a significantly lower restenosis rate compared with the thick-strut group (28.5% vs. 36.6%; $p = 0.009$). When three subgroups were defined (2.50 mm or smaller, 2.51 to 2.75 mm, and 2.76 to 2.99 mm), strut thickness influenced restenosis only in the 2.76- to 2.99-mm subgroup [23.5% (thin) vs. 37%; $p = 0.006$]. By logistic regression analysis, predictors of restenosis were stent length, strut thickness, and diabetes.

Drug Studies

157. **Schwartz L,** et al. Aspirin and dipyridamole in the prevention of restenosis after PTCA. *N Engl J Med* 1988;318:1714–1719.

Prospective, randomized, double-blind, placebo-controlled, multicenter study of 376 patients undergoing coronary angioplasty. Patients received aspirin, 330 mg/day, and dipyridamole, 75 mg 3 times daily (started 24 hours before angioplasty), or placebo. Dipyridamole was given by continuous intravenous infusion (10 mg/hr) from 16 hours before the procedure until 8 hours after. Among 249 patients who underwent follow-up angiography, similar restenosis rates [37.7% vs. 38.6% (placebo)] were observed. The drug therapy group had 77% fewer periprocedural Q-wave MIs (1.6% vs. 6.9%; $p = 0.01$).

158. **Serruys PW,** et al. Coronary Artery Restenosis Prevention on Repeated Thromboxane Antagonism (**CARPORT**). Prevention of restenosis after percutaneous transluminal coronary angioplasty with thromboxane A_2-receptor blockade. *Circulation* 1991;84:1568–1580.

Prospective, randomized, double-blind, placebo-controlled, parallel-group study of 697 patients who underwent successful balloon angioplasty of a *de novo* native coronary artery lesion. Patients received the thromboxane A_2–receptor antagonist, GR32191B, 80 mg before angioplasty and 40 mg/day for 6 months, or aspirin, 250 mg intravenously, before angioplasty and placebo for 6 months. At 6-month follow-up angiography (575 patients), no significant differences were found between the groups in lumen diameter or clinical events.

159. **Faxon DP,** et al. Enoxaparin Restenosis after Angioplasty (**ERA**). Low molecular weight heparin in prevention of restenosis after angioplasty: results of enoxaparin restenosis (ERA) trial. *Circulation* 1994;90:908–914.

Prospective, randomized, double-blind, placebo-controlled, multicenter study of 458 patients who underwent successful angioplasty. Patient received enoxaparin, 40 mg s.c. once daily for 1 month, or placebo. At 6 months, restenosis rates were similar in the two groups [51% (placebo) vs. 52%; $p = 0.63$]. Clinical event rates also were similar, except for minor bleeding, which was more frequent in the enoxaparin group.

160. **Weintraub WS,** et al. Lack of effect of lovastatin on restenosis after coronary angioplasty. *N Engl J Med* 1994;331:1331–1337.

Prospective, randomized, double-blind, placebo-controlled, multicenter study of 404 patients undergoing successful elective coronary angioplasty of native coronary vessels. Patients received lovastatin, 40 mg twice daily, started 7 to 10 days before angioplasty, or placebo. At 6-month angiography (321 patients), no significant reduction between the groups in luminal diameter was noted (preangioplasty, 64% vs. 63%; at 6 months, 44% vs. 46%; $p = 0.50$).

161. **Maresta A,** et al. Studio Trapidil versus Aspirin nella Restenosi Coronarica (**STARC**). Trapidil (triazolopyrimidine), a platelet-derived growth factor antagonist, reduces restenosis after PTCA. *Circulation* 1994;90:2710–2715.

Prospective, randomized, comparative study of 254 patients younger than 75 years undergoing coronary angioplasty of *de novo* lesions. Patients received trapidil, 300 mg orally every 8 hours, or acetylsalicylic acid, 100 mg 3 times daily for 6 months. At 6-month angiography, the trapidil group had a significantly lower restenosis rate (24.2% vs. 39.7%; $p < 0.01$). Clinical events were similar in the two groups, except that recurrent angina occurred less frequently with trapidil (25.8% vs. 43.7%).

162. Multicenter American Research with Cilazapril after Angioplasty to Prevent Transluminal Obstruction and Restenosis (**MARCATOR**). Effect of high-dose ACE inhibition on restenosis: final results of MARCATOR study, a multicenter, double-blind, placebo-controlled trial of cilazapril. *J Am Coll Cardiol* 1995;25:362–369.

Prospective, randomized, double-blind, multicenter study of 1,436 patients undergoing coronary angioplasty. Patients received cilazapril, 1.0 or 2.5 mg after angioplasty, and then 1, 5, or 10 mg twice daily for 6 months, or placebo. All received aspirin. At follow-up angiography, no differences were seen between any groups in change in MLD. A similar study of 693 patients enrolled at European sites (MERCATOR) showed no significant differences in MLD and major events at 6 months between cilazapril and placebo groups (see *Circulation* 1992;86:100).

163. **Serruys PW,** et al., the **HELVETICA** Investigators. A comparison of hirudin with heparin in the prevention of restenosis after coronary angioplasty. *N Engl J Med* 1995;333:757–763.

Prospective, randomized, double-blind, multicenter study of 1,141 unstable angina patients in three groups. Group 1, heparin, 10,000-U bolus, continuous infusion for 24 hours, and then s.c. placebo twice daily for 3 days; group 2, hirudin, 40 mg, i.v. infusion for 24 hours, and then s.c. placebo twice daily for 3 days; group 3, same as group 2, except hirudin, 40 mg s.c. twice daily for 3 days. Hirudin-treated patients had decreased early (96-hour) cardiac events (7.9% and 5.6% vs. 11%), but no significant differences were seen in the primary end point of event-free survival at 7 months (67.3%, 63.5%, 68%). Mean MLDs at 6-month follow-up angiography were 1.54, 1.47, and 1.56 mm, respectively ($p = 0.08$).

164. Subcutaneous Heparin and Angioplasty Restenosis Prevention Trial (**SHARP**). The SHARP trial: results of a multicenter randomized trial investigating the effects of high dose unfractionated heparin on angiographic restenosis and clinical outcome. *J Am Coll Cardiol* 1995;26:947–954.

Prospective, randomized, parallel-group, open-label, multicenter study of 339 patients who had undergone successful coronary angioplasty of *de novo* lesions. Patients received heparin, 12,500 U s.c. twice daily for 4 months, or no treatment. At follow-up angiography (mean, 4.2 months), no significant differences were found between treatment groups in change in mean lumen diameter.

165. **Savage MP,** et al., for the Multi-Hospital Eastern Atlantic Restenosis Trial (**M-HEART II**) Study Group. Effect of thromboxane A_2 blockade on clinical outcome and restenosis after coronary angioplasty. *Circulation* 1995;92:3194–3200.

This prospective, randomized, double-blind, placebo-controlled, multicenter study enrolled 752 patients undergoing elective angioplasty. Patients received aspirin, 325 mg once daily; sulotroban, 800 mg 4 times daily; or placebo, started 1 to 6 hours before PTCA and continued for 6 months. The aspirin group had less angiographic restenosis (by lesion) than did the sulotroban group (39% vs. 53%; $p = 0.006$).

166. **Cairns JA,** et al. Enoxaparin MaxEPA Prevention of Angioplasty Restenosis (**EMPAR**). Fish oils and low-molecular-weight heparin for the reduction of restenosis after percutaneous transluminal coronary angioplasty. *Circulation* 1996;94:1553–1560.

Prospective, randomized, partially open, multicenter study of 814 patients undergoing elective angioplasty of *de novo* lesions. Patients received maxEPA, 18 capsules/day (5.4-g n-3 fatty acids) or placebo started a median 6 days before angioplasty and continued for 18 weeks. After sheath removal, 653 patients had one successfully dilated lesion and were randomized to enoxaparin, 30 mg s.c. twice daily or control (no treatment) for 6 weeks. At follow-up angiography (18 $\pm$ 2 weeks), no significant differences were observed in restenosis rates per patient and per lesion (fish oils, 46.5% vs. 39.7%; placebo, 44.7% vs. 38.7%; enoxaparin, 45.8% vs. 38.0%; control, 45.4% vs. 40.4%).

167. **Karsch KR,** et al. Reduction of Restenosis after PTCA: early Administration of Reviparin in a Double-blind, Unfractionated Heparin and Placebo-controlled Evaluation (**REDUCE**). Low-molecular weight heparin (reviparin) in percutaneous transluminal coronary angioplasty. *J Am Coll Cardiol* 1996;28:1437–1443.

Prospective, randomized, double-blind, multicenter study of 625 stable or unstable angina patients with single lesions suitable for elective PTCA. Patients received reviparin, 7,000 U, before PTCA, followed by 10,500 U over a 24-hour period, and then 3,500 U twice daily for 28 days, or heparin, 10,000 U over a 24-hour period, and then s.c. placebo. At 30 weeks, no significant differences were seen between groups in the primary composite end point of death, MI, reintervention, or CABG surgery [33.3% (reviparin) vs. 32%], loss of lumen diameter, and bleeding. The reviparin group had fewer acute events (3.9% vs. 8.2%; $p < 0.03$).

168. **Lablanche J-M,** et al. Angioplastie Coronaire Corvasal Diltiazem (**ACCORD**). Effect of the direct nitric oxide donors linsidomine and molsidomine on angiographic restenosis after coronary balloon angioplasty. *Circulation* 1997;95:83–89.

This prospective, multicenter trial randomized 700 patients 12 to 24 hours before angioplasty to linsidomine infusion followed by oral molsidomine or oral diltiazem, 60 mg 3 times daily for 6 months. The nitric oxide donor group had a better mean luminal diameter (initial, 1.94 vs. 1.81 mm; $p = 0.001$; 3 months, 1.54 vs. 1.38; $p = 0.007$) and lower restenosis rate (38% vs. 46.5%; $p = 0.026$). However, no significant differences in major clinical events were observed (32.2% vs. 32.4%).

169. **Bertrand ME,** et al. Prevention of Restenosis by Elisor after Transluminal Coronary Angioplasty Trial (**PREDICT**). Effect of pravastatin on angiographic restenosis after coronary balloon angioplasty. *J Am Coll Cardiol* 1997;30:863–869.

Prospective, randomized, double-blind, placebo-controlled, multicenter study of 695 patients with total cholesterol, 200 to 310 mg/dL, undergoing elective angioplasty. Patients received pravastatin, 40 mg/day, or placebo for 6 months. No significant difference in mean lumen diameter was observed between the two groups [1.54 mm (pravastatin) vs. 1.54 mm; $p = 0.21$]. Late loss and net gain did not differ significantly between groups. Restenosis rates also were similar [39.2% (pravastatin) vs. 43.8%; $p = 0.26$].

170. **Tardif JC,** et al., for the Multivitamins and Probucol (**MVP**) Study Group. Probucol and multivitamins in the prevention of restenosis after coronary angioplasty. *N Engl J Med* 1997;337:365–372 (editorial, 418–419).

Design: Prospective, randomized, double-blind, placebo-controlled, multicenter study. Primary end point was reduction in MLD.

Purpose: To evaluate whether the antioxidant probucol, multivitamins (vitamins E and C and β-carotene), or the combination reduce restenosis after angioplasty.

Population: 317 patients undergoing elective PTCA of *de novo* lesion(s) in native vessels.

Treatment: Probucol, 500 mg, multivitamins (vitamin C, 500 mg; vitamin E, 700 IU; β-carotene, 30,000 IU), or both twice daily, started 1 month before to PTCA and continued for 6 months after. Twelve hours before PTCA, an extra 1 g of probucol, 2,000 IU of vitamin E, both, or placebo were given.

Results: Probucol therapy resulted in a significantly smaller mean reduction in luminal diameter: 0.12 vs. 0.22 mm (combined treatment), 0.33 mm (multivitamins), and 0.38 mm (placebo) ($p = 0.006$ for those receiving vs. those not receiving probucol). The probucol group had less restenosis per segment: 20.7% vs. 28.9%, 40.3%, and 38.9% ($p = 0.003$ for probucol vs. no probucol). Probucol also was associated with less repeated angioplasty (11.2% vs. 16.2%, 24.4%, and 26.6%; $p = 0.009$). HDLs decreased by more than 40% in the probucol group.

171. **Yokoi H,** et al. Probucol Angioplasty Restenosis Trial (**PART**). Effectiveness of an antioxidant in preventing restenosis after percutaneous transluminal coronary angioplasty: the Probucol Angioplasty Restenosis Trial. *J Am Coll Cardiol* 1997;30:855–862.

This prospective, randomized study of 101 patients showed that probucol, started well before elective angioplasty, appears to reduce restenosis rates. Patients received probucol, 1,000 mg/day, or control (no lipid-lowering) therapy starting 4 weeks before angioplasty, and continued until follow-up angiography at 24 weeks. Angiographic restenosis rate was (60% lower in probucol group: 23% vs. 58%; $p = 0.001$).

172. **Kosuga K,** et al. Effectiveness of tranilast on restenosis after directional coronary atherectomy. *Am Heart J* 1997;134:712–718.

This nonrandomized study was composed of 192 patients who underwent successful DCA. After the procedure, 40 patients were given oral tranilast for 3 months, and 152 were not. Angiographic follow-up at 3 and 6 months showed that the tranilast patients had a significantly lower MLD (2.08 vs. 1.75 mm; $p = 0.004$; 2.04 vs. 1.70 mm; $p = 0.003$). The restenosis rate at 3 months was more than 50% lower in the tranilast group (11% vs. 26%; $p = 0.03$). At 1 year, the tranilast group also had experienced fewer clinical events ($p = 0.013$).

173. **Kastrati A,** et al. Restenosis after coronary stent placement and randomized to a 4-week combined antiplatelet or anticoagulant therapy. *Circulation* 1997;96:462–467 (editorial, 383–385).

This analysis of 432 ISAR patients who underwent 6-month angiography showed no favorable effects on restenosis in patients receiving an antiplatelet regimen. Antiplatelet versus anticoagulant therapy showed no significant differences in restenosis rate (26.8% vs. 28.9%), mean luminal diameter (1.95 vs. 1.90 mm), late lumen loss (1.10 vs. 1.15 mm), or TVR (14.6% vs. 15.6%). The accompanying editorial points out that this analysis was poorly powered to detect a restenosis difference.

174. **Lablanche J-M,** et al. Fraxiparine Angioplastie Coronaire Transluminale (**FACT**). Effect of nadroparin, a low-molecular-weight heparin, on clinical and angiographic restenosis after coronary balloon angioplasty. *Circulation* 1997;96:3396–3402.

Prospective, randomized, double-blind, placebo-controlled, multicenter study of 354 patients ≤75 years undergoing elective angioplasty of *de novo* lesions. Patients received daily s.c. nadroparin (0.6 mL of 10,250 anti-Xa IU/mL) or placebo injections started 3 days before angioplasty and continued for 3 months. At follow-up angiography (3 months), no significant differences were noted between groups in mean lumen diameter and mean residual stenosis (1.37 vs. 1.48 mm; 51.9% vs. 48.8%) or major cardiac events.

175. **Ohsawa H,** et al. Preventive effects of an antiallergic drug, pemirolast potassium, on restenosis after percutaneous transluminal coronary angioplasty. *Am Heart J* 1998;136:1081–1087.

This prospective, randomized trial was composed of 205 patients with restenosis in native vessels. Patients received pemirolast, 20 mg/day, starting 1 week before PTCA until 4-month follow-up angiography. The pemirolast group had a significantly lower restenosis rate (24.0% vs. 46.5% of patients, 18.6% vs. 35.3% of lesions; both $p < 0.01$). At 8-month follow-up, the pemirolast group also had lower incidences of death, MI, bypass surgery, and repeated PTCA (18.3% vs. 36.6%; $p = 0.013$).

176. **Dwens JA,** et al. Usefulness of nisoldipine for prevention of restenosis after percutaneous transluminal coronary angioplasty (results of the nisoldipine in Coronary Disease in Leuven (**NICOLE**) study). *Am J Cardiol* 2001;87:28–33.

This randomized, double-blind, placebo-controlled, single-center trial enrolled 826 patients who underwent successful intervention in native coronary arteries. Patients were randomized to nisoldipine (20 mg/day for 2 weeks and then 40 mg/day for 3 years) or placebo. At 6 months, no significant difference was found between groups in MLD, initial gain, late loss, diameter stenosis, or binary restenosis. The nisoldipine group had a lower incidence of unscheduled coronary angiography ($p = 0.006$), CABG surgery ($p = 0.012$), and repeated target lesion PTCA ($p = 0.017$), which was likely driven by the lower incidence of recurrent angina in nisoldipine-treated patients (12% vs. 21%; $p = 0.004$).

177. **Tamai H,** et al. Impact of tranilast on restenosis after coronary angioplasty: tranilast restenosis following angioplasty trial (**TREAT**). *Am Heart J* 1999;138:968–975.

This prospective, randomized, double-blind, placebo-controlled, multicenter trial of 255 patients examined the use of tranilast in reducing restenosis in *de novo* lesions. Patients received 600 mg/day of tranilast, 300 mg/day, or placebo for 3 months after successful angioplasty. It is unclear whether aspirin was mandatory and whether stents and GP IIb/IIIa inhibitors were allowed. Restenosis rates were 17.6% in the 600-mg/day tranilast group, 38.6% in the 300-mg/day tranilast group, and 39.4% in the placebo group ($p = 0.005$ for 600 mg/day tranilast vs. placebo).

178. **Tsuchikane E,** et al. Impact of cilostazol on restenosis after percutaneous coronary balloon angioplasty. *Circulation* 1999;100:21–26.

A total of 211 patients with 273 lesions who had successful PTCA was randomized to cilostazol (200 mg/day for 3 months) or aspirin (250 mg/day). At follow-up angiography (193 patients), the cilostazol group had significantly lower restenosis and TVRs compared with the aspirin group (17.9% vs. 39.5%; $p < 0.001$; 11.4% vs. 28.7%; $p < 0.001$).

179. Coronary Angioplasty Restenosis Trial (**CART**). n-3 Fatty acids do not prevent restenosis after coronary angioplasty: results from the CART study. *J Am Coll Cardiol* 1999;33:1619–1626.

Prospective, randomized, double-blind, placebo-controlled study of 500 patients undergoing elective coronary angioplasty. Patients received n-3 fatty acids, 5.1 g/day, or corn oil (placebo) starting at least 2 weeks before and continued for 6 months after angioplasty. The restenosis rates were similar in the two groups (defined as MLD, less than 40%): 40.6% in the n-3 fatty acid group and 35.4% in the placebo group ($p = 0.21$).

180. **Gimple LW,** et al. Usefulness of subcutaneous low molecular weight heparin (ardeparin) for reduction of restenosis after percutaneous transluminal coronary angioplasty. *Am J Cardiol* 1999;83:1524–1529.

Prospective, randomized, double-blind, placebo-controlled, multicenter study of 565 patients older than 25 years who had undergone successful PTCA of one or two *de novo* lesions. Patients received ardeparin s.c. twice daily (50 or 100 antiXa μL/kg) or placebo for 3 months. At follow-up angiography (3 to 5 months), ardeparin had no effect on the incidence of angiographic restenosis (41.5% vs. 42.1%).

181. Evaluation of Reopro and Stenting to Eliminate Restenosis (**ERASER**) Investigators. Acute platelet inhibition with abciximab does not reduce in-stent restenosis. *Circulation* 1999;100:799–806.

This prospective, multicenter, double-blind, placebo-controlled trial randomized 225 patients undergoing primary stent implantation to abciximab (12- or 24-hour infusion) or placebo. Target lesions were *de novo* 60% stenoses in native vessels with 3.0 mm to 3.5 mm diameter. At 6-month follow-up, no significant differences between groups were found in in-stent volume obstruction (primary end point).

182. **Serruys PW,** et al. A randomized placebo-controlled trial of fluvastatin for prevention of restenosis after successful coronary balloon angioplasty; final results of the fluvastatin angiographic restenosis (**FLARE**) trial. *Eur Heart J* 1999;20:58–69.

This prospective trial randomized 1,054 patients to either placebo or fluvastatin, 40 mg twice daily, starting 2 to 4 weeks before planned PTCA and after successful PTCA only (no stent) for 6 months. The fluvastatin group had 33% reduction in LDL cholesterol at 26 weeks. The loss in MLD (primary end point) was similar in both groups [0.23 mm (fluvastatin) vs. 0.23 (placebo)], and no significant differences in binary restenosis rates were seen (fluvastatin, 28%; placebo, 31%) or the composite clinical end point of death, MI, CABG surgery, or repeated PCI at 40 weeks (22.4% vs. 23.3%).

183. **Jorgensen B,** et al. Restenosis and clinical outcome in patients treated with amlodipine after angioplasty: results from the Coronary AngioPlasty Amlodipine REStenosis Study (**CAPARES**). *J Am Coll Cardiol* 2000;35:592–599.

This prospective, randomized, double-blind, placebo-controlled, multicenter study enrolled 585 patients. Patients received amlodipine (5 to 10 mg/day) or placebo started 2 weeks before the procedure. Nonstudy calcium channel blockers were prohibited. Stenting was allowed only for bailout or unsatisfactory PTCA results (15.6%). At follow-up angiography, no significant differences were noted between groups in primary end point of mean loss in mean luminal diameter [0.30 mm (amlodipine) vs. 0.29 mm (placebo)]. At 4 months, the amlodipine group had a lower incidence of death, MI, CABG surgery, and repeated PTCA [9.4% vs. 14.5% (placebo group); $p = 0.049$]; this difference was primarily owing to fewer repeated PTCAs [3.1% vs. 7.3% (placebo group); $p = 0.02$].

184. **Meneveau N,** et al. Local delivery of nadroparin for the prevention of neointimal hyperplasia following stent implantation: results of the **IMPRESS** trial, a multicentre, randomized, clinical, angiographic and intravascular ultrasound study. *Eur Heart J* 2000;21:1767–1775.

Prospective, randomized, open-label, multicenter study of 250 patients who underwent PTCA followed by stenting. Patients were assigned to no local drug delivery (control group) or intramural delivery of nadroparin (2 mL of 2,500 anti-Xa-units/mL). Local nadroparin delivery was not associated with an increase in stent thrombosis, coronary artery dissection, side-branch occlusion, distal embolization, or abrupt arterial closure. At 6-month angiography, no significant differences were noted between groups in primary end point of late loss in lumen diameter [0.84 mm (control) vs. 0.88 mm (nadroparin)] and binary restenosis rate [20% (control) vs. 24% (nadroparin)]. An IVUS substudy found that the average area of neointimal tissue within the stent was similar between the groups (2.86 mm vs. 2.90 mm). MACE rates also were similar.

185. **Serruys PW,** et al. Carvedilol for prevention of restenosis after directional coronary atherectomy: final results of the European Carvedilol Atherectomy Restenosis (**EUROCARE**) Trial. *Circulation* 2000;101:1512–1518.

This prospective, double-blind, randomized, placebo-controlled trial enrolled 406 patients; 377 underwent attempted DCA with a 50% diameter stenosis achieved in 89% without stent use. Patients received carvedilol, 25 mg twice daily, starting 24 hours before scheduled DCA and for 5 months after a successful procedure, or placebo. At follow-up angiography (mean, 6 months), no significant differences were seen between the placebo and carvedilol groups in MLD (1.99 mm vs. 2.00 mm) or angiographic restenosis (23.4% vs. 23.9%). TLR and event-free survival also were similar at 7 months (16.2% vs. 14.5%; 79.2% vs. 79.7%).

186. **Meurice T,** et al. Effect of ACE inhibitors on angiographic restenosis after coronary stenting (**PARIS**): a randomised, double-blind, placebo-controlled trial. *Lancet* 2001;357:1321–1324.

The ACE I/D polymorphism was characterized in 345 consecutive patients undergoing coronary stenting. Fifteen had the DD genotype and were randomized to quinapril, 40 mg daily, or placebo, started within 48 hours of stenting and continued for 6 months. At 6-month follow-up angiography (done in 79 patients), the quinapril group had a significantly higher late loss in MLD compared with the control group (mean, 1.11 mm vs. 0.76 mm; $p = 0.018$).

187. **Neumann F,** et al. Treatment of *Chlamydia pneumoniae* infection with roxithromycin and effect on neointima proliferation after coronary stent placement (**ISAR-3**): a randomised, double-blind, placebo-controlled trial. *Lancet* 2001;357:2085–2089.

Prospective, randomized, double-blind trial of 1,010 consecutive patients who underwent successful stenting. Patients received roxithromycin, 300 mg once daily for 28 days, or placebo. No difference was found between the groups in the primary end point of angiographic restenosis [31% (roxithromycin group) vs. 29%; $p = 0.43$] as well as TVR (19% vs. 17%; $p = 0.30$). Interestingly, in patients with high serum titers of *C. pneumoniae,* roxithromycin use was associated with a significantly lower restenosis rate [adjusted ORs at a titer of 1:512 were 0.44 (0.19 to 1.06) and 0.32 (0.13 to 0.81), respectively].

188. **Schnyder G,** et al. Decreased rate of coronary restenosis after lowering of plasma homocysteine levels. *N Engl J Med* 2001;345:1593–1600.

Design: Prospective, randomized, double-blind, placebo-controlled, multicenter study. Primary end point was 50% or more restenosis at follow-up examination.
Purpose: To evaluate the effect of lowering homocysteine on the rate of restenosis after PTCA with or without stents.
Population: 205 patients with successful angioplasty of at least one coronary stenosis of 50% or greater.
Exclusion Criteria: Unstable angina, MI in previous 2 weeks, significant left main disease, creatinine greater than 1.8 mg/dL, and current multivitamin use.
Treatment: Folic acid, 1 mg/day; vitamin B_{12}, 400 μg/day; AND pyridoxine, 10 mg/day, or matching placebo. Use of stents and antiplatelet agents was at operator discretion. QCA was performed at baseline, when clinically necessary, or routinely at 6 months.
Results: Treatment was associated with a lowering of homocysteine levels from 11.1 μm/L to 7.2 μm/L ($p < 0.001$). The treatment group had a significantly lower binary restenosis rate (19.6% vs. 37.6%; $p = 0.01$) as well as a decreased need for TVR (10.8% vs. 22.3%; $p = 0.047$). At angiographic follow-up, the treatment group had a larger mean MLD (1.72 mm vs. 1.45 mm; $p = 0.02$), and less severe mean stenosis (39.9% vs. 48.2%; $p = 0.01$). No difference was found in other coronary events. The benefit was predominantly in those with PTCA without stenting.
Comments: The optimal dose of folic acid is not clear, nor is the added benefit or detriment of vitamin B_{12} and pyridoxine. Because HATS results (see Chapter 1)

found that certain vitamin supplements may counteract the beneficial effects of lipid lowering in patients with a low HDL, it would be helpful to examine the separate contributions of each component of the treatment arm used in this study.

189. **Tamai H,** et al. The impact of tranilast on restenosis after coronary angioplasty: the Second Tranilast Restenosis Following Angioplasty Trial (**TREAT-2**). *Am Heart J* 2002;14:506–513.

This prospective, randomized, double-blinded, placebo-controlled, multicenter trial enrolled 297 patients with 329 lesions to tranilast or placebo for 3 months after successful PTCA for both *de novo* and restenotic lesions. At 3-month angiography, the tranilast group had significantly lower binary restenosis (25.9% vs. 41.9%; $p = 0.012$). In restenotic lesions, the restenosis rate also was significantly lower in the tranilast subgroup.

190. **Holmes DR Jr,** et al. Results of Prevention of REStenosis with Tranilast and its Outcomes (**PRESTO**) trial. *Circulation* 2002;106:1243–1250.

Design: Prospective, randomized, placebo-controlled, double-blind, multicenter study. Primary composite end point of death, MI, or ischemia-driven TVR at 9 months.
Purpose: To determine whether tranilast reduces restenosis and major coronary events compared with placebo in patients undergoing successful PCI.
Population: 11,484 patients who underwent successful PCI and had no evidence of MI.
Treatment: Tranilast, 300 or 450 mg twice daily, for 1 or 3 months (four groups) or placebo.
Results: At 9 months, the incidence of the composite primary end point coronary was similar in the three groups (1-month tranilast group, 15.5%; placebo, 15.8%; 3-month tranilast group, 16.1%). In an angiographic substudy of 2,018 patients, the follow-up mean MLDs were similar (placebo, 1.76-mm group; tranilast, 1.72 mm to 1.78 mm); binary restenosis (greater than 50%) rates also were similar (32% to 35%). In an IVUS substudy of 1,107 patients, plaque volume was not different between the placebo and tranilast groups (39.3 vs. 37.5 to 46.1 mm^3, respectively; $p = 0.16$ to 0.72).

191. **FACIT** (Folate After Coronary Intervention Trial). Preliminary results presented at 52nd ACC Scientific Sessions, Chicago, IL: March 2003.

This prospective, randomized trial enrolled 626 patients who underwent successful stenting. Patients received 1.2 mg folic acid, 4.8 mg pyridoxine and 0.06 mg vitamin B12, or placebo. The folate group had a smaller average minimal luminal diameter (primary end point: 1.59 mm vs. 1.74 mm) and a higher target vessel revascularization rate (15.8% vs. 10.6%).

Radiation
Gamma Radiation
192. **Teirstein PS,** et al., Scripps Coronary Radiation to Inhibit Proliferation Post-Stenting (**SCRIPPS**). Catheter-based radiotherapy to inhibit restenosis after coronary stenting. *N Engl J Med* 1997;336:1697–1703 (editorial, 1748–1749).

Fifty-five patients with restenosis (in-stent, 62%) were randomized to ^{192}Ir (20- to 45-minute exposure; dose of 800 to 3,000 cGy) or placebo. The iridium group had less diabetes mellitus. Angiographic follow-up in 53 patients at 6.7 ± 2.2 months showed that the iridium group had a larger mean luminal diameter (2.43 vs. 1.85 mm; $p = 0.02$) and an impressive 69% lower restenosis rate (17% vs. 54%; $p = 0.01$). No apparent complications were seen with iridium use, although long-term follow-up is necessary. At 2-year follow-up (see *Circulation* 1999;99:243), the incidence of death, MI, or TLR was 55% lower in the radiation group (23.1% vs. 51.7%; $p = 0.03$). Most of this benefit was owing to a 75% lower TLR rate (15.4% vs. 44.8%; $p < 0.001$).

193. Washington Radiation for In-Stent Restenosis Trial (**WRIST**). *Circulation* 2000;101:2165–2171.

Design: Prospective, randomized, blinded, placebo-controlled study. Primary clinical end point was cumulative composite of death, MI, repeated TLR.

Purpose: To evaluate the effectiveness of gamma radiation as adjunctive therapy for patients with ISR.

Population: 130 patients with ISR in native coronary arteries ($n = 100$) and saphenous vein grafts ($n = 30$) with reference diameter 3.0 mm to 5.0 mm and lesion length less than 47 mm.

Treatment: Catheter-delivered gamma radiation (^{192}Ir source; mean dwell time, 22 minutes) or placebo.

Results: At 6 months, the radiation therapy group had a significant reduction in the primary composite end point of death, MI, and TLR (29.2% vs. 67.6%; $p < 0.001$), primarily owing to a lower TLR rate (13.8% vs. 63.1%; $p < 0.001$). The deaths rates were in 4.6% in radiated group and 6.2% in the nonradiated groups; no patients had Q-wave infarcts. TLR also was lower in the radiation group (13.8%) versus the placebo group (63.1%), and the same pattern was seen at 12 months.

Most restenosis in the radiation group occurred at the edges of the stent.

194. **Leon MB,** et al., **GAMMA-1.** Localized intracoronary gamma-radiation therapy to inhibit the recurrence of restenosis after stenting. *N Engl J Med* 2001;344:250–256.

Design: Prospective, randomized, double-blind, multicenter study. Primary composite end point was death, MI, emergency CABG, or need for TLR at 9 months.

Purpose: To assess whether gamma radiation can prevent ISR.

Population: 252 patients with 60% restenosis of stented native vessels 2.75 mm to 4 mm in diameter and lesion length ≤ 45 mm.

Exclusion Criteria: Included MI in prior 72 hours, visible thrombus, ejection fraction less than 40%, and anticipated abciximab administration (actual use, less than 10%).

Treatment: Gamma radiation by using an ^{192}Ir ribbon or placebo. Lesions were irradiated with 800 to 3,000 cGy used (6, 10, or 14 seeds); delivery device dwell time was approximately 20 minutes. Most treated lesions (more than 70%) were complex (type B2 or C).

Results: Radiation group had a 58% lower stent restenosis rate ($p < 0.001$). At 9 months, the radiation group also had a significantly lower incidence of primary composite end point compared with the placebo group (28.2% vs. 43.8%; $p = 0.02$). Late thrombosis occurred in 5.3% (^{192}Ir) versus 0.8% (placebo; $p = 0.07$). A subsequent cost-effectiveness study found that initial costs were increased by nearly $4,100 per patient ($15,724 vs. $11,675; $p < 0.001$) and by $2,200 per patient at 1 year. However, if late thrombosis can be eliminated with extended antiplatelet therapy, long-term medical care costs will likely be lower with brachytherapy (see *Circulation* 2002;106:691–697).

195. **Waksman R,** et al., **WRIST PLUS.** Prolonged antiplatelet therapy to prevent late thrombosis after intracoronary gamma-radiation in patients with in-stent restenosis. *Circulation* 2001;103:2332–2335.

A total of 120 consecutive patients with diffuse ISR in native coronary arteries and vein grafts with lesions smaller than 80 mm underwent PCI, including stenting in 28.3%. After PCI, gamma radiation was administered (^{192}Ir seeds; 14 Gy to 2 mm). All received clopidogrel for 6 months. Late occlusion and thrombosis rates were compared with the 125 gamma radiation–treated patients and 126 placebo patients from WRIST and LONG WRIST (only 1 month of antiplatelet therapy). At 6 months, prolonged antiplatelet therapy resulted in total occlusion in 5.8%, and late thrombosis, in 2.5%; these rates were lower than those in the active gamma radiation group and similar to those in the placebo historical control group.

196. **SCRIPPS II** (Scripps Coronary Radiation to Inhibit Proliferation Post Stenting) results presented at AHA 2001.

Design: Prospective, randomized, blinded, multicenter study. Primary end point was MACE at 9 months.

Purpose: To determine whether gamma radiation with ^{192}Ir can reduce restenosis rates after angioplasty for diffuse ISR.

Population: 100 patients with a restenotic lesion shorter than 65 mm in native coronary or vein graft with a 3.0 mm to 3.5 mm diameter.

Treatment: ^{192}Ir gamma emitter versus placebo. Intracoronary ultrasound used for dosimetry; target farthest from source received 800 cGy, whereas closest target received 3,000 cGy or less. Mean radiation dose at 2 mm was 1,397 cGy.

Results: At 9-month follow-up, radiation group had a 33% lower TVR rate compared with placebo (42% vs. 63%). TVR decreased significantly as radiation dose increased, with a dose of less than 1,200 cGy at 2 mm from the source associated with 66% TVR probability, whereas more than 1,500 cGy resulted in a TVR probability of 25%.

Comments: SCRIPPS II was *not* designed to be a dose-finding study, and the number of patients receiving ^{192}Ir was rather small.

197. **SCRIPPS III** (Scripps Coronary Radiation to Inhibit Proliferation Post Stenting III). *N Engl J Med* 2001;344:297–299 (editorial; also see *J Am Coll Cardiol* 2001;37(suppl A): 60A (abstract)).

Design: Registry study of patients from SCRIPPS III and WRIST-Plus. Primary end points were stent thrombosis and mortality.

Purpose: To determine whether longer term antiplatelet therapy is needed after stenting and beta-radiation brachytherapy to prevent late stent thrombosis.

Population: 500 patients with restenotic lesions within a stented area of a native coronary or bypass graft with vessel diameter of 2.75 mm to 4.0 mm and lesion length less than 80 mm. Of note, 25% in SCRIPPS-III and 29% in WRIST-Plus received new stents at the time of brachytherapy.

Treatment: Patients who received a 14-Gy fixed dose of beta radiation were given clopidogrel for 6 months. If a new stent was placed at the time of irradiation, clopidogrel was given for 12 months.

Results: At the time of the review of the Checkmate device for premarketing approval, 534 patients were registered in the two studies, of whom 206 (38.6%) had been followed up for 7 months. Late thrombosis had occurred in only three patients. In the combined population of these registries, the thrombosis-free survival rate was 99%.

198. **Waksman R,** et al., **WRIST 12.** Twelve versus six months of clopidogrel to reduce major cardiac events in patients undergoing gamma-radiation therapy for in-stent restenosis. *Circulation* 2002;106:776–778.

A total of 120 consecutive patients with diffuse ISR underwent PCI, including additional stent placement in 33%, followed by gamma radiation (^{192}Ir; 14 Gy at 2 mm). All patients received clopidogrel for 12 months. Clinical event rates at 15 months were compared with those of WRIST PLUS patients who received clopidogrel for 6 months. Late thrombosis rates were not significantly different [3.3% (12 months vs. 4.2%); $p = 0.72$]; no cases in the 12-month group were seen between 12 and 15 months. The 12-month group did have a significantly lower incidence of MACE (21% vs. 36%; $p = 0.01$) and TLR (20% vs. 35%; $p = 0.009$).

199. **Waksman R,** et al., **SVG WRIST.** Intravascular gamma radiation for in-stent restenosis in saphenous-vein bypass grafts. *N Engl J Med* 2002;346:1194–1199.

Design: Prospective, randomized, placebo-controlled, double-blind study. Primary end points were death from cardiac causes, Q-wave MI, TVR, and a composite of these events at 12 months.

Purpose: To examine the effects of i.v. gamma radiation in patients with ISR of saphenous vein grafts.

Population: 120 patients with angina and evidence of ISR in saphenous vein grafts who underwent successful PTCA with provisional stenting, laser, or atherectomy.

Treatment: Gamma radiation (^{192}Ir source; 14 to 15 Gy in 2.5-mm to 4.0-mm vessels, and 18 Gy if diameter greater than 4.0 mm), or placebo.

Results: At 6 months, the gamma-radiation group had more than a 50% relative reduction in restenosis compared with placebo (21% vs. 44%; $p = 0.005$). Restenosis rates were significantly lower in all segments (i.e., stented, injured, irradiated). No significant differences were found between the groups in the incidence of death or Q-wave MI, but the radiation group had much lower revascularization rates (1 year TVR, 17% vs. 57%; $p < 0.001$). Late thrombosis rates were similar (both 1.7%).

200. **GAMMA II.** Preliminary results.

The GAMMA II trial was a safety and efficacy registry of 125 patients who received brachytherapy with [192]Ir (14 Gy) to treat ISR. Source trained lengths used were 23, 39, and 55 mm (six, 10, and 14 seeds). In contrast to GAMMA I, a fixed dosimetry model of 14 Gy at 2-mm radius was used. This registry experience was compared in a nonrandomized fashion with that of the 121 patients in the GAMMA I placebo arm. The average lesion length was 19 mm, and the reference vessel diameter was 2.7 mm. Angiographic follow-up was available in 86% at 9 months and showed a 52% lower ISR rate ($p < 0.001$) and a 40% lower in-lesion restenosis rate ($p < 0.001$) compared with the GAMMA I placebo group. A 48% decrease in the TLR rate was noted ($p = 0.001$). The incidence of late stent thrombosis was 6%, similar to the rate seen in GAMMA I.

201. **LONG WRIST.** Waksman R, et al. Intracoronary radiation therapy improves the clinical and angiographic outcomes of diffuse in-stent restenotic lesions. *Circulation* 2003;107:1744–1749.

Design: Prospective, randomized, placebo-controlled; registry group: open label. Primary 1 year clinical end point: deaths MI, target lesion revascularization.
Purpose: To determine the safety and efficacy of vascular brachytherapy for the treatment of diffuse in-stent restenosis.
Population: 120 patients with lesions 36 to 88 mm in length; additional 120 patients were treated with 18 Gy (registry patients).
Treatment: [192]Ir with 15 Gy at 2 mm or placebo; registry group: 18 Gy.
Results: At 6 months, binary restenosis rates were 73%, 45%, and 38% in placebo, 15 Gy, and 18 Gy groups. One year primary event rates were 63% in placebo group compared to 42% in 15 Gy group ($p < 0.05$) and only 22% with 18 Gy.

Beta Radiation
202. **King SB III,** et al., Beta Energy Restenosis Trial (**BERT**). Endovascular beta-radiation to reduce restenosis after coronary balloon angioplasty. *Circulation* 1998;97:2025–2030.

This small study (23 patients) demonstrated the safety and feasibility of beta radiation after angioplasty. A ^{90}Sr/Y source was used to deliver 12, 14, or 16 Gy at 2 mm. Source delivery was successful in 21 (91%) of 23 patients. No in-hospital morbidity or mortality occurred, and follow-up angiography in 20 patients showed a late lumen loss of only 0.5 mm and restenosis in 15%. A larger, randomized, double-blind study is ongoing. Subsequent 6-month follow-up data on 64 patients showed an overall restenosis rate of 14% (20% in the 12-Gy group and 11% in the 14- and 16-Gy groups).

203. **Waksman R,** et al. **BETA-WRIST.** Intracoronary β-radiation therapy inhibits recurrence of in-stent restenosis. *Circulation* 2000;101:1895–1898.

This small prospective study enrolled 50 patients with in-stent stenosis greater than 50%; lesion length, less than 47 mm; vessel diameter, 2.5 mm to 4.0 mm; and who had successful primary treatment (less than 30% residual stenosis without complications). Exclusion criteria were recent acute MI (less than 72 hours), ejection fraction less than 20%, angiographic thrombus, and multiple lesions in the same vessel. Patients received beta radiation with yttrium 90 at a dose of 20.6 Gy at 1.0 mm. At 6 months, the binary angiographic restenosis rate was 22%, the TLR rate was 26%, and the TVR rate was 34%.

204. **Serruys PW,** et al. Safety and performance of 90-strontium for treatment of *de novo* and restenotic lesions: the **BRIE** Trial (Beta Radiation in Europe). *Circulation* 2000;102:II-750.

This prospective, randomized, multicenter study enrolled 150 patients with *de novo* lesions. Patients were treated with the Novoste Betacath system (30-mm source) after angioplasty/stenting. At follow-up **(6 months)**, angiographic restenosis had occurred in 33.6% and TVR in 15.4%. Geographic miss occurred in 41% of the patients and led to increased rates of restenosis (16.3% vs. 4.3%), especially at the edges of treated area (see *J Am Coll Cardiol* 2001;38:415–420). Geographic miss of stent-injured segments resulted in increased restenosis rates, whereas geographic miss of balloon-injured segments did not statistically increase restenosis.

205. **Raizner AE,** et al. Inhibition of restenosis with beta-emitting radiotherapy: report from the Proliferative Reduction with Vascular Energy Trial (**PREVENT**). *Circulation* 2000;102:951–958.

This prospective, randomized, sham-controlled study enrolled 105 patients with *de novo* (70%) or restenotic (30%) stenoses. Stenting was performed in 39% and PTCA in only 39%. Patients received 0 (control), 16, 20, or 24 Gy. At 6 months, angiography demonstrated significantly lower binary restenosis rates in the radiotherapy patients at the target site (8% vs. 39%; $p = 0.012$) and at the target site plus adjacent segments (22% vs. 50%; $p = 0.018$). The radiotherapy patients also had a lower TLR rate (6% vs. 24%; $p < 0.05$).

206. **Verin V,** et al., for the **Beta-Radiation Dose-Finding Study** Group. Endoluminal beta-radiation therapy for the prevention of coronary restenosis after balloon angioplasty. *N Engl J Med* 2001;344:243–249.

Design: Prospective, randomized, multicenter study. The primary end point was the MLD at 6 months.
Purpose: To determine the lowest dose that can prevent restenosis after coronary angioplasty.
Population: 181 patients who underwent successful balloon angioplasty of a previously untreated coronary stenosis
Exclusion Criteria: Included recent MI, cancer within 5 years, prior mediastinal irradiation.
Treatment: Radiation, 9, 12, 15, or 18 Gy, was delivered by a centered ^{90}yttrium source. Adjunctive stenting was required in 28% of the patients. Beta-radiation not performed if there was urgent need for stent implantation or if GP IIb/IIIa–receptor blocker had been given.
Results: At follow-up coronary angiography, mean MLD was 1.67 mm in the 9-Gy group, 1.76 mm in the 12-Gy group, 1.83 mm in the 15-Gy group, and 1.97 mm in the 18-Gy group ($p = 0.06$ for 9 Gy vs. 18 Gy). Restenosis rates were 29%, 21%, 16%, and 15%, respectively ($p = 0.14$ for 9 Gy vs. 18 Gy). In 130 patients treated with balloon angioplasty alone, restenosis rates were 28%, 17%, 16%, and 4%, respectively ($p = 0.02$ for 9 Gy vs. 18 Gy). Among these patients, there was a dose-dependent enlargement of the lumen in 28%, 50%, 45%, and 74% of patients, respectively ($p < 0.001$ for 9 Gy vs. 18 Gy). The rate of repeated revascularization was 18% with 9 Gy and 6% with 18 Gy ($p = 0.26$).

207. **Waksman R,** et al. Use of localised intracoronary beta radiation in treatment of in-stent restenosis: the **INHIBIT** (Intimal Hyperplasia Inhibition with Beta In-stent Trial) randomised controlled trial. *Lancet* 2002;359:551–557.

Design: Prospective, randomized, blinded, multicenter study. Primary composite safety end point was death, Q-wave MI, and TLR at 9 months. Angiographic end point was binary restenosis.
Purpose: To evaluate whether beta-radiation brachytherapy with a P-32 source can reduce MACE and restenosis after treatment of ISR.
Population: 332 patients who underwent PTCA for single native vessel ISR. Reference vessel diameter was 2.4 to 3.7 mm, and lesion length, less than 45 mm.
Exclusion Criteria: Acute MI in previous 72 hours, previous radiation treatment to chest, thrombus by angiogram, multiple lesions in target vessel.
Treatment: P-32 beta emitter versus placebo delivered through a centering catheter via an automatic afterloader.
Results: The P-32 beta-irradiation group had a 56% reduction compared with the control group in the composite end point of death, Q-wave MI, and TLR (15% vs.

31%; $p = 0.0006$) and a 50% reduction in the angiographic binary restenosis rate (26% vs. 52% control; $p < 0.0001$).

208. **START** (Sr90 Treatment of Angiographic Restenosis). Preliminary results presented at 49th ACC Annual Scientific Session, Anaheim, CA, March 2000.

This prospective, randomized, placebo-controlled, multicenter study enrolled 476 patients with native coronary ISR in lesions shorter than 20 mm. After angioplasty, patients were assigned to either 16 or 20 Gy of beta radiation (depending on diameter of vessel) or placebo. Primary end points at 8 months were restenosis, TLR, TVR, and MACE. Beta radiation was associated with significantly lower restenosis rates compared with placebo (in-stent 14% vs. 41%, analysis segment 29% vs. 45%). Radiation group also had improved clinical outcomes (TLR, 13% vs. 22%; TVR, 16% vs. 24%; and MACE, 18% vs. 26%).

209. **BETA CATH.** Results presented at the 50th ACC Annual Scientific Session, Orlando, FL, March 2001.

This prospective, randomized, placebo-controlled, multicenter study enrolled 1,455 patients with a single *de novo* or restenotic lesion with 60% to 100% diameter stenosis and shorter than 20 mm and in 2.7 mm to 4.0 mm diameter vessel. All patients were treated with PTCA and approximately 50% received stents (allowed for suboptimal PTCA result). Patients received strontium 90 beta radiation (30-mm source; 14 Gy for 2.7-mm to 3.35-mm vessels, 18 Gy for 3.35-mm to 4.0-mm vessels) or placebo. Early in the trial, it was mandated that antiplatelet therapy with clopidogrel be extended to at least 3 months, which resulted in the late thrombosis rate decreasing from 6.3% to 1.3% by the end of the trial. At 8 months, the radiation group had nonsignificant reductions compared with the placebo group in the incidence of TLR [12% relative risk reduction (RRR)], TVR (10% RRR), and MACE (9% RRR). Among PTCA-only–treated patients, radiation was associated with significant reductions in all three main measures (35%, 28%, and 30% for TLR, TVR, and MACE, respectively). In contrast, among stented patients, radiation was associated with a *higher* incidence of these events (14%, 9%, and 13%, respectively). It has been suggested that geographic miss was responsible for adverse outcomes in the stented patients receiving radiation.

Drug-eluting Stents
210. **Morice M-C,** et al., for the **RAVEL** (Randomized BX VELocity) Study Group. Randomized comparison of a sirolimus-eluting stent with a standard stent for coronary revascularization. *N Engl J Med* 2002;346:1773–1780.

Design: Prospective, randomized, double-blind, multicenter study. Primary end points were mean lumen diameter and late lumen loss at 6 months.
Purpose: To determine whether implantation of a sirolimus-eluting stent in *de novo* lesions will result in decreased restenosis compared with a bare stent.
Population: 238 patients with stable or unstable angina pectoris or silent ischemia who needed treatment of a single *de novo* lesion in a native vessel (2.5 to 3.5 mm or larger) that could be covered by a single 18-mm stent.
Exclusion Criteria: Included evolving MI, left main stenosis, ostial lesion location, calcified lesion that could not be completely dilated before stenting, angiographically visible thrombus within target lesion, ejection fraction less than 30%.
Treatment: Sirolimus-eluting stent or uncoated Bx Velocity balloon-expandable stent. All received ticlopidine or clopidogrel for 2 months.
Results: Rapamycin group had a mean late loss of 0.01 mm compared with 0.80 mm in the control group ($p < 0.0001$). Restenosis occurred in none of the rapamycin patients versus 26% of controls ($p < 0.0001$). Freedom from MACE (death, MI, repeated PCI, and CABG) was 96.7% in the rapamycin group compared with 72.9% in the control group ($p < 0.0001$). No cases of subacute stent thromboses were found.

211. **SIRIUS** (Sirolimus-Eluting Stent in Coronary Lesions) Trial. Results presented at the Course on Revascularization in Paris, France, May 2002, and Transcatheter Cardiovascular Therapeutics, Washington, DC, September 2002.

Design: Prospective, randomized, double-blind, placebo-controlled, study. Primary end point was target vessel failure defined as cardiac death, MI, or TVR at 9 months.

Purpose: To establish the safety and efficacy of the sirolimus-eluting BX Velocity stent in decreasing target vessel failure in *de novo* native coronary artery lesions compared with the uncoated BX Velocity stent.

Population: 1,058 patients requiring single-vessel treatment of *de novo* higher-risk lesions (2.5 mm to 3.5 mm diameter and 15 mm to 30 mm long) in native vessels. Of note, 26% had diabetes, and 42% had multivessel disease. Most lesions were type B2 or C.

Exclusion Criteria: Included recent MI (less than 24 hours), unprotected left main disease, ostial location, total occlusion, angiographic evidence of thrombus, calcified lesion that could not be predilated; LVEF less than 25%, impaired renal function, pretreatment with devices other than balloon angioplasty, prior or planned intervention within 30 days.

Treatment: Sirolimus-eluting stent or uncoated stent. Antiplatelet therapy for given for 3 months.

Results: Target vessel failure (primary end point) was reduced by nearly 60% in the sirolimus group compared with the bare metal stent group (from 21.0% to 8.6%; $p < 0.001$). The sirolimus stent group had a 91% reduction in ISR compared with bare metal stents (3.2% vs. 35.4%; $p < 0.001$). ISR, which included the 5-mm segments proximal and distal to the stent, was reduced by 75% in the sirolimus group (8.9% vs. 36.3%; $p < 0.001$). Among diabetics, restenosis in the stent and in the segment was 8.3% and 17.6%, respectively, for sirolimus, compared with 48.5% and 50.5% for the bare stent. The distal margin had an equal treatment effect to that seen within the stent, whereas there was less intense effect but still significant effect in the proximal margin (late loss, 0.17 mm vs. 0.33 mm; $p < 0.001$). ISR increased by 13% for every additional 10 mm of implanted stent length in controls, compared with only 1.6% in the sirolimus group. Aneurysms occurred in two (0.6%) patients in the sirolimus group and in four (1.1%) patients in the control group. Stent thrombosis rates were also similar (0.6% and 1.1%). An IVUS study of 141 patients found an overall 90% reduction in neointimal volume in the coated-stent group; the lowest reduction was seen at the proximal margin in smaller vessels.

Comments: SIRIUS cohort had more patients with clinical characteristics associated with higher rates of restenosis as well as more complex lesions than the RAVEL cohort. However, several types of lesions were still excluded (see earlier), and ongoing studies are addressing these issues. The proximal margin findings suggest that balloon injury in this area is associated with pre/post dilation or stent delivery.

212. **ASPECT** (Asian Paclitaxel-Eluting Stent Clinical Trial). Park SJ, et al. A paclitaxel-eluting stent for the prevention of coronary restenosis. *N Engl J Med* 2003;348:1537–1545.

This prospective, randomized, triple-blind, multicenter study enrolled 177 patients with discrete coronary lesions (<15 mm in length, 2.25 to 3.25 mm in diameter). Patients received a low dose (1.3 mcg/mm^2) or high dose (3.1 mcg/mm^2) paclitaxel mounted on a nonpolymerized stent, or a bare metal stent. At 4 to 6 month angiographic follow-up, the high-dose group had better results for the degree of stenosis (mean 14% vs. 39%, $p < 0.001$), late loss of luminal diameter (0.29 mm vs. 1.04 mm, $p < 0.001$), and binary restenosis (4% vs. 27%, $p < 0.001$). Of note, the larger DELIVER trial found benefit with this type of stent (see below).

213. **TAXUS II.** Preliminary results presented at Transcatheter Cardiovascular Therapeutics, Washington, DC, September 2002.

This prospective, randomized, multicenter trial enrolled a total of 402 patients and compared a bare stent with two formulations of a paclitaxel-eluting stent [slow-release (drug released over a 1-month period) or moderate-release (most released in the first 2 days)]. Lesions were standard-risk *de novo* lesions (average length, approximately 10 mm; average reference vessel diameter, approximately 2.75 mm). Patients received aspirin and clopidogrel for 6 months. Both paclitaxel-eluting stents demonstrated substantial reductions in the primary end point, percentage of in-stent net volume obstruction (by IVUS), compared with the bare stent group (60% reduction with slow-release and 62% with moderate-release version). At 6 months, MACE was significantly reduced with the drug-eluting stents [slow release, 8.5% vs. 19.5% (control); $p = 0.013$; moderate release, 7.8% vs, 20%; $p = 0.006$]. These reductions were driven by lower rates of TVR and TLR. Binary restenosis rates were significantly reduced versus controls in both the slow-release and moderate-release cohorts [in-stent, 2.3% (slow release) vs. 17.9%; $p = 0.0002$; 4.7% (moderate-release) vs. 202.%; $p < 0.0001$]. Importantly, no sign of edge effect was found, with nonsignificant *reductions* seen both in the proximal and distal segments of the segment with the drug-eluting stents versus controls.

214. **DELIVER** Preliminary results (released by Guidant 1-3-03). The prospective, randomized, multicenter trial enrolled 1,042 patients. Patients received a paclitaxel-coated ACHIEVE stent or bare DENTA stent. The paclitaxel group had a nonsignificant reduction in 9-month incidence of target vessel failure (11% to 12% vs.14% to 15%) and binary restenosis (16% to 17% vs. 21% to 22%).

CABG Surgery

Review Articles, Meta-Analyses

215. **Kirklin JW,** et al., ACC/AHA Guidelines. Guidelines and indications for coronary artery bypass graft surgery; a report of the ACC/AHA Task Force on Assessment of Diagnostic and Therapeutic Cardiovascular Procedures (Subcommittee on CABG Surgery). *J Am Coll Cardiol* 1991;17:543–589.

216. **Yusuf S,** et al. Effect of coronary artery bypass graft surgery on survival: overview of 10-year results from randomised trials by the CABG Trialists Collaboration. *Lancet* 1994;344:563–570.

This review of data focuses on 1,324 patients assigned to CABG surgery and 1,325 patients who received medical management. The CABG group had a significantly lower mortality rate at 5 years (10.2% vs. 15.8%; OR, 0.61; $p = 0.0001$), 7 years (15.8% vs. 21.7%; OR, 0.68; $p < 0.001$), and 10 years (26.4% vs. 30.5%; OR, 0.83; $p = 0.03$). The risk reduction was most marked in patients with left main CAD and three-vessel disease or one- or two-vessel disease [ORs, 0.32, 0.58 vs. 0.77 (two- and one-vessel disease)]. High-risk patients (defined as those with two of following: severe angina, history of hypertension, prior MI, and ST-segment depression at rest) had a 29% mortality reduction at 10 years compared with a 10% reduction in patients at moderate risk and a nonsignificant trend toward higher mortality in low-risk patients [no risk factors (except ST depression) allowed].

217. **Nwasokwa ON.** Coronary artery bypass graft disease. *Ann Intern Med* 1995;123:528–545.

This thorough review of the literature showed only an approximate 50% patency of saphenous vein grafts at 10 years after bypass surgery versus more than 90% patency achieved with IMA grafts. The use of IMA grafts leads to less frequent symptoms, better LV function, decreased need for reoperation, and improved survival. The role of antiplatelet agents in decreasing graft occlusion rates also is reviewed.

218. **Pocock SJ,** et al. Meta-analysis of randomised trials comparing coronary angioplasty with bypass surgery. *Lancet* 1996;346:1184–1189.

This analysis of data was derived from 3,771 patients in eight trials (CABRI, RITA, EAST, GABI, MASS, ERACI, Toulouse, Lausanne). The average follow-up period was 2.7 years. No differences were demonstrated in overall cardiac mortality between PTCA and CABG. However, CABG patients had 90% fewer first-year reinterventions (3.3% vs. 33.7%) and less angina. A CABG was performed in 18% of PTCA patients within 1 year. The impact of longer follow-up is unknown (e.g., increased saphenous venous graft disease).

219. **Roach G,** et al. Adverse cerebral outcomes after coronary bypass surgery. *N Engl J Med* 1996;335:1857–1863.

This prospective study was composed of 2,108 patients, 6.1% with cerebral events: type I, 3.1% [focal injury, or stupor or coma at hospital discharge (D/C); 55 of 66 had nonfatal strokes] or type II, 3% (deterioration in intellectual function, memory deficit, or seizures). Events were associated with increased in-hospital mortality [21% (type I) and 10% vs. 2%], longer hospital stay (25 days, 21 days, 10 days), and more patients discharged to intermediate or long-term care (47%, 30%, 8%). Type I predictors included proximal aortic atherosclerosis, history of neurologic disease, and age; type II predictors included age, hypertension, pulmonary disease, and alcohol consumption.

Studies
CABG versus Medical Therapy
220. European Coronary Surgery Study (**ECSS**) Group. Long-term results of prospective randomised study of coronary artery bypass surgery in stable angina pectoris. *Lancet* 1982;320:1173–1180.

Design: Prospective, randomized, open study. Primary end point was all-cause mortality. Follow-up period was 5 to 8 years.
Purpose: To compare CABG surgery with initial medical management in patients with angina and multivessel CAD.
Population: 768 men aged ≤65 years with mild to moderate angina, ≥50% stenosis in two major vessels, and good LV function.
Treatment: CABG surgery or medical therapy.
Results: Surgery was beneficial in the total population (88.6% survival vs. 79.9% at 8 years), although most of the benefit was seen in patients with proximal LAD artery stenoses (10-year survival, 76% vs. 66%). No benefit was present if left main disease was present. Independent predictors of surgical benefit were abnormal rest ECG, ST depression 1.5 mm with exercise, peripheral vascular disease, and increased age.

221. Coronary Artery Surgery Study (**CASS**) Principal Investigators and their associates. Myocardial infarction and mortality in the CASS randomized trial. *N Engl J Med* 1984;310:750–758.

Design: Prospective, randomized, open, parallel-group study. Primary end point was all-cause mortality. Mean follow-up period was 6 years.
Purpose: To determine whether CABG surgery reduces mortality and MI rates in patients with mild angina and angiographically documented CAD.
Population: 780 patients aged ≤65 years with coronary artery stenosis ≥70%.
Exclusion Criteria: Prior CABG, unstable angina, heart failure (NYHA class III or IV).
Treatment: CABG surgery or medical therapy.
Results: Lower mortality trend was observed with CABG (1.1%/year vs. 1.6%/year), strongest in patients with EF ≤50% ($p = 0.085$) and three-vessel disease and EF ≤50% ($p = 0.063$). Among patients with three-vessel disease and EF of 35% to 49%, a significant mortality difference was found at subsequent follow-up [12% (CABG) vs. 35% mortality; $p = 0.009$; see *N Engl J Med* 1985;312:1665]. At 10-year follow-up (see *Circulation* 1990;82:1629), CABG had been performed in 40% of medical patients, and no overall survival difference was noted (medical group, 79%; surgical group, 82%). However, the results of CABG were significantly better than medical therapy in patients with an EF less than 50% (79% vs. 61%; $p = 0.01$).
Comments: Long-term follow-up in 912 patients with left main equivalent disease (e.g., severe proximal LAD and left circumflex disease) showed that surgery prolongs life (13.1 vs. 6.2 years), but not if normal LV function is present (15-year survival, 63% vs. 54%; $p = $ NS), even with right coronary artery stenosis ≥70% (see *Circulation* 1995;91:2335).

222. **VA** Coronary Artery Bypass Surgery Cooperative Study Group. Eleven year survival in Veterans Affairs randomized trial of coronary bypass surgery for stable angina. *N Engl J Med* 1984;311:1333–1339.

Design: Prospective, randomized, multicenter, open study. Primary end point was all-cause mortality. Average follow-up was 11.2 years.

Purpose: To compare CABG with medical therapy in patients with stable angina.

Population: 686 patients with stable angina pectoris of longer than 6 months' duration.

Exclusion Criteria: MI in prior 6 months, unstable angina, DBP greater than 100 mm Hg, uncompensated congestive heart failure.

Treatment: CABG surgery or medical therapy.

Results: Overall, a significant mortality difference was observed between groups at 7 years (77% survival in CABG group vs. 70%; $p = 0.043$) but not at 11 years (57% vs. 58%). Surgery was beneficial in the following subgroups: (a) three-vessel disease plus LV dysfunction (per angiography), 50% versus 38% survival at 11 years ($p = 0.026$); (b) clinically high-risk patients (at least two of the following: resting ST depression, history of MI, history of hypertension), 49% versus 36% survival ($p = 0.015$); and (c) combined angiographic and clinically high risk, 54% versus 24% ($p = 0.005$). Patients with LV dysfunction (EF, less than 45%; end-diastolic pressure, more than 14 mm Hg; or any contraction abnormality) benefited from surgery at 7 years (survival, 74% vs. 63%; $p = 0.049$) but not at 11 years (53% vs. 49%).

Comments: Subsequent 18-year follow-up report showed no benefit of surgery, even in the high-risk subgroups. Overall, the benefits of surgery began to diminish after 5 years, a time course that parallels the development of graft disease.

Coronary Artery Bypass Graft Surgery versus Percutaneous Transluminal Coronary Angiography

223. Coronary angioplasty vs coronary artery bypass surgery: the Randomised Intervention Treatment of Angina (**RITA**) trial. *Lancet* 1993;341:573–580.

Design: Prospective, randomized, multicenter study. Primary end point was death and MI. Mean follow-up period was 2.5 years.

Purpose: To compare bypass surgery with coronary angioplasty in patients in whom equivalent myocardial revascularization could be achieved by either treatment method.

Population: 1,011 patients with multivessel coronary disease (55% with at least two diseases of the coronary arteries).

Exclusion Criteria: Left main disease, prior coronary angioplasty or bypass surgery, and significant valve disease.

Treatment: CABG surgery or PTCA.

Results: No difference was observed in the primary composite end point of death or MI at 5 years (8.6% vs. 9.8%; RR, 0.88; 95% CI, 0.59 to 1.29). CABG patients had a longer recovery but fewer additional measures. At 2 years, repeated angiography was performed in 7% versus 31% ($p < 0.001$), and revascularization or a primary event occurred in 11% vs. 38% ($p < 0.001$). CABG patients also had less angina (22% vs. 31% at 2 years). A subsequent report showed that the PTCA group had a higher out-of-work rate at 2 years (26% vs. 22%) (see *Circulation* 1996;94: 135).

224. **Rodriguez A,** et al. Estudio Randomizado Argentino de Angioplastia versus Cirugia (**ERACI**). Argentine randomized trial of PTCA vs coronary artery bypass surgery in multivessel disease: in-hospital results and one year follow-up. *J Am Coll Cardiol* 1993;22:1060–1067.

In this prospective, single-center study, 127 patients were randomized to angioplasty or bypass surgery. No differences were seen in in-hospital deaths, periprocedural MIs, emergency revascularization, or 1-year mortality rate. However, CABG patients had less angina and fewer reinterventions and combined cardiac events (83.5% vs. 63.7%; $p < 0.005$).

225. **Hamm CW,** et al. German Angioplasty Bypass Surgery Investigation (**GABI**). A randomized study of coronary angioplasty compared with bypass surgery in patients with symptomatic multivessel coronary disease. *N Engl J Med* 1994;331:1037–1043.

Design: Prospective, randomized, multicenter study. Primary end point was freedom from angina at 1 year.

Purpose: To compare the clinical efficacy of bypass surgery with balloon angioplasty in patients with symptomatic multivessel CAD.

Population: 8,981 patients younger than 75 years were screened, and 359 were enrolled (total revascularization of at least two major vessels needed and feasible technically).

Exclusion Criteria: Totally occluded vessels, left main stenosis greater than 30%, MI in prior 4 weeks, and prior bypass or angioplasty.

Treatment: CABG surgery or PTCA.

Results: CABG group had longer hospitalization (19 vs. 5 days) and more MIs (8.1% vs. 2.3%; $p = 0.022$) owing to procedures. However, CABG patients had similar in-hospital mortality rates (2.5% vs. 1.1%), fewer interventions (6% vs. 44%; $p < 0.001$), and less angina at hospital discharge (7% vs. 18%; no difference at 1 year), and fewer patients were taking antianginal medications (12% vs. 22%; $p = 0.041$).

226. **King SB,** et al. Emory Angioplasty vs Surgery Trial (**EAST**). A randomized trial comparing coronary angioplasty with coronary bypass surgery. *N Engl J Med* 1994;331:1044–1050 (editorial, 1086–1087).

Design: Prospective, randomized, multicenter study. Composite primary end point was death, Q-wave MI, and large defect on thallium scan at 3 years.

Purpose: To compare outcomes of bypass surgery with angioplasty in patients with multivessel disease.

Population: 392 patients with two- or three-vessel CAD (5,118 patients screened; 842 eligible).

Exclusion Criteria: Prior bypass surgery or coronary angioplasty, recent myocardial infarction (less than 5 days), old chronic occlusions (more than 8 weeks), left main stenosis greater than 30%, and EF, less than 25%.

Treatment: CABG surgery or PTCA.

Results: No significant difference was observed between groups in 3-year mortality (7.1% vs. 6.3%) or primary composite end points (28.8% vs. 27.3%). However, CABG patients required fewer repeated CAGB surgeries (1% vs. 22%; $p < 0.001$) and fewer angioplasties (13% vs. 41%; $p < 0.001$), and reported less angina (12% vs. 20%).

227. CABRI Trial Participants. First year results of **CABRI** (Coronary Angioplasty vs Bypass Revascularization Investigation). *Lancet* 1995;346:1179–1184.

Design: Prospective, randomized, multicenter, open study. Primary outcomes were 1-year mortality and symptom status (based on angina class) at 1 year.

Purpose: To compare bypass surgery with angioplasty in patients with multivessel coronary disease requiring intervention.

Population: 1,054 patients aged ≤75 years with multivessel disease and typical angina or unstable angina, 62% with class III angina.

Treatment: CABG surgery or PTCA.

Exclusion Criteria: MI in prior 10 days; EF, less than 35%; and prior PTCA or CABG.

Results: At 1-year follow-up, mortality rates were similar between groups (2.7% for CABG, 3.9% for PTCA). The CABG group had 81% fewer reinterventions (6.5% vs. 33.6%; $p < 0.001$) and 35% less angina, and patients were taking fewer medications. The 1-year mortality rate was highest in patients with grade IV angina or unstable angina (5% vs. 2.7%).

Comments: Complete revascularization was not required, and patients with total occlusions were not excluded.

228. **Hueb WA,** et al. Medicine, Angioplasty or Surgery Study (**MASS**): a prospective, randomized trial of medical therapy, balloon angioplasty or bypass surgery for single proximal left anterior descending stenoses. *J Am Coll Cardiol* 1995;26:1600–1605.

This prospective, randomized, multicenter study was composed of 214 patients with stable angina, normal LV function, and more than 80% proximal LAD stenosis. Patients were randomized to CABG, PTCA, or medical therapy alone. At an average follow-up of 3 years, no CABG patients needed revascularization (vs. eight and seven patients; $p = 0.019$) and only 3% [vs. 24% (PTCA), $p = 0.0002$; and vs. 17%, $p = 0.006$]

had experienced a primary end point (death, Q-wave MI, or large ischemic defect on thallium scan at 3 years). However, no significant difference in mortality or infarction rates was found. CABG and PTCA groups had greater symptom relief and decreased ischemia on treadmill.

229. **Frye RL,** et al. Bypass Angioplasty Revascularization Investigation (**BARI**). Comparison of coronary bypass surgery with angioplasty in patients with multivessel disease. *N Engl J Med* 1996;335:217–225 (editorial, 275–276).

Design: Prospective, randomized, multicenter study. Primary end point was all-cause mortality. Follow-up period was 5.4 years.
Purpose: To compare outcomes of bypass surgery with angioplasty in patients with multivessel disease and severe angina or ischemia.
Population: 1,829 patients; 41% had three-vessel CAD.
Treatment: CABG surgery or PTCA.
Results: CABG and PTCA groups had similar in-hospital mortality rates [1.3% (CABG) vs. 1.1%] and 5-year survival rates (89% vs. 86%; $p = 0.19$). The CABG group had more in-hospital Q-wave MIs (4.6% vs. 2.1%; $p < 0.01$) but had an 85% lower 5-year revascularization rate (8% vs. 54%) and 44% better 5-year survival in patients with diabetes (19% of enrolled patients; 81% vs. 66%; $p = 0.003$). The PTCA group had a 31% 5-year CABG rate.
Comments: Accompanying editorial reports that combining data from the BARI, EAST, and CABRI trials, CABG is associated with nonsignificant 14% mortality reduction (95% CI, +16% to −37%). A subsequent cost and quality-of-life analysis of 934 patients showed that the initial costs were 35% lower in the PTCA group but only 5% lower at 5 years ($56,000 vs. $58,900; $p = 0.047$). The cost of surgery was −$26,000/year of life added, and surgical patients returned to work 5 weeks later but had better functional status at 3 years (see *N Engl J Med* 1997;336:92). Another analysis showed that more lesions were favorable for revascularization by CABG (92% vs. 78%; $p < 0.001$), especially 99% to 100% lesions (78% vs. 22%) (see *Am J Cardiol* 1996;77:805).

230. **SIMA** (Stenting vs. Internal Mammary Artery). Preliminary results. *Circulation* 1998;98(suppl I):I-349.

The European SIMA trial randomized 123 patients with proximal LAD stenoses in vessels greater than 3 mm diameter to either stenting or CABG surgery. Six patients in the surgical group underwent minimally invasive CABG surgery. Procedural success was 98% in both groups. Acute complications were more frequent in the stent group (7% vs. 4%). One patient died 2 days after stenting because of subacute stent closure. Three stent patients and one surgical patient had a non–Q-wave MI, whereas one patient in the CABG group had a Q-wave MI at home while awaiting surgery. The CABG had more minor complications (10% vs. 3%), primarily because of arrhythmias. Hospitalization was significantly shorter with stenting (2.6 vs. 13 days). At 6 months, the CABG group had a lower reintervention rate (none vs. 13%) and were more likely to be symptom free (96% vs. 77%).

231. **Rodriguez A,** et al., ERACI II Investigators. Argentine Randomized Study: Coronary Angioplasty with Stenting versus Coronary Bypass Surgery in patients with Multiple-Vessel Disease (**ERACI II**): 30-day and one-year follow-up results. *J Am Coll Cardiol* 2001;37:51–58.

Design: Prospective, randomized, double-blind, placebo-controlled, multicenter study. Primary end point: death, MI, repeated revascularization procedures, and stroke at 30 days.
Purpose: To compare PTCR with stent implantation with conventional CABG surgery in symptomatic patients with multivessel CAD.
Population: 450 patients with multivessel CAD (2,759 screened) and an indication for revascularization.
Treatment: PTCR (225 patients) or CABG (225 patients).
Results: At 30 days, the PTCR group had fewer major adverse events compared with the CABG group (3.6% vs. 12.3%; $p = 0.002$), including a significantly lower

mortality (0.9% vs. 5.7%; $p < 0.013$). At follow-up (mean, 18.5 months), the PTCR had a persistent mortality benefit (3.1% vs. 7.5%; $p < 0.017$). However, as seen in prior trials of similar design, the PTCR group had a much higher revascularization rate than did the CABG group (16.8% vs. 4.8%; $p < 0.002$).

232. **Serruys PW,** et al., for the Arterial Revascularization Therapies Study (**ARTS**) Group. Comparison of coronary-artery bypass surgery and stenting for the treatment of multivessel disease. *N Engl J Med* 2001;344:1117–1124.

Design: Prospective, randomized, double-blind, placebo-controlled, parallel-group study. Primary end point: Freedom from death, MI, any cerebrovascular event, and any repeated coronary revascularization at 1 year.

Purpose: To compare coronary artery stenting with CABG surgery in patients with multivessel disease.

Population: 1,205 patients (average age, 61 years) who had not undergone bypass surgery or angioplasty with stable angina, unstable angina, or silent ischemia AND ≥two *de novo* lesions in different vessels and territories that were amenable to stenting. The average interval between randomization and treatment was 27 days for patients in surgery group and 11 days for the stenting group.

Exclusion Criteria: LVEF, 30% or less; overt congestive heart failure; history of cerebrovascular accident (CVA); transmural MI in previous week; severe hepatic or renal disease; diseased saphenous veins; neutropenia or thrombocytopenia; intolerance or contraindication to aspirin or ticlopidine; need for major surgery.

Treatment: Stenting or CABG surgery (randomized *after* a cardiac surgeon and an interventional cardiologist concurred that the same extent of revascularization could be achieved with either technique. The average interval between randomization and treatment was 27 days for patients in the surgery group and 11 days for the stenting group. Fewer than 4% were treated with GP IIb/IIIa inhibitors.

Results: At 1 year, no significant differences were seen between the two groups in death, stroke, or MI. Surgery was associated with a higher event-free survival compared with stenting (87.8% vs. 73.8%; $p < 0.001$). This difference was due to primarily to the much higher rate of repeated revascularization in the stenting group; among those without a stroke or MI, the incidence was 16.8% versus 3.5% in the surgery group. No significant difference was noted between the two groups in the incidence of death (2.8% vs. 2.5%), stroke (2.0% vs. 1.5%), or MI (4.0% vs. 5.3%). The costs for the initial procedure were $4,212 less per patient for the stenting group, but this difference narrowed to $2,973 per patient by 1-year follow-up. Among CABG patients, an elevated CK-MB was observed in 61%, and an increase to more than 5 times normal in 12%, and was an independent predictor of adverse clinical events. A subsequent report (see *Circulation* 2001;104:533) found that diabetics who underwent stenting had the lowest event-free survival (63.4% vs. 84.4% diabetes and CABG, 76.2% no-diabetes and stenting, and 88.4% no diabetes plus CABG); this was owing to an increased incidence of repeated revascularization. A nonsignificant trend toward a lower mortality rate was seen in the diabetic CABG group compared with the diabetic stenting group (3.1% vs. 6.3%).

Comments: GP IIb/IIIa inhibitors were used infrequently in this trial; higher use may have decreased the 2.8% stent thrombosis rate and the 30% CK-MB release in the stent group. Outcomes in the modern era of GP IIb/IIIa inhibition, clopidogrel, and coated stents and with longer follow-up to detect late graft failure are not known.

233. **Morrison DA,** et al., for the Investigators of the Department of Veterans Administration Affairs Cooperative Study 385, the Angina with Extremely Serious Operative Mortality Evaluation (**AWESOME**). Percutaneous coronary intervention vs. coronary artery bypass graft surgery for patients with medically refractory myocardial ischemia and risk factors for adverse outcomes with bypass: a multicenter, randomized trial. *J Am Coll Cardiol* 2001;38:143–149.

Design: Prospective, randomized, multicenter study. Primary end point was survival. Secondary end points were unstable angina, repeated hospitalization, repeated catheterization, and repeated revascularization with CABG or PCI.

Purpose: To compare PCI with CABG in high-risk patients with medically refractory MI.

Population: 554 patients (22,662 screened) with evidence of medically refractory MI and one or more of five high-risk clinical characteristics for CABG including prior open heart surgery, older than 70 years, LVEF less than 35, MI within 7 days, or intraaortic balloon pump requirement.

Treatment: PCI or CABG surgery. The use of left IMA grafting increased from 57% in 1995 to 78% in 2000 (average, 70%), whereas stent use increased from 26% to 88% (average, 54%) and GP IIb/IIIa inhibitor use from 1% to 52% (average, 11%).

Results: The in-hospital and 30-day survival rates were 96% and 95%, respectively, for CABG, and 99% and 97% for PCI. At 6-month follow-up, the small difference in survival rates was still present (90% for CABG and 94% for PCI), whereas at 3-year follow-up, survival rates were similar (79% for CABG and 80% for PCI; $p = 0.46$). No significant differences were noted between the groups in freedom from unstable angina [65% (CABG) vs. 59%; $p < 0.16$], whereas freedom from unstable angina and repeated revascularization was significantly better with CABG compared with PCI (61% vs. 48%; $p = 0.001$).

234. **SoS** (Stent or Surgery). SoS Investigators. Coronary artery bypass surgery versus percutaneous coronary intervention with stent implantation in patients with multivessel coronary artery disease (the Stent or Surgery Trial): a randomised controlled trial. *Lancet* 2002;360:965–970.

Design: Prospective, randomized, open, multicenter study. Primary outcome measure was rate of repeat revascularization. Median follow-up was 2 years.

Purpose: To assess the effect of stent-assisted PCI versus CABG in multivessel CAD patients.

Population: 988 patients with symptomatic multivessel CAD.

Exclusion Criteria: Previous CABG or PCI, acute MI in prior 48 hours, intervention of valves, myocardium, great vessels, carotids, or aorta scheduled for index revascularization procedure.

Treatment: Angioplasty with stenting (PCI) or CABG surgery; in PCI arm, mean number of vessels treated was 2.2, with 78% of lesions receiving stents.

Results: The PCI group had a higher revascularization rate compared with the CABG group (21% vs. 6%, $p < 0.0001$). The incidence of death or MI at 2 years was similar in both groups (PCI 9%, CABG 10%). Though the mortality rate was significantly lower in the surgery group (2% vs. 5%, $p = 0.01$).

Comments: Although the revascularization rate was higher in the stent arm, the rates were about half those seen in the BARI and EAST trials.

235. **Diegeler A,** et al. Comparison of stenting with minimally invasive bypass surgery for stenosis of the left anterior descending coronary artery. *N Engl J Med* 2002;347:561–566.

A total of 220 symptomatic patients with high-grade proximal LAD lesions of the coronary artery were randomized to minimally invasive surgery (thoracotomy; no cardiopulmonary bypass) or stenting. At 6 months, the surgery group had a lower incidence of MACEs, consisting of cardiac death, MI, and TLR, compared with the stenting group (15% vs. 31%; $p = 0.02$). The difference was primarily owing to higher TLR for restenosis after stenting (29% vs. 8%; $p = 0.003$), as the combined rates of death and MI did not differ significantly between groups [6% (surgery) vs. 3%; $p = 0.50$]. The surgery group had more patients free from angina after 6 months compared with the stenting group (79% vs. 62%; $p = 0.03$). It should be noted that the stent group did not receive GP IIb/IIIa inhibitors.

Graft and Patency Studies

236. **Loop FD,** et al. Influence of the internal mammary graft on 10 year survival and other cardiac events. *N Engl J Med* 1986;314:1–6.

This retrospective analysis focused on 5,931 patients who underwent CABG from 1971 to 1979; 3,625 patients had saphenous vein grafts only. IMA patients had better survival. Ten-year rates were 93.4% versus 88% ($p = 0.05$) for one-vessel disease; 90%

vs. 79.5% ($p < 0.0001$) for two-vessel disease; and 82.6% versus 71% ($p < 0.001$) for three-vessel disease. A Cox multivariate analysis was performed, and for the saphenous vein graft group, the RR of death was 1.61; late MI RR, 1.14; hospitalization for cardiac events RR, 1.25; and cardiac reoperation RR, 2.0.

237. **Cameron A,** et al. Coronary bypass surgery with internal thoracic artery grafts: effects on survival over a 15-year period. *N Engl J Med* 1996;334:216–219 (editorial, 263–265).

This analysis focused on 5,637 CASS registry patients, including 749 patients who received arterial grafts. In multivariate analysis, internal thoracic artery patients had a 27% lower mortality rate at 15-year follow-up. Benefit was seen in all major subgroups, with the mortality difference widening over time. The accompanying editorial refers to specific situations in which internal thoracic artery grafting is contraindicated: radiation damage, extensive brachiocephalic atherosclerosis, and subclavian steal.

238. **Fitzgibbon GM,** et al. Coronary bypass graft fate and patient outcome: angiographic follow-up of 5065 grafts related to survival and reoperation in 1388 patients during 25 years. *J Am Coll Cardiol* 1996;28:616–626.

This retrospective analysis focused on 1,388 patients (mostly male veterans) who underwent surgery between 1969 and 1994; 91% of grafts were venous. Saphenous vein graft patency was 88% at early angiography, 81% at 1 year, 75% at 5 years, and 50% at 15 years. At 15 years, 44% had more than 50% stenoses. Arterial patency rates were significantly better: early, 95%; late (5 years), 80%. Reoperative mortality (6.6% vs. 1.4% for isolated first CABG) and morbidity were mostly owing to vein graft atheroembolism.

239. **Goldman S,** et al. Predictors of graft patency 3 years after coronary artery bypass graft surgery. *J Am Coll Cardiol* 1997;29:1563–1568.

This retrospective analysis focused on 266 male VA patients with 656 grafts patent at 7 to 10 days. Multivariate analysis predictors of 3-year patency (related to operative technique vs. antiplatelet therapy) included total cholesterol $\leq$225 mg/dL ($p = 0.024$), no more than two proximal anastomoses ($p = 0.032$), vein preservation solution temperature $\leq$5°C ($p = 0.004$), and recipient artery diameter more than 1.5 mm ($p = 0.034$).

Transmyocardial Revascularization

240. **Schofiel PM,** et al. Transmyocardial laser revascularization in patients with refractory angina: a randomised controlled trial. *Lancet* 1999;353:519–524.

In this prospective trial, 188 patients were randomized to surgical TMR plus normal medication(s) or medical management alone. The perioperative mortality rate in TMR patients was 5%. One-year survival was 89% in the TMR group and 96% in the medical management group ($p = 0.14$). Most of the excess mortality in the TMR group was owing to perioperative deaths. At 1 year, the TMR group did not have a significantly longer mean exercise treadmill time (+40 seconds; $p = 0.152$) or greater mean 12-minute walk distance (+33 meters; $p = 0.108$). The TMR group had a significant improvement in Canadian Cardiovascular Society Angina score: 25% of patients had a two-class improvement (at 1 year) versus only 4% of medical management patients ($p < 0.001$). Necropsy reports of three patients showed dense fibrous scarring and no open channels.

241. **Burkhoff D,** et al. The Angina Treatments-Lasers and Normal Therapies in Comparison (**ATLANTIC**) Investigators. Transmyocardial laser revascularisation compared with continued medical therapy for treatment of refractory angina pectoris: a prospective randomized trial. *Lancet* 1999;354:885–890.

This prospective, randomized, open, multicenter study was composed of 182 patients with Canadian Cardiovascular Society Angina (CCSA) score of III or IV, reversible ischemia, and incomplete response to other therapies. Patients were assigned to TMR and continued medication, or continued medication alone. At 1 year, the TMR group had improved exercise tolerance (+65 seconds vs. −46 seconds; $p < 0.0001$) and better CCSA scores (II or lower in 47.8% vs. 14.3%; $p < 0.001$).

242. **Oesterle SN,** et al. Percutaneous transmyocardial laser revascularisation for severe angina: the **PACIFIC** randomised trial: Potential Class Improvement From Intramyocardial Channels. *Lancet* 2000;356:1705–1710.

This prospective, randomized, open study enrolled 221 patients with stable class III or IV angina symptoms refractory to medical therapy who were not PTCA or CABG candidates, reversible ischemia on thallium stress test, and an EF less than 30%. Patients underwent percutaneous TMR (PTMR) plus medical treatment or medical treatment alone. At 3 and 6 months, PTMR patients had a significant angina improvement (average, −1.3 and −1.4 Canadian Cardiovascular Society classes). The PTMR group also had significantly better exercise tolerance at 6 months (+30%; $p = 0.0002$). Complications of PTMR included bradycardia (three episodes, one requiring a permanent pacemaker), VT (one episode), myocardial perforation (three episodes, one requiring pericardiocentesis), CVA (two episodes), TIA (one episode) and vascular-access complications (two episodes). At 1-year follow-up, a nonsignificant trend toward a higher mortality rate was found in the PTMR group (eight deaths vs. three in the medical group; $p = 0.12$). Investigator bias in favor of PTMR was seen when comparing investigator assessment and masked assessment of angina. Thus despite the randomized design, it is possible that the beneficial effects of PTMR on exercise were due to a placebo effect.

243. **Aaberge L,** et al. Transmyocardial revascularization with CO_2 laser in patients with refractory angina pectoris: clinical results from the Norwegian randomized trial. *J Am Coll Cardiol* 2000;35:1170–1177.

Prospective, randomized, open study of 100 patients with refractory angina not eligible for conventional revascularization. Patients underwent continued optimal medical treatment (MT) or transmyocardial revascularization (TMR) with CO_2-laser and MT. At 3 and 12 months, TMR was associated with significant relief in angina symptoms compared with baseline. At 3 and 6 months, the TMR group had longer times to exercise-induced angina (+78 seconds compared with baseline, $p =$ NS; +66 seconds, $p < 0.01$). However, the TMR had no significant changes in total exercise time or MVO_2. The MT group had no significant changes in any of the measures. Perioperative mortality was 4%, whereas all-cause mortality at 1 year was 12% in the TMR group and 8% in MT group ($p =$ NS). At longer-term follow-up (mean, 43 months), the TMR group still had significantly improved angina symptoms and 55% fewer unstable angina hospitalizations ($p < 0.001$), whereas LVEF and mortality were similar (see *J Am Coll Cardiol* 2002;39:1588).

244. **Stone GW,** et al. A prospective, multicenter, randomized trial of percutaneous transmyocardial laser revascularization in patients with nonrecanalizable chronic total occlusions. *J Am Coll Cardiol* 2002;39:1581–1587.

This prospective, randomized, blinded trial enrolled 141 patients with class III or IV angina caused by one or more chronically occluded native coronary arteries in which PCI failed. Patients underwent PTMR plus maximal medical therapy (MMT) or MMT alone. At 6 months, no significant differences were seen between the two groups in angina improvement [more than two classes; 49% (PTMR) vs. 37%; $p = 0.33$], increase in exercise duration (64 seconds vs. 52 seconds; $p = 0.73$), death (8.6% vs. 8.8%), MI (4.3% vs. 2.9%), or any revascularization (4.3% vs. 2.9%).

245. **DIRECT** (Direct Myocardial Revascularization in Regeneration of Endocardial Channels Trial). Results presented at 73rd Scientific Sessions of AHA, New Orleans, LA, November 2000.

This prospective, randomized, double-blind, placebo-controlled trial enrolled 298 patients with refractory angina patients (CCS class III or IV) who were not candidates for PTCA or CABG surgery. Patients underwent low- or high-energy direct myocardial revascularization (DMR) with a percutaneous holmium:YAG laser-tipped catheter to generate channels in subendocardium OR placebo procedure (catheter was placed against the ventricular wall but not fired). At 6 months, similar improvements were noted in exercise tolerance (primary end point) in all three groups. No significant differences were found between the three groups in improvement of two or more angina classes (as rated by blinded investigators; low-dose DMR, 39%; high-dose DMR, 28%; placebo, 33%). At 30 days, DMR was associated with a higher incidence of adverse events, but at 6 months, no significant difference was noted between the groups. In summary, these data suggest that benefits observed in other trials with this technique may be due to the placebo effect.

3. UNSTABLE ANGINA/NON–ST ELEVATION MI

EPIDEMIOLOGY

Each year in the United States, approximately 1,400,000 persons are admitted to hospitals for unstable angina and non–ST-elevation myocardial infarction (UA/NSTEMI), and 2 million to 2.5 million, worldwide. UA precedes myocardial infarction (MI) in approximately half of the cases.

PATHOPHYSIOLOGY

UA/NSTEMIs are typically the result of nonocclusive coronary artery thrombus due to ruptured plaque(s). Other causes include vasoconstriction (e.g., Prinzmetal's angina, microcirculatory angina); progressive mechanical obstruction; and secondary causes (e.g., tachycardia, fever, thyrotoxicosis, anemia, and hypotension). Substantial data now also support the role of inflammation.

Two recent reports suggest that acute coronary syndrome (ACS) patients also have significant inflammation and plaque instability in nonculprit lesions and vessels, suggesting a widespread process. In an intravascular ultrasound of ACS patients, plaque ruptures were evident in other lesions and vessels in more than 70% of cases (4). A second study examined neutrophil myeloperoxidase (NMP) levels in several types of patients and found that the UA subset had evidence of widespread inflammation [i.e., right and left coronary circulations low NMP levels (indicative of enzyme depletion due to neutrophil activation)] (5).

CLASSIFICATION

Unstable Angina

Canadian Cardiovascular Society (CCS) and Braunwald classifications (see *Circulation* 2000;102:118–122; *JAMA* 1995;273:136) are the most commonly used classifications systems. In the CCS scale, class I is angina only with strenuous activity; class II is slight limitation with vigorous activity; class III patients have marked limitation with normal activity; and class IV patients are unable to perform activities of daily living and have episodes of rest angina. The Braunwald system is multitiered; severity of angina consists of three classes: class I, new-onset (less than 2 months), severe, or accelerated, with no rest pain in the preceding 2 months; class II, subacute (angina at rest more than 48 hours to 1 month previously); and class III, acute (at least one episode in the preceding 48 hours). Patients also are assigned a clinical class as follows: class A, secondary unstable angina (e.g., triggered by anemia, infection, thyrotoxicosis); class B, primary UA; class C, postinfarction UA (less than 2 weeks after documented MI). Class IIIB patients are further subdivided into troponin-negative and troponin-positive patients. The third tier of the system is intensity of therapy: 1, absence of or minimal therapy; 2, occurring in the presence of standard therapy for chronic stable angina (e.g., oral β-blockers, nitrates, calcium antagonists); and 3, occurring despite maximal therapy [oral therapy and intravenous (i.v.) nitroglycerin (NTG)].

Non–ST-elevation Myocardial Infarction

One third to one half of patients in UA trials actually had an NSTEMI. Of NSTEMI patients, Q waves develop in 15% to 25%.

CLINICAL AND LABORATORY FINDINGS

History and Symptoms

Chest discomfort typically occurs at rest or with increasing frequency and lasts 5 to 20 minutes but can last several hours. Temporary/incomplete relief is provided by sublingual NTG. Most chest-pain episodes respond to sublingual NTG.

Electrocardiogram

In UA/NSTEMI, ST-segment depression is seen in approximately 20% to 30% of cases, and transient ST-segment elevation, in 2% to 5%; these changes are predictive of adverse outcomes. T-wave inversions occur in approximately 20%; if present in five or more leads, they are associated with higher risk (see *Circulation* 1998;98:2004).

Cardiac Enzymes

Creatine Kinase and Creatine Kinase-MB
These markers of myocardial necrosis are elevated in patients with NSTEMI. Both levels will typically increase approximately 6 hours after onset of ischemic symptoms and normalize within 48 hours.

Troponins T and I
An elevated troponin is now considered a qualifying criterion for myocardial infarction. Because these markers are more sensitive than creatine kinase (CK) and CK-MB, the new MI definition will lead to higher MI rates, as one in three patients previously diagnosed with UA have had a small NSTEMI (some have called these "microinfarctions"). In a meta-analysis of 21 published studies, the two types of troponins were found to be equally sensitive and specific (see *Am J Cardiol* 1998;81:1405). In one study of patients with rest pain, troponin T was detected in 39%, whereas CK-MB was elevated in fewer than 10% (56). Troponin levels begin to increase within 4 to 6 hours after symptom onset, remain elevated for several days, and thus are a reliable marker for diagnosing MI within the preceding 2 to 7 days. For the same reason, however, CK-MB levels are necessary to diagnose reinfarction within the first several days of an index infarction.

Myoglobin
Usefulness is limited by lack of cardiac specificity and period of brief elevation (less than 24 hours). However, in conjunction with other data, a negative myoglobin can be helpful in ruling out MI.

Estimation of Early Risk at Presentation
The Thrombolysis in Myocardial Infarction (TIMI) Risk Score consists of seven predictor variables (each worth 1 point): age older than 65 years; three or more coronary artery disease (CAD) risk factors; prior coronary stenosis of more than 50%; ST-segment deviation on initial ECG; two or more anginal events in prior 24 hours; use of aspirin in prior 7 days; and elevated serum cardiac markers. With TIMI 11B and Efficacy and Safety of Subcutaneous Enoxaparin in Non-Q-wave Coronary Events (ESSENCE) data, the event rate (death, new or recurrent MI, ischemia requiring urgent revascularization) at 14 days increased from 4.7%, with a TIMI risk score of 0 or 1, to 40.9% for a score of 6 or 7 (**Fig. 3.1**; 65). This score has been validated in eight studies including the TIMI III Registry (see *Am J Cardiol* 2002;90:303), PRISM-PLUS (see *Eur Heart J* 2002;23:223), and CURE (see *Circulation* 2002;106:1622), where a higher risk also predicted greater benefit from glycoprotein (GP) IIb/IIIa inhibition. In a prespecified analysis in TACTICS-TIMI 18, those with higher TIMI risk scores were those found to have a significantly greater benefit from an early invasive strategy, whereas those with TIMI risk score of 0 to 2 had similar outcomes with an invasive or conservative strategy. In summary, this score with broad applicability is easily

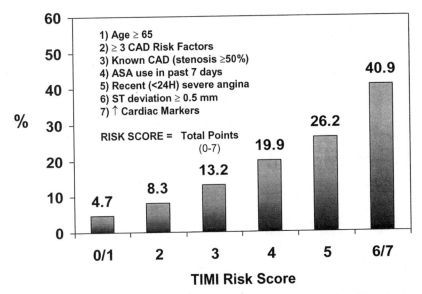

FIG. 3.1. This risk score is derived from data on TIMI-11B and ESSENCE patients, and shows a clear gradation of increasing risk with a higher risk score. [Adapted from Antman EM, et al. (ref. 65)].

calculated and identifies patients with different responses to treatments for UA/NSTEMI (53).

Boersma et al. (see *Circulation* 2000;101:2557) also developed a risk-estimation score based on analysis of PURSUIT trial data. The most important baseline features associated with death were age, higher heart rate, lower systolic blood pressure (SBP), ST-segment depression, signs of heart failure, and elevated cardiac markers.

Treatment

Aspirin
Aspirin (160 to 325 mg initially then 81 to 325 mg daily) has been shown to reduce the risk of fatal or nonfatal MI by 50% to 70% during the acute phase in patients with UA or NSTEMI and by 50% to 60% at 3 months to 3 years (6,7). For chronic treatment, low dose aspirin (e.g., 75 to 81 mg) has lower bleeding risk and similar efficacy compared with higher doses (9).

Thienopyridines
Two thienopyridines are commercially available, ticlopidine and clopidogrel, but clopidogrel is the preferred agent because of a lower incidence of side effects, especially neutropenia (0.1% or less risk vs. 1% risk with ticlopidine).

In one early study of UA patients, ticlopidine (250 mg twice daily) reduced cardiovascular mortality and reinfarction rates by nearly 50% (8). Clopidogrel was evaluated in the recent Clopidogrel in Unstable Angina to Prevent Recurrent Events (CURE) trial, which randomized 12,662 patients with unstable or NSTEMI to aspirin alone or clopidogrel, 300 mg loading dose and 75 mg once daily, and aspirin (9). At follow-up (mean, 9 months), the clopidogrel group had a significant 20% reduction in cardiovascular death, MI, or stroke compared with the aspirin-only group. An initial loading dose of clopidogrel (300 mg) was given, and the events curves separated within 2 hours.

The clopidogrel group had a higher incidence of major bleeding at 1 year (3.7% vs. 2.7%).

Based on these results, the American College of Cardiology (ACC)/American Heart Association (AHA) Guidelines (**Table 3.1**) have been modified and now advocate that clopidogrel should be given in addition to aspirin for at least 9 months.

TABLE 3.1. ACC/AHA GUIDELINE RECOMMENDATIONS FOR ANTIPLATELET AND ANTICOAGULANT THERAPY FOR UA/NSTEMI

Class I

1. Antiplatelet therapy should be initiated promptly. ASA should be administered as soon as possible after presentation and continued indefinitely (Level of Evidence: A).
2. Clopidogrel should be administered to hospitalized patients who are unable to take ASA because of hypersensitivity or major gastrointestinal intolerance (Level of Evidence: A).
3. In hospitalized patients in whom an early noninterventional approach is planned, clopidogrel should be added to ASA as soon as possible on admission and administered for ≥1 mo (Level of Evidence: A) and for ≤9 mo (Level of Evidence: B).
4. In patients in whom PCI is planned, clopidogrel should be started and continued for ≥1 mo (Level of Evidence: A) and in ≥9 mo in patients who are not at high risk for bleeding (Level of Evidence: B).
5. In patients taking clopidogrel in whom elective CABG is planned, the drug should be withheld for 5 to 7 d (Level of Evidence: B).
6. Anticoagulation with subcutaneous LWMH or intravenous unfractionated heparin (UFH) should be added to antiplatelet therapy with ASA and/or clopidogrel (Level of Evidence: A).
7. A platelet GP IIb/IIIa antagonist should be administered, in addition to ASA and heparin, to patients in whom catheterization and PCI are planned. The GP IIb/IIIa antagonist also may be administered just before PCI (Level of Evidence: A).

Class IIa

1. Eptifibatide or tirofiban should be administered, in addition to ASA and LMWH or UFH, to patients with continuing ischemia, an elevated troponin level, or with other high-risk features in whom an invasive management strategy is *not* planned (Level of Evidence: A).
2. Enoxaparin is preferable to UFH as an anticoagulant in patients with UA/NSTEMI, unless CABG is planned within 24 hr (Level of Evidence: A).
3. A platelet GP IIb/IIIa antagonist should be administered to patients already receiving heparin, ASA, and clopidogrel, in whom catheterization and PCI is planned. The GP IIb/IIIa antagonist also may be administered just before PCI (Level of Evidence: B).

Class IIb

1. Eptifibatide or tirofiban, in addition to ASA and LMWH or UFH, to patients without continuing ischemia who have no other high-risk features and in whom PCI is not planned (Level of Evidence: A).

Class III

1. Intravenous fibrinolytic therapy in patients without acute ST-segment elevation, a true posterior MI, or a presumed new left bundle branch block (Level of Evidence: A).
2. Abciximab administration in patients in whom PCI is not planned (Level of Evidence: A).

ACC, American College of Cardiology; AHA, American Heart Association; UA, unstable angina; NSTEMI, non–ST elevation myocardial infarction; ASA, aspirin; PCI, percutaneous coronary intervention; CABG, coronary artery bypass graft; LWMH, low-molecular-weight heparin; GP, glycoprotein.

Heparin

In a meta-analysis of six trials, unfractionated heparin [UFH; 60-U/kg to 70-U/kg bolus, and then 12 to 15 U/kg/h; goal activated partial thromboplastin time (aPTT), 1.5 to 2.0 times control] showed a strong trend toward reducing rates of reinfarction and recurrent ischemia when used with aspirin [odds ratio (OR), 0.67; 95% confidence interval (CI) 0.44 to 1.02] (15). After discontinuation of heparin infusion, a rebound phenomenon occurs, with patients at increased risk of reactivation of UA and MI (12).

Low-molecular-weight Heparins

The Efficacy and Safety of Subcutaneous Enoxaparin in Non–Q-wave Coronary Events (ESSENCE) and Thrombolysis In Myocardial Infarction (TIMI-IIB) trials showed enoxaparin (1 mg/kg subcutaneously twice daily) to be superior to UFH, resulting in 15% to 20% fewer major events (death, MI, and urgent revascularization) at 6 weeks (20,22). In the smaller EVET trial, enoxaparin was directly compared with another low-molecular-weight heparin (LWMH), tinzaparin; the enoxaparin group had a significantly lower incidence of recurrent UA or need for revascularization (see *J Am Coll Cardiol* 2001;37:365).

In the Fragmin during Instability in CAD (FRISC) trial (18), dalteparin (120 IU/kg subcutaneously twice daily for 6 days, and then 7,500 IU/day for 35 to 45 days) showed a significant reduction in death and MI at 6 days compared with placebo, whereas the Fragmin in Unstable Coronary Artery Disease (FRIC) trial showed equivalence between dalteparin and i.v. UFH (19). In FRISC II (21), extended use of dalteparin (120 IU/kg twice daily for 3 months) was associated with a significant reduction in death or MI at 30 days, but the reduction did not remain significant at 3 months.

In the Fraxiparine in Ischemic Syndrome (FRAXIS) trial (23), fraxiparine showed no benefit compared with UFH; this study enrolled many low-risk patients.

It is not clear why enoxaparin is the only agent with a clear benefit, but it does have a higher ratio of anti–factor Xa to antithrombin activity (3.8:1.0) than dalteparin or fraxiparine. The current ACC/AHA Guidelines have a class I recommendation for either LWMH or UFH as treatment for UA/NSTEMI, and a class IIa recommendation that enoxaparin is the preferred agent to UFH (**Table 3.1**).

Recent evidence demonstrates that LWMH can be used in conjunction with GP IIb/IIIa inhibitors. In the Integrelin and Enoxaparin Randomized Assessment of Acute Coronary Syndrome Treatment (INTERACT) trial, 746 UA/NSTEMI patients receiving eptifibatide were randomized to heparin or enoxaparin, and the enoxaparin group had a significantly lower incidence of death and MI at 30 days (24). In the Antithrombotic Combination Using Tirofiban and Enoxaparin (ACUTE II) study, UFH and enoxaparin were compared in UA/NSTEMIs receiving tirofiban, and a trend toward fewer adverse events was noted in the enoxaparin group, and bleeding rates were similar (see *Circulation* 2000;102(suppl II):II-826). Other smaller studies have found similar findings [see *J Invasive Cardiol* 2000;12(suppl):E14–E18 [enoxaparin + abciximab in elective percutaneous coronary intervention (PCI)], *Am Heart J* 2001;141:358 (dalteparin + abciximab)].

A to Z was the first large trial to compare enoxaparin with UFH in a patient population which all received IIb/IIIa inhibitors and mainly involved a noninvasive approach. A total of 3,987 high-risk ACS patients, all of whom received aspirin and tirofiban, were randomized to enoxaparin or UFH; 60% of patients underwent angiography. The enoxaparin group had a 12% reduction in death, MI, or refractory ischemia compared to UHF (8.4% vs. 9.4%), which fulfilled the trial's noninferiority goal but did not demonstrate superiority ($p = 0.23$). Finally, the ongoing 8,000 patient SYNERGY is comparing the two agents in patients who are all going to the cath lab; also, crossover from enoxaparin to UFH in the cath lab is not allowed.

LMWHs stimulate platelets less than UFHs (see *Circulation* 1998;97:251) and have a lower incidence of heparin-induced thrombocytopenia (HIT; see *N Engl J Med* 1995;332:1330). All these agents also are associated with a higher incidence of minor bleeding compared with UFH.

Glycoprotein IIb/IIIa Inhibitors
Intravenous Agents
The current ACC/AHA guidelines recommend (class IA) the use of an i.v. GP IIb/IIIa antagonist in UA/NSTEMI patients in whom catheterization and PCI are planned. In patients with continuing ischemia, an elevated troponin level, or with other high-risk features in whom an invasive strategy is *not* planned, the use of eptifibatide or tirofiban is considered class IIa (**Table 3.1**).

1. Tirofiban: In the Platelet Receptor Inhibition in Ischemic Syndrome Management in Patients Limited by Unstable Signs and Symptoms (PRISM-PLUS) trial (30), tirofiban (0.4 μg/kg/min for 30 minutes, and then 0.10 μg/kg/min for 48 to 72 hours), heparin, and aspirin resulted in decreased death, MI; and refractory ischemia at 7 days compared with heparin alone (29), and death and MI were decreased by approximately 30% at 30 days.
2. Eptifibatide: In the large Platelet Glycoprotein IIb/IIIa in Unstable Angina Receptor Suppression Using Integrelin Therapy (PURSUIT) trial, eptifibatide (180 μg/kg bolus, and then 2.0 μg/kg/min) showed an approximately 10% reduction in death and MI at 30 days (33).
3. Abciximab (0.25 μg/kg bolus, and then 0.10 μg/min for 12 hours). The Evaluation of 7E3 for the Prevention of Ischemic Complications (EPIC), Evaluation in PTCA to Improve Long-term Outcome with Abciximab Glycoprotein IIb/IIIa Blockade (EPILOG), and c7E3 Fab Antiplatelet Therapy in Unstable Refractory Angina (CAPTURE) trials were interventional studies that enrolled some UA patients, and all showed substantial reductions (30% to 60%) at 30 days in the rates of death, MI, and ischemia-provoked intervention or revascularization (see Chapter 2). The 6-month results of the Evaluation of Platelet IIb/IIIa Inhibitor for Stenting (EPISTENT) trial, another interventional study comparing stenting alone versus stenting plus abciximab versus balloon angioplasty plus abciximab, showed a 10% absolute reduction in death and MI in the subgroup of patients with UA. However, the large GUSTO IV-ACS trial, which enrolled all ACS patients (7,800), abciximab was associated with no reduction in death or MI at 30 days compared with placebo, and the mortality rate was actually higher in the first 48 hours in the abciximab groups (38). Based on these results, abciximab is contraindicated (class III) in ACS patients in whom PCI is not planned.

A recent meta-analysis of six large trials (PRISM, PRISM-PLUS, PARAGON A, PARAGON B, PURSUIT, GUSTO IV) with 31,402 ACS patients found a significant absolute reduction in 30-day mortality of 1% with GP IIb/IIa inhibitor use ($p = 0.015$) (40). However, another analysis found that this benefit was restricted to the diabetic patients (1.6% absolute mortality reduction, 26% relative risk reduction), with no significant benefit seen in the 23,072 nondiabetic patients (39). Among diabetic patients undergoing PCI, in-hospital mortality was 70% lower in those receiving a GP IIb/IIIa inhibitor.

Oral Agents
In contrast to the i.v. agents, several oral agents have shown an *increased* risk of death or bleeding events (see *Circulation* 2002;106:375, *Am J Med* 2002;112:647). The OPUS-TIMI 16 trial was terminated early because of an increased 30-day mortality in one of the orbofiban arms (34). In the SYMPHONY trial (36), sibrafiban was comparable to aspirin for major events but was associated with increased bleeding; these results prompted the early termination of the larger SYMPHONY II trial (37).

Direct Thrombin Inhibitors
In the Global Utilization of Strategies to Open Occluded Arteries (GUSTO) IIb trial, hirudin use in patients with ACSs [chest pain with electrocardiographic (ECG) changes] resulted in a nonsignificant 11% reduction in death and MI at 30 days compared with heparin (43). In the Organization to Assess Strategies for Ischemic Syndromes (OASIS-2) trial, medium-dose hirudin (0.4 mg/kg bolus and then 0.15 mg/kg/h) resulted in a nonsignificant 16% reduction in cardiovascular death and MI at 7 days (3). A meta-analysis of the GUSTO IIb, TIMI 9B, OASIS 1, and OASIS 2 trials

found that hirudin was associated with a significant 10% lower risk of death or MI at 35 days compared with heparin ($p = 0.015$) (45). Hirudin is currently indicated only for anticoagulation in patients with HIT, but these data show that additional trials of the direct antithrombins are warranted.

Thrombolytic Therapy

Thrombolytic therapy was not found to be beneficial in the TIMI III and the Unstable Angina Study Using Eminase (UNASEM) trials (46,47). Use was associated with increased bleeding and MI rates, and no benefit of adjunctive intracoronary thrombolytic therapy was observed during percutaneous transluminal coronary angioplasty (PTCA) in the Thrombolysis and Angioplasty in Unstable Angina (TAUSA) trial (48).

Antiischemic Medications

β-Blockers

Limited randomized trial data are available on the use of β-blockers in UA/NSTEMI (see *Circulation* 1986;73:331). However, given the significant benefit demonstrated in acute MI, recent MI, heart failure, and stable angina with daily life ischemia, it is appropriate to extrapolate to UA/NSTEMI. Specific medication choices include metoprolol (5 mg i.v. every 5 minutes for three doses, and then 25 to 50 mg orally every 6 hours), propranolol (0.5 to 1.0 mg i.v., and then 40 to 80 mg orally every 6 to 8 hours), and atenolol (5 mg i.v., and then 50 to 100 mg orally daily). Contraindicated if marked first-degree atrioventricular (AV) block [PR interval, more than 0.25 seconds; any second- or third-degree block in the absence of a pacemaker; asthma; severe left ventricular dysfunction with congestive heart failure (CHF); heart rate (HR) less than 50; and SBP, less than 90 mm Hg].

Nitrates

Nitrates are useful for treating episodes of recurrent ischemia (reducing both left ventricular end-diastolic pressure and SBP). If no relief is gained from three sublingual NTG tablets, i.v. NTG (5 to 200 μg/min) should be started. If nitrates do not provide adequate relief or if acute pulmonary congestion is found, consider morphine administration. Nitrates are contraindicated if a patient has taken sildenafil (Viagra) within 24 hours.

Calcium-channel Blockers

Calcium-channel blockers are as effective in relieving symptoms, but an overview of randomized trials showed no reduction in mortality or MI rates (see *Br Med J* 1989;299:1887). Diltiazem confers a possible benefit in non–Q-wave MI patients (majority with NSTEMI). In the Diltiazem Reinfarction Study, diltiazem use (90 mg, 4 times daily) was associated with a significant reduction in in-hospital mortality (26). However, no overall benefit was observed by the Multicenter Diltiazem Postinfarction Trial Research Group (60 mg, 4 times daily), although a *post hoc* analysis showed benefit in patients without evidence of left ventricular dysfunction.

3-Hydroxy-3-Methylglutaryl Coenzyme A Reductase Inhibitors (Statins)

In the Myocardial Ischemia Reduction with Aggressive Cholesterol Lowering (MIRACL) study, 3,086 conservatively managed UA/NSTEMI patients were randomized to high-dose atorvastatin (80 mg once daily) or placebo (58). In the atorvastatin group, mean low-density lipoprotein (LDL) cholesterol decreased from 124 mg/dL to 72 mg/dL, and a significantly lower incidence of death, nonfatal MI, cardiac arrest with resuscitation, or ischemia requiring rehospitalization was found. Data from the CHAMP study found that if a statin was started in hospital, 91% were taking a statin at 1 year versus only 10%, and 58% had an LDL less than 100 mg/dL versus only 6% prior to institution of the quality improvement program (see *Am J Cardiol* 2001;87: 819).

Miscellaneous

Potassium adenosine triphosphate (KATP) channel openers are promising agents with beneficial hemodynamic and cardioprotective effects. In the placebo-controlled (Clinical European Studies in Angina and Revascularization (CESAR 2) study of 245 UA patients (56), the addition of nicorandil to conventional treatment significantly reduced epidoses of ischemia (mostly silent) and arrhythmias. In the larger GUARd During Ischemia Against Necrosis (GUARDIAN) study (57), 11,590 UA/NSTEMI patients undergoing high-risk percutaneous or surgical revascularization, high-dose cariporide had a nonsignificant 10% reduction in death or MI compared with placebo ($p = 0.12$). However, among coronary artery bypass graft (CABG) patients, a significant 25% reduction was noted, driven by fewer non–Q-wave MIs. Further studies of this class of agents are ongoing.

Invasive Strategy
Coronary Angiography
With coronary angiography, multivessel disease is found in 40% to 50%, single-vessel disease in 30% to 35%, left main disease in 5% to 10%, and no critical obstruction in 10% to 20%.

The routine use of angiography has now been studied in nine randomized trials, with the five most recent studies all showing a significant benefit associated with an invasive strategy. The first trial, TIMI IIIB, showed that early angiography followed by revascularization (if indicated) did not reduce major cardiac events but did result in fewer hospital readmissions (49), whereas the Veteran Affairs Non–Q-wave Infarction Strategies in Hospital (VANQWISH) study, which enrolled medium- to high-risk patients, showed no benefit of an invasive strategy and a trend toward higher mortality (50). The invasive group in the VANQWISH study had a high CABG operative mortality rate (12%). Both the TIMI IIIB and VANQWISH trials were performed before GP IIb/IIIa inhibitors and coronary stenting were commonly used.

The FRagmin and Fast Revascularization during InStability in Coronary artery disease study reported a significantly lower incidence of death or MI with an invasive strategy compared with a noninvasive strategy (at 6 months, 9.4% vs. 12.1%; $p = 0.031$) (52). A subgroup analysis showed that this benefit was restricted to men.

The Treat Angina with Aggrastat and Determine Cost of Therapy with an Invasive or Conservative Strategy (TACTICS)-TIMI 18 study enrolled 2,220 patients with at least one high-risk feature [ECG changes, elevated cardiac markers, or a history of CAD (prior catheterization, revascularization, or MI)] (53). Patients randomized to an early invasive strategy (routine catheterization within 4 to 48 hours and revascularization as appropriate) had a 22% lower incidence of death, nonfatal MI, and rehospitalization for an ACS at 6 months compared with a more conservative strategy (catheterization only if recurrent ischemia or abnormal stress test). Patients with an elevated troponin T had an even larger 39% reduction in the primary end point.

In the Randomised Intervention Trial of unstable Angina (RITA) trial (54), 1,810 UA/NSTEMI patients were randomized to an early intervention or a conservative strategy. The intervention group had a 34% lower incidence of death, MI, or refractory angina at 4 months. Two other smaller randomized studies also found significant benefits with an early invasive strategy (TRUCS; see *Eur Heart J* 2000;21:1954; VINO, see *Eur Heart J* 2002;23:230).

In summary, TACTICS-TIMI 18 and RITA-3 reexamined management strategy in the current era, and the data resulted in changes to the ACC/AHA guidelines. The latest version now considers an early invasive strategy a class I indication if any of the following high-risk features are present: (a) recurrent angina/ischemia at rest or low-level activity despite intensive therapy; (b) elevated troponin T or troponin I; (c) new or presumably new ST-segment depression; (d) recurrent angina with CHF symptoms, S_3 gallop, pulmonary edema, worsening rales, new or worsening mitral regurgitation; (e) high-risk findings on noninvasive stress testing; (f) ejection fraction, less than 40%; (g) hemodynamic instability; (h) sustained ventricular tachycardia (VT); (i) PCI within previous 6 months; or (j) prior CABG surgery.

Percutaneous Coronary Intervention
The success rate of PCI is 90% to 95%. Ischemic complications are reduced by concomitant administration of i.v. GP IIb/IIIa inhibitor (see earlier).

Coronary Artery Bypass Graft Surgery
The operative mortality rate with CABG surgery is typically 3% to 4% in patients with refractory unstable angina (vs. approximately 2% for patients with chronic stable

angina). Improved survival has been demonstrated in patients with left main disease and three-vessel disease with significant left ventricular dysfunction (see Chapter 2). An intraaortic balloon pump may be needed for stabilization before surgery.

One observational study showed that patients treated by cardiologists (vs. internists) tended to have lower mortality rates ($p = 0.06$). Cardiologists prescribed more appropriate medications and ordered more-invasive testing (59).

Noninvasive Evaluation

Exercise Treadmill Test
Treadmill testing should not be performed in the acute phase. In low-risk patients free of rest or low-level ischemia and CHF, the exercise treadmill test (ETT) can be performed after a minimum of 12 to 24 hours. In intermediate-risk patients, the wait should be at least 2 or 3 days. If the patient is high risk (e.g., ≥2-mm ST-segment depression), catheterization should be considered in place of ETT.

Exercise Treadmill Testing with Nuclear Imaging
The ACC/AHA Guidelines have a class I recommendation for the following patient subsets: baseline ST-segment abnormalities, bundle branch block, left ventricular hypertrophy, intraventricular conduction delay, paced rhythm, preexcitation, and digoxin effect. Imaging also adds sensitivity to low-level/nondiagnostic ETT tests. The size of perfusion defect(s) is predictive of mortality and major cardiac events.

Pharmacologic Stress Testing with Imaging
Pharmacologic stress testing with imaging is indicated in patients with severe physical limitations.

Echocardiography
In patients with chest pain but no ECG changes or an obscured ECG picture [left bundle branch block (LBBB), paced rhythm], echocardiography can be used to evaluate whether a wall-motion abnormality is present.

Prognosis

Unstable Angina
The hospital mortality rate is 1% to 2%; 1-year mortality rate, 7% to 10%; and 1-month reinfarction rate, approximately 5%. Twenty percent to 25% of patients are rehospitalized within 1 year. Recurrent ischemia is associated with a nearly threefold higher mortality (75).

Non–ST-Elevation Myocardial Infarction
The in-hospital mortality rate is 3% to 4%; reinfarction rate, 8% to 10%; and 1-year mortality rate, 10% to 15%. (The latter is similar to that of ST-elevation patients.)

Prior Aspirin Use (Aspirin Failures)
Prior aspirin use is associated with an increased risk of death or MI at 30 days (64).

Electrocardiography
A TIMI III Registry analysis showed an increased risk of death and MI at 1 year with LBBB on admission ECG [relative risk (RR), 2.8] and 0.5 mm of ST deviation (RR, 2.5). T-wave inversion alone was not associated with increased risk (82).

Echocardiography
Transthoracic echocardiography is a widely available method to assess left ventricular function and is generally recommended in the ACC/AHA Guidelines.

Troponin Levels

Troponin levels have been shown to provide substantial prognostic information. TIMI IIIB and FRISC analyses showed a strong correlation between troponin T levels and adverse outcomes (68,69). In the FRISC trial, the benefit of LMWH over aspirin was limited to patients with elevated troponin T levels (68). In four trials (CAPTURE, PRISM, PRISM-PLUS, Paragon B), the benefit of GP IIb/IIIa inhibition was magnified (50% to 70%) in patients with elevated troponin-T levels, with no benefit in troponin-negative patients (72,73; also see *J Thromb Thrombolysis* 2001;11:211, *Circulation* 2001;103:2891). In the TACTICS-TIMI 18 trial, an elevated troponin level was associated with a 40% reduction in major cardiac events in the early invasive group versus conservative strategy group, whereas patients with normal levels (troponin I less than 0.1 ng/mL or troponin T less than 0.01 ng/mL) had no significant benefit from an early invasive strategy (74).

C-Reactive Protein

Elevated levels of C-reactive protein (CRP) are found in patients who die. A TIMI IIA analysis showed patients at highest risk of subsequent adverse events if both CRP and troponin were elevated (77).

Von Willebrand Factor, Fibrinogen

Analysis of a small group of ESSENCE patients showed lower von Willebrand factor levels among enoxaparin-treated patients; further studies are needed. High fibrinogen levels were associated with increased mortality in a FRISC analysis (76) and higher incidence of death, MI, and spontaneous ischemia in a TIMI IIIB analysis (76).

B-Type Natriuretic Peptide

Brain (B-type) natriuretic peptide (BNP) is a neurohormone synthesized predominantly in ventricular myocardium.

A substudy of 2,525 ACS patients in the OPUS-TIMI 16 trial measured BNP in plasma samples at a mean of 40 ± 20 hours after the onset of symptoms (78). Baseline BNP level more than 80 pg/mL was significantly correlated with an increased risk of death, heart failure, and new or recurrent MI at 30 days and 10 months. A more recent analysis of 1,676 TACTICS-TIMI 18 patients found similar findings; in addition, BNP was shown to add significant incremental prognostic information to troponin I measurement (see *J Am Coll Cardiol* 2003;41:1264).

REFERENCES

Review Articles and Pathophysiology

1. **Braunwald E.** Unstable angina: an etiologic approach to management. *Circulation* 1998;98:2219–2222.

   This editorial describes five different, though not mutually exclusive, causes of UA: (a) nonocclusive thrombus on preexisting plaques (most common); (b) dynamic obstruction (e.g., Prinzmetal's variant angina, microcirculatory angina); (c) progressive mechanical obstruction; (d) inflammation and/or infection; and (e) secondary causes (e.g., fever, thyrotoxicosis, hypotension).

2. **Cannon CP, Turpie AG.** Unstable angina and non-ST-elevation myocardial infarction: initial antithrombotic therapy and early invasive strategy. *Circulation* 2003;107:2640–2645.

   This review discusses the pathophysiology, clinical presentation, diagnosis, and risk assessment of unstable angina. Acute medical therapy is then reviewed in detail with an emphasis on major clinical studies, invasive versus conservative strategies, and improvements in PCI.

3. **Braunwald E,** et al. ACC/AHA guideline update for the management of patients with unstable angina and non-ST segment elevation myocardial infarction: a report

of the American College of Cardiology/American Heart Association Task Force on Practice Guidelines (Committee on the Management of Unstable Angina). 2002. Available at http://www.acc.org/clinical/guidelines/unstable/unstable.pdf.

4. **Rioufol G,** et al. Multiple atherosclerotic plaque rupture in acute coronary syndrome: a three-vessel intravascular ultrasound study. *Circulation* 2002;106:804–808.

A total of 24 patients who underwent PCI after a first ACS with troponin-I elevation underwent intravascular ultrasound of the three major coronary arteries. Fifty plaque ruptures (mean, 2.08 per patient) were diagnosed by the association of a ruptured capsule with intraplaque cavity. Plaque rupture on the culprit lesion was seen in nine (37.5%) patients. At least one plaque rupture was found somewhere other than on the culprit lesion in 19 (79%) patients, and these lesions were in a different artery than the culprit artery in 70.8%. Thus although one single lesion is clinically active at the time of ACS, the syndrome appears associated with overall coronary instability.

5. **Buffon A,** et al. Widespread coronary inflammation in unstable angina. *N Engl J Med* 2002;347:5–12.

Results from this provocative study argue against the concept of a single vulnerable plaque in unstable coronary syndromes. NMP levels were measured from blood in the aorta, femoral vein, and great cardiac vein [latter drains blood from the left but not the right coronary artery (RCA)]. Patients had unstable angina and a left anterior descending artery (LAD) stenosis (24) or RCA stenosis (nine), chronic stable angina (13), or variant angina and recurrent ischemia (13); there were six controls. The NMP content of aortic blood was similar in the unstable angina groups [−3.9 and −5.5 (negative values indicative of enzyme depletion due to neutrophil activation)] and significantly lower than in the other three groups ($p < 0.05$). NMP levels from the great cardiac vein also were significantly lower in UA groups [−6.4 (left coronary lesion) and −6.6 (RCA lesion)], but not in the other patient groups and controls.

Drugs and Studies

Aspirin
6. **Lewis HD Jr,** et al. **VA Cooperative Study.** Protective effects of aspirin against acute MI and death in men with unstable angina. *N Engl J Med* 1983;309:396–403.

Design: Prospective, randomized, double-blind, placebo-controlled, multicenter study. Primary end point was death or MI at 12 weeks.
Purpose: To determine whether aspirin can decrease death and acute MI in patients with UA.
Population: 1,266 men with pain at rest, beginning within the previous month, and present within the last week and evidence of CAD, defined as one or more of the following: history of MI, ST depression ≥1 mm, angiogram showing 75% stenosis of at least one vessel, exercise test with ≥1 mm ST depression, and exertional angina relieved by NTG within 5 minutes.
Exclusion Criteria: Included new Q-waves or ST elevation, elevated enzymes (more than twice normal level), severe heart failure (NYHA class IV), ventricular arrhythmia, oral anticoagulation, bleeding diathesis, allergy or intolerance to aspirin, recent aspirin ingestion (on more than 3 days of the previous 7), MI within the previous 6 weeks, bypass surgery in the previous 12 weeks, and cardiac catheterization in the prior week.
Treatment: Buffered aspirin, 324 mg once daily, or placebo for 12 weeks.
Results: At 12 weeks, the aspirin group had a 51% lower incidence of death and MI (5% vs. 10%; $p < 0.0005$), with both death and nonfatal MI being reduced by 51% (3.4% vs. 6.9%; $p = 0.005$; 1.6% vs. 3.3%, $p = 0.054$). No difference was observed in gastrointestinal symptoms or evidence of blood loss between the two treatment and placebo groups.

7. **Cairns JA,** et al. Aspirin, sulfinpyrazone, or both in unstable angina: results of a Canadian multicenter trial. *N Engl J Med* 1985;313:1369–1375.

Design: Prospective, randomized, double-blind, placebo-controlled, multicenter study. Primary end point was cardiac death and nonfatal MI. Mean follow-up period was 18 months.

Purpose: To evaluate the efficacy of aspirin, sulfinpyrazone, or both in the acute management of unstable angina.

Population: 555 patients aged 70 years with evidence of myocardial ischemia (exertional angina, transient ST- or T-wave changes with pain, or relief with sublingual NTG in less than 10 minutes on at least three occasions in hospital) and unstable pain pattern (crescendo pain or pain 15 minutes in duration).

Exclusion Criteria: Included MI in preceding 12 weeks, contraindications to study medications, new Q waves on ECG, severe chest pain lasting ≥ 30 minutes, and elevated [more than twice the upper limit of normal (ULN)] enzymes (at least two of following: serum aspartate aminotransferase, lactic dehydrogenase, CK), with positive CK-MB fraction or MB more than 5%.

Treatment: Aspirin, 325 mg 4 times daily; sulfinpyrazone, 200 mg 4 times daily; both; or neither.

Results: Aspirin groups had 51% less cardiac death and MI than did nonaspirin groups (8.6% vs. 17%; $p = 0.008$). The aspirin groups also had 71% lower all-cause mortality rates (3.0% vs. 11.7%; $p = 0.004$). Intention-to-treat analysis showed aspirin groups to have 30% lower rates of cardiac death and nonfatal MI ($p = 0.072$), 56% fewer cardiac deaths ($p = 0.009$), and 43% lower all-cause mortality rate ($p = 0.035$). Sulfinpyrazone showed no benefit for any outcome event.

Thienopyridines

8. **Balsano F,** et al. Antiplatelet therapy with ticlopidine in unstable angina: controlled, multicenter clinical trial. *Circulation* 1990;82:17–26 (editorial, 296–298).

In this randomized trial, 652 patients received conventional therapy (without aspirin) or ticlopidine, 250 mg twice daily. At 6 months, the ticlopidine group had 46% fewer primary end points, consisting of vascular death or nonfatal MI (7.3% vs. 13.6%; $p = 0.009$). A 53% reduction in risk of fatal or nonfatal MI was found (5.1% vs. 10.9%; $p = 0.006$).

9. The Clopidogrel in Unstable Angina to Prevent Recurrent Events (**CURE**) Trial Investigators. Effects of clopidogrel in addition to aspirin in patients with acute coronary syndromes without ST segment elevation. *N Engl J Med* 2001;345:494–502).

Design: Prospective, randomized, double-blind, placebo-controlled, multicenter trial. Primary end-point composite was cardiovascular death, MI, or stroke. Mean follow-up was 9 months (range, 3 to 12 months).

Purpose: To evaluate the efficacy and safety of the antiplatelet agent clopidogrel when given with aspirin in ACSs without ST-segment elevation.

Population: 12,562 patients with unstable angina or NSTEMI with ECG changes, positive serum cardiac markers, or history of CAD, and seen within 24 hours of symptom onset.

Exclusion Criteria: Age younger than 60 years, contraindication to antithrombotic therapy, ST elevation, high bleeding or CHF risk, oral anticoagulation, coronary revascularization in previous 3 months, GP IIb/IIIa inhibitor in previous 3 days.

Treatment: Aspirin (75 to 325 mg once daily) and clopidogrel (300 mg loading dose, and then 75 mg once daily) or aspirin and placebo.

Results: The clopidogrel group had a 20% relative reduction in cardiovascular death, nonfatal MI, or stroke at 1 year compared with the placebo group (9.3% vs. 11.4%; $p < 0.001$). Clopidogrel group also had a significantly lower incidence of the primary composite end point or refractory ischemia (16.5% vs. 18.8%; RR, 0.86; $p < 0.001$; at 24 hours: 1.4% for clopidogrel vs. 2.1%; 34% RR reduction; $p = 0.002$). The incidence of in-hospital refractory or severe ischemia, heart failure, and revascularization procedures were also significantly lower with clopidogrel. The clopidogrel group experienced more major bleeding at 1 year than the placebo group (3.7% vs. 2.7%; RR, 1.38; $p = 0.001$), but no significant excess of life-threatening bleeding occurred (2.1% vs. 1.8%; $p = 0.13$) or hemorrhagic strokes. Bleeding was lower in patients treated with aspirin, 75 to 100 mg once daily, compared with aspirin, 200 to 325 mg once daily (2.0% vs. 4.0%, respectively, in aspirin-only group; 2.6% vs. 4.9% in clopidogrel and aspirin group), indicating that bleeding appeared lower with clopidogrel and low-dose aspirin versus 325 mg of aspirin alone.

Comments: Benefits associated with clopidogrel occurred within 2 hours. The benefits were consistent in low-, intermediate-, and high-risk patients, as stratified by TIMI risk score (see *Circulation* 2002;106:1622).

Unfractionated Heparin and Warfarin

10. **Theroux P,** et al., **Montreal Heart Study.** Aspirin, heparin, or both to treat acute unstable angina. *N Engl J Med* 1988;319:1105–1111.

Design: Prospective, randomized, double-blind, placebo-controlled, dual-center study. Major end points were death, MI, and refractory angina.

Purpose: To evaluate the usefulness of aspirin, i.v. heparin, and their combination in the early management of UA.

Population: 479 patients aged ≤75 years with accelerating pattern of chest pain occurring at rest or with minimal exercise, or pain lasting 20 minutes with the last episode in the previous 24 hours. Their ECG changes had to be consistent with ischemia; if absent, diagnosis had to be confirmed by two cardiologists. CK levels had to be less than twice the ULN.

Exclusion Criteria: Included regular use of aspirin, contraindications to heparin or aspirin, coronary angioplasty within the previous 6 months, and bypass surgery within the previous 12 months (or scheduled).

Treatment: Aspirin, 325 mg twice daily, or i.v. heparin, 1,000 U/hour (given for average 6 days).

Results: Incidence of MI was significantly reduced in groups receiving aspirin [3% vs. 12% (placebo); $p = 0.01$], heparin (0.8%; $p < 0.001$); and aspirin plus heparin (1.6%; $p = 0.003$). No deaths occurred in these three treatment groups. Heparin was associated with a trend toward refractory angina compared with aspirin (RR, 0.47; 95% CI, 0.21 to 1.05; $p = 0.06$). Combination therapy was associated with more serious bleeding [3.3% vs. 1.7% (heparin alone)].

Comments: An additional 245 patients were randomized to either aspirin or heparin to allow an adequately powered comparison (see *Circulation* 1993;88:2045). A total of 484 patients was randomized to these two treatments, and the heparin group demonstrated a 78% lower MI rate at 5.7 ± 3.3 days (0.8% vs. 3.7%; $p = 0.035$). Only one death occurred (aspirin patient).

11. **Wallentin LW,** et al. Research on Instability in CAD (**RISC**) Risk of MI and death during treatment with low dose aspirin and intravenous heparin in men with unstable coronary artery disease. *Lancet* 1990;336:827–830.

Design: Prospective, randomized, double-blind, placebo-controlled, 2 × 2 factorial, multicenter study. Primary end point was death and MI.

Purpose: To evaluate the efficacy of aspirin and/or heparin in acute treatment of unstable and non–Q-wave MI and to assess the long-term effects of aspirin compared with placebo in these patients.

Population: 796 men younger than 70 years with non–Q-wave MI or increasing angina within the previous 4 weeks, with the last episode of pain within 72 hours and ischemia on resting ECG or predischarge exercise test.

Exclusion Criteria: Included Q-wave MI, myocardial dysfunction due to prior MI, previous CABG surgery, LBBB or pacemaker, concurrent anticoagulant or aspirin therapy, and increased bleeding risk.

Treatment: Aspirin, 75 mg daily for 1 year, or placebo, and i.v. heparin boluses (10,000 U every 6 hours for four doses, and then 7,500 U every 6 hours for 4 days), or placebo alone.

Results: Trial was stopped early due to publication of ISIS-2 results (minimum follow-up reduced to 3 months vs. 12 months). Aspirin patients had a markedly reduced risk of MI and death at 5 days (OR, 0.43; $p = 0.033$), 1 month (OR, 0.31; $p < 0.0001$), and 3 months (OR, 0.36; $p < 0.0001$). No benefits were seen with heparin alone. The aspirin and heparin group had fewer events in the first 5 days [1.4% vs. 3.7% (aspirin alone); $p = $ NS; 5.5% (heparin alone), $p = 0.045$; 6.0% (both placebos), $p = 0.027$]. Gastrointestinal symptoms with aspirin became more frequent after 3 months.

12. **Theroux P,** et al. Reactivation of unstable angina after the discontinuation of heparin. *N Engl J Med* 1992;327:141–145.

This study demonstrated a clear rebound effect with discontinuation of heparin in patients not taking aspirin. Four hundred three patients were randomized to i.v. heparin, aspirin, both, or neither, and completed 6 days of treatment without refractory angina or MI. After discontinuation of therapy, heparin-only patients had more frequent reactivation of unstable angina or MI in the subsequent 96 hours: 14 of 107 patients versus only five patients in each of the other three groups ($p < 0.01$). Eleven of 14 of these reactivations required urgent interventions (thrombolysis, angioplasty, or bypass surgery) versus only two in the other groups combined ($p < 0.01$).

13. **Cohen M,** et al. Antithrombotic Therapy in Acute Coronary Syndromes **(ATACS).** Prospective comparison of unstable angina vs non-Q wave MI during antithrombotic therapy. *J Am Coll Cardiol* 1993;22:1338–1343.

Design: Prospective, randomized, open, parallel-group, multicenter study. Primary end point was death, MI, and recurrent ischemia at 12 weeks.
Purpose: To evaluate whether the combination of aspirin and anticoagulant therapy is superior to either agent alone in reducing ischemic events in patients with UA or non–Q-wave MI.
Population: 358 patients older than 21 years with ischemic pain for 10 minutes at rest and within the past 48 hours and definite evidence of underlying ischemic heart disease (ECG changes during chest pain, history of prior MI, positive exercise test result, angiography with $\geq$50% stenosis).
Exclusion Criteria: Included evolving Q-wave MI, LBBB or permanent pacemaker, balloon angioplasty in the prior 6 months, CABG surgery in the past 12 months, and contraindications to anticoagulation.
Treatment: Aspirin, 162.5 mg, or aspirin plus heparin (100 U/kg bolus, and then continuous infusion for 3 to 4 days), and then aspirin plus warfarin [target international normalized ratio (INR), 2.0 to 3.0].
Results: At 12 weeks, the non–Q-wave MI group had a higher incidence of MI (11% vs. 4%; $p < 0.01$) and death and MI (16% vs. 7%), whereas a trend toward more frequent recurrent angina was seen in the unstable angina group (20% vs. 11%; $p = 0.10$).
Comments: Subsequent analysis of 214 nonprior aspirin users showed that the combination-therapy group had 61% fewer ischemic events at 14 days (10.5% vs. 27%; $p = 0.004$) and nonsignificant reduction at 12 weeks (13% vs. 25%; $p = 0.06$) (see *Circulation* 1994;89:81).

14. **Serneri GGN,** et al., Studio Eparina Sottocutanea nell Angina Instabile Refrattaria **(SESAIR).** Randomised comparison of subcutaneous heparin, intravenous heparin and aspirin in unstable angina. *Lancet* 1995;345:1201–1204.

This prospective, randomized trial was composed of 108 patients refractory to 24 hours of antianginal therapy. Patients received i.v. heparin (aPTT, 1.5 to 2.0 times normal), subcutaneous heparin (5,000 to 7,500 U every 8 hours; goal aPTT, 1.5–2.0 times normal), or aspirin, 325 mg once daily for 3 days (after which treatment could be discontinued or dosage modified). Over the first 3-day period, the heparin groups had a 91% reduction in frequency of angina, 46% fewer silent ischemic episodes, and 66% shorter overall duration of ischemia. In the subcutaneous group, reductions were 86%, 46%, and 61%, respectively. No significant effects were seen with aspirin. Favorable effects remained evident at 1 month.

15. **Oler A,** et al. Adding heparin to aspirin reduces the incidence of MI and death in patients with unstable angina: a meta-analysis. *JAMA* 1996;276:811–815.

This meta-analysis was derived from six randomized trials enrolling 1,353 patients. Aspirin and heparin tended to be preferable to aspirin alone (RR of death and MI, 0.67; 95% CI, 0.44 to 1.02). Combination therapy also was associated with nonsignificant reduction in recurrent ischemia (RR, 0.82; 95% CI, 0.40 to 1.17). No difference in revascularization rates was observed (RR, 1.03; 95% CI, 0.74 to 1.43), whereas aspirin and heparin were associated with a nonsignificant increase in major bleeding (RR, 1.99; 95% CI, 0.52 to 7.65).

16. Organization to Assess Strategies for Ischemic Syndromes (**OASIS**) Investigators. Comparison of the effects of two doses of recombinant hirudin compared with heparin in patients with acute myocardial ischemia without ST elevation. *Circulation* 1997;96:769–777.

Design: Prospective, randomized, open, multicenter study. Primary end point was cardiovascular death, MI, or refractory angina at 7 days.
Purpose: To compare the effects of a 3-day treatment with hirudin versus heparin on clinical outcomes in unstable angina and NSTEMI patients.
Population: 909 patients with unstable angina or suspected NSTEMI within 12 hours of the most recent episode of chest pain and with either ECG evidence of ischemia or previous objective documentation of CAD.
Exclusion Criteria: Included PTCA within 6 months, planned thrombolysis, stroke in the previous year, creatinine greater than 2.0 mg/dL, age older than 85 years, body weight more than 110 kg, cardiogenic shock, need for long-term oral anticoagulation.
Treatment: UFH (5,000 IU bolus + 1,000 to 1,200 U/hr), low-dose hirudin (0.2 mg/kg bolus and then 0.10 mg/kg/hr infusion), or medium-dose hirudin (0.4 mg/kg bolus and then 0.15 mg/kg/hr infusion) for 72 hours.
Results: At 7 days, cardiovascular death, new MI, or refractory angina (primary outcome) occurred in 6.5% in heparin group, 4.4% in low-dose hirudin group, and 3.0% medium-dose hirudin group ($p = 0.27$ heparin vs. low-dose hirudin; $p = 0.047$ heparin vs. medium-dose hirudin). The incidence of new MI was lower in the hirudin groups: 2.6% and 1.9% versus 4.6% ($p = 0.14$ heparin vs. low-dose hirudin; $p = 0.046$ heparin vs. medium-dose hirudin). An increase in ischemic events was seen in the low-dose hirudin group at around 24 hours after treatment cessation and at approximately 5 days in the medium-dose group, but the differences between hirudin and heparin persisted at 180 days.

17. **Anand SS,** et al. Long-term oral anticoagulant therapy in patients with unstable angina or suspected non-Q-wave myocardial infarction: organization to assess strategies for ischemic syndromes (**OASIS**) pilot study results. *Circulation* 1998;98:1064–1070.

Design: Prospective, randomized, open, multicenter study. Primary end point was cardiovascular death, nonfatal MI, and refractory angina.
Purpose: To evaluate the efficacy, feasibility, and safety of fixed-dose, low-intensity warfarin and moderate-intensity warfarin in patients with acute ischemic syndromes without ST-segment elevation.
Population: Phase 1: 309 patients seen within 12 hours of an episode of chest pain suspected to be due to unstable angina or MI without ST elevation. Phase 2: 197 patients seen within 48 hours of onset of symptoms.
Exclusion Criteria: Included major bleeding in previous 48 hours, requirement for coumadin, or CABG planned before or within 1 week of hospital discharge.
Treatment: Phase 1: Fixed-dose warfarin for 180 days [started on days 5 to 7 (after 72 hours of heparin or hirudin) with 10-mg loading dose, and then 3 mg once daily]. Phase 2: Adjusted-dose warfarin for 3 months (started 24 hours after initiation of heparin or hirudin; target INR, 2.0 to 3.0). Aspirin was recommended for all patients (actual rates, 85% to 87%).

Results: Phase 1: At 6 months, the fixed-dose warfarin group had nonsignificantly higher rates of cardiovascular death, MI, and refractory angina (6.5% vs. 3.9%; RR, 1.66; $p = 0.31$), and death, new MI, and stroke (6.5% vs. 2.6%; RR, 2.48; $p = 0.10$). The warfarin group had a significant excess of minor bleeds (RR, 5.46; $p = 0.001$). Phase 2: Mean INR was 2.3. At 3 months, the warfarin group tended toward reductions in primary end points (5.1% vs. 12.1%; RR, 0.42; $p = 0.08$) and death, MI, and stroke [5.1% vs. 13.1%; RR, 0.39 (95% CI, 0.14 to 1.05); $p = 0.05$]. The warfarin group had significantly fewer rehospitalizations for unstable angina (7.1% vs. 17.2%; RR, 0.42; $p = 0.03$) and more minor bleeding episodes (28.6% vs. 12.1%; RR, 2.36; $p = 0.004$).

Low-molecular-weight Heparins

18. **Wallentin L,** et al. Fragmin during Instability in CAD **(FRISC).** Low molecular weight heparin during instability in coronary artery disease. *Lancet* 1996; 347:561–568.

Design: Prospective, randomized, double-blind, placebo-controlled, multicenter study. Primary end point was death or MI at 6 days.

Purpose: To evaluate whether subcutaneous dalteparin provides an additive benefit to that provided by aspirin and antianginal drugs in patients with unstable angina or non–Q-wave MI.

Population: 1,506 patients (men aged 40 years, women more than 1 year after menopause) with chest pain in the previous 72 hours. All had newly developed or increasing angina or angina at rest during the previous 2 months or persisting chest pain with a suspicion of MI and ST depression ≥ 1 mm or T-wave inversion ≥ 1 mm in two adjacent leads without Q waves in ischemic leads.

Exclusion Criteria: Included increased bleeding risks (e.g., cerebral bleeding in the previous 3 months, gastrointestinal bleeding in the prior 5 years, platelet count less than 100,000, oral anticoagulation), creatinine more than 200 μM, new Q waves in ischemic leads, indications for thrombolysis, LBBB or pacemaker, and PCI or bypass surgery planned before admission or in prior 3 months.

Treatment: Dalteparin, 120 IU/kg subcutaneously twice daily for 6 days, and then 7,500 IU daily for 35 to 45 days; or placebo.

Results: At 6 days, the dalteparin group had a 63% lower rate of death and new MI (1.8% vs. 4.8%; $p = 0.001$); a nonsignificant reduction was observed at 40 days (8% vs. 10.7%; $p = 0.07$).

Comments: Subsequent analysis showed the additive value of troponin T to predischarge ETT in providing risk stratification (see *Eur Heart J* 1997;18:762).

19. **Klein W,** et al. Fragmin in Unstable Coronary Artery Disease. **(FRIC)** Comparison of low molecular weight heparin with unfractionated heparin acutely and with placebo for 6 weeks in the management of unstable coronary artery disease. *Circulation* 1997;96:61–68 (editorial, 3–5).

Design: Prospective, randomized, partially open-label, parallel, multicenter, study. Primary end point was death, MI, or recurrent angina.

Purpose: To compare the efficacy and safety of weight-adjusted subcutaneous dalteparin with UFH in the acute treatment of unstable angina or non–Q-wave MI and the value of prolonged dalteparin compared with placebo in those initially given anticoagulants.

Population: 1,482 patients with chest pain in the preceding 72 hours and admission ECG with temporary or persistent ST depression ≥ 1 mV in at least two adjacent leads and/or temporary or persistent T-wave inversion ≥ 1 mm in two adjacent leads.

Exclusion Criteria: Included new Q waves, LBBB, indication for thrombolytic therapy, oral anticoagulation, diastolic blood pressure (DBP) greater than 120 mm Hg or SBP less than 90 mmHg, bleeding diathesis or recent surgery, and history of cerebrovascular event.

Treatment: Phase 1 (open label, days 1 to 6): Dalteparin, 120 IU/kg subcutaneously twice daily, or i.v. UFH. Phase 2 (double-blind, days 6 to 45): Dalteparin, 7,500 IU subcutaneously once daily, or placebo.

Results: In the first 6 days, no significant differences were observed between groups in death, MI, or recurrent angina [7.6% (heparin) vs. 9.3% (dalteparin); 95% CI, 0.84 to 1.66]; death and MI (3.6% vs. 3.9%), or revascularization (5.3% vs. 4.8%). For days 6 to 45, similar incidences of composite end points (both 12.3%) and revascularization [14.2% (placebo) vs. 14.3%] were observed. The dalteparin group had a higher phase 1 mortality rate (11 vs. three deaths; RR, 3.37; 95% CI, 1.01 to 11.24).

Comments: Lack of benefit with dalteparin may be due to the low ratio of anti–Factor Xa to antithrombin activity (only 2.0).

20. **Cohen M,** et al. Efficacy and Safety of Subcutaneous Enoxaparin in Non-Q wave Coronary Events **(ESSENCE).** A comparison of low molecular weight heparin with unfractionated heparin for unstable coronary artery disease. *N Engl J Med* 1997;337:447–452 (editorial, 492–494).

Design: Prospective, randomized, double-blind, placebo-controlled, parallel-group, multicenter study. Primary end point was death, MI, or recurrent angina at 14 days.

Purpose: To compare the efficacy and safety of enoxaparin with UFH in patients with unstable angina or non–Q-wave MI.

Population: 3,171 patients with rest pain 10 minutes in the preceding 24 hours accompanied by one of the following: (a) new ST depression ≥1 mm, transient ST elevation, or T-wave changes in at least two contiguous leads; (b) documented prior MI or revascularization procedure; or (c) noninvasive or invasive tests suggesting ischemic heart disease. Only about one third had ST-segment changes on admission.

Exclusion Criteria: Included LBBB or pacemaker, persistent ST elevation, angina with an established precipitating cause (e.g., heart failure), contraindications to anticoagulation, and creatinine clearance less than 30 mL/min.

Treatment: Enoxaparin, 1 mg/kg subcutaneously twice daily, or UFH for 2 to 8 days (mean duration, 2.8 days).

Results: Enoxaparin group had a 16% lower rate of death, MI, and recurrent angina at 14 days (16.6% vs. 19.8%; *p* = 0.019); at 30 days, the benefit persisted (19.8% vs. 23.3%; *p* = 0.016). Enoxaparin also was associated with a lower 30-day revascularization rate (27% vs. 32.2%; *p* = 0.001). Similar rates of major bleeding were observed at 30 days (6.5% vs. 7.0%), but overall bleeding was higher in the enoxaparin group (18.4% vs. 14.2%; *p* = 0.001) because of injection-site ecchymoses.

21. FRagmin and Fast Revascularization during InStability in coronary artery disease **(FRISC II)** Investigators. Long-term, low-molecular-mass heparin in unstable coronary artery disease: FRISC II prospective randomized multicenter study. *Lancet* 1999;354:701–707.

Design: Prospective, randomized, partially blinded parallel group, multicenter study. Primary end point was death or MI at 3 months.

Purpose: To assess the effects of long-term treatment with dalteparin compared with a placebo in patients undergoing a noninvasive treatment strategy.

Population: 2,267 patients (median age, 67 years) with ischemic symptoms in the previous 48 hours accompanied by ECG changes (ST depression or T-wave inversion ≥0.1 mV) or elevated markers (e.g., CK-MB, more than 6 mg/L; troponin T, more than 0.10 mg/L).

Exclusion Criteria: Included angioplasty in previous 6 months, indication for or treatment with thrombolysis in past 24 hours, scheduled revascularization procedure.

Treatment: After 5 or more days of open-label dalteparin, patients randomized to subcutaneous dalteparin, 120 IU/kg twice daily, or placebo for 3 months.

Results: At 30 days, the dalteparin group had a significant reduction in death or MI (3.1% vs. 5.9%; *p* = 0.002), but at 3 months, the reduction was nonsignificant (6.7% vs. 8.0%; *p* = 0.17). A significant reduction was found in the 3-month incidence of death, MI, or revascularization (29.1% vs. 33.4%; *p* = 0.031), but this benefit did not persist at 6 months (38.4% vs. 39.9%; *p* = 0.50). Mortality was significantly reduced at 1 year (*Lancet* 2000;356:9).

22. **Antman E,** for the **TIMI 11B** Investigators. Enoxaparin prevents death and cardiac ischemic events in unstable angina/non–Q-wave MI: results of the TIMI 11B trial. *Circulation* 1999;100:1593–1601.

Design: Prospective, randomized, double-blind, placebo-controlled, multicenter study. Primary end point was death, MI, or urgent revascularization at 8 and 43 days.

Purpose: To evaluate the benefits of an extended course of enoxaparin compared with standard UFH for preventing death and cardiac events in patients with UA or non–Q-wave MI.

Population: 3,910 patients with ischemic discomfort at rest within the past 24 hours and ST-segment deviation or positive CK-MB or troponin.

Exclusion Criteria: Included planned revascularization within 24 hours, treatable cause of angina, evolving Q-wave MI, CABG surgery within 2 months, or PTCA within 6 months, UFH infusion for more than 24 hours before enrollment, history of heparin-associated thrombocytopenia (HIT), contraindications to anticoagulation.

Treatment: Enoxaparin [1 mg/kg subcutaneously twice daily (acute phase), and then 60 mg ($\geq$65 kg) or 40 mg (less than 65 kg) twice daily] during both acute (2 to 8 days) and chronic phases (through day 43) OR i.v. UFH (acute phase only).

Results: Enoxaparin-treated patients had a significant 12% reduction in the primary composite end point of death, MI, or urgent revascularization at day 43 (17.3% vs. 19.7%; $p = 0.048$). This benefit was apparent by day 8 (12.4% vs. 14.5%; $p = 0.048$). During the first 72 hours and entire initial hospitalization, no difference was noted in the major bleeding rates between the treatment groups. However, long-term enoxaparin treatment was associated with an increase in the rate of major hemorrhage (spontaneous and instrumented; 2.9% vs. 1.5%; $p = 0.021$). At 1-year follow-up, a persistent significant benefit was associated with enoxaparin therapy (incidence of primary composite end point, 32.0% vs. 35.7%; $p = 0.022$; see *J Am Coll Cardiol* 2000;36:693).

Comments: When these results are pooled with the ESSENCE data, a significant reduction in death and MI is found at day 8 (4.1% vs. 5.3%), day 14 (5.2% vs. 6.5%), and day 43 (7.1% vs. 8.6%).

23. Comparison of two treatment durations (6 days and 14 days) of a low molecular weight heparin with a 6-day treatment of UFH in the initial management of unstable angina or non-Q wave myocardial infarction: **FRAXIS** (FRAxiparine in Ischaemic Syndrome). *Eur Heart J* 1999;20:1553–1562.

This prospective, randomized, controlled study enrolled 3,468 patients with UA and non–Q-wave MI (angina within 48 hours and ST depression, T-wave inversion, or ST elevation not justifying thrombolysis). Patients received nadroparine for a short course (6 days) or long course (14 days) or UFH (6 $\pm$ 2 days). At 14 days, the incidence of the primary composite end point, consisting of cardiovascular death, recurrent angina, and recurrence of UA, was similar in the three treatment groups (heparin, 18.1%; short-course fraxiparine, 17.8%; long-course fraxiparine, 20%). A higher incidence of hemorrhage was seen in the long-course fraxiparine group [at 14 days, 3.5% vs. 1.6% (UFH) and 1.5% (short-course nadroparin)].

24. Integrelin and Enoxaparin Randomized Assessment of Acute Coronary Syndrome Treatment (**INTERACT**). Goodman SG, et al. INTERACT Investigators. Randomized evaluation of the safety and efficacy of enoxaparin versus unfractionated heparin in high-risk patients with non–ST-segment elevation acute coronary syndromes receiving the glycoprotein IIb/IIIa inhibitor eptifibatide. *Circulation* 2003;107:238–244.

This prospective, randomized, open-label, multicenter trial enrolled 746 patients with ischemic chest discomfort without ST-segment elevation. Patients received UFH or enoxaparin. All aspirin (160-mg loading dose and then 80 to 325 mg/day) and the GP IIb/IIIa inhibitor eptifibatide (180-μg/kg i.v. bolus, and then 2.0 μg/kg/min for 48 hours); cardiac catheterization and/or coronary revascularization decisions were left to the discretion of the investigator. The incidence of the primary end point, non-CABG TIMI major bleeding at 96 hours, occurred less frequently in the enoxaparin group than in the UFH group (1.8% vs. 4.6%; $p = 0.03$). The enoxaparin group also had a significantly lower incidence of death and nonfatal MI at 30 days (5.0% vs. 9.0%; $p = 0.031$). Limitations of this study include the open-label design and the long time to coronary revascularization (median, 101 hours vs. 21 hours in TACTICS-TIMI 18). The ongoing SYNERGY trial is examining the same issue among 8,000 patients treated with GP IIb/IIIa inhibitors.

25. **A to Z.** Preliminary results Presented at the 52nd ACC Scientific Sessions, Chicago, IL: March 2003.

This prospective, randomized, open, multicenter trial enrolled 3,987 high-risk ACS patients (ST segment changes or positive cardiac marker). All patients received aspirin and tirofiban: 60% of patients underwent angiography, Crossover from enoxaparin to UFH in the cath lab was allowed. Patients were randomized to enoxaparin (1 mg/kg every 12 hours) or weight-adjusted UFH. The enoxaparin had a nonsignificant 12% reduction in death, MI, or refractory ischemia compared to UFH (8.4% vs. 9.4%, $p = 0.23$); however, the trial was designed to demonstrate noninferiority and this goal was met.

β-Blockers, Calcium Antagonists, and Nitrates

26. **Gibson RS,** et al., Diltiazem Reinfarction Study Group. Diltiazem and reinfarction in patients with non–Q-wave MI. *N Engl J Med* 1986;315:423–429.

Design: Prospective, randomized, double-blind, multicenter study. Primary end point was reinfarction at 14 days.
Purpose: To determine whether diltiazem would reduce the incidence of early reinfarction in patients recovering from a non–Q-wave MI.
Population: 576 patients with non–Q-wave MI [elevated CK-MB and either ischemic pain for 30 minutes or ST-segment deviation (elevation or depression ≥1 mm or T-wave inversions in at least two leads)].
Exclusion Criteria: Included new Q waves, HR less than 50 beats/min, advanced heart block, cardiogenic shock or sustained SBP less than 100 mm Hg, coronary bypass surgery in the past 3 months, therapy with a calcium-channel blocker.
Treatment: Randomized at 24 to 72 hours to diltiazem, 90 mg every 6 hours, or placebo.
Results: Diltiazem patients had a significantly lower 14-day reinfarction rate (5.2% vs. 9.3%; $p = 0.03$) and 50% less refractory angina (3.5% vs. 6.9%; $p = 0.03$). No significant difference was observed in mortality rates (3.1% vs. 3.8%). Adverse reactions were common in the diltiazem group [overall, 24% vs. 6% (AV block, 6% vs. 2%; SBP less than 90 mm Hg, 8% vs. 2%)], but only 4.9% of the diltiazem patients stopped therapy because of the adverse effects.

27. Interuniversity Nifedipine/Metoprolol Trial (**HINT**) Research Group. Early treatment of unstable angina in the coronary care unit: a randomised, double blind, placebo controlled comparison of recurrent ischaemia in patients treated with nifedipine or metoprolol or both. *Br Heart J* 1986;56:400–413.

This prospective, randomized, double-blind, placebo-controlled, multicenter trial enrolled 515 patients with unstable angina, of whom 338 were not pretreated with a β-blocker. In patients not pretreated with a β-blocker, no significant differences were found between the three groups (nifedipine, metoprolol, or both) in the incidence of recurrent ischemia or MI at 48 hours. However, a trend was seen toward a higher incidence of MI in the nifedipine group (RR, 1.51; 95% CI, 0.87 to 2.74). In patients already taking a β-blocker, the addition of nifedipine was beneficial (RR, 0.68; 95% CI, 0.47 to 0.97). These results suggest that in patients not taking previous β-blockade, metoprolol has a beneficial short-term effect on UA, and that nifedipine alone may be detrimental.

28. **Gheorghiade M,** et al. Effects of propranolol in non–Q-wave acute MI in the β-blocker heart attack trial. *Am J Cardiol* 1990;66:129–133.

This retrospective analysis focused on the 601 β-Blocker Heart Attack Trial patients (17%) with a non–Q-wave MI. Patients in this trial were randomized to propranolol,

180 to 240 mg/day, or placebo. At follow-up (median, 24.6 months), similar mortality, sudden death, and reinfarction rates were observed.

29. **Doucet S,** et al. Randomized trial comparing intravenous nitroglycerin and heparin for treatment of unstable angina secondary to restenosis after coronary artery angioplasty. *Circulation.* 2000;101:955.

This prospective, randomized, double-blind, single-center study enrolled 200 patients hospitalized for UA within 6 months after angioplasty alone (no stenting). Patients received i.v. NTG, heparin, their combination, or placebo for 63 ± 30 hours. Recurrent angina occurred less frequently in the NTG groups [42.6% (NTG alone), 41.7% (NTG + heparin) vs. 75% (placebo and heparin-alone groups); $p < 0.003$]. Refractory angina requiring angiography occurred less often with NTG (4.3%, 4.2%, 22.9%, and 29.2%, respectively; $p < 0.002$). No deaths or MIs were found. These results suggest that smooth muscle cell proliferation and increased vasoreactivity are more important roles than thrombus formation in restenosis-related UA.

Glycoprotein IIb/IIIa Inhibitors

30. Platelet Receptor Inhibition in Ischemic Syndrome Management in Patients Limited by Unstable Signs and Symptoms (**PRISM-PLUS**) Investigators. Inhibition of the platelet glycoprotein IIb/IIIa receptor with tirofiban in unstable angina and non–Q-wave myocardial infarction. *N Engl J Med* 1998;338:1488–1497 (editorial, 1539–1541).

Design: Prospective, randomized, double-blind, multicenter study. Primary end point was death, MI, or refractory ischemia at 7 days.

Purpose: To investigate the clinical efficacy of tirofiban, a short-acting, nonpeptide GP IIb/IIIa inhibitor, in the prevention of acute ischemic events in patients with UA and non–Q-wave MI.

Population: 1,915 patients with prolonged anginal pain or repetitive episodes of angina at rest or during minimal exercise in the previous 12 hours and new ST-T changes [$\geq$1-mm elevation or depression, $\geq$3-mm T-wave inversion on at least three limb leads or precordial leads (excluding V_1), or pseudonormalization $\geq$?///////mm] or an elevated CK or CK-MB.

Exclusion Criteria: Included ST elevation longer than 20 minutes, thrombolysis in the previous 48 hours, angioplasty in the past 6 months, or CABG surgery in the previous month, stroke in the prior year, active bleeding or high bleeding risk, history of thrombocytopenia or platelet count less than 150,000, and creatinine more than 2.5 mg/dL.

Treatment: (a) Tirofiban, 0.6 μg/kg/min for 30 minutes, and then 0.15 μg/kg/min and placebo heparin; (b) tirofiban, 0.4 μg/kg/min for 30 minutes, and then 0.1 μg/kg/min, plus heparin; or (c) heparin plus placebo tirofiban.

Results: The tirofiban-plus-heparin group had a significant reduction compared with the heparin-alone group in the 7-day composite end points (12.9% vs. 17.9%; RR, 0.68; $p = 0.004$). This difference persisted at 30-day and 6-month follow-up (18.5% vs. 22.3%; $p = 0.03$; 27.7% vs. 32.1%; $p = 0.02$). The tirofiban-plus-heparin group also had a significant reduction in death or MI at 7 days and 30 days (4.9% vs. 8.3%; $p = 0.006$; 8.7% vs. 11.9%; $p = 0.03$).

Comments: Benefit was seen regardless of treatment strategy: medical therapy group with 25% reduction in death or MI at 30 days, PCI group with 34% reduction, and CABG group with 30% reduction. The troponin substudy also showed that the combination of tirofiban plus heparin reduced infarct size, as measured by peak troponin [see *J Am Coll Cardiol* 1998;31(suppl A):229A]. Angiographic study (1,491 patients) found a lower thrombus burden with tirofiban + heparin compared with heparin alone (OR, 0.65; $p = 0.002$) and higher TIMI grade 3 flow rate (82% vs. 74%) (see *Circulation* 1999;100:1609).

31. Platelet Receptor Inhibition in Ischemic Syndrome Management (**PRISM**) Study Investigators. A comparison of aspirin plus tirofiban with aspirin plus heparin for unstable angina. *N Engl J Med* 1998;338:1498–1505 (editorial, 1539–1541).

Design: Prospective, randomized, multicenter study. Primary end point was death, MI, and refractory ischemia at 48 hours.

Purpose: To compare i.v. tirofiban with i.v. UFH for the treatment of UA in patients receiving aspirin.

Population: 3,232 patients with rest or accelerating chest pain within 24 hours of randomization and at least one of the following criteria: (a) ST depression ≥ 1 mm in at least two contiguous leads, transient (less than 20 minutes) ST elevation, or T-wave inversion; (b) elevated cardiac enzymes; and (c) history of MI, revascularization more than 6 months earlier, coronary surgery more than 1 month earlier, positive exercise or pharmacologic stress test result, or more than 50% stenosis on prior angiogram.

Exclusion Criteria: Included thrombolytic therapy in previous 48 hours, creatinine greater than 2.5 mg/dL, increased bleeding risks, history of thrombocytopenia, SBP more than 180 mm Hg, and DBP more than 110 mm Hg.

Treatment: Tirofiban, 0.6 μg/kg/min for 30 minutes, and then 0.15 μg/kg/min through 48 hours, with placebo heparin, or UFH (5,000-U bolus, and then 1,000 U/h for 48 hours, adjusted if necessary based on aPTT at 6 and 24 hours). All patients were taking aspirin, 300 to 325 mg daily.

Results: Tirofiban group had a 32% reduction in the composite primary end points at 48 hours: 3.8% vs. 5.6% (RR, 0.67; $p = 0.01$). At 30 days, a similar frequency of composite end points was observed (15.9% vs. 17.1%; $p = 0.34$). At 7 days, the tirofiban group had a significantly lower mortality rate (2.3% vs. 3.6%; $p = 0.02$) and tended toward a reduction in death and MI (5.8% vs. 7.1%; $p = 0.11$). Tirofiban was associated with increased thrombocytopenia (1.1% vs. 0.4%; $p = 0.04$). Identical major bleeding rates were observed (0.4%). At 30 days, death or MI occurred in 13.0% of troponin I–positive patients compared with 4.9% for troponin I–negative patients ($p < 0.0001$), and 13.7% compared with 3.5% for troponin T ($p < 0.001$) (see ref. 72). In troponin I–positive patients, tirofiban substantially lowered the risks of death [adjusted hazard ratio (HR), 0.25 (95% CI, 0.09 to 0.68), $p = 0.004$] and MI [HR, 0.37 (0.16 to 0.84), $p = 0.01$].

32. Platelet IIb/IIIa Antagonism for the Reduction of Acute Coronary Syndrome Events in a Global Organization Network **(PARAGON),** The PARAGON Investigators. International, randomized, controlled trial of lamifiban (a platelet GP IIb/IIIa inhibitor), heparin, or both in unstable angina. *Circulation* 1998;97:2386–2395.

This prospective, randomized, partial factorial (2×2), controlled (heparin alone), multicenter study enrolled 2,282 patients with chest discomfort in the prior 12 hours associated with transient or persistent ST depression (≥ 0.5 mm) or T-wave inversion or transient (less than 30 minutes) ST elevation (≥ 0.5 mm). Patients were randomized to five groups: lamifiban placebo plus heparin (control); lamifiban (300-μg bolus, and then 1 μg/min), with and without heparin; and lamifiban (750-μg bolus, and then 5 μg/min), with and without heparin. Lamifiban was given for 3 to 5 days. All patients received aspirin daily (160 mg recommended). A similar incidence of death and MI was found at 30 days (primary end point) with heparin alone, low-dose lamifiban, and high-dose lamifiban (11.7%, 10.6%, 12.0%; $p = 0.668$). At 6 months, low-dose lamifiban was associated with fewer events compared with heparin alone [13.7% vs. 17.9%; $p = 0.027$; 16.4% (high-dose lamifiban); $p = 0.45$]. Low-dose lamifiban yielded the best results with heparin: the 6-month ischemic event rate was 12.6% versus 17.9% without heparin ($p = 0.025$), and bleeding rates were similar.

33. Platelet Glycoprotein IIb/IIIa in Unstable Angina Receptor Suppression Using Integrelin Therapy **(PURSUIT)** Trial Investigators. Inhibition of platelet glycoprotein IIb/IIIa with eptifibatide in patients with acute coronary syndromes. *N Engl J Med* 1998;339:436–443.

Design: Prospective, randomized, double-blind, placebo-controlled, multicenter study. Primary end point was death or nonfatal MI at 30 days.

Purpose: To determine if the addition of eptifibatide to heparin and aspirin provides additional benefit in patients with acute coronary syndromes without ST elevation.

Population: 10,948 patients with ischemic chest pain lasting 10 minutes in the prior 24 hours (median, 11 hours) and ECG changes (transient or persistent ST-segment depression more than 0.5 mm, transient ST-segment elevation more than 0.5 mm, or T-wave inversion more than 1 mm within 12 hours before or after chest pain), or serum CK-MB above the ULN.

Exclusion Criteria: Included persistent ST elevation more than 1 mm, SBP more than 200 mm Hg or DBP more than 100 mm Hg, major surgery within the prior 6 weeks, nonhemorrhagic stroke in the prior 30 days, or any history of hemorrhagic stroke, renal failure, planned used of thrombolytic or GP IIb/IIIa inhibitors, and thrombolysis in the prior 24 hours.

Treatment: Eptifibatide, 180-μg/kg bolus, and then 1.3 or 2.0 μg/kg/min for 72 hours (up to 96 hours if intervention was near the end of a 72-hour period), or placebo; 1.3-μg/kg/min infusion was dropped after 3,218 patients enrolled. No protocol-mandated strategy of catheterization and revascularization was undertaken.

Results: Eptifibatide was associated with a 9.6% relative reduction in death or MI at 30 days (14.2% vs. 15.7%; $p = 0.04$); this effect was apparent by 72 hours. Among patients undergoing early (less than 72 hours) PCI, eptifibatide was associated with a 32% benefit (also see *Circulation* 1999;99:2371). Eptifibatide was associated with increased major bleeding (10.6% vs. 9.1%; $p = 0.02$) and higher transfusion rates (11.6% vs. 9.2%; RR, 1.3; 95% CI, 1.1 to 1.4). The eptifibatide group also had more cases of profound thrombocytopenia (platelet count less than 20,000): RR, 5.0 (nine vs. two patients; 95% CI, 1.3 to 32.4). Eptifibatide was not associated with increased incidence of bleeding in those undergoing CABG surgery. Stroke occurred in 79 (0.7%) patients, 66 of whom were nonhemorrhagic, and no significant differences in stroke rates were found between patients who received placebo and those assigned high-dose eptifibatide (see *Circulation* 1999;99:2371).

Comments: Among the 87% of patients who did not undergo early PCI, only a non-significant trend was seen toward fewer primary events with eptifibatide (14.6% vs. 15.6%; $p = 0.23$). The finding of no extra bleeding risk in those undergoing CABG surgery is consistent with the short half-life of eptifibatide.

34. **Cannon CP,** et al. Oral glycoprotein IIb/IIIa inhibition with orbofiban in patients with unstable coronary syndromes (**OPUS-TIMI 16**) trial. *Circulation* 2000;102:149–156.

Design: Prospective, randomized, double-blind, multicenter study. Primary end point was death, MI, recurrent ischemia requiring rehospitalization, urgent revascularization, or stroke.

Purpose: To determine whether prolonged oral GP IIb/IIIA inhibition with orbofiban provides additional reduction in recurrent ischemic events.

Population: 10,288 patients with ACSs defined as ischemic rest pain within 72 hours and one or more of the following: new ST-segment deviation of 0.5 mm or more, T-wave inversion of 3 mm or more in three leads or LBBB, positive cardiac markers, or (for the first 3,000 patients only) history of MI, PCI, CABG surgery, coronary stenosis of 50% or more, age 65 years or older, and a history of angina or positive stress test, prior peripheral arterial or cerebrovascular disease, or diabetes mellitus.

Exclusion Criteria: Included serious illness, PCI in the previous 6 months, CABG surgery in the previous 2 months, need for warfarin or daily nonsteroidal anti-inflammatory drugs (NSAIDs), more than two doses of ticlopidine/clopidogrel in the previous 48 hours or abciximab within 24 hours, creatinine more than 1.6 mg/dL, increased bleeding risk [prior intracranial hemorrhage (ICH), peptic ulcer within 6 months, etc.]

Treatment: Orbofiban, 50 mg twice daily (50/50 group); orbofiban, 50 mg twice daily for 30 days followed by 30 mg orbofiban twice daily (50/30 group), or placebo.

Results: Trial was terminated early because of increased 30-day mortality in the 50/30 orbofiban group. At 10 months, mortality was 3.7% in the placebo group versus 5.1% in the 50/30 group ($p = 0.008$) and 4.5% in the 50/50 group ($p = 0.11$). No differences were found between the three groups in the incidence of the primary composite end point (22.9%, 23.1%, and 22.8%, for the placebo, 50/30, and 50/50 groups, respectively). The orbofiban groups had a significantly higher incidence of major or severe bleeding (but not ICH) compared with placebo [3.7% (50/30) and 4.5% (50/50) vs. 2.0%). The subgroup of patients undergoing PCI had a lower mortality and primary event rate with orbofiban [23.9% (50/30), 21.8% (50/50), 27.5% (placebo)].

35. **PARAGON B** (Platelet IIb/IIIA Antagonist for the reduction of Acute Coronary Syndrome Events in a Global Organization Network B). Preliminary results presented at 49th ACC Meeting, Anaheim, CA, March 2000.

This prospective, randomized, double-blind, placebo-controlled, multicenter trial enrolled 5,225 patients with non-ST elevation ACSs within 12 hours of onset of symptoms. Patients received lamifiban (500-μg bolus, and then i.v. infusion for 72 hours) or placebo. All were given aspirin and heparin. At 30 days, no significant difference was seen between groups in the primary end point of death, MI, or urgent revascularization [11.8% (lamifiban) vs. 12.8% (placebo); $p = 0.329$]. Bleeding occurred more often in the lamifiban group ($p = 0.002$), but no difference was found in major bleeding (1.3% vs. 0.9%) or in lamifiban patients undergoing CABG surgery. Subgroup analysis revealed that lamifiban significantly reduced primary events in those undergoing PCI (11.6% vs. 18.5%) and with a positive troponin (11% vs. 19%; $p = 0.018$; see *Circulation* 2001;103:2891)

36. The **SYMPHONY** Investigators, Sibrafiban versus Aspirin to Yield Maximum Protection from Ischemic Heart Events Post-acute Coronary Syndromes. Comparison of sibrafiban with aspirin for prevention of cardiovascular events after acute coronary syndromes: a randomised trial. *Lancet* 2000;355:337–345.

Design: Prospective, randomized, double-blind, multicenter study. Primary end point was death, MI, or severe recurrent ischemia at 90 days.
Purpose: To compare the efficacy, safety, and tolerability of long-term administration of the oral GP IIb/IIIa inhibitor sibrafiban with aspirin in ACSs
Population: 9,233 patients seen within 7 days of an ACS, clinically stable for 12 hours or more, and Killip class 1 or 2
Exclusion Criteria: Serious illness, predisposition to bleeding, major surgery, previous stroke or ICH, thrombocytopenia, renal failure, treatment with oral anticoagulants, antiplatelet agents, or NSAIDs.
Treatment: Aspirin, 80 mg, low-dose sibrafiban (4.5 or 3 mg, depending on creatinine and body weight), high-dose oral sibrafiban (6, 4.5, or 3 mg depending on creatinine and body weight). All were taken every 12 hours.
Results: No differences were found between the three groups in the incidence of the primary composite end point [9.8% (aspirin), 10.1% (low-dose sibrafiban), 10.1% (high-dose sibrafiban); OR for aspirin vs. both the low- and high-dose sibrafiban, 1.03; 95% CI, 0.87 to 1.21]. Death or MI rates also were similar (7.0%, 7.4%, and 7.9%, respectively). Large MIs (CK-MB more than 5 times the ULN) occurred less frequently in the aspirin group (37.4%) than in the sibrofiban groups [45.3% (low dose), 49.7% (high dose)]. The aspirin group had a significantly lower incidence of bleeding (13.0% vs. 18.7% and 25.4%), whereas major bleeding occurred in 3.9%, 5.2%, and 5.7%, respectively.

37. **SYMPHONY II** Investigators. Randomized trial of aspirin, sibrafiban, or both for secondary prevention after acute coronary syndromes. *Circulation* 2001;103:1727–1733.

Design: Prospective, randomized, double-blind, multicenter study. Primary end point was death, MI, and severe recurrent ischemia.
Purpose: To assess whether longer treatment (12 to 18 months) with low-dose sibrafiban in combination with aspirin or high-dose sibrafiban alone was more effective for secondary prevention than is aspirin alone
Population: Same inclusion criteria as SYMPHONY I; 6,671 patients completed a median of 90 days of follow-up (original design, 8,400 patients)
Exclusion Criteria: See SYMPHONY I.
Treatment: Aspirin alone (80 mg twice daily), low-dose sibrafiban (LDS) + aspirin, or high-dose sibrafiban (HDS). Average time from qualifying event to first dose was 94 hours (range, 63 to 132 hours).

Results: Study terminated after SYMPHONY I results were reported. No difference was noted between the three groups in the incidence of the primary composite end point (aspirin, 9.3%; LDS + aspirin, 9.2%; HDS, 10.5%). The HDS group had a higher incidence of death or MI compared with the aspirin-alone group (6.1% vs. 8.6%), whereas major bleeding occurred more frequently in the LDS + aspirin group compared with the aspirin-alone group (5.7% vs. 4.0%).

Comments: Some evidence suggests that the increased thrombosis seen with oral GP IIb/IIIa inhibitors is due to enhanced receptor activity during the hours when the drugs are less active or not available.

38. **Simoons ML, GUSTO IV-ACS** Investigators. Effect of glycoprotein IIb/IIIa receptor blocker abciximab on outcome in patients with acute coronary syndromes without early coronary revascularisation: the GUSTO IV-ACS randomised trial. *Lancet* 2001;357:1915–1924.

Design: Prospective, randomized, open, multicenter study. Primary end point was death or MI at 30 days.

Purpose: To study the effect of the GP IIb/IIIa blocker abciximab in ACS patients not undergoing early revascularization.

Population: 7,800 patients with UA or NSTEMI. Eligible if chest pain longer than 5 minutes within the last 24 hours, 0.5-mm or more ST-segment depression, OR positive troponin T or I.

Exclusion Criteria: Included ST elevation or new LBBB, PCI within the past 2 weeks, planned PCI/CABG in the next 30 days, active bleeding or bleeding disorder, recent trauma or surgery, gastrointestinal (GI)/genitourinary (GU) bleeding in the prior 6 weeks, intracranial neoplasm/aneurysm, stroke in the past 2 years or with residual defect, oral anticoagulation, platelet count less than 100,000.

Treatment: Abciximab for 24 hours, or abciximab for 48 hours, or placebo. All received aspirin and either UFH or LMWH.

Results: No significant differences were observed between the groups in the incidence of death or MI at 30 days (abciximab for 24 hours, 8.2%; abciximab for 48 hours, 9.1%; placebo, 8.0%; p = NS). No differences were noted among those with a positive troponin or in any other subgroups. The mortality rate was actually higher in first 48 hours in both abciximab groups compared with the placebo group [0.7% and 0.9% vs. 0.3%; ORs, 2.3 (p = 0.048) and 2.9 (p = 0.007)]. In particular, no benefit was seen in patients with increased cardiac troponin T or I concentrations at enrollment, although these patients had a strongly increased risk of subsequent events. Bleeding rates were low but were higher with abciximab, particularly in the 48-hour group. Thrombocytopenia also was more common in the abciximab groups

Comments: Based on these results, abciximab for ACS patients not undergoing planned PCI is contraindicated (class III recommendation).

39. **Roffi M,** et al. Platelet glycoprotein IIb/IIIa inhibitors reduce mortality in diabetic patients with non-ST-segment-elevation acute coronary syndromes. *Circulation* 2001;104:2767–2771.

This meta-analysis examined patients enrolled in six large GP IIb/IIIa inhibitor trials (PRISM, PRISM-PLUS, PARAGON A, PARAGON B, PURSUIT, GUSTO IV). Among the 6,458 diabetic patients, GP IIb/IIIa inhibitor use was associated with a significant lower 30-day mortality compared with no GP inhibition (4.6% vs. 6.2%; OR, 0.74; 95% CI, 0.59 to 0.92; p = 0.007). The largest benefit was seen in the subgroup of 1,279 diabetic patients who underwent PCI during the index hospitalization; they had a 70% lower mortality with GP inhibitor use (1.2% vs. 4.0%; OR, 0.30; 95% CI, 0.14 to 0.69; p = 0.002). In contrast, among the 23,072 nondiabetic patients, no survival benefit was associated with GP inhibitor use (3.0% in both groups). The interaction between GP IIb/IIIa inhibition and diabetic status was statistically significant (p = 0.036).

40. **Boersma E,** et al. Platelet glycoprotein IIb/IIIa inhibitors in acute coronary syndromes: a meta-analysis of all major randomised clinical trials. *Lancet* 2002;359:189–198.

This meta-analysis examined the same six trials (see preceding) that randomized 31,402 ACS patients to various GP IIb/IIIa inhibitors versus placebo or control. The meta-analysis of all end points was performed by using Cochrane-Mantel-Haenszel, Breslow-Day, and Kaplan-Meier methods. The 30-day pooled incidence of death or MI showed a significant absolute reduction of 1% with GP inhibitor use [10.8% vs. 11.8% (placebo or control); OR, 0.91; $p = 0.015$). A significant benefit also was seen at 5 days (5.7% vs. 6.9%; OR, 0.84; $p = 0.0003$). The benefits were seen in all important subgroups, such as age, diabetics, and prior cardiac history. GP IIb/IIIa inhibitor use was associated with an increased risk of bleeding (OR, 1.62), but no increased rate of intracranial hemorrhage or stroke was seen. Gender difference favored treatment of men with GP IIb/IIIa inhibitors, but women benefited when controlled for baseline troponin. No benefit is apparent with GP inhibitor use when patients do not have a positive troponin test.

Direct Thrombin Inhibitors

41. **Topol EJ,** et al. Recombinant hirudin for unstable angina pectoris: a multicenter, randomized angiographic trial. *Circulation* 1994;89:1557–1566.

This randomized, open-label, multicenter, angiographic trial was composed of 163 patients with rest pain, abnormal ECG, and angiography demonstrating 60% stenosis of a major epicardial artery. Patients were randomized to one of two heparin groups (targeted aPTT of 65 to 90 or 90 to 110 seconds) or one of four hirudin groups (0.05, 0.1, 0.2, or 0.3 mg/kg/hr) in a dose-escalating protocol. Repeated angiography was performed at 72 to 120 hours. A higher proportion of hirudin-treated patients had an aPTT within a 40-second range (71% vs. 16%). Hirudin patients tended to have a lower cross-sectional area of culprit lesion (primary efficacy variable; $p = 0.08$) and significant reduction in minimal luminal diameter ($p = 0.028$).

42. **Fuchs J,** et al. Thrombolysis in MI **(TIMI-7).** Hirulog in the treatment of unstable angina: results of TIMI-7 trial. *Circulation* 1995;92:727–733.

In this prospective, randomized trial, 410 patients were randomized to aspirin (325 mg daily) plus hirulog for 72 hours at one of four dosages (0.02, 0.25, 0.5, or 1.0 mg/kg/hr). Fewer deaths and nonfatal MIs through hospital discharge were observed in the three higher-dose groups (3.2% vs. 10%; $p = 0.008$). Only two patients had a major hemorrhage.

43. **Topol EJ,** et al. Global Utilization of Strategies to Open Occluded Arteries **(GUSTO IIb):** a comparison of recombinant hirudin with heparin for the treatment of acute coronary syndromes. *N Engl J Med* 1996;335:775–782.

Design: Prospective, randomized, double-blind, multicenter study. Primary end point was death or nonfatal MI (or reinfarction) at 30 days.

Purpose: To compare the clinical effectiveness of hirudin with that of heparin in patients with all types of ACSs.

Population: 12,142 patients with chest pain in the prior 12 hours accompanied by persistent ST elevation or depression ≥ 0.5 mm ($n \geq 4,131$) or T-wave inversion ($n \geq 8,011$).

Exclusion Criteria: Included oral anticoagulation, active bleeding, history of stroke, serum creatinine more than 2.0 mg/dL, contraindication to heparin, and SBP more than 200 mm Hg or DBP more than 110 mm Hg.

Treatment: Patients were randomized to heparin or hirudin [0.1 mg/kg i.v. bolus, and then 0.1 mg/kg/hr (vs. 0.6 then 0.2 in GUSTO IIa)].

Results: At 30 days, the hirudin group had a nonsignificant 11% reduction in death and MI (8.9% vs. 9.8%; $p = 0.06$). *Post hoc* analysis showed that the hirudin group had a significant reduction in death and MI at 24 hours (1.3% vs. 2.1%; $p = 0.001$). Hirudin patients had more moderate (but not severe) bleeds (8.8% vs. 7.7%). Patients with ST elevation were younger and had fewer cardiac risk factors but a higher 30-day mortality rate (6.1% vs. 3.8%).

44. Organization to Assess Strategies for Ischemic Syndromes **(OASIS-2)** Investigators. Effects of recombinant hirudin (lepirudin) compared with heparin on death, MI, refractory angina, and revascularization procedures in patients with acute myocardial ischaemia without ST elevation: a randomised trial. *Lancet* 1999;353:429–438 (editorial, 423–424).

Design: Prospective, randomized, multicenter, double-blind, double-dummy study. Primary end point was cardiovascular death or new MI at 7 days.

Purpose: To evaluate whether hirudin is superior to heparin in reducing major cardiac events in patients with UA or suspected NSTEMI.

Population: 10,141 patients aged 21 to 85 years with UA (abnormal ECG required if younger than 60 years) or suspected acute MI without ST elevation.

Exclusion Criteria: Included PTCA within the prior 6 months, planned thrombolysis or primary PTCA, and history of stroke in the prior year.

Treatment: Heparin, 5,000-U bolus, and then 15 U/kg/hr for 72 hours, or hirudin, 0.4-mg/kg bolus, and then 0.15 mg/kg/hr for 72 hours.

Results: Hirudin group had a nonsignificant 16% RR reduction in cardiovascular death and MI at 7 days (3.6% vs. 4.2%; $p = 0.077$). The hirudin group also had a significant 18% RR reduction in cardiovascular death, MI, and refractory angina at 7 days (5.6% vs. 6.7%; $p = 0.0125$). Most of the differences between the groups were observed during the first 72 hours: cardiovascular death or MI RR, 0.76 ($p = 0.039$), and cardiovascular death, MI, and refractory angina RR, 0.78 ($p = 0.019$). The hirudin group had an excess of major bleeding (1.2% vs. 0.7%; $p = 0.01$) but no excess of life-threatening bleeds.

45. The Direct Thrombin Inhibitor Trialists' Collaborative Group. Direct thrombin inhibitors in acute coronary syndromes: principal results of a meta-analysis based on individual patients' data. *Lancet* 2002;359:294–302.

This meta-analysis included 35,970 patients from 11 randomized trials that enrolled 200 or more patients and assigned up to 7 days of treatment with a direct thrombin inhibitor or heparin and had a 30-day or longer follow-up. Compared with heparin, direct thrombin inhibitors were associated with a lower risk of death or MI at the end of treatment [4.3% vs. 5.1%; OR, 0.85 (95% CI, 0.77 to 0.94); $p = 0.001$] and at 30 days [7.4% vs. 8.2%; 0.91 (0.84 to 0.99); $p = 0.02$]. This was driven by fewer MIs [2.8% vs. 3.5%; 0.80 (0.71 to 0.90); $p < 0.001$]. Subgroup analyses revealed a benefit of direct thrombin inhibitors on death or MI in both ACS and PCI trials. A reduction in death or MI was evident with hirudin and bivalirudin but not with univalent agents (argatroban, efegatran, inogatran). Compared with heparin, an increased risk of major bleeding was found with hirudin, but a reduction, with bivalirudin.

Thrombolytics
46. **Bar FW,** et al. Unstable Angina Study Using Eminase **(UNASEM).** Thrombolysis in patients with unstable angina improves the angiographic but not clinical outcome: results of UNASEM, a multicenter, randomized, placebo-controlled, clinical trial with anistreptilase. *Circulation* 1992;86:131–137.

Prospective, randomized, double-blind, placebo-controlled, multicenter study of 159 patients aged 30 to 70 years with angina of recent onset (less than 4 weeks) or of the crescendo type with the last episode within 12 hours of admission and ischemic ST changes (ST depression, $\geq$1 mm; T-wave inversion, $\geq$2 mm). After coronary angiography, patients were randomized to anistreptlase, 30 U over 5 minutes, or placebo; repeated angiography was performed at 12 to 28 hours. All patients were given heparin and aspirin, 300 mg/day (started after second catheterization). Anistreptlase group had a significant decrease in stenosis diameter between the first and second angiograms [11% (from 70% to 59%) vs. 3% (from 66% to 63%); $p = 0.008$]. No difference was observed in clinical outcome between the groups (e.g., infarct size, MI rate), but more bleeding complications occurred with anistreptlase (32% vs. 11%; $p = 0.001$).

47. Thrombolysis in Myocardial Ischemia **(TIMI IIIA)** Investigators. Early effects of tissue-type plasminogen activator added to conventional therapy on the culprit

coronary lesion in patients presenting with ischemic cardiac pain at rest: results of the TIMI IIIA trial. *Circulation* 1993;87:38–52.

Design: Prospective, randomized, open, parallel-group, multicenter study. Primary end point was 10% reduction of stenosis and improvement of two TIMI flow grades.

Purpose: To evaluate the effects of tissue-type plasminogen activator (tPA) added to conventional therapy on the culprit coronary lesion in patients with UA or non–Q-wave MI

Population: 306 patients aged 22 to 75 years with chest pain at rest lasting 5 minutes to 6 hours and accompanied by ECG changes or documented CAD.

Exclusion Criteria: Included CABG surgery, MI in the prior 21 days, PTCA in the prior 6 months, cardiogenic shock, and oral anticoagulation requirement.

Treatment: Front-loaded tPA (maximum, 80 mg) or placebo plus conventional antianginal therapy. All patients received heparin (5,000-U bolus and infusion for 18 to 48 hours) and aspirin, 325 mg daily.

Results: The tPA group had more frequent improvement of TIMI flow by two grades or reduction of stenosis by 20% on repeated angiography at 18 to 48 hours (15% vs. 5%; $p = 0.003$). The tPA benefit was most marked in patients with thrombus-containing lesions (36% vs. 15%; $p < 0.01$) and non–Q-wave MI (33% vs. 8%; $p < 0.005$).

Comments: Only modest angiographic improvement was observed.

48. **Ambrose JA,** et al. Thrombolysis and Angioplasty in Unstable Angina **(TAUSA).** Adjunctive thrombolytic therapy during PTCA for ischemic rest angina. *Circulation* 1994;90:69–77.

Design: Prospective, randomized, double-blind, multicenter study.

Purpose: To assess the role of intracoronary urokinase during angioplasty for UA or postinfarction rest angina.

Population: 469 patients aged ≤80 years with ischemic rest pain accompanied by ST-segment or T-wave changes and an angiogram demonstrating 70% stenosis.

Exclusion Criteria: Included normal baseline ECG, blood pressure greater than 180/110, prior stroke, recent (within fewer than 10 days) major surgery, bleeding diathesis, active GI or GU bleeding.

Treatment: Intracoronary urokinase (250,000 or 500,000 U) or placebo. All patients received aspirin and heparin.

Results: No significant differences in incidence of post-PTCA thrombi were observed [13.8% (urokinase) vs. 18%; $p = $ NS], but the urokinase group had a higher acute closure rate (10.2% vs. 4.3%, $p < 0.02$; most of difference was in the in 500,000-U group) and more adverse outcomes (ischemia, MI, CABG surgery; 6.3% vs. 2.9%, $p < 0.02$).

Comments: Possible explanations of adverse effects of urokinase include increased hemorrhagic dissection, lack of intimal sealing, and procoagulant or platelet-activating effects.

49. Thrombolysis in MI **(TIMI IIIB).** Effects of tissue plasminogen activator and a comparison of early invasive and conservative strategies in unstable angina and non–Q-wave MI. *Circulation* 1994;89:1545–1556.

Design: Prospective, randomized (2 × 2 factorial design), double-blind, placebo-controlled, multicenter study. Primary end point was death, MI, or failure of treatment at 6 weeks (for tPA comparison), and death, MI, or positive ETT (for strategy comparison).

Purpose: To evaluate the use of thrombolytic therapy in UA and non–Q-wave MI and to compare an early invasive with a conservative strategy.

Population: 1,473 patients aged 21 to 76 years within 24 hours of ischemic discomfort at rest consistent with UA or non–Q-wave MI.

Exclusion Criteria: Included treatable cause of unstable angina, MI in the prior 21 days, coronary angiography in the prior 30 days, PTCA within 6 months, history of CABG, SBP higher than 180 mm Hg or DBP higher than 100 mm Hg, and contraindication to thrombolysis.

Treatment: tPA, 0.8 mg/kg over a 90-minute period (maximum, 80 mg; mean, 63 mg), including one third of dose as an i.v. bolus (up to 20 mg); or placebo. The early invasive strategy involved catheterization 18 to 48 hours after randomization, and revascularization, if feasible. Conservative strategy allowed catheterization for recurrent ischemia at rest with ECG changes or other failure of medical therapy.

Results: No difference was observed between invasive and conservative strategies in combined primary end points (16.2% vs. 18.1%), but the early invasive strategy was associated with a shorter hospital stay and lower incidence of rehospitalization. tPA was not shown to be beneficial and may be harmful (e.g., four intracranial hemorrhages vs. none with placebo; $p = 0.06$).

Comments: One-year results (see *J Am Coll Cardiol* 1995;26:1643) showed similar death and nonfatal reinfarction rates between tPA and placebo (12.4% vs. 10.6%; $p = 0.24$) and early invasive versus early conservative groups (10.8% vs. 12.2%; $p = 0.42$). The early invasive group had a higher revascularization rate (64% vs. 58%; $p < 0.001$), primarily because of more PTCAs (39% vs. 32%), but fewer readmissions (26% vs. 33%; $p < 0.001$).

Invasive versus Conservative Management (see also 48)

50. **Boden WE,** et al., for the Veteran Affairs Non–Q-Wave Infarction Strategies in Hospital **(VANQWISH)** Trial Investigators. Outcomes in patients with acute non–Q-wave MI randomly assigned to an invasive as compared with a conservative strategy. *N Engl J Med* 1998;338:1785–1792 (editorial, 1838–1839).

Design: Prospective, randomized, controlled, multicenter study. Primary end point was death or MI.

Purpose: To compare a conservative with an invasive strategy on the incidence of clinical outcomes in non–Q-wave MI.

Population: 920 patients with an evolving MI characterized by no Q waves on serial ECGs and CK-MB more than 1.5 times the ULN.

Exclusion Criteria: Persistent or recurrent ischemia at rest despite intensive medical therapy, severe heart failure despite i.v. diuretics and/or vasodilators, and serious coexisting conditions.

Treatment: Patients were assigned within 24 to 72 hours to invasive strategy (routine angiography followed by revascularization, if feasible) or conservative strategy [medical therapy, noninvasive testing (radionuclide left ventriculography and symptom-limited ETT with thallium scintigraphy, and invasive procedures only in a setting of spontaneous or inducible ischemia]. All patients received aspirin (325 mg daily) and diltiazem (180 to 300 mg/day).

Results: Only 9% were excluded secondary to high-risk ischemic complications. Only 29% of the conservative group (vs. 64% in TIMI-IIIB) underwent catheterization within 30 days. At follow-up (average, 23 months), the two groups had a similar incidence of death and MI [152 events (invasive, 32.9%) vs. 139 (conservative, 30.3%); $p = 0.35$]. The conservative group showed a nonsignificant trend toward lower mortality (HR, 0.72; 95% CI, 0.51 to 1.01). Fewer patients treated conservatively had death plus MI or death at hospital discharge (36 vs. 15 patients; $p = 0.004$; 21 vs. six; $p = 0.007$), at 1 month (48 vs. 26; $p = 0.012$; 23 vs. 9; $p = 0.021$), and at 1 year (111 vs. 85; $p = 0.05$; 58 vs. 36; $p = 0.025$). The invasive group had a higher CABG surgery mortality rate [11.6% vs. 3.4% (11 vs. three patients in the conservative group)].

51. **McCullough PA,** et al. Medicine vs. Angioplasty in Thrombolytic Exclusion **(MATE).** A prospective, randomized trial of triage angiography in acute coronary syndromes ineligible for thrombolytic therapy. *J Am Coll Cardiol* 1998;32:596–605.

Design: Prospective, randomized, controlled, multicenter study. Primary composite end point was death and recurrent ischemic events.

Purpose: To determine whether early triage with revascularization, if indicated, favorably affects clinical outcomes in patients with suspected acute MI who are ineligible for thrombolysis.

Population: 201 patients seen within 24 hours with an acute chest syndrome consistent with acute MI (high clinical suspicion with or without immediate enzymatic confirmation) and considered ineligible for thrombolysis because of lack of ECG changes (68% without ST elevation), symptoms for more than 6 hours, or increased bleeding or stroke risks.

Exclusion Criteria: Included symptoms for more than 24 hours or an absolute indication or contraindication to cardiac catheterization.

Treatment: Early triage angiography and subsequent therapies based on the angiogram versus conventional medical therapy consisting of aspirin, i.v. heparin, NTG, β-blockers, and analgesics.

Results: Acute MI was confirmed in 51% and 54% of triage angiography and conservative patients, respectively. The triage angiography group had a significant reduction in the primary end points of recurrent ischemic events and death (13% vs. 34%; RR, 45%; 95% CI, 27% to 59%; $p = 0.0002$). In the triage angiography group, 58% received revascularization, whereas in the conservative group, 60% subsequently underwent nonprotocol angiography because of recurrent ischemia, and 37% received revascularization ($p = 0.004$). The mean time to revascularization was substantially shorter in the triage angiography group (27 vs. 98 hours; $p = 0.0001$). No differences were seen in length of stay or hospital costs. At long-term follow-up (median, 21 months), no significant differences in late revascularization, recurrent MI, or all-cause mortality were observed.

Comments: This was a low-risk study group (in-hospital mortality rate only 2%) and was powered to show reduction in long-term recurrent MI and death. Troponin testing was not used in making the decision to use early angiography.

52. FRagmin and Fast Revascularization during InStability in coronary artery disease **(FRISC II)** Investigators. Invasive compared with noninvasive treatment in unstable coronary artery disease: FRISC II prospective randomized multicenter study. *Lancet* 1999;354:708–715.

Design: Prospective, randomized, partially open (strategy assignment), multicenter study. Primary end point was death or MI at 6 months.

Purpose: To compare an early invasive with a noninvasive strategy in patients with unstable coronary disease in addition to optimal background antithrombotic medication.

Population: 2,457 patients with ischemic symptoms in the previous 48 hours accompanied by ECG changes (ST depression or T-wave inversion ≥ 0.1 mV) or elevated markers (e.g., CK-MB greater than 6 mg/L; troponin T, greater than 0.10 mg/dL).

Exclusion Criteria: See reference 21.

Treatment: Early invasive or noninvasive treatment strategy (coronary angiography within 7 days performed in 96% and 10%, and revascularization in first 10 days, in 71% and 9%). Patients also received dalteparin or placebo for 3 months.

Results: The invasive group had a significantly lower incidence of death or MI at 6 months [9.4% vs. 12.1% (noninvasive group); $p = 0.031$]. A significant decrease in MI alone was noted (7.8% vs. 10.1%; $p = 0.045$), whereas the reduction in mortality was nonsignificant (1.9% vs. 2.9%; $p = 0.10$). Subgroup analysis showed that these benefits were restricted to men (RRs of death or MI at 6 months, 0.64 and 1.26 in men and women, respectively). Invasive strategy also was associated with 50% lower recurrent angina and hospital readmission rates. At 1-year follow-up, a persistent reduction in the incidence of death or MI was seen in the invasive group (10.4% vs. 14.1%; RR, 0.74; $p = 0.005$); 52% of the noninvasive group had undergone coronary angiography (see *Lancet* 2000;354:9).

53. **Cannon CP,** et al. for the Treat Angina with Aggrastat and Determine Cost of Therapy with an Invasive or Conservative Strategy **(TACTICS)-TIMI 18** Investigators. Comparison of early invasive versus early conservative strategies in patients with unstable angina and non-ST elevation myocardial infarction treated with early glycoprotein IIb/IIIa inhibition. *N Engl J Med* 2001;344:1879–1887.

Design: Prospective, randomized, multicenter study. Primary end point composite of death, nonfatal MI, and rehospitalization for an ACS at 6 months.

Purpose: To compare an early invasive strategy with an early conservative strategy in patients with UA and NSTEMI treated with early GP IIb/IIIa inhibition.

Population: 2,220 patients with UA and NSTEMI who had one of more of the following: ECG changes, elevated levels of cardiac markers, or a history of CAD (prior cardiac catheterization, revascularization, or MI).

Exclusion Criteria: Included persistent ST elevation, secondary angina, PTCA or CABG within 6 months, history of GI bleeding, platelet disorder, thrombocytopenia or hemorrhagic cerebrovascular disease, nonhemorrhagic stroke or transient ischemic attack (TIA) within 1 year, severe CHF or cardiogenic shock, serum creatinine greater than 2.5 mg/dL, treatment with abciximab within 96 hours, or current long-term treatment with ticlopidine, clopidogrel, or warfarin.

Treatment: Early invasive strategy (routine catheterization within 4 to 48 hours and revascularization as appropriate), or more conservative strategy [catheterization only if patient had objective evidence of recurrent ischemia (ECG changes, positive markers) or an abnormal stress test]. All patients were treated with aspirin, heparin, and tirofiban, 0.4 μg/kg/min for 30 minutes.

Results: At 6 months, the early invasive strategy had a significantly lower incidence of the primary end point compared with the conservative strategy (15.9% vs. 19.4%; OR, 0.78; $p = 0.025$). The early invasive group also had a lower rate of death or nonfatal MI at 6 months (7.3% vs. 9.5%; OR, 0.74; $p < 0.05$). The invasive strategy provided a significantly greater benefit in the patients with baseline ST-segment changes (p for interaction ≥ 0.006). In patients with a troponin T level greater than 0.01 ng/mL, a 39% relative reduction in the primary end point with the invasive strategy was noted, compared with the conservative strategy ($p < 0.001$), whereas patients with a troponin T level of 0.01 ng/mL or more had similar outcomes with either strategy. In a prespecified analysis that used the TIMI risk score (see *JAMA* 2000;284:835), the benefits of the invasive strategy were observed in intermediate-risk and high-risk patients (75% of the study population).

Comments: Both the TIMI IIIB and VANQWISH trials were performed before GP IIb/IIIa inhibitors and coronary stenting were commonly used. TACTICS reexamines management strategy in the current era, and the compelling data support wider use of early GP IIb/IIIa inhibition in combination with an early invasive strategy.

54. **Fox KAA**, et al., for the Randomized Intervention Trial of unstable Angina (RITA) Investigators. Interventional versus conservative treatment for patients with unstable angina or non–ST-elevation myocardial infarction: the British Foundation **RITA 3** randomised trial. *Lancet* 2002;360:743–751.

Design: Prospective, randomized, open, multicenter trial. Co-primary end points were death, MI, or refractory angina at 4 months and death or MI at 1 year. Median follow-up was 2.0 years.

Purpose: To determine whether routine early angiography with myocardial revascularization (as clinically indicated) is better than a conservative strategy in UA/NSTEMI patients.

Population: 1,810 patients with non–ST-elevation ACSs

Exclusion Criteria: Included probable evolving MI, CK or CK-MB twice the ULN before randomization, planned PCI within 72 hours, MI in the previous month, PCI in the previous year, or CABG at any time.

Treatment: Early intervention (angiography with PCI if indicated) or conservative strategy [ischemia-driven or symptom-driven angiography (performed in 48% at 1 year)]. Antithrombin agent in both groups was enoxaparin. Approximately 25% received a GP IIb/IIIa inhibitor.

Results: At 4 months, the early intervention group had a 34% lower incidence of death, MI, or refractory angina compared with the conservative strategy group (9.6% vs. 14.5%; $p = 0.001$). This benefit was driven primarily driven by a 53% reduction in refractory angina in the intervention group. Refractory angina required occurrence of ischemic pain, at rest or with minimal exertion, despite maximal medical treatment, associated with ECG changes, and prompting revascularization within 24 hours. At 1 year, the incidence of death or MI was similar in both groups (7.6% vs. 8.3%; $p = 0.58$). Using the ESC/ACC MI definition, death or MI at 1 year was reduced (12.5% vs. 17.1%, $p = 0.007$). The interventional group had a significant reduction in symptoms of angina and use of antianginal medications ($p < 0.0001$).

Miscellaneous
55. **Gurfinkel E,** et al., for the **ROXIS** Study Group. Randomised trial of roxithromycin in non–Q-wave coronary syndromes: ROXIS pilot study. *Lancet* 1997;350:404–407 (editorial, 378–379).

This prospective, randomized, double-blind, placebo-controlled, multicenter study was composed of 202 patients with rest pain lasting more than 10 minutes in the previous 48 hours and ischemic ECG changes (ST depression, transient ST elevation ≥1 mm, T-wave inversion in at least two contiguous leads). Patients received roxithromycin, 150 mg twice daily, or placebo for 30 days. The antibiotic group had fewer primary events (death, MI, recurrent angina) from 72 hours to 31 days (2% vs. 9%; adjusted $p = 0.032$). No significant difference was seen in incidence of death or MI (none vs. 2%). The accompanying editorial points out that the study failed to measure markers of inflammation, thrombogenesis, and endothelial dysfunction and did not report response based on *Chlamydia* seropositivity (48%). The ACADEMIC trial, which examined azithromycin in stable CAD patients, had similar negative results (see Chapter 1).

56. **Patel DJ,** et al. Cardioprotection by opening of the K(ATP) channel in unstable angina: Is this a clinical manifestation of myocardial preconditioning? Results of a randomized study with nicorandil: **CESAR 2** investigation (Clinical European Studies in Angina and Revascularization). *Eur Heart J* 1999;20:51–57.

This prospective, randomized, double-blind, parallel-group, placebo-controlled, multicenter study enrolled 245 UA patients [43 retrospectively excluded with an index diagnosis of MI (elevated troponin T)]. Patients received oral nicorandil, 20 mg twice daily, or a matching placebo, for a minimum of 48 hours. Continuous Holter ECG monitoring was performed for 48 hours to assess the frequency and duration of transient MI and any tachyarrhythmia. Significantly fewer nicorandil patients experienced an arrhythmia compared with those taking placebo (6.7% vs. 17.2%; $p = 0.04$). The nicorandil group also had fewer episodes of transient MI (mostly silent; 12.4% vs. 21.2%; $p = 0.12$ patients; $p = 0.0028$ episodes). No significant differences were found between groups in the rates of death or MI.

57. **Théroux P,** et al., for the GUARd During Ischemia Against Necrosis (**GUARDIAN**) Investigators. Inhibition of the sodium-hydrogen exchange with cariporide to prevent myocardial infarction in high-risk ischemic situations. *Circulation* 2000;102:3032–3038.

A total of 11,590 patients with UA or NSTEMI or undergoing high-risk percutaneous or surgical revascularization were randomized to receive placebo or cariporide (20 mg, 80 mg, or 120 mg every 8 hours). At 36 days, no significant difference was noted between the groups in death or MI (primary outcome). The 120-mg cariporide group had a nonsignificant 10% risk reduction compared with placebo ($p = 0.12$); however, among these patients undergoing bypass surgery, a significant 25% risk reduction ($p = 0.03$) was noted, driven by fewer non–Q-wave MIs. No effect was found on mortality. The incidence of Q-wave MI was 32% lower in the three cariporide groups compared with placebo (1.8% vs. 2.6%; $p = 0.03$). The incidence of non–Q-wave MI was reduced only in cariporide-treated patients undergoing surgery (3.8% vs. 7.1%; $p = 0.005$). No increases occurred in clinically serious adverse events.

58. **Schwartz GG,** et al., Myocardial Ischemia Reduction with Aggressive Cholesterol Lowering (**MIRACL**) Study Investigators. Effects of atorvastatin on early recurrent ischemic events in acute coronary syndromes: the MIRACL study: a randomized controlled trial. *JAMA* 2001;285:1711–1718.

Design: Prospective, randomized, double-blind, placebo-controlled, multicenter trial. Primary composite end point was death, nonfatal acute MI, cardiac arrest with resuscitation, or recurrent symptomatic MI with objective evidence and requiring emergency rehospitalization.

Purpose: To determine whether treatment with high-dose atorvastatin initiated 24 to 96 hours after an ACS reduces death and nonfatal ischemic events.

Population: 3,086 conservatively managed patients with UA/NSTEMI. Patients had chest pain for more than 15 minutes at rest or with minimal exertion in the previous 24 hours and a change from a previous pattern of angina, new or dynamic ST- or T-wave changes, or new wall-motion abnormality, or positive noninvasive test; troponin or CK-MB less than twice the ULN for unstable angina, or more than twice the ULN for non–Q-wave MI.

Exclusion Criteria: Included serum cholesterol more than 270, Q-wave MI in the prior 4 weeks, CABG surgery in the prior 3 months, PCI in the prior 6 months, LBBB or paced rhythm, lipid-lowering drugs other than niacin at doses greater than 500 mg daily, vitamin E unless at doses of less than 400 IU daily, liver dysfunction [alanine aminotransferase (ALT) greater than twice the ULN], insulin-dependent diabetes.

Treatment: Atorvastatin, 80 mg once daily, or matching placebo, in addition to standard therapy.

Results: The atorvastatin group had a significantly lower incidence of the composite primary end point compared with the placebo group (14.8% vs. 17.4%; RR, 0.84; $p = 0.048$). No significant differences were found between the groups in death, nonfatal MI, or cardiac arrest, although the atorvastatin group had less symptomatic recurrent ischemia with objective evidence and requiring emergency rehospitalization (6.2% vs. 8.4%; $p = 0.02$) and fewer strokes (12 vs. 24 events; $p = 0.045$). In the atorvastatin group, mean LDL cholesterol level decreased from 124 mg/dL (3.2 mM) to 72 mg/dL (1.9 mM). Abnormal liver transaminases (more than 3 times ULN) were more common in the atorvastatin group than in the placebo group (2.5% vs. 0.6%; $p < 0.001$); no cases of rhabdomyolysis were observed.

Prognosis and Assessment

Clinical or General Analyses

59. **Scirica BM,** et al., for the Thrombolysis in angocardial ischemia III Registry investigators. Prognosis in the Thrombolysis in angocardial ischemia III Registry according to the Braunwald unstable angina pectoris classification. *Am J Cardiol* 2002;90:821–826.

The Braunwald classification of unstable angina (see page 159) was prospectively validated in the TIMI III Registry. Of 3,318 patients, rates of death or MI at 1 year were lowest in those with "primary" UA, 9.7%, versus 16.7% for those with "secondary" UA and 19.7% for those with post-MI UA ($p < 0.001$). Patients with "secondary" UA had similar extent of disease at angiography as primary UAP. Patients with class I (non-rest pain) UA had lower rates of death on MI at 1 year than patients wih UAP at rest (8.2 % vs. 12.5%, $p = 0.004$). Patients with ST-segment duration and those already receiving antianginal medication had worse outcomes. Thus, the Braunwald UA classification was well correlated with prognosis; patients with secondary UA, post-MI UA, and patients with pain at rest. Who have higher risk for death or recurrent cardiac events, and thus deserve aggressive treatment.

60. **Schreiber TL,** et al. Cardiologist vs internist management of patients with unstable angina: treatment patterns and outcomes. *J Am Coll Cardiol* 1995;26:577–582 (editorial, 583–584).

This study showed that cardiologists more frequently prescribe appropriate medications and order more invasive testing compared with internists. The study population was composed of 890 consecutive UA patients (225 treated by internists, 665 by cardiologists) at community-based Michigan hospitals. Internists used less aspirin, heparin, and β-blockers (68% vs. 78%; 67% vs. 84%; 18% vs. 30%). They also ordered more exercise tests (37% vs. 22%) but fewer catheterizations and angioplasties (27% vs. 61%; 7% vs. 40%). The cardiologist-treated group showed a trend toward lower mortality (4% vs. 1.8%; $p = 0.06$), despite being higher risk patients (increased prior

MI, balloon angioplasty, and bypass surgery). The accompanying editorial points out that fewer studies by internists could be the result of less prior cardiac disease (53% vs. 80%). More studies also do not guarantee better outcome, as seen in TIMI III.

61. **Armstrong PW,** et al. Acute coronary syndromes in the GUSTO-IIb trial: prognostic insights and impact of recurrent ischemia. *Circulation* 1998;98:1860–1868.

Recurrent ischemia was approximately 50% more common in non–ST-elevation patients than in ST-elevation patients (35% vs. 23%; $p < 0.001$). This may explain why the non–ST-elevation group had a lower mortality rate at 30 days (3.8% vs. 6.1%; $p < 0.001$) but a similar rate by 1 year (8.8% vs. 9.6%). Compared with UA patients, NSTEMI patients had higher rates of reinfarction at 6 months (9.8% vs. 6.2%) and higher 6-month and 1-year mortality rates (8.8% vs. 5.0%; 11.1% vs. 7.0%).

62. **Farkouh ME,** et al. A clinical trial of a chest-pain observation unit for patients with unstable angina. *N Engl J Med* 1998;339:1882–1888.

This community-based, prospective study of 424 UA patients showed that a chest-pain observation unit located in the emergency department can be safe, effective, and result in cost savings. Patients with rest angina lasting longer than 20 minutes, new-onset angina on exertion (CCS class 3 or higher), and postinfarction angina were eligible. High-risk patients were excluded (e.g., ST-segment depression in several ECG leads). Eligible patients were randomized to routine hospital admission (monitored bed on cardiology service) or admission to the chest-pain observation unit. No significant difference was found in the rate of cardiac events between the two groups (OR for chest-pain observation unit group, 0.50; 95% CI, 0.20 to 1.24). At 6 months, chest-pain observation unit patients had used less resources ($p = 0.003$ by rank-sum test).

63. **Stone PH,** et al. Influence of race, sex and age of management of unstable angina and non–Q-wave MI (TIMI III registry). *JAMA* 1996;275:1104–1112.

This prospective analysis of 3,318 patients showed disparities in care among blacks, women, and the elderly. Compared with nonblacks, blacks were less likely to be treated with intensive antiischemic therapy and to undergo invasive procedures (RR, 0.65; $p < 0.001$). However, of those who had angiography (45% of blacks and 61% of nonblacks), blacks had less extensive and severe coronary stenoses. Blacks also had less recurrent ischemia. Women also were less likely to receive intensive antiischemic therapy and to undergo angiography (RR, 0.71; $p < 0.001$) and had less severe and extensive coronary disease; however, they had a similar risk of experiencing an adverse cardiac event by 6 weeks. Elderly patients (older than 75 years) received less-aggressive therapy and had less-frequent angiography (RR, 0.65; $p < 0.001$) and fewer revascularization procedures (RR, 0.79; $p = 0.002$) despite having more-extensive disease. At 6 weeks, the elderly had a higher incidence of adverse cardiac events (RR, 1.91; $p < 0.001$).

64. **Zaacks SM,** et al. Unstable angina and non–Q-wave MI: does the clinical diagnosis have therapeutic implications? *J Am Coll Cardiol* 1999;33:107–118.

This review of published literature asserts that the distinction between UA and non–Q-wave MI is no longer adequate to identify high-risk patients. Instead, such individuals are best identified by using patients' characteristics (e.g., age), specific ECG changes, newer biochemical markers (e.g., troponins), and angiographic findings.

65. **Alexander JH,** et al. Prior aspirin use predicts worse outcomes in patients with non-ST elevation acute coronary syndromes. *Am J Cardiol* 1999;83:1147–1151.

This analysis of 9,461 PURSUIT trial patients found that prior aspirin users had a higher rate of death or MI at 30 days and 6 months (16.1% vs. 13.0%; $p = 0.001$; 19.9% vs. 15.9%; $p = 0.001$) despite a lower incidence of an index MI (vs. unstable angina; 43.9% vs. 48.8%; $p = 0.001$). After adjustment for all significant, independent baseline predictors, prior aspirin users remained less likely to have an index MI (OR,

0.88; 95% CI, 0.79–0.97) and more likely to have MI or death at 30 days (OR, 1.16; 95% CI, 1.00 to 1.33) but not at 6 months (OR, 1.14; 95% CI, 0.98 to 1.33).

66. **Antman EM,** et al., The **TIMI Risk Score** for Unstable Angina/Non–ST Elevation MI. A method for prognostication and therapeutic decision making. *JAMA* 2000;284:835–842.

This retrospective analysis of the TIMI IIB and ESSENCE trials (see references) developed a simple risk score that has broad applicability, is easily calculated, and identifies patients with different responses to treatments for UA/NSTEMI. The test cohort was the 1957 TIMI IIB patients who received UFH, whereas the three validation cohorts were the UFH group from ESSENCE and both enoxaparin cohorts. Outcomes were TIMI risk score for developing at least one component of the primary end point (all-cause mortality, new or recurrent MI, or ischemia requiring urgent revascularization at 14 days). The seven TIMI risk score predictor variables were age older than 65 years, more than three CAD risk factors, prior coronary stenosis of more than 50%, ST-segment deviation on initial ECG, more than two anginal events in the prior 24 hours, use of aspirin in the prior 7 days, and elevated serum cardiac markers. As the TIMI risk score increased in the test cohort, event rates increased: 4.7% for a score of 0/1; 8.3% for 2; 13.2% for 3; 19.9% for 4; 26.2% for 5; and 40.9% for 6/7 ($p < 0.001$ by χ^2 for trend). The pattern of increasing event rates with increasing TIMI risk score was confirmed in all three validation groups ($p < 0.001$). The enoxaparin groups had a slower rate of increase in event rates with an increasing TIMI risk score.

Troponins

67. **Hamm CW,** et al. The prognostic value of serum troponin T in unstable angina. *N Engl J Med* 1992;327:146–150 (editorial, 192–194).

This prospective, multicenter analysis focused on 109 consecutive UA patients (84 with rest angina and 25 with accelerated or subacute angina) who had CK, CK-MB, and troponin T sampled every 8 hours for 2 days after hospital admission. Troponin T was detected (range, 0.20 to 3.64 μg/L) in 39% of the 84 patients with rest angina; only three of these patients had an elevated CK-MB (one of three with negative troponin T). Positive troponin-T patients had high event rates, with MI occurring in 30%, and in-hospital death, in 15%. In contrast, only one of 51 patients with rest angina and a negative troponin T had an MI ($p < 0.001$), and this patient died ($p = 0.03$). Troponin T was not detected in any of the 25 patients with accelerated or subacute angina.

68. **Lindahl B,** et al. Relation between troponin T and the risk of subsequent cardiac events in unstable coronary artery disease. *Circulation* 1996;93:1651–1657.

This prospective analysis of 976 FRISC patients showed that 5-month rates of cardiac death and MI correlate with troponin T. In the first quintile (maximum troponin T in first 24 hours, less than 0.06 μg/L), the incidence of death and MI was 4.3%; the second quintile (0.06 to 0.18 μg/L), 10.5%; the top three quintiles, 16.1%. In multivariate analysis, independent predictors of death and MI included troponin T (other predictors were age, hypertension, number of antianginal drugs, and rest ECG changes). A subsequent analysis (see *J Am Coll Cardiol* 1997;29:43) showed that the dalteparin group had a lower rate of death and MI only if troponin T was $\geq$0.1 μg/L (7.4% vs. 14.2%; $p < 0.01$).

69. **Antman E,** et al. Cardiac-specific troponin I levels to predict the risk of mortality in patients with acute coronary syndromes. *N Engl J Med* 1996;335:1342–1349 (editorial, 1388–1389).

This analysis focused on 1,404 TIMI IIIB patients. Troponin I was elevated ($\geq$0.4 ng/mL) in 573 patients and associated with a significantly increased 42-day mortality rate (3.7% vs. 1.0%; $p < 0.001$). Each 1-ng/mL increase in troponin I was associated with a mortality increase: $\leq$0.4, 1%; 0.4 to 0.9, 1.7%; 1 to 1.9, 3.4%; 2 to 4.9, 3.7%; 5 to 8.9, 6%; and $\geq$9, 7.5%. If no CK-MB elevation was present (948 patients), a troponin

I elevation was still associated with increased mortality: 2.5% vs. 0.8% (RR, 3.0; 95% CI, 0.97 to 9.2).

70. **Galvani M,** et al. Prognostic influence of elevated values of cardiac troponin I in patients with unstable angina. *Circulation* 1997;95:2053–2059.

This prospective cohort study was composed of 91 patients with rest chest pain within 48 hours of admission and ECG changes but normal CK in the first 16 hours. Seven patients had an elevated troponin I level on admission, compared with 15 at 8 hours. The elevated troponin group had an increased 30-day rate of death and MI (27.3% vs. 5.8%; $p = 0.02$) and an increased 1-year event rate (32% vs. 10%; $p = 0.01$).

71. **Luscher MS,** et al. Applicability of cardiac troponin T and I for early risk stratification in unstable coronary artery disease. *Circulation* 1997;96:2578–2585.

This analysis of 516 TRIM study patients with suspected unstable CAD showed that troponins independently predict cardiac death. Elevated troponin T (≥ 0.10 μg/L) was associated with increased risk of cardiac death at 30 days compared with that in patients with normal levels (3.2% vs. 0.4%; $p = 0.014$). Similarly, elevation of troponin I (more than 2.0 μg/L) was associated with increased cardiac death (3.2% vs. 0.7%; $p = 0.026$).

72. **Hamm CW,** et al. Benefit of abciximab in patients with refractory unstable angina in relation to serum troponin T levels. *N Engl J Med* 1999;340:1623–1629.

This analysis focused on 890 CAPTURE trial patients with UA who had serum samples drawn at the time of randomization to abciximab or placebo. Patients with postinfarction angina were excluded. Among placebo-treated patients, the incidence of death or nonfatal MI at 6 months was threefold higher in patients with elevated troponin-T levels (more than 0.1 ng/mL; 23.9% vs. 7.5%; $p < 0.001$), whereas no difference was found among abciximab-treated patients (9.5% vs. 9.4%). The lower incidence of death or MI in elevated troponin-T patients receiving abciximab compared with placebo (RR, 0.32; $p = 0.002$) was owing to the significant reduction in MI rate (OR, 0.23; $p < 0.001$). In patients without elevated troponin-T levels, no significant benefit was associated with abciximab treatment.

73. **Heescham C,** et al. Troponin concentrations for stratification of patients with acute coronary syndromes in relation to therapeutic efficacy of tirofiban: PRISM Study Investigators. Platelet Receptor Inhibition in Ischemic Syndrome Management. *Lancet* 1999;354:1757–1762.

A total of 629 (28.3%) patients had troponin-I concentrations higher than the diagnostic threshold of 1.0 μg/L, and 644 (29.0%) had troponin-T concentrations higher than 0.1 μg/L. At 30 days, death or MI occurred in 13.0% of troponin-I–positive patients compared with 4.9% for troponin-I–negative patients ($p < 0.0001$), and 13.7% compared with 3.5% for troponin T ($p < 0.001$). At 30 days, in troponin-I–positive patients, tirofiban lowered the risk of death [adjusted HR, 0.25 (95% CI, 0.09 to 0.68); $p = 0.004$] and MI [HR, 0.37 (0.16 to 0.84); $p = 0.01$]. By contrast, no treatment effect was seen for troponin-I–negative patients. Similar benefits were seen for troponin-T–positive patients.

74. **Morrow DA,** et al., for the TACTICS-TIMI 18 Investigators. Ability of minor elevations of troponin I and T to predict benefit from an early invasive strategy in patients with unstable angina and non-ST elevation myocardial infarction: results from a randomized trial. *JAMA* 2001;286:2405–2412

This prospective study obtained baseline troponin-level data in 1,821 ACS patients (of 2,220 total). An elevated cTnI level (0.1 ng/mL or greater; $n \geq 1,087$) was associated with a significant reduction in death, MI, or rehospitalization for ACS at 6 months with the invasive versus conservative strategy (15.3% vs. 25.0%; OR, 0.54; 95% CI, 0.40 to 0.73). Low-level cTnI elevations (0.1 to 0.4 ng/mL) also were associated with a benefit of an invasive strategy (30-day incidence of composite end point, 4.4% vs. 16.5%; OR, 0.24; 95% CI, 0.08 to 0.69). Patients with cTnI levels less than 0.1 ng/mL had no significant benefit from an early invasive strategy (16.0% vs. 12.4%;

OR, 1.4; 95% CI, 0.89 to 2.05; $p < 0.001$ for interaction). Similar results were observed with cTnT.

Inflammatory Markers

75. **Haverkate F,** et al. Production of C-reactive protein and risk of coronary events in stable and unstable angina. *Lancet* 1997;349:362–366.

This analysis focused on 2,121 outpatients with angina (1,030 unstable, 743 stable, 348 atypical); all had baseline angiography. At 2-year follow-up, patients with CRP in the fifth quintile (more than 3.6 mg/L) had a twofold higher risk of a coronary event. Thus acute-phase responses are probably not due to myocardial necrosis.

76. **Toss H,** et al. Prognostic influence of increased fibrinogen and C-reactive protein levels in unstable coronary artery disease. *Circulation* 1997;96:4204–4210.

This analysis of 965 FRISC study patients with unstable angina or non–Q-wave MI showed the independent predictive value of fibrinogen and CRP. Fibrinogen and CRP were measured at inclusion and related to outcomes at 5 months. Fibrinogen by tertiles (less than 3.38, 3.38 to 3.99, and more than 4.0 g/L) was associated with death in 1.6%, 4.6%, and 6.9% ($p = 0.005$) and death and MI in 9.3%, 14.2%, and 19.1% of patients ($p = 0.002$). CRP by tertiles (less than 2, 2 to 10, and more than 10 mg/L) was associated with death in 2.2%, 3.6%, 7.5% of patients ($p = 0.003$). In multiple logistic regression analysis, increased fibrinogen levels were independently associated with death and death and/or MI ($p = 0.013$), and CRP was independently associated with death ($p = 0.012$).

77. **Morrow DA,** et al. C-reactive protein is a potent predictor of mortality independent of and in combination with troponin T in acute coronary syndromes: a TIMI-II substudy. *J Am Coll Cardiol* 1998;31:1460–1465.

A total of 437 UA/non–Q-wave MI patients had quantitative CRP and rapid troponin-T assays performed. CRP was higher among patients who died than in survivors (7.2 vs. 1.3 mg/dL; $p = 0.0038$). Patients with CRP = 1.55 mg/dL and an early positive troponin-T assay result (≥ 10 minutes) had the highest mortality rates, followed by those with either CRP = 1.55 or early positive troponin-T assay results, whereas those with a low CRP and negative troponin-T assay results were at very low risk (9.10% vs. 4.65% vs. 0.36%; $p = 0.0003$).

B-type Natriuretic Peptide

78. **de Lemos JA,** et al. The prognostic value of B-type natriuretic peptide in patients with acute coronary syndromes. *N Engl J Med* 2001;345:1014–1021.

This substudy of 2,525 ACS patients in the OPUS-TIMI 16 trial measured B-type natriuretic peptide (BNP) in plasma samples obtained at mean of 40 ± 20 hours after the onset of symptoms. Baseline BNP level was significantly correlated with the risk of death, heart failure, and new or recurrent MI at 30 days and 10 months. The unadjusted rate of death increased in a stepwise fashion among patients in increasing quartiles of baseline BNP levels ($p < 0.001$). This mortality association was significant in the major patient subgroups [STEMI ($p = 0.02$), NSTEMI ($p < 0.001$), and unstable angina ($p < 0.001$)]. After risk-factor adjustment, the ORs for death at 10 months in the second, third, and fourth quartiles of BNP were 3.8 (95% CI, 1.1 to 13.3), 4.0 (95% CI, 1.2 to 13.7), and 5.8 (95% CI, 1.7 to 19.7).

Specific Tests: Laboratory, ECG, and Invasive

79. **Dewood MA,** et al. Coronary arteriographic findings soon after non-Q wave MI. *N Engl J Med* 1986;315:417–423.

In this angiography study, 341 non–Q-wave MI patients were divided into three groups: angiography at ≤ 24 hours, 24 to 72 hours, more than 72 hours for 7 days. Frequency of total occlusion and visible collateral vessels both increased with time [26% at ≤ 24 hours vs. 42% at ≥ 72 hours ($p < 0.05$); 27% vs. 42% ($p < 0.05$)]. The subtotal occlusion rate decreased with time.

80. **Becker RC,** et al. Relation between systemic anticoagulation as determined by activated thromboplastin and heparin measurements and in-hospital clinical events in unstable angina and non–Q-wave MI. *Am Heart J* 1996;131:421–433.

This prospective observational study of 1,473 TIMI IIIB patients showed a lower than expected optimal aPTT range. No differences were observed between treatment groups in median aPTTs for the 72- to 96-hour infusion period. Time-dependent covariate analyses failed to identify changes in aPTT or heparin levels between patients with and without in-hospital events ($p = 0.27$). No difference in events was observed between those with optimal anticoagulation (all aPTTs more than 60 seconds and heparin levels more than 0.2 U/mL) and those with values below these thresholds. This study suggests that the optimal aPTT range is 45 to 60 seconds.

81. **Langer A,** et al. Late assessment of thrombolytic efficacy (LATE) study: prognosis in patients with non–Q-wave MI. *J Am Coll Cardiol* 1996;27:1327–1332 (editorial, 1333–1334).

This *post hoc* analysis focused on 4,759 of 5,711 patients with documented MI, 1,309 with a non–Q-wave MI. Non–Q-wave MI versus Q-wave MI was associated with a lower 1-year mortality rate (13.3% vs. 17.1%; $p = 0.001$) and a similar reinfarction rate (8.6% vs. 7.9%; $p = 0.7$). Overall, no difference in rt-PA versus placebo was observed in patients with ST elevation, but rt-PA patients treated at less than 3 hours after admission had a lower 1-year mortality rate (15.8% vs. 19.6%; $p = 0.028$). Patients with greater than 2-mm ST depression demonstrated a significant benefit from thrombolysis (20.1% vs. 31.9%; $p = 0.006$). The accompanying editorial points out the need for more detailed analysis of LATE to see if any subgroup at longer than 6 hours benefits from thrombolysis. It is unclear what percentage of ST depression larger than 2 mm occurred in anterior leads, which could represent reciprocal changes from posterior MI due to an occluded left circumflex artery.

82. **Cannon CP,** et al. The electrocardiogram predicts one year outcome of patients with unstable angina and non–Q-wave MI: results of TIMI III Registry Ancillary Study. *J Am Coll Cardiol* 1997;30:133–140.

This prospective study focused on 1,416 patients, 14.3% with new ST deviation ≥ 1 mm; 21.9% had isolated T-wave inversion, and 9% had LBBB. The incidence of death and MI at 1 year was 11% in the group with ST changes [$p < 0.001$ (vs. no ST deviation)], 6.8% with T-wave inversion, and 8.2% without ECG changes. Two high-risk groups were identified: one with LBBB [22.9%; RR, 2.80 (multivariate analysis)], and the other with 0.5-mm ST changes (16.3%; RR, 2.45).

83. **Al-Khatib SM,** et al. Sustained ventricular arrhythmias among patients with acute coronary syndromes with no ST-segment elevation. *Circulation* 2002;106: 309–312.

Data analyzed from 26,416 patients in GUSTO-IIb, PURSUIT, PARAGON-A, and PARAGON-B trials. Independent predictors of in-hospital ventricular fibrillation included prior MI, prior hypertension, chronic obstructive pulmonary disease, and ST-segment changes at presentation. In-hospital VT was predicted by prior MI, COPD, and ST changes. In Cox proportional-hazards modeling, in-hospital VF and VT were independently associated with markedly higher rates of 30-day mortality (HR, 23.2; 95% CI, 18.1 to 29.8) for VF; and HR, 7.6; 95% CI, 5.5 to 10.4 for VT) and 6-month mortality (HR, 14.8; 95% CI, 12.1 to 18.3, for VF; and HR, 5.0; 95% CI, 3.8 to 6.5, for VT). After exclusion of heart failure patients, those in cardiogenic shock, and those who died within 24 hours of enrollment, these differences remained significant.

4. MYOCARDIAL INFARCTION

EPIDEMIOLOGY

In the United States, in approximately 1.1 million patients, an acute myocardial infarction (AMI) develops each year; 40% to 50% are accompanied by ST-segment elevation. Between 25% and 30% of nonfatal MIs are unrecognized by the patient and are discovered by routine electrocardiogram (ECG) or at postmortem examination. The overall associated early mortality rate ranges from 5% to 30%, depending on patient characteristics, with half of the deaths [most of them due to ventricular fibrillation (VF)] occurring before the patient receives medical attention. Among those who arrive at a hospital, approximately 25% of deaths occur in the first 48 hours. Men typically experience a first MI 10 years earlier in life than do women.

PATHOGENESIS

ST-elevation MI (STEMI) is the result of thrombotic coronary artery occlusion in more than 90% of patients. Nonatherosclerotic causes include emboli (atrial fibrillation, endocarditis), cocaine, trauma/contusion, arteritis, spasm, and dissection. Non–STEMIs are typically the result of nonocclusive thrombus over an underlying stenosis (see Chapter 3). Approximately two thirds of MIs occur in plaques with less than 50% underlying stenosis. Inflammation appears to play a role in plaque rupture (see *Circulation* 1988;78:1157). Extent of damage is related to the site and duration of occlusion and the presence or absence of adequate collateral supply.

DIAGNOSIS

Even with a strong clinical suspicion of MI based on history and physical examination, MI is subsequently confirmed in only 85% to 90% of patients. The revised World Health Organization (WHO) criteria require two of the following: ischemic chest pain, serial ECG changes, and increase and decrease in serum markers (now including cardiac troponins). MI also was redefined by a Joint European Society of Cardiology (ESC)/American College of Cardiology (ACC) Committee, which also includes troponins: "maximal concentration of troponin T or I exceeding the decision limit (99th percentile of values for a reference control group) on at least one occasion during the first 24 hours after the index clinical event" (see *J Am Coll Cardiol* 2000;36:959).

Pain

The pain of MI typically lasts for more than 30 minutes. In one study, the probability of MI (or unstable angina) was very low if (a) the pain was sharp or stabbing, (b) the pain was reproducible by palpation or was pleuritic or positional, and (c) the patient had no history of angina or MI (2).

Electrocardiography

Early ECG may show only hyperacute T waves. ST elevation 1 mm or more in two contiguous leads is highly sensitive, but also can be seen in left ventricular (LV) hypertrophy, early repolarization, and pericarditis. New left bundle branch block (LBBB) should raise strong clinical suspicion of MI. Approximately 75% of STEMIs evolve Q waves.

With right ventricular (RV) infarction, ST elevation is seen in the V_4R lead with a sensitivity of approximately 90% and specificity of approximately 80% (188). With posterior infarction, precordial ST-segment depression is seen in leads V_1 and V_2 and/or ST elevation in leads V_7 to V_9 (8,194; see also *Am J Cardiol* 1999;83:323).

Echocardiography

Echocardiography is useful if the ECG results have been nondiagnostic and in those with suspected aortic dissection. Areas of abnormal wall motion are typically observed in patients with AMI, especially those with transmural involvement.

Serum Markers

Creatine kinase (CK)-MB and troponin I (TnI) and troponin T (TnT) exceed normal ranges within 4 to 8 hours, and levels peak at 24 hours (CK-MB peak occurs sooner with successful thrombolysis). CK-MB levels normalize by 48 to 72 hours, whereas TnI remains elevated for up to 7 to 10 days, and TnT for up to 14 days, allowing detection of MI days before, but reducing their value in the diagnosis of recurrent MI within this time frame. TnI and TnT are cardiac specific, and levels strongly correlate with mortality (13). Myoglobin peak levels are reached earlier (within 1 to 4 hours), with a rapid increase indicative of successful reperfusion (15). Myoglobin also has an excellent negative predictive value (10).

TREATMENT (See Table 4.1)

Aspirin

In the second International Study of Infarct Survival (ISIS-2) (23), aspirin (162 mg chewed, to ensure rapid therapeutic blood levels) use was associated with a 23% lower mortality rate, as well as significantly fewer reinfarctions and strokes. Aspirin and thrombolytic therapy have an additive benefit (42% lower mortality rate in ISIS-2). If a patient has an aspirin allergy, clopidogrel (75 mg daily) can be substituted because it showed a slight benefit compared with aspirin in more than 8,000 patients with a recent MI (CAPRIE trial; see Chapter 1).

β-Blockers

Metoprolol, 5 mg i.v., may be given every 2 to 5 minutes for three doses along with 25 mg orally, and then, if tolerated, up to 50 mg every 6 hours (ultimately converted to twice-daily dosing). Alternatively, atenolol, 5 to 10 mg, may be administered intravenously (i.v.), and then 100 mg/day orally; or carvedilol can be started, initially 6.25 mg once daily, and titrated up to 25 mg twice daily over a 4- to 6-week period.

Contraindications to the use of β-blockers include hypotension [systolic blood pressure (SBP) less than 100 mm Hg], bradycardia [heart rate (HR) less than 60 beats/min], severe left ventricular (LV) failure, PR interval greater than 0.24 seconds, second- or third-degree heart block, severe chronic obstructive pulmonary disease (COPD), asthma, and insulin-dependent diabetes with frequent hypoglycemia. If β-blockade is still desired, the clinician should consider using esmolol (500 μg/kg/min for 1 minute, and then 50 to 200 μg/kg/min).

TABLE 4.1. TREATMENT OF ST-ELEVATION MYOCARDIAL INFARCTION

Beneficial	Limited Data or no Benefit	Special Situations	Harmful
Aspirin	Heparin	Coumadin	Nifedipine
β-Blockers	Nitrates	Vasopressors	Lidocaine
Thrombolytics	Magnesium	Diuretics	
Primary PCI	Verapamil	Insulin	
ACE inhibitors	Direct thrombin inhibitors	Intraortic balloon pump	
GP IIb/IIIa inhibitors	Amiodarone Adenosine	Surgery	

PCI, percutaneous coronary intervention; ACE, angiotensin-converting enzyme; GP, glycoprotein.

Early randomized trials showed mortality benefits with timolol, propranolol, and metoprolol (53,54,60). In the large ISIS-1 trial (56), use of atenolol (5 to 10 mg i.v., and then 100 mg/day orally) was associated with a 15% mortality benefit. In the Thrombolysis in MI (TIMI IIB) trial (57), immediate initiation of β-blockade was shown to be superior to delayed initiation (at 6 to 8 days). A meta-analysis of randomized trials (most completed before the widespread use of thrombolysis and aspirin) showed a 13% mortality reduction with early initiation of a β-blocker agent. However, even delayed therapy provides substantial benefit, as shown in the early placebo-controlled trials (53,54). β-Blockade also was associated with a decreased incidence of cardiac rupture and ventricular fibrillation (VF) (61). One analysis showed that the benefits of β-blockade are independent of thrombolytic and angiotensin-converting enzyme (ACE) inhibitor use (63).

The new agent carvedilol, which is both a β and a α antagonist, has shown significant promise in AMI patients and is now indicated for use in post-MI patients with left ventricular dysfunction. In the CAPRICORN trial (59), which enrolled 1,959 patients with an ejection fraction (EF) of 40% or less, long-term use of carvedilol was associated with a 23% relative reduction in all-cause mortality compared with placebo. These beneficial effects are additive to those provided by ACE inhibitors.

Angiotensin-converting Enzyme Inhibitors

Captopril, 6.25 to 50 mg, 3 times daily (rapidly titrated); lisinopril, 5 to 20 mg daily; and ramipril, 2.5 to 5 mg twice daily are used most commonly. Early initiation of ACE inhibition was found to decrease mortality in two large placebo-controlled trials. In GISSI-3 (142), use of lisinopril (5 to 10 mg daily) was associated with a 12% mortality reduction, whereas in ISIS-4 (144), use of captopril (initially 6.25 mg, titrated to maximum 50 mg) was associated with a 7% mortality reduction (greatest benefit in those with anterior MI). Among patients with LV dysfunction, mortality was reduced by approximately 20% to 30% by oral ACE inhibition [Survival and Ventricular Enlargement (SAVE), Acute Infarction Ramipril Efficacy (AIRE), and Trandolapril Cardiac Evaluation (TRACE) trials (139,141,146)]. Intravenous administration was used in the Cooperative New Scandinavian Enalapril Survival Study (CONSENSUS II) and was deemed harmful (140). A meta-analysis of 15 trials with more than 100,000 patients showed a 7% relative risk reduction (RRR), with the majority of benefit seen in anterior MIs (1.2% absolute mortality benefit vs. 0.1% for inferior MIs) (138). Approximately one third of the benefit of ACE inhibition is seen in the first few days after MI. Based on these data, current class I indications are as follows: (a) within 24 hours with anterior ST elevation or evidence of congestive heart failure (CHF); and (b) LVEF less than 40% or evidence of CHF during or after recovery.

Results from trials of angiotensin II–receptor blockers (ARBs) confirm that ACE inhibitors should remain first-line therapy in high-risk AMI patients. For example, in the OPTIMAAL study (148), losartan was compared with captopril in 5,477 MI patients within 10 days of presentation, and a nonsignificant trend toward an increased incidence of mortality was found with losartan (18.2% vs. 16.4%; $p = 0.069$). In patients who cannot tolerate ACE inhibitors, ARBs appear beneficial. The large ongoing VALIANT study is examining higher doses of ARBs and combination ARB-ACE inhibitor therapy in post-MI patients.

Thrombolytic Therapy

Thrombolytic therapy confers a 20% to 25% mortality benefit. Time to treatment is important: a 6.5% absolute mortality benefit if given in the first hour versus 2% to 3% if given after 1 to 6 hours (66) (**Fig. 4.1**). No benefit results if thrombolytic therapy is given after 12 hours (90). The largest absolute benefit is seen in those with LBBB and anterior MI (**Fig. 4.2**).

Indications for Thrombolysis

Thrombolysis should be considered if ST elevation is 1 mm or more in contiguous precordial leads in anatomically related limb leads, or if new LBBB is present. Thrombolysis is underused, given to only 65% to 70% of eligible patients (68).

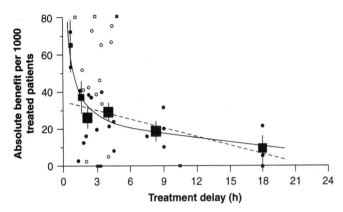

FIG. 4.1. Absolute 35-day mortality reduction versus treatment delay. ●, Information from trials included in Fibrinolytic Therapy Trialists (FTT) analysis, which found a linear relation between treatment delay and absolute mortality benefit (*dotted line*). ○, Information from additional trials. □, Data beyond scale of x/y cross. ■, Average effects in six time-to-treatment groups. (Areas of squares are inversely proportional to variance of absolute benefit described.) Analysis by Boersma et al., of randomized trials with 100 or more patients (50,246 patients) yielded a nonlinear regression curve (*solid line*), suggesting greatest benefit with time saved early after symptom onset. (Adapted from Boersma E, et al. Early thrombolytic therapy in acute MI: reappraisal of the golden hour. *Lancet* 1996;348:771–775, with permission.)

Contraindications

Contraindications include substantial gastrointestinal (GI) bleeding, aortic dissection (known or suspected), prolonged cardiopulmonary resuscitation (CPR), intracranial neoplasm/aneurysm/arteriovenous malformation, trauma or surgery in the prior 2 weeks, pregnancy, prior hemorrhagic stroke, or any stroke within the prior year.

Relative contraindications include nonhemorrhagic stroke more than 1 year earlier, active peptic ulcer disease, coumadin use, bleeding diathesis, prolonged CPR, SBP 180 mm Hg or higher, or diastolic BP, 110 mm Hg or higher.

Advanced age is not a contraindication (class IIa if older than 75 years). These patients have increased complications (especially intracranial hemorrhage) but a substantial absolute mortality reduction.

Prehospital administration has been shown to confer a benefit in several trials (88,89). A systematic overview showed a significant 17% mortality reduction. The magnitude of benefit correlates with time saved; in the ER-TIMI 19 trial, the median time saved was 32 minutes (93).

Common Agents (See Table 4.2)

Streptokinase
Intravenous streptokinase (SK) regimens proved superior to placebo in the trial of the Gruppo Italiano per lo Studio della Sopravvivenza nell' Infarto Miocardico (GISSI-1; 18% lower mortality) (83) and ISIS-2 (25% lower mortality) (84). SK was comparable with tissue plasminogen activator (tPA) in GISSI-2 and ISIS-3 (70,71), but was inferior to it in the Global Utilization of Strategies to Open Occluded Arteries (GUSTO-I) study (72; see tPA section later).

Tissue Plasminogen Activator
A clear mortality benefit with tPA compared with placebo was shown in the Anglo-Scandinavian Study of Early Thrombolysis (ASSET) (86). When compared with SK in the large GISSI-2 and ISIS-3 trials, mortality rates were similar. However, the

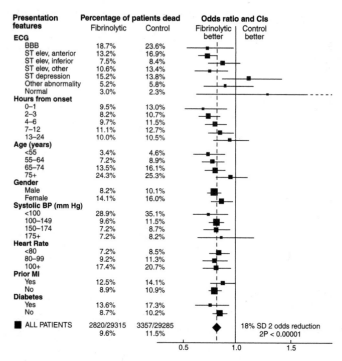

FIG. 4.2. Mortality differences during days 0 to 35 subdivided by presentation features in a collaborative overview of nine thrombolytic trials. Absolute mortality rates are shown for the fibrinolytic and control groups in the center portion of the figure for each of the clinical features at presentation listed on the left side of the figure. The ratio of the odds of death in the fibrinolytic group to that in the control group is shown for each subdivision (■), along with its 99% confidence interval (*horizontal line*). The summary odds ratio at the bottom of the figure corresponds to an 18% proportional reduction in 35-day mortality and is highly statistically significant. The absolute reduction is nine deaths per 1,000 patients treated with thrombolytic agents. (Adapted from Fibrinolytic Therapy Trialists (FTT) Collaborative Group. Indications for fibrinolytic therapy in suspected acute MI: collaborative overview of early mortality and major morbidity results from all randomised trials of >1000 patients. *Lancet* 1994;343:311–322, with permission.)

front-loaded tPA regimen was not used, and tPA was given without heparin or with subcutaneous (s.c.) heparin. The now widely used front-loaded regimen (15-mg bolus, and then 50 mg over a 30-minute period, and 35 mg over the final 60 minutes) was shown to achieve earlier patency with better TIMI grade 3 flow at 60 and 90 minutes (96). This also was demonstrated in TIMI-4 (74) and the GUSTO Angiography substudy (73).

In the GUSTO-I trial (72), the tPA and intravenous heparin group had the best outcome: 6.3% 30-day mortality versus 7.2% and 7.4% in the SK groups ($p < 0.001$). The greatest benefit was seen in those patients with large anterior MIs.

In the Continuous Infusion versus Double-Bolus Administration of Alteplase (COBALT) study (92), a double-bolus regimen [50 mg × 2 (30 minutes apart)] yielded clinically worse outcomes compared with a front-loaded tPA regimen (mortality, +0.44%; intracranial hemorrhage, +0.3%). Statistically, outcomes also were not equivalent to those with front-loaded tPA.

TABLE 4.2. CHARACTERISTICS OF COMMONLY USED FIBRINOLYTIC AGENTS

Agent	Dosage	90-Minute TIMI Grade 3 Flow	Heparin	Allergy	Cost
SK	1.5 million U over 60 min	30%–35%	No	Yes	Low
tPA	15-mg bolus, 0.75 mg/kg over 30 min, then 0.5 mg/kg over 60 min (max, 100 mg)	54%–60%	Yes	No	High
TNK	Bolus over 5–10 min (30 mg if <60 kg, 35 mg if 60–69 kg, 40 mg if 70–79 kg, 45 mg if 80–89 kg, 50 mg if ≥90 kg)	~60%	Yes	No	High
rPA	10 U + 10 U given 30 min apart	~60%	Yes	No	High

TIMI, Thrombolysis In Myocardial Infarction; tPA, tissue plasminogen activator; TNK, tenecteplase; rPA, reteplase. (From refs. 70, 71, 74.)
From Gruppo Italiano per lo Studio della Streptochinasi nell' Infanto Miocardico (GISSI–2). GISSI–2: a factorial randomised trial of alteplase vs. streptokinase and heparin vs. no heparin among 12,490 patients with acute MI. *Lancet* 1990;336:65–71, IS1S–3 Collaborative Group. A randomised comparison of streptokinase versus tissue plasminogen activator versus anistreplase and of heparin versus aspirin alone among 41,299 cases of suspected acute MI. *Lancet* 1992;339:753–770, and Cannon CP et al., TIMI-4. Comparison of front-loaded recombinant tissue plasminogen activator, anistreplase, and combination thrombolytic therapy for acute MI. *J Am Coll Cardiol* 1994;24: 1602–1610, with permission.

Reteplase
A double-bolus regimen of reteplase (rPA) was approved for use by the U.S. Food and Drug Administration (FDA) based on demonstrated equivalence to SK in the International Joint Efficacy Comparison of Thrombolytics (INJECT) trial (76). In the RAPID II angiographic trial (77), rPA showed better TIMI grade 3 flow at 90 minutes compared with front-loaded tPA (60% vs. 45%; $p = 0.01$); however, mortality was similar to that with tPA in the large GUSTO-III study (78).

Tenecteplase
Tenecteplase (TNK) is another single-bolus thrombolytic that achieves TIMI grade 3 flow similar to or slightly higher than that of tPA alone (see *Circulation* 1997;95:351). The Assessment of the Safety and Efficacy of a New Thrombolytic: TNK (ASSENT II) trial enrolled 16,949 patients and showed TNK to be equivalent to tPA alone (30-day mortality rates, 6.17% and 6.15%) (80). A potential benefit of bolus administration is ease of administration. [In GUSTO-I, incorrect dosing of tPA was associated with higher mortality (7.7% vs. 5.5% for correct dosing; $p < 0.0001$).] Intracranial hemorrhage rates were similar, whereas noncerebral bleeding occurred less frequently with TNK (26.4% vs. 29.0%).

Reduced-dose Thrombolysis in Conjunction with Glycoprotein IIb/IIIa Inhibitors
See later section, Intravenous Glycoprotein IIb/IIIa Inhibitors.

Prognostic Indicators
1. Early infarct-related artery (IRA) patency. Ninety-minute patency (TIMI grade 2 or 3 flow) correlates strongly with outcome: greater than twofold higher 1-year mortality rate in those with persistent occlusion at 90 minutes in TIMI 1 and similar

findings in subsequent studies (227). Subsequent analyses showed TIMI grade 3 flow to be associated with significantly better outcomes than TIMI grade 2 flow (227,228,231). The corrected TIMI frame count, which treats flow as a continuous variable, appears to provide an even more accurate prognostic assessment (233).

2. Microvascular reperfusion. The TIMI myocardial perfusion (TMP) grade classification is as follows: TMP grade 1 indicates presence of myocardial blush but no clearance from the microvasculature (blush or a stain was present on the next injection); TMP grade 2 blush clears slowly (blush is strongly persistent and diminishes minimally or not at all during three cardiac cycles of the washout phase); and TMP grade 3 indicates that blush begins to clear during washout (blush is minimally persistent after three cardiac cycles of washout). Analyses of angiographic cinefilms from the TIMI 10B (thrombolysis) (234) and ESPRIT trials (PCI trial, see Chapter 2) demonstrate that a TMP grade 0/1 is associated with frequent adverse outcomes even in patients with optimal epicardial flow (TIMI grade 3), whereas the lowest mortality is seen in patients with both TMP grade 3 and TIMI 3 flow. In a multivariate model, TIMI flow, TMP grade (TMPG), and TIMI frame count were all predictors of mortality (235).

3. Time to treatment. Lower mortality is achieved with early administration of thrombolytic agents, especially within the first "golden" hour (57).

4. Reocclusion. A 4% to 10% incidence is observed at 2 to 4 weeks. Although approximately 50% of cases are not accompanied by clinical reinfarction or ischemia (i.e., silent), reocclusion is associated with a more than twofold higher mortality rate (269). Revascularization appears to be helpful (see *N Engl J Med* 1992;327: 1825).

5. Reinfarction is associated with a two- to threefold higher mortality rate.

Percutaneous Coronary Intervention

Primary Angioplasty

The 1999 American Heart Association (AHA)/ACC class I indications for primary percutaneous transluminal coronary angioplasty (PTCA) are as follows: (a) within 12 hours or after 12 hours if ischemic symptoms persist, and when performed in a timely fashion by an experienced operator (more than 75 PTCA cases/year) and supported by experienced personnel in an appropriate laboratory environment (more than 200 procedures/year and cardiac surgical capability); (b) within 36 hours if shock, younger than 75 years, and in whom PTCA can be done within 18 hours of onset of shock (see cardiogenic shock section later). The 1999 ACC/AHA PCI Guidelines have a class IIb recommendation for primary PCI without surgical backup.

Procedural Volume Studies

Substantial data on operator and hospital volume have now been accumulated. An analysis of New York State data found that primary PTCA performed by a high-volume operator (11 or more cases/year) was associated with a 57% lower in-hospital mortality compared with those treated by low-volume operators (one to ten cases/year) (99). Primary PTCA performed in high-volume hospitals (57 or more cases/year) was associated with a 44% lower in-hospital mortality reduction compared with that in low-volume hospitals. As for hospital volume, one large analysis of 62,299 patients found that primary PCI was superior to thrombolytic therapy for treatment of acute STEMI at hospitals with intermediate (17 to 48 procedures/year) and high volume (more than 49/year), whereas no significant mortality difference was found between the treatments at low-volume hospitals (98). Another analysis of 98,898 Medicare patients found that those admitted to hospitals in the lowest quartile of volume of invasive procedures had a 17% higher in-hospital mortality rate compared with patients at highest-volume-quartile hospitals [hazard ratio (HR), 1.17; 95% confidence interval (CI), 1.09 to 1.26; $p < 0.001$] (97).

Primary Angioplasty versus Thrombolysis

A meta-analysis of ten trials through 1997 showed a significant mortality benefit of primary angioplasty compared with thrombolysis: odds ratio (OR), 0.66 (95% CI, 0.46

to 0.94) (100). An updated meta-analysis of 23 studies published in 2003 confirmed primary PCI had lower short-term mortality than thrombolytic therapy (7% vs. 9%) (101).

PTCA had a lower associated mortality rate in the Primary Angioplasty in MI (PAMI) trial (2.6% vs. 6.5%) (98), and a nonsignificant trend toward lower mortality were observed in the larger GUSTO-IIb trial (104). However, no mortality difference was found in a subsequent study of 19 Seattle hospitals (103).

More recent studies compared primary PCI with thrombolysis, including two that included facilities without PCI capability (i.e., transfer required for the PCI group). In the second Danish Trial in Acute MI (DANAMI-2), primary PCI was associated with a 45% lower incidence of death, reinfarction, or disabling stroke, primarily because of less reinfarction [1.6% vs. 6.3% (tPA)] (108). In PRAGUE-2, primary PCI was associated with a nonsignificant mortality reduction compared with SK (6.8% vs. 10%); however, a significant mortality reduction was seen in those seen at 3 to 12 hours (6% vs. 15.3%) (109). The rapid transfer and door-to-balloon times in these two trials are likely not typical of the usual community setting. In the Air PAMI study, all enrolled patients arrived in hospitals without on-site PTCA; despite long transfer delays, the emergency transfer for the primary PCI group had a nonsignificant 38% reduction in major events compared with on-site thrombolysis (106). Finally, in the Atlantic Cardiovascular Patient Outcomes Research team (C-PORT) study, sites without a *de novo* primary PCI program had one developed (without on-site surgery). The primary PCI group had significantly lower incidence of death, recurrent MI, or disabling stroke compared with those given tPA (107).

In summary, primary PCI is superior to thrombolysis when performed at experienced centers that can achieve a short door-to-balloon time.

Rescue Angioplasty
Rescue angioplasty (i.e., after failed thrombolytic therapy) reduces postinfarct angina, and pooled data from small randomized trials showed a trend toward lower mortality (OR, 0.38; 95% CI, 0.13 to 1.06) (see *Circulation* 1999;91:476). Failed rescue angioplasty is associated with high mortality (approximately 30% in GUSTO-I analysis) (127).

Routine Immediate Percutaneous Transluminal Coronary Angioplasty (after Thrombolysis) versus Delayed or Conservative Management
Most trials performed in the mid 1980's showed immediate PTCA to be associated with increased bleeding and an overall trend toward increased mortality [Thrombolysis and Angioplasty in MI (TAMI), TIMI-2A, and European Cooperative Study Group (ECSG-4)] (114,115). Based on these data, the 1999 ACC/AHA Guidelines considered as class III the use of PTCA in those who receive thrombolysis and are symptom free. However, observational data from recent trials reveal a potential benefit of early PCI (122; see also *Am Heart J* 2001;141:592), suggesting that randomized trials of an early invasive strategy after thrombolysis in the current management era are warranted (also see "Facilitated" PCI later).

Routine Delayed Percutaneous Transluminal Coronary Angioplasty (after Thrombolysis) versus Conservative Management
Similar mortality and reinfarction rates and EFs were reported in older studies [TIMI IIB and the Should We Intervene Following Thrombolysis (SWIFT) study] (57,117). In TIMI IIB, the subgroup with a prior MI had a lower 6-week mortality rate. The recent GRACIA trial compared routine angiography within 24 hours of thrombolysis with an ischemia-guided approach (121). Preliminary results showed that the routine invasive group had a significantly lower incidence of death, reinfarction, or revascularization (0.8% vs. 3.7%; $p = 0.003$). This trial suggests that routine coronary angiography and revascularization after thrombolytic therapy now is safe and associated with fewer major events at 30 days. These findings require validation in larger studies.

"Facilitated" Percutaneous Coronary Intervention
Recent trial data indicate that "facilitated" PCI (thrombolysis followed by immediate angiography and PCI *only* if indicated) may be safe and indicated in certain

situations. The Plasminogen activator Angioplasty Compatibility Trial (PACT) evaluated precatheterization thrombolysis (tPA, 50-mg bolus) or placebo followed by immediate angiography; if TIMI grade 3 flow was present, a second bolus of tPA, 50 mg, was administered, whereas PCI was performed if TIMI grade 0 to 2 flow was present (119). As expected, the tPA group had much higher initial TIMI grade 3 flow (32.8% vs. 14.8%). After angioplasty, TIMI flow grade was similar between the two groups, indicating that tPA administration did not adversely affect procedural outcomes. No significant differences were noted in bleeding rates, suggesting that immediate angioplasty could be performed safely after reduced-dose tPA. Further studies of this and other pharmacologic regimens (e.g. 6 p IIb/IIIa inhibitors) are needed.

Cardiogenic Shock
The Should We Emergently Revascularize Occluded Coronaries for Cardiogenic Shock (SHOCK) trial found that emergency revascularization (ERV; balloon angioplasty or bypass surgery) did not result in improved 30-day survival (primary end point) compared with aggressive medical management [e.g., thrombolysis, intraaortic balloon pump (IABP)] (129). However, at 6 months, mortality was lower with ERV (50.3% vs. 63.1%; $p = 0.027$). Among patients younger than 75 years, ERV was significantly better than medical therapy (30-day mortality, 41% vs. 57%; $p < 0.01$; 6 months, 48% vs. 69%; $p < 0.01$). Based on these results, the 1999 ACC/AHA Guidelines consider primary PTCA a class I indication in those within 36 hours of symptom onset in whom cardiogenic shock develops, are younger than 75 years, and in whom revascularization can be performed within 18 hours of onset of shock.

Stenting
Before the identification of an effective antiplatelet regimen to prevent stent thrombosis, stent use was typically avoided in the patient with AMI. However, several studies then showed that stenting in the AMI was safe and efficacious (130,131). The STAT and STOPAMI-2 trials demonstrated superior outcomes with stenting compared with fibrinolytic therapy (133,134). The larger Stent PAMI study compared primary PTCA alone with heparin-coated Palmaz-Schatz stenting in 900 patients (132). At 6 months, stenting was associated with a significant reduction in the 6-month composite primary end point (12.6% vs. 20.1%; $p < 0.01$), primarily because of a lower rate of ischemia-driven target vessel revascularization (TVR; 7.7% vs. 17%; $p < 0.001$). The Controlled Abciximab and Device Investigation to Lower Late Angioplasty Complications (CADILLAC) trial enrolled 2,082 patients and compared PTCA alone, PTCA plus abciximab, stenting alone, and stenting plus abciximab in 2,082 patients (47). At 6 months, the stent groups had a lower incidence of death, reinfarction, disabling stroke, and ischemia-driven TVR [11.5% (stent alone) and 10.2% vs. 20% (PTCA alone) and 16.5% (PTCA plus abciximab)]. As in Stent PAMI, the benefit was owing to a lower TVR-rate benefit, whereas no difference in mortality rates was found. These lower TVR rates are the result of the lower restenosis rates seen with PTCA compared with angioplasty alone.

In summary, these data demonstrate that in experienced centers, stent implantation (with or without an i.v. glycoprotein IIb/IIIa inhibitor) should be considered the preferred reperfusion strategy.

Antithrombotic/Antiplatelet Agents

Heparin
Intravenous heparin should be used in conjunction with tPA, or rPA or TNK (GUSTO data show the optimal partial thromboplastin time (PTT) range to be 50 to 70 seconds; see *Circulation* 1996;93:870). Heparin is optimal if the patient is not also receiving a thrombolytic agent. A meta-analysis of prethrombolytic trials showed an approximately 20% mortality benefit (21). Another meta-analysis of trials comprising approximately 70,000 patients showed borderline benefit when used with thrombolytics (6% lower mortality; $p = 0.03$) (22). Subcutaneous administration showed no benefit in reducing death or reinfarction (ISIS-3 and GISSI-2) (70,71).

Low-Molecular-Weight Heparins

Low-molecular-weight heparins have now been evaluated in several studies and appear safe and efficacious in the acute STEMI setting. In the Assessment of the Safety and Efficacy of a New Thrombolytic Regimen (ASSENT)-3 trial, those treated with enoxaparin and TNK had significantly fewer major events compared with the unfractionated heparin (UFH) and TNK group (11.4% vs. 15.4%; $p < 0.001$); bleeding events were similar in both groups. In the smaller ENTIRE-TIMI 23 trial, TIMI grade 3 flow rates were similar between enoxaparin- and UFH–treated patients (28). However, among patients receiving full-dose TNK, the enoxaparin group had a lower incidence of death or recurrent MI at 30 days (4.4% vs. 15.9%; $p = 0.005$). Another angiographic study, the second Heparin and Aspirin Reperfusion Therapy (HART II) trial, randomized 400 tPA-treated patients to enoxaparin or UFH (27). The enoxaparin group had a nonsignificantly higher TIMI grade 3 flow rate (52.9% vs. 47.6%; $p =$ NS) as well as a lower reocclusion rate at 5 to 7 days. Finally, in the AMI-SK study, patients treated with SK were randomized to enoxaparin or placebo for 3 to 8 days, and the enoxaparin group had significantly better ST-segment resolution and angiographic patency, as well as fewer major clinical events, indicating less reocclusion (see *Eur Heart J* 2002;16:1282). The large EXTRACT TIMI-25 trial is comparing enoxaparin and UFH with all lytic agents.

Direct Thrombin Inhibitors

Trials using hirudin showed no significant advantage [TIMI-5, TIMI-9B (30), GUSTO-IIb (104)]. In the Hirulog Early Perfusion/Occlusion (HERO) trial (31), hirulog showed better TIMI grade 3 flow compared with SK. In the larger HERO-2 trial (17,073 patients), bivalirudin was compared with UFH in patients receiving SK (32). No mortality difference occurred between the two groups. The bivalirudin group had a 30% reduction in the reinfarction rate, but it also was associated with an increased bleeding rates.

Warfarin

In the Aspirin/Anticoagulants Following Thrombolysis with Eminase in Recurrent Infarction (AFTER) trial, patients treated with warfarin had similar cardiac outcomes compared with aspirin-treated patients, but warfarin was associated with an increased incidence of bleeding (37). In the Warfarin Reinfarction Study (WARIS), a 24% lower mortality rate versus placebo was observed (15.5% vs. 20.3%; $p = 0.03$) (35). Based on these data, it was recommended that warfarin could be used in aspirin-intolerant patients. It also should be considered in those at high risk of LV thrombus formation (large anterior MI, EF less than 20%), or with atrial fibrillation. In one analysis of 11 studies, anticoagulation was associated with 68% lower rate of embolization (276).

Several recent studies examined warfarin plus aspirin with various intensities of anticoagulation. In the large Combination Hemotherapy and Mortality Prevention (CHAMP) study, lower-intensity anticoagulation [international normalized ratio (INR), 1.5 to 2.5] plus aspirin had outcomes similar to those with aspirin alone, whereas major bleeding occurred more frequently with combination therapy (39). In the Antithrombotics in the Prevention of Reocclusion in Coronary Thrombolysis (APRICOT)-2 trial, aspirin plus moderate-intensity warfarin (goal INR, 2.0 to 3.0) was associated with less reocclusion compared with aspirin alone (15% vs. 28%; $p = 0.02$), as well as a lower incidence of death, reinfarction, or revascularization (14% vs. 34%; $p < 0.01$) (42). No increased incidence of bleeding events was observed. In the Antithrombotics in the Secondary Prevention of Events in Coronary Thrombosis-2 (ASPECT-2) study, high-dose oral anticoagulation alone (target INR, 3.0 to 4.0) and the combination of aspirin and moderate-dose anticoagulation (target INR, 2.0 to 3.0), resulted in a lower incidence of death, MI, or stroke compared with low-dose aspirin (80 mg once daily) (40). Bleeding rates were similar in all groups. The Warfarin-Aspirin Reinfarction Study-2 (WARIS-2) examined high-intensity anticoagulation (INR, 2.8 to 4.2) as well as moderate-dose anticoagulation (INR, 2.0 to 2.5) plus low-dose aspirin and low-dose aspirin alone (75 mg/day) (41). Both warfarin groups had a lower incidence of death, nonfatal MI, and stroke compared with aspirin alone. The warfarin plus aspirin group also had a significantly lower mortality than did aspirin alone ($p = 0.003$). However, the warfarin groups had more major bleeding, but these rates were relatively low (0.58/100 patient years and 0.52/100 patient years vs. 0.15/100 patient years for aspirin).

In summary, these data suggest that with careful monitoring of INR, the combination of warfarin (INR, 2.0 to 3.0) plus low-dose aspirin or warfarin alone (INR, 3.0 to 4.5), reduces major events compared with aspirin alone. However, given the slight increased bleeding risk and frequent monitoring required, the routine use of long-term warfarin will not likely supplant the current antiplatelet therapy regimen. These studies did not evaluate long-term warfarin regimens compared with dual antiplatelet therapy (e.g., aspirin and clopidogrel).

Intravenous Glycoprotein IIb/IIIa Inhibitors
Abciximab
Abciximab alone (i.e., with heparin but no thrombolytic) achieved TIMI grade 3 flow at 90 minutes in 32% in TIMI-14 (48). Abciximab in conjunction with PCIs has been shown to reduce subsequent ischemic events. The Reopro and Primary PTCA Organization and Randomized Trial (RAPPORT) showed that abciximab use in conjunction with primary PTCA resulted in a significant reduction in death, MI, and urgent revascularization at 30 days (105). [See also EPIC and GUSTO-III subgroup analyses (*J Am Coll Cardiol* 1998;31:191A).] The Abciximab before Direct Angiography and Stenting in MI Regarding Acute and Long-term Follow-up (ADMIRAL) trial showed that abciximab use in conjunction with stenting resulted in a nearly 50% reduction in the incidence of death, MI, and urgent revascularization (46). The larger Controlled Abciximab and Device Investigation to Lower Late Angioplasty Complications (CADILLAC) trial compared PTCA alone, PTCA plus abciximab, stenting alone, or stenting plus abciximab (47). At 6 months, death, reinfarction, disabling stroke, and ischemia-driven TVR occurred in 20.0% of the PTCA-alone group, 16.5% with PTCA plus abciximab, 11.5% with stenting, and 10.2% with stenting plus abciximab ($p < 0.001$). The differences in the incidence of this composite end point were primarily owing to varying TVR rates (15.7% with PTCA alone, 13.8% with PTCA + abciximab, 8.3% with stenting, and only 5.2% with stenting + abciximab; $p < 0.001$).

Glycoprotein IIb/IIIa Inhibition Plus Reduced-dose Thrombolysis
Reduced-dose thrombolysis in conjunction with i.v. glycoprotein IIb/IIIa administration is being intensely evaluated.

Eptifibatide (Integrilin)
In IMPACT-AMI (43), the highest dose of integrelin (180 μg/kg i.v. bolus and then 0.75 μg/kg/min) with full-dose tPA was associated with better TIMI grade 3 flow at 90 minutes compared with full-dose tPA alone; no significant difference was seen between the groups in major in-hospital events. The INTEGRETI trial (52) used optimal eptifibatide dosing [two 180-μg/kg boluses (10 minutes apart); infusion rate, 2.0 μg/kg/min] and found that eptifibatide plus full-dose TNK, compared with TNK alone, tended to achieve better TIMI 3 flow (59% vs. 49%; $p = 0.15$), arterial patency (85% vs. 77%; $p = 0.17$), and ST-segment resolution (71% vs. 61%; $p = 0.08$). Combination therapy was associated with increased rates of noncerebral bleeding. This regimen is being examined further in larger, ongoing phase III studies.

Abciximab
TIMI-14 found that a combination of abciximab and tPA (15-mg bolus and then 35 mg over a 60-minute period) resulted in better TIMI grade 3 flow at 60 and 90 minutes compared with tPA alone (72% vs. 43%; $p = 0.0009$; 77% vs. 62%, $p = 0.02$) (48). The Strategies for Patency Enhancement in the Emergency Department (SPEED) trial evaluated a regimen of abciximab plus reteplase (49). TIMI grade 3 flow rates were 54% with abciximab and reteplase, 5 U + 5 U, compared with 47% reteplase only (10 U + 10 U; $p = 0.32$). The INTRO-AMI trial evaluated a regimen of eptifibatide and tPA; the highest TIMI grade flow rates were seen with eptifibatide, 180/90-μg/kg

boluses (30 minutes apart) and 1.33-μg/kg/min infusion plus 50 mg tPA (51). None of these three studies was powered to detect differences in major events.

The Assessment of the Safety and Efficacy of a New Thrombolytic Regimen (ASSENT)-3 trial evaluated abciximab and TNK as well as comparing UFH and enoxaparin (82). The half-dose TNK and abciximab group had a lower incidence of death, in-hospital MI, or in-hospital refractory ischemia compared with full-dose TNK and UFH (11.1% vs. 15.4%) and similar to TNK and enoxaparin (11.4%). Of concern, the abciximab group had nearly twice the risk of major hemorrhage compared with the UFH group (4.3% vs. 2.2%; $p = 0.0002$; enoxaparin group, 3.0%; $p = $ NS vs. UFH).

The 16,558-patient GUSTO-V trial (50) compared standard-dose reteplase (two 10-U boluses, 30 minutes apart) with half-dose reteplase (two 5-U boluses) and full-dose abciximab. No significant differences were seen between the two groups in 30-day mortality. The combination therapy group had significantly lower rates of death and reinfarction (7.4% vs. 8.8%; $p = 0.0011$) and reinfarction (at 7 days, 2.3% vs. 3.5%) but was associated with higher rate of non–intracranial bleeding complications.

Additional studies are required to determine whether these combinations are beneficial compared with primary "facilitated" PCI.

Nitrates

Nitrates are indicated for relief of persistent pain and treatment of heart failure or hypertension [sublingual nitroglycerin (NTG), 0.4 mg every 5 minutes for three doses, or i.v. NTG, 10 to 200 μg/min]. A meta-analysis of data on approximately 2,000 patients treated in the prereperfusion era demonstrated a 35% mortality reduction with nitrate use. However, in the large GISSI-3, ISIS-4, and CCS-1 trials (142,144,145), routine use of i.v. and oral nitrates after MI conferred no mortality benefit.

Nitrates should not be used in patients with inferior MI complicated by RV involvement (reduces preload).

Calcium-Channel Blockers

Nifedipine has been associated with increased mortality [Trial of Early Nifedipine in Acute MI (TRENT), and Secondary Prevention Reinfarction Israel Nifedipine Trials I and II (SPRINT-I and -II) (155,158). In the Multicenter Diltiazem Post-Infarction Trial (MDPIT) (156), diltiazem was deemed harmful in those with pulmonary congestion and low EF (41% increase in cardiac events). A meta-analysis performed in 1993 of 24 trials of all types of calcium-channel blockers showed a nonsignificant 4% increase in mortality (171). Verapamil appears to be safe; a meta-analysis of verapamil studies showed a significant 19% lower reinfarction rate and nonsignificant 7% mortality reduction (159). These agents should be considered only in patients with clear contraindication(s) to β-blockade and good LV function.

Antiarrhythmics

Prophylactic use of lidocaine appears to be harmful, with a meta-analysis showing a 12% higher mortality rate (172). However, lidocaine (1 to 3 mg/min) can be used in patients who have had ventricular tachycardia (VT) or VF.

In the Cardiac Arrhythmia Suppression Trials (CAST I and II) (165,166), the routine use of type I agents (e.g., encainide, flecainide, moricizine) was associated with significantly higher all-cause mortality rates.

In the Basel Antiarrhythmic Study of Infarct Survival (BASIS) (164), amiodarone (1 g for 5 days, and then 200 mg daily) in patients with complex ventricular ectopy was associated with 61% lower 1-year mortality rates ($p < 0.05$). However, in two large trials [the European MI Amiodarone Trial (EMIAT) and Canadian Amiodarone MI Arrhythmia Trial (CAMIAT) (168,169)], when given to patients with frequent ventricular ectopy and LV dysfunction, amiodarone (vs. placebo) showed no overall mortality benefit, although arrhythmic deaths were decreased.

The Survival with Oral D-sotalol (SWORD) trial showed 65% increased mortality with D-sotalol (167).

Magnesium

Initial studies suggested a mortality benefit [second Leicester Intravenous Magnesium Intervention Trial (LIMIT-2) (161)], and an early meta-analysis showed 54% lower mortality (see *Circulation* 1992;86:774). However, in the ISIS-4 megatrial (162), magnesium had no mortality benefit and was associated with excess hypotension. Proponents of magnesium argued that it could be beneficial in high-risk patients and perhaps when given before thrombolytic therapy to prevent reperfusion injury. However, the large 6,213-patient National Heart, Lung, and Blood Institute (NHLBI)-sponsored MAGIC trial examined these hypotheses and found no benefit associated with magnesium administration (163).

Adenosine

Results with this agent have been mixed. In the Acute Myocardial Infarction Study of Adenosine (AMISTAD) trial, 236 patients were enrolled, and adenosine-treated patients were found to have reduced infarct size (180). In the larger AMISTAD II trial (2,118 patients), adenosine was associated with a nonsignificant trend toward a reduction in death and CHF at 6 months (181).

Glucose-Insulin-Potassium

Results with this combination therapy have been promising, but further study is needed to clearly identify the subgroups of patients in which it provides benefit. A meta-analysis performed several years ago of nine randomized, placebo-controlled, prethrombolytic era trials with 1,932 patients (all prethrombolytic era) found that glucose-insulin-potassium (GIK) was associated with lower hospital mortality (16.1% vs. 21%; OR, 0.72; $p = 0.004$). A 48% reduction was seen in the four trials using high-dose GIK (to suppress free fatty acid levels maximally). The more recent Estudios Cardiologicos Latinoamerica (ECLA) trial enrolled 407 patients and found that GIK-treated patients had nonsignificant reductions in major events, but among the 252 patients (61.9%) treated with reperfusion strategies, GIK resulted in a significant 66% reduction in in-hospital mortality (179). The preliminary findings of the GIPS trial, which enrolled 940 patients undergoing primary PCI, are that there was a nonsignificant trend toward a reduction in the combined end point of death, reinfarction, and repeated revascularization in GIK group (8.0% vs. 9.9%; $p = 0.08$) (182). In a subgroup analysis, a significant reduction was found in the primary end point among those without heart failure symptoms.

OTHER MODES OF TREATMENT

Analgesia

Morphine sulfate may be administered, 2 to 5 mg i.v., repeated every 5 to 15 minutes (some patients require up to 30 mg for adequate pain relief). It is particularly helpful in patients with pulmonary edema due to vasodilatory effect.

Diuretics

Intravenous furosemide (Lasix) is indicated in severe CHF but should be avoided in an inferior MI complicated by RV infarction.

Vasopressors/Inotropes

Vasopressors/inotropes are useful in the treatment of cardiogenic shock (SBP, less than 90 mm Hg; cardiac index, 2.2 L/kg/m^2 or less). Initial choices include dopamine

(5 to 20 μg/kg/min) and dobutamine (2.5 to 20 μg/kg/min; an ideal agent if BP is adequate but cardiac output is poor). If SBP is less than 60 mm Hg, norepinephrine should be considered.

Temporary Pacing

Class I indications are as follows: (a) asystole; (b) symptomatic bradycardia including sinus block with hypotension and Mobitz type I second-degree block with hypotension unresponsive to atropine; (c) bilateral BBB (alternating BBB or RBBB with alternating left anterior fascicular block/left posterior fascicular block); (d) new or indeterminate-age bifascicular block with first-degree atrioventricular (AV) block; or (e) Mobitz-type II second-degree block.

Insulin

Aggressive serum glucose control in diabetics with insulin drip resulted in a significant mortality benefit in the Diabetic Insulin-Glucose Infusion in Acute MI (DIGAMI) trial (177).

Intraaortic Balloon Pump

A balloon pump appears useful in the treatment of cardiogenic shock (trend toward lower mortality in GUSTO-I) (168) and after emergency catheterization [IABP Trial (173)]. Contraindications include the presence of aortic regurgitation and severe peripheral vascular disease. Vascular complications occur in 5% to 20% of cases (173–176).

Emergency Coronary Artery Bypass Graft Surgery

Emergency coronary artery bypass graft (CABG) surgery should be considered if PTCA fails and results in persistent pain or hemodynamic instability, or left main disease is present. Acute mitral regurgitation and ventricular septal defect typically require immediate surgical intervention.

SPECIAL CASE

Right Ventricular Infarction

RV infarction is typically caused by right coronary artery occlusion proximal to the acute marginal branch and is associated with 20% to 50% of inferior MIs (188–193). If the right coronary artery is occluded, RV infarction is 6 times more likely in the absence of preinfarction angina (193).

Diagnosis
1. Triad of hypotension, clear lung fields, and elevated jugular venous pressure is highly specific, but only 25% sensitive.
2. Hemodynamics. Right atrial pressure is more than 10 mm Hg and within 1 to 5 mm Hg of pulmonary capillary wedge pressure (73% sensitivity, 100% specificity).
3. ECG. ST elevation is present in lead V_4R (sensitivity, 80% to 100%, 80% to 100% specificity) and resolves quickly. In one study, ST elevation resolved in 48% of patients within 10 hours (see *Br Heart J* 1983;49:368). RBBB and complete heart block may be observed.
4. Echocardiography. Typical features are RV dilatation, RV wall asynergy, and abnormal interventricular septal motion. Tricuspid regurgitation, ventricular septal defect, and/or early pulmonary valve opening also may be seen.

Complications
High-degree AV block is present in up to 50% of patients, and atrial fibrillation, in up to one third. A high incidence of pericarditis is seen, mostly because of transmural

involvement of the thin-walled right ventricle. Less common complications include rupture of the interventricular septum, RV free-wall rupture, pulmonary embolism, right atrial infarction, and right-to-left shunting across a patent foramen ovale.

Treatment
Diuretics and nitrates should be avoided (i.e., to not decrease preload). Beneficial measures include:

1. Volume loading (2 to 4 L of normal saline is commonly needed);
2. Inotropic support (dobutamine) if volume does not improve cardiac output;
3. Temporary wire placement if complete heart block develops and AV sequential pacing if hemodynamics is poor;
4. Cardioversion if atrial fibrillation is present; and
5. Thrombolysis significantly reduces mortality (190).

Unsuccessful PTCA is associated with high mortality [58% vs. 2% in one study (191)].

COMPLICATIONS

Early

1. Pump failure/cardiogenic shock: incidence, 3% to 7%; most common if more than 40% of myocardium involved; hospital mortality is very high: 50% to 70%; prompt IABP insertion can be useful as a bridge to revascularization.
2. Postinfarct angina: more frequent after thrombolysis than after primary PCI.
3. Reinfarction: more frequent after thrombolysis, and if non–Q-wave MI; should be treated as initial MI with medical therapy and intervention.
4. Arrhythmias.
   a. Ventricular tachycardia: incidence, 5%; associated with larger infarcts/LV dysfunction; nonsustained VT occurring beyond 24 to 48 hours after MI portends poorer prognosis (210) and is an indication for an EP study and implantable cardioverter defibrillator (ICD) implantation.
   b. Ventricular Fibrillation (VF): declining incidence (now less than 1%); primary VF occurs in 85% to 90% of cases in the first 24 hours, 60%, in the first 6 hours; secondary VF: occurs at 1 to 4 days, often associated with pump failure/shock; poor prognosis (40% to 60% in-hospital mortality).
   c. Asystole: associated with high mortality; transcutaneous or transvenous pacing is indicated.
   d. Atrial fibrillation (254): incidence, 5% to 15%; treated with anticoagulation, rate control (β-blockers, calcium-channel blockers, digoxin), cardioversion if hemodynamically unstable, or amiodarone if multiple episodes occur.
   e. Heart block: common with inferior MI (increased vagal tone, AV node ischemia): first-degree heart block typically progresses to Mobitz I and then to third degree; anterior MI (His-Purkinje system affected): BBB progresses to Mobitz II and then third degree (advanced block associated with mortality rate of more than 40%); temporary pacer indicated for high-degree block that develops via Mobitz II mechanism or bifascicular block.
   f. Accelerated idioventricular rhythm: occurs more frequently in patients with early reperfusion; temporary pacing is not indicated.
   g. Premature ventricular contractions: incidence approximately 75%; routine suppression with lidocaine associated with increased mortality.
   h. Sinus tachycardia: if it persists, may signify evolving CHF.
5. Cholesterol embolization: more common with thrombolytic therapy (see *Circulation* 1990;81:477).

Intermediate

1. LV thrombus: incidence, 4% to 20%; most common in anterior MI; treatment: anticoagulation (usually warfarin for 3 to 12 months); decreases the risk of emboliza-

tion (275); primary prevention: consider anticoagulation if EF is less than 30% to 35%.

2. Rupture: causes a higher percentage of deaths in patients undergoing thrombolysis [12% vs. 6% (255)]; risk factors include first MI, female gender, age older than 60 years, no LV hypertrophy, hypertension, and possibly thrombolysis after 12 hours [while primary PTCA appears protective (259)].

   a. Free wall: incidence approximately 5%; lower risk after thrombolysis and with use of β-blockers; although most die immediately, treatment includes emergency pericardiocentesis and fluids, followed by immediate surgical repair.
   b. Septum: incidence, 0.5% to 2.0%; new murmur with palpable thrill in up to 90%; surgical mortality, 20% to 30% (higher if inferior MI and/or cardiogenic shock) versus 80% to 90% with medical therapy (278).
   c. Papillary muscle: incidence approximately 1%; murmur is only 50%; occurs primarily with inferior MIs; posteromedial papillary muscle affected more often (6 times) than anterolateral; best treatment is surgery (mortality, approximately 10%).

3. Fibrinous pericarditis: most common after Q-wave MI; treated with aspirin and analgesics [avoid nonsteroidal antiinflammatory drugs (NSAIDs) and steroids; both may impair healing].

Late

1. Ventricular aneurysm: usually do not rupture, but often complicated by mural thrombi and severe CHF; treated with surgical resection if complicated by CHF, severe arrhythmias, thromboemboli; primary prevention is early ACE inhibition.
2. Pseudoaneurysm: contained rupture of myocardium; surgical resection usually recommended.
3. Dressler syndrome (late pericarditis): usually occurs at 4 to 6 weeks; incidence, approximately 1%; treated with NSAIDs (if they fail, steroids).
4. Sudden Cardiac Death is increased in patients with reduced ejection fraction. The MAD IT 2 Trial showed a 31% reduced mortality at 2 years with prophylactic ICD implantations in patients with EF < 30%.

PROGNOSIS AND RISK STRATIFICATION AFTER MYOCARDIAL INFARCTION

The majority of hospitalized patients with MI are at low risk for adverse outcomes. Age is a strong predictor of outcome. In a multivariate analysis of GUSTO-I data, mortality ranged from 1.1% in those younger than 45 years to 20.5% in those older than 75 (245). Other factors associated with mortality included lower SBP, higher Killip class, elevated HR, and anterior infarct. These five factors contributed to approximately 90% of prognostic information (**Fig. 4.3**). Another analysis of 3,339 TIMI-2 patients identified a low-risk group (26%; none of eight risk factors) that had a 6-week mortality rate of 1.5%. Patients with one risk factor (age 70 years, female gender, diabetes, prior MI, anterior MI, atrial fibrillation, SBP less than 100 mm Hg, HR more than 100 beats/min) had a 6-week mortality rate of 5.3% ($p < 0.001$), whereas those with four risk factors had a 17.2% mortality rate.

A more recently developed clinical score, the TIMI risk score, was derived based on an analysis of 11,114 patients from the InTIME II trial (200). Ten baseline variables accounted for 97% of the predictive capacity of the model. These included age older than 75 years (3 points); age 65 to 74 years (2 points); diabetes, hypertension, or angina (1 point); SBP less than 100 mm Hg (3 points); heart rate more than 100 beats/min (2 points); Killip class II to IV (2 points); weight less than 67 kg (1 point); anterior STEMI or LBBB (1 point); and time to treatment more than 4 hours (1 point). The risk score showed a more than 40-fold graded increase in mortality (less than 1% with a score of 0 vs. 35.9% for score more than 8 (see **Fig. 4.4**). This scoring system was then applied to 84,029 STEMI patients in NRMI-3, and it showed a similar strong prognostic capacity with a graded increase in mortality with increasing TIMI risk score (range, 1.1% to 30.0%; $p < 0.001$ for trend) (201). The risk score was equally predictive in those treated with thrombolytic therapy or primary PCI.

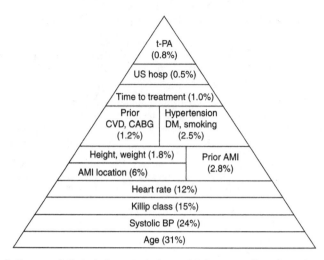

FIG. 4.3. Influence of clinical characteristics on 30-day mortality after myocardial infarction (MI) in patients treated with thrombolytic agents based on GUSTO-I data. Although much attention has been paid to optimizing thrombolytic regimens, the choice of the agent is far less important than are certain clinical variables with respect to mortality. This pyramid depicts the importance of such clinical characteristics, as calculated from a regression analysis in the GUSTO trial. Numbers in parentheses represent the proportion of risk for 30-day mortality associated with the particular characteristics. AMI, acute myocardial infarction; BP, blood pressure; CVD, cardiovascular disease; DM, diabetes mellitus; tPA, tissue-type plasminogen activator; US Hosp, patients treated in a United States hospital. (Modified from Braunwald EB. *Heart disease.* Philadelphia: WB Saunders, 1997:1218, with permission.)

Psychosocial predictors of adverse outcomes include depression (248) and living alone (247). Finally, an analysis of more than 8,000 Medicare patients showed that MI patients treated by cardiologists fared better than those treated by other types of physicians (249).

Uncomplicated Course

In patients treated with primary PCI, early hospital discharge has been shown to be safe and more cost effective. For a large STEMI not treated with PCI, the clinician should consider obtaining an echocardiogram, especially with a high clinical suspicion of LV dysfunction. Catheterization should be considered if the EF is less than 40%. If the EF is 40% or higher, the TIMI IIB study observed no difference in outcome between an early conservative approach when the patient undergoes an exercise treadmill test (ETT), versus an early invasive approach with routine angiography. Accordingly, the ACC/AHA Guidelines recommend an early conservative approach. If the result of the ETT is positive for ischemia, or patient has rest pain, the patient should undergo cardiac catheterization. One recent randomized pilot study (GRACIA), and other observational data from recent studies, suggest that in the current era of stenting and of glycoprotein IIb/IIIa inhibition, an early invasive approach may be superior, but larger trials are needed.

For a small MI, the patient should usually have a submaximal predischarge ETT. If results of this test are negative, medical therapy should be continued, with repeated symptom-limited ETT after several weeks. If the results are positive, catheterization is usually warranted (118).

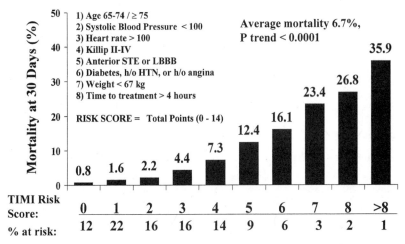

FIG. 4.4. TIMI Risk Score for STEMI. Derivation set based on InTIME II data. Ten baseline variables accounted for 97% of the predictive capacity of the model and compose the TIMI risk score. These included age older than 75 years (3 points); age 65 to 74 years (2 points); diabetes, hypertension, or angina (1 point); systolic blood pressure, <100 mm Hg (3 points); heart rate, >100 (2 points); Killip class II–IV (2 points); weight, <67 kg (1 point); anterior ST-elevation myocardial infarction or left bundle branch block (1 point); and time to treatment, >4 hours (1 point). The risk score showed a >40-fold graded increase in mortality (<1% with a score of 0 vs. 35.9% for score >8. (Modified from Morrow DA, et al. Evaluation of the time saved by prehospital initiation of reteplase for ST-elevation myocardial infarction: results of The Early Retavase-Thrombolysis in Myocardial Infarction (ER-TIMI) 19 trial. *J Am Coll Cardiol* 2002;40:71–77, with permission.)

Complicated Course

Examples of a complicated course include severe heart failure, cardiogenic shock, failed thrombolysis, recurrent ischemia, and VT or VF after 48 hours.

Treatment is composed of catheterization and PCI or CABG surgery, as indicated; for late VT/VF, electrophysiologic testing with possible defibrillator implantation should be considered.

Specific Tests

1. ETT: submaximal test (70% predicted maximal HR or 5 to 6 METS) can be performed at day 3 to 5, or a symptom-limited test can be performed at day 14 to 21 (often as a prelude to initiation of rehabilitation program). This test has an excellent safety record: 0.03% mortality in one review of 151,949 tests (212). The strongest predictors of poor outcome are limited exercise duration and hypotension. ST depression was predictive of death in only 43% of studies in one large overview. If no predischarge ETT is performed, it is associated with a poor prognosis (213). An ETT is not required if complete revascularization has been performed (i.e., successful PCI).
2. ETT with nuclear imaging may be used in patients who have baseline ECG abnormalities or who require localization of ischemia to guide planned PCI. Positive test results lead to angiography and revascularization, which reduce the future cardiac event rate.
3. Pharmacologic stress imaging is indicated in those who cannot exercise. It also is preferred to dobutamine stress echocardiography in those who had significant arrhythmia(s) (especially VT) and or with marked hypertension.

4. Echocardiography is useful in the assessment of LV function (218), which often guides decisions about the need for catheterization, coronary bypass surgery (mortality benefit if EF less than 35%, and three-vessel disease is present), prolonged ACE-inhibition therapy, and long-term anticoagulation. End-systolic volume may be a stronger predictor of survival than is LVEF (219).

5. Pharmacologic stress echocardiography is performed by using agents such as dobutamine, adenosine, and dipyridamole and typically is performed in higher-risk patients (219,220). Even a negative test result has been associated with subsequent moderate event rate.

REFERENCES

General Review Articles

1. **Ryan TJ,** et al. **ACC/AHA Guidelines** for the management of patients with acute myocardial infarction: a report of the American College of Cardiology/American Heart Association Task Force on Practice Guidelines (updated: *Circulation* 1999;100:1016–1030). *J Am Coll Cardiol* 1996;28:1328–1428.

Diagnosis

Chest Pain and Symptoms

2. **Lee TH,** et al. Acute chest pain in the emergency room: identification and examination of low-risk patients. *Arch Intern Med* 1985;145:65–69.

This analysis of 596 emergency department (ED) patients showed that no one variable could identify low-risk patients as efficiently as an ECG. However, a combination of three variables defined a group of patients (8%) in whom ECGs did not add accuracy, and the probability of MI/unstable angina was zero: (a) sharp or stabbing pain; (b) pain that was reproducible by palpation or was pleuritic or positional; and (c) no history of angina or MI (if just the first two variables, 3% probability of unstable angina, none of MI).

3. **Edmondstone WM.** Cardiac chest pain: does body language help the diagnosis? *BMJ* 1995;311:1660–1661.

This study was composed of 203 consecutive patients with chest pain. Among the patients in whom a cardiac etiology was established (68%), 80% used three types of hand movements—Levine sign (clenched fist to middle of chest), flat hand to center of chest, both hands placed flat in middle of chest and drawn outward—versus only 51% with noncardiac etiology ($p < 0.01$). Overall, sensitivity was 80%; specificity, 49%; positive predictive value, 77%; and negative predictive value, 53%.

4. **Douglas PS, Ginsburg GS.** The evaluation of chest pain in women. *N Engl J Med* 1996;334:1311–1315.

This review article discusses the major determinants of coronary artery disease (CAD) in women [chest pain (quality and incidence), hormonal status, diabetes, peripheral vascular disease], as well as intermediate determinants (hypertension, smoking, lipoproteins) and minor determinants (age older than 65 years, obesity, sedentary lifestyle, family history). The review concludes with a discussion of diagnostic testing.

5. **Goldman L,** et al. Prediction of the need for intensive care in patients who come to emergency departments with chest pain. *N Engl J Med* 1996;334:1498–1504.

This study was composed, in part, of a derivation set (10,682 patients) used to identify clinical predictors of major complications: ST elevation or Q waves, other ECG changes indicating myocardial ischemia, low SBP, pulmonary rales above bases, or an exacerbation of known ischemic heart disease. The validation set (4,676 patients) stratified patients into four groups with risk of major complications ranging from 0.15% to 8%. After 12 hours, the probability was updated based on whether the patient had a complication or confirmed MI. Patients with intermediate events (e.g., heart block, pulmonary edema without hypotension, recurrent ischemia not requiring CABG or PTCA within 72 hours) or confirmed MI had 3.5% to 7.5% risk of a major event per 24-hour period. Authors recommended intensive care unit (ICU) admission in this group. Echocardiographic, serum marker, or stress imaging data were not incorporated into this risk-stratification algorithm.

6. **Panju AA,** et al. Is this patient having a myocardial infarction? *JAMA* 1998;280: 1256–1263.

Case-based discussion of history, physical, and ECG findings that are suggestive of the diagnosis of MI. Likelihood ratios are provided for these features; the most powerful predictors (or nonpredictors) of MI include new ST elevation (likelihood ratio range, 5.7 to 53.9), new Q-wave (5.3 to 24.8), chest pain radiating to both arms simultaneously (7.1), positional chest pain (0.3), chest pain reproduced by palpation (0.2 to 0.4), pleuritic chest pain (0.2), and a normal ECG (0.1 to 0.3).

Electrocardiography

7. **Sgarbossa EB,** et al. Electrocardiographic diagnosis of evolving acute MI in the presence of left bundle branch block. *N Engl J Med* 1996;334:481–487 (editorial, 528–529).

Three ECG criteria were derived from an analysis of 131 GUSTO patients: (a) ST elevation of 1 mm concordant with QRS complex; (b) ST depression of 1 mm in V_1, V_2, or V_3; and (c) ST elevation of 5 mm discordant with QRS. Odds ratios for confirmed MI were 25.2, 6.0, and 4.3. If the index score was 3 (a, n = five patients; b, n = three patients; c, n = two patients), sensitivity was 78%, and specificity, 90%. However, sensitivity was only 36% in the validation group of 45 patients. The authors assert that the low sensitivity is an intrinsic property of ST elevation. The reported sensitivity and specificity depend on a 50% prevalence of MI (i.e., high index of suspicion of MI necessary). A retrospective cohort analysis of 83 patients with LBBB and symptoms suggestive of MI found that the sensitivity of this algorithm was only 10% (see *JAMA* 1998;281:714).

8. **Casas RE,** et al. Value of leads V_7–V_9 in diagnosing posterior wall acute MI and other causes of tall R waves in V_1–V_2. *Am J Cardiol* 1997;80:508–509.

This large retrospective analysis found that 250 of approximately 17,000 hospital patients had leads V_7 to V_9 assessed because of a tall R in V_1 and/or suspicion of posterior MI. Among this selected group, 110 patients had evidence of new or old posterior MI, and in 25% of cases, V_7 to V_9 were the only leads diagnostic of MI.

Serum Markers

9. **Puleo PR,** et al. Use of rapid assay of subforms of CK-MB to diagnosis or rule out acute MI. *N Engl J Med* 1994;331:561–566.

This prospective analysis focused on 1,110 evaluated patients with chest pain in the preceding 24 hours. Diagnosis of MI was confirmed in 121 patients. If $CK-MB_2$ was 1.0 U/L or more and $CK-MB_2/CK-MB_1$ was 1.5 or more in the first 6 hours, then sensitivity was 95.7% (vs. 48% for CK-MB), and specificity 93.9% (vs. 94%). The test requires 6 minutes to perform.

10. **deWinter RJ,** et al. Value of myoglobin, troponin T and CK-MB in ruling out an acute MI in the emergency room. *Circulation* 1995;92:3401–3407.

This prospective analysis focused on 309 consecutive patients with chest pain. At 3 to 6 hours after symptoms, myoglobin yielded the best negative predictive value (89% at 4 hours). The negative predictive value of CK-MB reached 95% at 7 hours. The markers were found to increase fastest with large MIs.

11. **Stubbs P,** et al. Prognostic significance of admission troponin T concentration in patients with MI. *Circulation* 1996;94:1291–1297.

This prospective study was composed of 240 patients showing any detectable TnT on admission associated with worse prognosis (median follow-up, 3 years). Admission TnT of 0.2 ng/mL was associated with a higher risk of subsequent cardiac death ($p = 0.0002$) and death plus MI ($p = 0.00006$). Most of this excess risk was confined to those with ST-segment elevation on admission ECG.

12. **Ohman EM,** et al. Cardiac troponin T levels for risk stratification in acute myocardial ischemia. *N Engl J Med* 1996;335:1333–1341.

This analysis focused on 801 GUSTO-IIa patients, of whom 72% had an MI. An elevated TnT (more than 1 ng/mL) was associated with a threefold higher 30-day mortality rate (11.9% vs. 3.9%; $p < 0.001$). Overall, the top mortality predictors were an elevated TnT (x^2, 21; $p < 0.001$), ECG category (ST change or T-wave inversion; x^2, 14; $p = 0.003$), and CK-MB (x^2, 11; $p = 0.004$). TnT was still predictive in a model incorporating all three of these factors (x^2, 9.2; $p = 0.027$). Proposed explanations of the increased mortality with elevated TnT included (a) later presentation; (b) higher in cases of reocclusion, which is known to be associated with increased mortality; and (c) patients who died had larger infarcts (also earlier release). TnT also had predictive prognostic value, even in patients with ST elevation.

13. **Antman E,** et al. Cardiac-specific TnI levels to predict the risk of mortality in patients with acute coronary syndromes. *N Engl J Med* 1996;335:1342–1349.

This analysis focused on 1,404 TIMI IIIB patients. TnI was elevated (0.4 ng/mL or more) in 573 patients and associated with a significantly increased 42-day mortality rate (3.7% vs. 1.0%; $p < 0.001$). Even after adjustments for ST depression and age 65 years or older (the two independent mortality predictors), each 1-ng/mL increase in TnI was associated with a mortality increase: 0.4 or less, 1%; 0.4 to 0.9, 1.7%; 1 to 1.9, 3. 4%; 2 to 4.9, 3.7%; 5 to 8.9, 6%; and 9, 7.5%. TnI provided more prognostic information in patients with a late presentation (more than 6 hours to 24 hours): mortality 4% (TnI, 0.4 ng/mL or more) vs. 0.4% (relative risk, 9.5). In contrast, in patients seen early, the relative risk was only 1.8 (3.1% vs. 1.7%; p = NS). If no CK-MB elevation was present (948 patients), a TnI elevation was still associated with increased mortality: 2.5% versus 0.8% (relative risk, 3.0; 95% CI, 0.97 to 9.2). The elevated-TnI group had more ST deviation and less stenosis on angiography at 18 to 48 hours after symptom onset. However, few had angiography within hours of symptom onset.

14. **Newby LK,** et al. Value of serial TnT measures for early and late risk stratification in patients with acute coronary syndromes. *Circulation* 1998;98:1853–1859.

This GUSTO-IIa substudy of 734 patients showed the usefulness of the addition of later cardiac TnT (cTnT) samples. All patients had cTnT samples drawn at baseline, 8 hours, and 16 hours. At baseline, 260 patients were cTnT positive (more than 0.01 ng/mL), 323 became positive later, and 151 remained negative. The mortality rates were 10% in the baseline-positive group, 5% in the late-positive group, and none in negative patients; thus late positive patients are at intermediate risk. After adjustment for baseline characteristics, any positive cTnT result predicted 30-day mortality. Only age and ST-segment elevation were stronger predictors than baseline cTnT. Most of the mortality difference between cTnT-positive and -negative patients occurred in the first 30 days.

15. **Tanasijevic MJ,** et al. Myoglobin, creatine-kinase-MB and cardiac troponin I 60-minute ratios predict infarct-related artery patency after thrombolysis for acute MI: results from TIMI 10B. *J Am Coll Cardiol* 1999;34:739–747.

This study was composed of 442 TIMI 10B patients who had CK-MB and cTnI measured immediately before and 60 minutes after TNK administration. Patent IRA (TIMI grade 2 or 3 flow) at 60 minutes was demonstrated in 77.8%. The diagnostic performance of the three assays was similar: area under receiver-operating characteristic (ROC) curve for diagnosis of occlusion was 0.71, 0.70, and 0.71 for myoglobin, cTnI, and CK-MB. Sixty-minute ratios (concentration at 60 minutes/concentration at baseline) of 4.0 or more for myoglobin, 3.3 or more for CK-MB, and more than 2.0 for cTnI yielded probabilities of patency of 90%, 88%, and 87%, respectively. Authors assert that early invasive interventions to establish IRA patency may not be needed in these patients with high 60-minute ratios.

Emergency Department Evaluation
16. **Goldman L,** et al. A computer protocol to predict MI in emergency department patients with chest pain. *N Engl J Med* 1988;318:797–803.

This prospective study was composed of 4,770 MI patients. Treatment decisions based on computer protocol had a higher specificity (74% vs. 71%) and similar sensitivity (88% vs. 87.8%) than did those based on physician judgment. Computer protocol–based decisions would have resulted in 11.5% fewer cardiac care unit admissions without MI (thus, cost savings). Whether physicians who are aided by the protocol would perform better than unaided physicians was not assessed.

17. **Gibler WB,** et al. A rapid diagnostic and treatment center for patients with chest pain in the emergency department. *Ann Emerg Med* 1995;25:1–8.

This analysis focused on 1,010 patients with possible acute ischemic heart disease (patients directly admitted if known CAD, hemodynamic instability, ST-segment changes greater than 1 mm, or ongoing chest pain). Serial CK-MB sampling was done at 0, 3, 6, and 9 hours, and continuous ECG monitoring was done for 9 hours. Two-dimensional echocardiography was performed at 9 hours if these tests were negative. If the echocardiogram was then negative, the patient underwent a graded exercise test. Overall, 82% of patients were discharged from the ED. Of the admitted patients, a substantial portion (34%) was found to have cardiac causes.

18. **Gomez MA,** et al., for the Rapid Rule-Out of Myocardial Ischemia Observation (**ROMIO**) study group. An emergency department-based on protocol for rapidly ruling out myocardial ischemia reduces hospital time and expense: result of a randomized study (ROMIO). *J Am Coll Cardiol* 1996;28:25–33.

This study randomized 100 low-risk patients to ED rule-out or hospital care. The ED protocol consisted of enzyme tests at 0, 3, 6, and 9 hours, serial ECGs with continuous ST-segment monitoring, and, if results were negative, predischarge exercise testing. The protocol group had a shorter hospital stay and incurred fewer costs. The routine-care group included more MI and unstable angina patients, but among patients ruled out, the protocol still was associated with decreased stay and cost (12 vs. 23 hours; $p = 0.0001$; initial stay, $890 vs. $1,350; 30 days, $900 vs. $1,520; $p < 0.0001$).

19. **Jesse RL, Kontos MC.** Evaluation of chest pain in the emergency department. *Curr Probl Cardiol* 1997;22:154–236.

This review discusses the differential diagnosis of chest pain, presenting symptoms, and ECG analysis, and the role of serum markers and noninvasive testing. It concludes with a discussion of the role of guidelines, protocols, and pathways.

20. **Kontos MC,** et al. Comparison of myocardial perfusion imaging and cardiac troponin I in patients admitted to the emergency department with chest pain. *Circulation* 1999;99:2073–2078.

This study was composed of 620 patients considered at low to moderate risk for acute coronary syndromes who underwent gated single-photon emission Tc sestamibi imaging and serial measurements of CK, CK-MB, and TnI over an 8-hour period. The incidence of MI was 9%; significant CAD was demonstrated in 13%; and revascularization was performed in 9%. Perfusion imaging was more sensitive but less specific than TnI in identifying patients who were revascularized [sensitivity, 81% vs. 26% (TnI, 1.0 ng/mL); specificity, 74% vs. 96%].

Treatment

General Meta-analysis

21. **Lau JL,** et al. Cumulative meta-analysis of therapeutic trials for MI. *N Engl J Med* 1992;327:248–254.

This overview showed that significant mortality reduction was associated with aspirin (19,077 patients; OR, 0.77; $p < 0.001$), β-blockers (31,669 patients; OR, 0.88; $p = 0.$ 024), thrombolytics (OR, 0.75; $p < 0.001$), intravenous vasodilators (2,170 patients; OR, 0.57; $p < 0.001$), magnesium (only 1,304 patients; OR, 0.44; $p < 0.001$), and anticoagulation (4,975 patients; OR, 0.78; $p < 0.001$). Calcium-channel blockers and prophylactic lidocaine were both associated with a nonsignificant increase in mortality (6,420 patients: OR, 1.12; 8,745 patients: OR, 1.15). For secondary prevention, a protective effect was seen with β-blockers (20,138 patients; OR, 0.81; $p < 0.001$), anticoagulation (4,975 patients; OR, 0.78; $p < 0.001$), cholesterol-lowering drugs (10,775 patients; OR, 0.86; $p < 0.001$), and antiplatelet agents (18,411 patients; OR, 0.90; $p = 0.051$). Rehabilitation programs were beneficial (5,022 patients; OR, 0.80; $p = 0.012$). No benefit was seen with calcium-channel blockers (13,114 patients; OR, 1.10), and class I antiarrhythmics were harmful (4,336 patients; OR, 1.28; $p = 0.03$).

Antithrombotic Agents

General Reviews

22. **Collins R,** et al. Clinical effects of anticoagulation therapy in suspected acute MI: systemic overview of randomised trials. *BMJ* 1996;313:652–659.

This analysis focused on 26 randomized studies (GUSTO not included). No aspirin was used in 5,000 patients, whereas routine aspirin was given in approximately 68,000 patients. In the absence of aspirin, anticoagulation reduced mortality by 25% (and fewer strokes occurred). With aspirin use, heparin was associated with 6% lower mortality (five deaths/1,000; $p = 0.03$) but excess bleeding (+3/1,000). It was unclear whether heparin provides benefit if no thrombolytic agent is administered.

Aspirin

23. Second International Study of Infarct Survival (**ISIS-2**). Randomised trial of intravenous streptokinase, oral, both, or neither among 17,187 cases of suspected acute MI. *Lancet* 1988;332:349–360.

This large trial clearly demonstrated the additive benefit of thrombolytic therapy and aspirin administration. Patients were randomized to streptokinase, 1.5 million U over 60 minutes; and/or aspirin, 162.5 mg; or placebo. The streptokinase and aspirin-alone groups had 25% and 23% lower 5-week vascular mortality, respectively [9.2% vs. 12.0% (placebo); $p < 0.00001$; 9.4% vs. 11.8%; $p < 0.00001$]. The streptokinase and aspirin group had a larger 42% mortality reduction (8% vs. 13.2%). Combination therapy also was effective in patients with LBBB (mortality, 14% vs. 27.7%). Aspirin reduced nonfatal reinfarction and stroke rates (1.0% vs. 2.0%; 0.3% vs. 0.6%).

24. **Roux S,** et al. Effect of aspirin on coronary reocclusion and recurrent ischemia after thrombolysis: a meta-analysis. *J Am Coll Cardiol* 1992;19:671–677.

This analysis of 32 studies (19 randomized, 13 nonrandomized) from 1980 to 1990 showed the impressive benefits of aspirin. In these studies, 3,209 of 4,930 patients were treated with aspirin. Among the 1,022 patients who underwent angiography, aspirin use was associated with a 56% lower reocclusion rate (11% vs. 25%; $p < 0.001$) and fewer recurrent ischemic events (25% vs. 41%; $p < 0.001$). This protective effect of aspirin was similar in trials with either streptokinase or recombinant tPA (rtPA).

Heparin

25. **Hsia J,** et al., for the Heparin Aspirin Reperfusion Trial (**HART**) Investigators. A comparison between heparin and low-dose aspirin as adjunctive therapy with tissue plasminogen activator for acute MI. *N Engl J Med* 1990;323:1433–1437.

Design: Prospective, randomized, open-label, multicenter study. Primary end point was IRA patency at 7 to 24 hours and 7 days.

Purpose: To compare the effects of heparin with aspirin after rtPA in patients with acute MI.

Population: 205 patients aged 75 years and older with acute STEMI (0.1 mm or more in at least two contiguous leads).

Exclusion Criteria: Severe hypotension, cerebrovascular disease, bleeding disorders, LBBB, prior CABG, recent surgery, and prolonged CPR.

Treatment: rtPA, 100 mg i.v. over a 6-hour period (6-mg bolus, 54 mg during hour 1, 20 mg in hour 2, 5 mg/hr for 4 hours) plus either aspirin, 80 mg/day, or heparin, 5,000 U i.v. bolus, and then 1,000 U/hr [adjusted to keep activated partial thromboplastin time (aPTT) within 1.5 to 2.0 times control]. Coronary angiography was performed 7 to 24 hours after rtPA infusion was started and again at 7 days.

Results: Heparin group had higher patency (TIMI grade 2 or 3 flow) at initial angiography (82% vs. 52%; $p < 0.0001$), but no significant difference was seen by the time of the second angiograms (88% vs. 95%). No significant differences were seen in hemorrhagic or recurrent ischemic events.

Comments: A retrospective analysis showed that patients with open arteries at early angiography had a higher mean PTT (81 vs. 54 seconds; $p < 0.02$). However, patients with a PTT of more than 100 at 8 hours had a higher rate of access-related hemorrhage (see *J Am Coll Cardiol* 1992;20:513).

Low-molecular-weight Heparin

26. **Kontny F,** et al., on behalf of the Fragmin in Acute MI (**FRAMI**) Study Group. Randomized trial of low molecular weight heparin (dalteparin) in prevention of left ventricular thrombus formation and arterial embolism after acute anterior MI: the FRAMI study. *J Am Coll Cardiol* 1997;30:962–969.

Design: Prospective, randomized, multicenter study. Primary outcomes were thrombus formation (echocardiography at 9 ± 2 days) and arterial embolism.

Purpose: To evaluate the efficacy and safety of dalteparin in the prevention of LV thrombus formation and arterial embolism after acute anterior MI.

Population: 776 patients seen at 15 hours or less after symptom onset with 2 mm or greater ST elevation in ECG leads V_1 to V_6 or 1 mm or more in leads I and aVL.

Exclusion Criteria: Prior anterior MI, ongoing treatment with or indication for heparin or warfarin, SBP greater than 210 mm Hg or DBP greater than 115 mm Hg, recent cerebrovascular events (2 months or less), and increased bleeding risks.

Treatment: Dalteparin, 150 IU/kg every 12 hours, or placebo; 91.5% of patients received a thrombolytic agent.

Results: Only 517 patients had echocardiograms available for analysis. The dalteparin group had a lower rate of thrombus formation and arterial embolism: 14.2% versus 21.9% ($p = 0.03$). Regarding individual end points, LV thrombus relative risk was 0.63 ($p = 0.02$); arterial embolism, six versus five patients ($p = NS$); and reinfarction, eight versus six patients ($p = NS$). In both groups, 23 patients died; however, dalteparin was associated with increased major and minor hemorrhage rates (2.9% vs. 0.3%; $p = 0.006$; 14.8% vs. 1.8%; $p < 0.001$).

27. **Ross AM,** et al. Randomized comparison of enoxaparin, a low-molecular-weight heparin with unfractionated heparin adjunctive to recombinant tissue plasminogen activator thrombolysis and aspirin: second trial of Heparin and Aspirin Reperfusion Therapy (**HART II**). *Circulation* 2001;104:648–652.

Design: Prospective, randomized, open-label, parallel group, international trial. Primary end point was IRA patency (TIMI grade 2 or 3 flow) at 90 minutes.

Purpose: To demonstrate noninferiority of enoxaparin compared with UFH as an adjunctive therapy during thrombolytic treatment for acute MI.

Population: 400 patients seen within 12 hours and with ST elevation 0.1 mV of more in two or more limb leads or ST elevation of 0.2 mV or more in two or more contiguous precordial leads.

Exclusion Criteria: Contraindications to thrombolysis, serum creatinine more than 2 mg/dL.

Treatment: Enoxaparin or UFH for at least 3 days. All received accelerated tPA regimen and aspirin.

Results: Patency rates at 90 minutes were 80.1% and 75.1% in the enoxaparin and UFH groups, respectively. TIMI grade 3 flow was observed in 52.9% and 47.6%, respectively. Reocclusion at 5 to 7 days from TIMI grade 2 or 3 to TIMI 0 or 1 flow and TIMI grade 3 to TIMI 0 or 1 flow, respectively, occurred in 5.9% and 3.1% of the enoxaparin group versus 9.8% and 9.1% in the UFH group. Bleeding and 30-day mortality rates were similar in both groups.

Comments: The results of this study complement the findings of the larger ASSENT-3 trial (83).

28. **Antman EM,** et al. Enoxaparin as adjunctive antithrombin therapy for ST-elevation myocardial infarction: results of the ENTIRE-Thrombolysis in Myocardial Infarction (**TIMI**) 23 Trial. *Circulation* 2002;105:1642–1649.

Design: Prospective, randomized, open, 2 × 2 factorial, multicenter trial. Primary end point: TIMI grade 3 flow at 60 minutes.

Purpose: To evaluate enoxaparin with full-dose TNK and half-dose TNK plus abciximab.

Population: 483 patients with STEMI seen less than 6 hours from symptom onset.

Exclusion Criteria: Included contraindications to thrombolysis, abciximab within the prior 7 days or eptifibatide or tirofiban within the prior 24 hours; treatment with any LMWH or UFH within 24 hours.

Treatment: Full-dose TNK and either UFH (60-U/kg bolus and then 12 U/kg/hr) or enoxaparin (1.0 mg/kg s.c. every 12 hrs ± initial 30-mg i.v. bolus) OR half-dose TNK plus abciximab and either UFH (40-U/kg bolus and then 7 U/kg/hr) or enoxaparin (0.3 to 0.75 mg/kg s.c. every 12 hours ± initial i.v. bolus of 30 mg).

Results: With full-dose TNK and UFH, TIMI grade 3 flow at 60 minutes was 52%, and was 48% to 51% with enoxaparin. With combination therapy, the TIMI 3 flow was achieved in 48% with UFH and 47% to 58% with enoxaparin. The rate of TIMI 3 flow among all UFH patients was 50% compared with 51% among enoxaparin patients. At 30 days, death or recurrent MI occurred with the full-dose TNK group in 15.9% of patients with UFH compared with only 4.4% with enoxaparin ($p = 0.005$). With combination therapy, the rates were 6.5% with UFH and 5.5% with enoxaparin. Major hemorrhage with full-dose TNK occurred in 2.4% with UFH and 1.9% with enoxaparin; with combination therapy, 5.2% with UFH and 8.5% with enoxaparin.

Comments: Major finding is that in patients receiving full-dose TNK, enoxaparin was associated with similar TIMI 3 flow rates but fewer ischemic events at 30 days compared with UFH.

29. **TETAMI** (Treatment with Enoxaparin and Tirofiban in Acute Myocardial Infarction). Preliminary results presented at AHA Scientific Session, Chicago, IL, November 2002.

This prospective, randomized, 2 × 2 factorial, multicenter trial enrolled 1,224 patients with STEMI considered ineligible for reperfusion therapy and seen within 24 hours of symptom onset. All patients received enoxaparin (30 mg i.v, and then 1 mg/kg s.c. twice daily) or UFH (70-U/kg bolus and then infusion); and tirofiban (100 μg/kg i.v., and then 0.1 μg/kg/min) or placebo. All received aspirin. At 30 days, no significant differences were found between the four groups in combined incidence of death, recurrent MI, or recurrent angina (enoxaparin, 15.4%; enoxaparin + tirofiban, 16.1%; UFH, 17.3%; UFH + tirofiban, 17.2%). In those seen within 12 hours, fewer primary events were seen; a small benefit was noted in favor of enoxaparin and tirofiban. The study was underpowered and confounded by 30% preuse of UFH.

Direct Thrombin Inhibitors

30. **Antman EM,** et al., for the **TIMI-9B** Investigators. Hirudin in AMI. *Circulation* 1996;94:911–921.

Design: Prospective, randomized, double-blind, parallel-group, multicenter study. Primary end point was 30-day incidence of death, nonfatal MI, severe CHF, and cardiogenic shock.

Purpose: To compare the safety and effectiveness of hirudin with heparin in patients undergoing thrombolysis for acute MI.

Population: 3,002 patients within 12 hours of onset of symptoms and with greater than 1-mm ST elevation in at least two contiguous ECG leads; mean age, 60 ± 12 years.

Exclusion Criteria: Contraindications to thrombolytic therapy, creatinine more than 2.0 mg/dL, cardiogenic shock, therapeutic anticoagulation (PT, 14 seconds; aPTT, 60 seconds).

Treatment: Heparin, 5,000-U i.v. bolus, and then 1,000 U/h, or hirudin, 0.1-mg/kg i.v. bolus, and then 0.1 mg/kg/h (maximum, 15 mg/h) for 96 hours. Infusions were started before or immediately after thrombolysis (front-loaded tPA or streptokinase) and adjusted to keep aPTT at 55 to 85 seconds. All patients were given thrombolysis.

Results: No significant difference in primary end points was observed: 12.9% (hirudin) versus 11.9%, nor were any differences observed in hemorrhage and intracranial hemorrhage rates (4.6% vs. 5.3; 0.4% vs. 0.9%). Target aPTT was achieved more frequently with hirudin.

31. **White HD,** et al., on behalf of the Hirulog Early Perfusion/Occlusion (**HERO**) Trial Investigators. Randomized, double-blind comparison of hirulog versus heparin in patients receiving streptokinase and aspirin for acute MI (HERO). *Circulation* 1997;96:2155–2161 (editorial, 2118–2120).

Design: Prospective, randomized, double-blind, multicenter study. Primary outcome was TIMI grade flow at 90 to 120 minutes.

Purpose: To evaluate and compare the safety and efficacy of two hirulog regimens with heparin in acute MI patients receiving streptokinase (SK).

Population: 412 patients seen within 12 hours of symptom onset and with 1-mm ST elevation or greater in at least two contiguous limb leads and/or V_4 to V_6 or 2 mm or more in V_1 to V_3.

Exclusion Criteria: Prior SK; cardiogenic shock; contraindicatiosn to thrombolysis.

Treatment: Heparin, 5,000-U i.v. bolus, and then 1,000 to 1,200 U/hr, low-dose hirulog (0.125-mg/kg i.v. bolus, 0.25 mg/kg/hr for 12 hours, and then 0.125 mg/kg/hr), or high-dose hirulog (0.25-mg/kg intravenous bolus, 0.5 mg/kg/hr for 12 hours, and then 0.25 mg/kg/hr).

Results: Hirulog groups had better TIMI grade 3 flow at 90 to 120 minutes (primary outcome): 46% and 48% versus 35% (heparin vs. hirulog, $p = 0.023$; heparin vs. high-dose hirulog, $p = 0.03$). However, no significant difference in rates of reocclusion was observed at 48 hours (5% and 1% vs. 7%) or death, shock, and reinfarction at 35 days (14% and 12.5% vs. 17.9%). Hirulog also was associated with less major bleeding: 14% and 19% versus 28% (low-dose hirulog vs. heparin, $p < 0.01$).

32. **Behar S,** et al., for the **ARGAMI-2** Study Group. Argatroban versus heparin as adjuvant therapy to thrombolysis for acute myocardial infarction.

This prospective, randomized, placebo-controlled study of 1,200 patients seen within 6 hours and with ST elevation in two or more leads. Exclusion criteria included CNS events, elevated creatinine, and increased bleeding risk(s). Patients were randomized to argatroban (60 μg + 2 μg/kg/min or 120 μg + 4 μg/kg/min for 72 hours) or heparin (5,000 IU + 1,000 IU/hr for 72 hours) with dose adjustment(s) to achieve aPTT of 55 to 85 seconds. All received aspirin and tPA or SK. Low-dose argatroban arm was closed after interim analysis of first 609 patients. At 30 days, no difference was found between the high-dose argatroban and heparin groups in total cardiovascular events, mortality, recurrent MI, heart failure/cardiogenic shock, need for revascularization, or stroke. The argatroban group had a lower incidence of major bleeding, intracranial hemorrhage, and stroke. Maintaining aPTT was easier with argatroban, with only 35% of having an aPTT value less than 55 seconds at 24 hours compared with 68% in the heparin group.

33. The Hirulog and Early Reperfusion or Occlusion **(HERO)-2** Trial Investigators. Thrombin-specific anticoagulation with bivalirudin versus heparin in patients receiving fibrinolytic therapy for acute myocardial infarction: the HERO-2 randomized trial. *Lancet* 2001;358:1855–1863.

Design: Prospective, randomized, open, multicenter study. Primary end point: 30-day mortality.

Purpose: To evaluate the effect on 30-day mortality of bivalirudin versus UFH in acute MI patients treated with SK.

Population: 17,073 patients with acute STEMI seen within 6 hours of symptom onset and with 1 mm or more of ST elevation in two limb leads or 2 mm or more in two contiguous precordial leads or presumed new LBBB.

Exclusion Criteria: Included contraindications to thrombolysis, LMWH therapy within 12 hours, and previous SK therapy.

Treatment: Bivalirudin (0.25-mg/kg bolus, and then 0.5 mg/kg/hr for 12 hours, and then 0.25 mg/kg/hr for 36 hours) or UFH. All received SK, 1.5 MU over a 30- to 60-minute period, and aspirin, 150 to 325 mg once daily.

Results: At 30 days, no significant difference appeared between the two groups in unadjusted mortality (bivalirudin, 10.8%; heparin, 10.9%) and adjusted mortality (10.5% vs. 10.9%). At 96 hours, the bivalirudin group had a 30% reduction in reinfarction compared with the heparin group (1.6% vs. 2.3%; $p = 0.001$). Nonsignificant trends were seen toward increased severe bleeding and intracerebral bleeding with bivalirudin (0.7% vs. 0.5%; $p = 0.07$; 0.6% vs. 0.4%; $p = 0.09$), whereas significant increased risks of both moderate and mild bleeding were noted (1.4% vs. 1.1%; $p = 0.05$; 12.8% vs. 9.0%; $p < 0.001$).

34. The **Direct Thrombin Inhibitor** Trialists' Collaborative Group. Direct thrombin inhibitors in acute coronary syndromes: principal results of a meta-analysis based on individual patients' data. *Lancet* 2002;359:294–302.

This meta-analysis examined 11 randomized trials (35,970 total patients) comparing a direct thrombin inhibitor (DTI; hirudin, bivalirudin, argatroban, efegatran, or inogatran) with heparin. Compared with heparin, DTIs were associated with a lower risk of death or MI at the end of treatment [4.3% vs. 5.1%; OR, 0.85 (95% CI, 0.77 to 0.94); $p = 0.001$] and at 30 days [7.4% vs. 8.2%; OR, 0.91 (CI, 0.84 to 0.99); $p = 0.02$]. This was due primarily to a reduction in MI [2.8% vs. 3.5%; OR, 0.80 (CI, 0.71 to 0.90); $p < 0.001$] with no significant effect on mortality [1.9% vs. 2.0%; OR, 0.97 (CI, 0.83 to 1.13); $p = 0.69$]. Subgroup analyses suggested a benefit of DTIs on death or MI in trials of both acute coronary syndromes and PCIs. Compared with heparin, an increased risk of major bleeding with hirudin was seen, but a reduction, with bivalirudin. No increased incidence of intracranial hemorrhage was found with DTIs.

Warfarin

35. **Smith P,** et al., Warfarin Reinfarction Study (**WARIS**). The effect of warfarin on mortality and reinfarction after MI. *N Engl J Med* 1990;323:147–152.

Design: Prospective, randomized, double-blind, placebo-controlled, multicenter study. Mean follow-up period was 37 months. Primary end point was all-cause mortality and reinfarction.

Purpose: To evaluate the effects of warfarin on mortality, reinfarction, and cerebrovascular events in post-MI patients.

Population: 1,214 patients aged 75 years or younger; mean time since index MI, 27 days.

Exclusion Criteria: Required anticoagulant use and significant bleeding risk.

Treatment: Warfarin dose adjusted to achieve target INR of 2.8 to 4.8; or placebo.

Results: Warfarin group had 24% lower all-cause mortality (15.5% vs. 20.3%; $p = 0.03$), 34% fewer reinfarctions (13.5% vs. 20.4%; $p < 0.001$), and 55% fewer cerebrovascular accidents (3.3% vs. 7.2%; $p = 0.0015$). Serious bleeding rate in the warfarin group was 0.6%/yr (intracranial hemorrhage rate, 0.2%/yr).

36. Anticoagulants in Secondary Prevention of Events in Coronary Thrombosis (**ASPECT**) Research Group. Effect of long-term anticoagulant treatment on mortality and cardiovascular morbidity after MI. *Lancet* 1994;343:499–503.

Design: Prospective, randomized, double-blind, placebo-controlled, multicenter study. Mean follow-up period was 37 months. Primary end point was all-cause mortality.

Purpose: To evaluate the impact of long-term anticoagulation in the secondary prevention of morbidity and mortality after acute MI.

Population: 3,404 patients with cardiac serum marker evidence of an acute MI (2× or more the upper limit of normal).

Exclusion Criteria: Need for long-term anticoagulation, anticoagulation therapy in the prior 6 months, increased bleeding tendency, and anticipated coronary revascularization procedure.

Treatment: Phenprocoumon or nicoumalone started within 6 weeks of hospital discharge to achieve an INR of 2.8 to 4.8; or placebo.

Results: No significant mortality difference was observed between groups [10% (anticoagulation) vs. 11.1%]. Anticoagulation was associated with a reduction in two secondary end points: more than 50% fewer recurrent MIs (6.7% vs. 14.2%) and approximately 40% fewer cerebrovascular events (2.2% vs. 3.6%). The anticoagulation group had more major bleeding complications (4.3% vs. 1.1%).

Comments: A *post hoc* analysis showed that the optimal INR was 3 to 4. The rate of major bleeding plus thromboembolic complications was 3.2 per 100 patient years (INR, less than 2, 8.0; 2 to 3, 3.9; 4 to 5, 6.6; more than 5, 7.7) (see *J Am Coll Cardiol* 1996;27:1349).

37. **Julian DG,** et al., for the Aspirin/Anticoagulants Following Thrombolysis with Eminase in Recurrent infarction (**AFTER**) Study Group. A comparison of aspirin and anticoagulation following thrombolysis for MI (the AFTER study): a multicentre unblinded randomised clinical trial. *BMJ* 1996;313:1429–1431.

Design: Prospective, randomized, unblinded, multicenter study. Follow-up period was 1 year. Primary end point was cardiac death and nonfatal MI at 30 days.

Purpose: To compare aspirin with heparin followed by oral anticoagulation therapy in MI patients undergoing thrombolysis with anistreplase.

Population: 1,036 patients treated with anistreplase within 6 hours of onset of symptoms (ECG criteria, 2-mm or more ST elevation in at least two adjacent precordial leads or 1 mm or more in at least two limb leads).

Treatment: Aspirin, 150 mg/day, or heparin, 1,000 U/h for 24 hours (started 6 hours after anistreplase, 30 U) followed by oral anticoagulation to achieve a target INR of 2.0 to 2.5. Therapy was discontinued after 3 months.

Results: Similar 30-day incidences of cardiac death and reinfarction were observed [11.2% (aspirin) vs. 11%]. The anticoagulation group had more severe bleeding and strokes: at 3 months, 3.9% vs. 1.7% ($p = 0.04$).

38. Coumadin Aspirin Reinfarction Study (**CARS**) Investigators. Randomised double-blind trial of fixed low-dose warfarin with aspirin after MI. *Lancet* 1997;350:389–396.

Design: Prospective, randomized, double-blind, multicenter study. Median follow-up period was 14 months. Primary end point was MI, stroke, and cardiovascular death.

Purpose: To compare long-term administration of aspirin alone with lower-dose aspirin in combination with fixed low-dose regimens of oral anticoagulation in acute MI patients.

Population: 8,803 patients aged 21 to 85 years with a documented MI 3 to 21 days before enrollment.

Exclusion Criteria: Included circulatory shock, heart failure (Killip class III or IV), rest angina refractory to medical therapy, history of bleeding or stroke (without full recovery), SBP higher than 180 mm Hg or DBP higher than 100 mm Hg.

Treatment: Aspirin, 160 mg/day, aspirin, 80 mg/day, and warfarin 1 mg/day, or aspirin, 80 mg/day, and warfarin, 3 mg/day.

Results: Average measured INRs at week 4 were 1.02 (aspirin alone), 1.05 (aspirin and warfarin, 1 mg/day), and 1.27 (aspirin and warfarin, 3 mg/day). No significant difference in primary end points (MI, stroke, or cardiovascular death) was observed [1-year rates, 8.6% (aspirin), 8.8% (aspirin and warfarin, 1 mg/day), 8.4% (aspirin and warfarin, 3 mg/day)]. However, the warfarin, 3 mg/day, group had a higher rate of spontaneous major hemorrhage versus aspirin alone: 0.74%/yr versus 1.4%/yr ($p = 0.014$).

39. **Fiore LD,** et al., for the Combination Hemotherapy and Mortality Prevention (**CHAMP**) Study Department of Veterans Affairs Cooperative Studies Program clinical trial comparing combined warfarin and aspirin with aspirin alone in survivors of acute myocardial infarction: primary results of the CHAMP Study. *Circulation* 2002;105:557–563.

Design: Prospective, randomized, open-label, multicenter. Primary end point was all-cause mortality. Median follow-up was 2.7 years.

Purpose: The determine if the combination of aspirin and warfarin is more effective than aspirin monotherapy in the secondary prevention of vascular events and death after acute myocardial infarction (AMI).

Population: 5,059 patients with AMI within 14 days. Diagnosis of AMI as defined by the presence of two of the following: (a) chest discomfort typical of AMI, (b) ECG changes typical of AMI, (c) blood enzyme changes typical of AMI.

Exclusion Criteria: Included more than 14 days after MI, ongoing bleeding or bleeding risk, alternative indication for anticoagulant therapy, treatment with high-dose aspirin or NSAID, hypersensitivity to aspirin or warfarin.

Treatment: Warfarin (target INR, 1.5 to 2.5) plus aspirin (81 mg once daily) or aspirin alone (162 mg once daily).

Results: At follow-up, all-cause mortality was similar in the two groups [17.6% (combination group) vs. 17.3% (aspirin only)]. No significant difference was seen between the groups in recurrent MI (13.3% vs. 13.1%, respectively; log-rank $p = 0.78$) or stroke (3.1% vs. 3.5%, respectively; log-rank $p = 0.52$). Major bleeding, primarily gastrointestinal, occurred more often in the combination-therapy group than in the aspirin group (1.28 vs. 0.72 events per 100 patient years, respectively; $p < 0.001$).

40. **van Es RF,** et al., for the Antithrombotics in the Secondary Prevention of Events in Coronary Thrombosis-2 (**ASPECT-2**) Research Group. Aspirin and coumadin after acute coronary syndromes (the ASPECT-2 study): a randomised controlled trial. *Lancet* 2002;360:109–113.

Design: Prospective, randomized, open-label, multicenter trial. The primary composite end point was MI, stroke, or death.

Purpose: To determine whether the combination of aspirin and oral anticoagulants provides a greater benefit than either of these agents alone, without excessive risk of bleeding.

Population: 999 patients with AMI or unstable in previous 8 weeks.

Exclusion Criteria: Included established indication(s) for oral anticoagulation or platelet inhibitors, planned revascularization, increased risk of bleeding, bleeding diathesis, history of stroke, pregnancy.

Treatment: Low-dose aspirin (80 mg), high-intensity oral anticoagulation (target INR, 3.0 to 4.0), or combined low-dose aspirin and moderate-intensity oral anticoagulation (target INR, 2.0 to 2.5).

Results: The anticoagulant and combination-therapy groups had a significantly lower incidence of the primary composite end point compared with the aspirin group [hazard ratio, 0.55 (95% CI, 0.30 to 1.00); $p = 0.0479$; hazard ratio, 0.50 (0.27 to 0.92); $p = 0.03$], respectively. Major bleeding was similar in the three groups (1% to 2%). Frequency of minor bleeding was 5%, 8% [1.68 (0.92 to 3.07); $p = 0.20$], and 15% [3.13 (1.82 to 5.37), $p \leq 0.0001$], in the aspirin, anticoagulant, and combination groups, respectively.

41. **Hureln M,** et al. Warfarin, aspirin, or both after myocardial infarction: **WARIS-II** (Warfarin-Aspirin Reinfarction Study). *N Engl J Med* 2002;347:969–974 (editorial, 1019–1022).

Design: Prospective, randomized, open-label, multicenter trial. Primary end point: death, nonfatal MI, and stroke. Mean follow-up, 4 years.

Purpose: To compare the efficacy and safety of long-term treatment with warfarin alone, aspirin alone, or the two combined in survivors of AMI.

Population: 3,630 patients aged 20 to 74 years with two or more of following: ischemic chest pain, ECG changes typical of AMI, CK greater than 250 U/L and/or aspartate aminotransferase greater than 50 U/L of probable cardiac origin.

Exclusion Criteria: Included history of serious bleeding or bleeding diathesis, spontaneous bleeding with aspirin or warfarin, and any contraindication to or indication for aspirin or warfarin.

Treatment: Randomized on hospital discharge to warfarin (target INR, 2.8 to 4.2) or aspirin (160 mg/day) or warfarin (target INR, 2.0 to 2.5) and aspirin (75 mg/day). The average INR was 2.8 in the warfarin-alone group and 2.2 in the warfarin + aspirin group; however, measured INRs were below target one third of the time.

Results: The incidence of death, nonfatal MI, and stroke was 20.0% in the aspirin-alone group compared with 16.7% in warfarin-alone group [relative risk ratio (RRR) compared with aspirin, 0.81 (95% CI, 0.67 to 0.98); $p = 0.028$] and 15.0% in the aspirin + warfarin group [RRR compared with aspirin, 0.71 (95% CI, 0.58 to 0.86); $p = 0.0005$]. The aspirin + warfarin group had a significantly higher cumulative probability of survival compared with the aspirin-alone group ($p = 0.0033$), whereas no significant difference was seen between the warfarin-alone and the warfarin + aspirin groups. However, major bleeding rates (bleeding requiring transfusion or surgical intervention) were higher in the warfarin groups (0.58/100 patient years with warfarin alone and 0.52/100 patient years in the warfarin + aspirin group) compared with aspirin alone (0.15/100 patient years in the aspirin group). Minor bleeding rates were 0.81, 2.16, and 2.75/100 patient years, respectively.

Comments: The exclusion of patients 75 years or older likely attenuated the excess warfarin-associated bleeding risk. Only 35% of patients underwent revascularization (PCI or CABG). The efficacy of warfarin as part of an early revascularization strategy and in conjunction with thienopyridine therapy is unknown.

42. **Brouwer MA,** et al. Aspirin plus coumarin versus aspirin alone in the prevention of reocclusion after fibrinolysis for acute myocardial infarction: results of the Antithrombotics in the Prevention of Reocclusion In Coronary Thrombolysis **(APRICOT)-2** Trial. *Circulation* 2002;106:659–665.

Design: Prospective, randomized, open, multicenter trial. Primary end point was angiographic reocclusion at 3 months.

Purpose: To evaluate a prolonged anticoagulation regimen as an adjunct to aspirin in the prevention of reocclusion and recurrent ischemic events after fibrinolysis for STEMI.

Population: 308 STEMI patients receiving aspirin and IVH and angiography within 48 hours showing TIMI grade 3 flow in IRA.

Treatment: Standard in-hospital heparinization and aspirin, or aspirin and coumarin for 3 months (target INR, 2.0 to 3.0; median achieved INR, 2.6).

Results: The incidence of reocclusion (TIMI grade 2 flow or less) at 3 months was significantly lower in aspirin and coumarin compared with aspirin alone (15% vs. 28%; RR, 0.55; 95% CI, 0.33 to 0.90; $p < 0.02$). TIMI grade 0 to 1 flow rates were 9% and 20%, respectively (RR, 0.46; 95% CI, 0.24 to 0.89; $p < 0.02$). Aspirin and coumarin was also associated with lower rate of death, reinfarction, and revascularization (14% vs. 34%; $p < 0.01$). Bleeding rates (TIMI major and minor) were similar (5% vs. 3%; $p = $ NS).

Glycoprotein IIb/IIIa Inhibitors
43. **Ohman EM,** et al., for the **IMPACT-AMI** Investigators. Combined accelerated tissue plasminogen activator and platelet glycoprotein IIb/IIIa integrelin receptor

blockade with integrelin in acute MI. *Circulation* 1997;95:846–854 (editorial, 793–795).

Design: Prospective, randomized, placebo-controlled, partially open (first 132 patients), partially blinded (last 48 patients), dose-ranging, multicenter study. Primary end point was TIMI flow grade 3 at 90 minutes.

Purpose: To determine the safety and efficacy of eptifibatide in conjunction with aspirin, heparin, and accelerated alteplase in AMI.

Population: 180 patients seen within 6 hours of onset of symptoms with chest pain lasting 30 minutes or more, ST elevation 1 mm or more in at least two inferior or precordial leads or leads I and aVL, ST depression in V_1 to V_6 consistent with posterior injury, or LBBB.

Exclusion Criteria: Included weight more than 125 kg, SBP greater than 200 mm Hg or DBP greater than 100 mm Hg, prior stroke, oral anticoagulation, recent (less than 6 weeks) bleeding, platelets fewer than 100,000, and creatinine more than 4.0 mg/dL.

Treatment: The 132 patients were assigned in 2:1 fashion to one of six doses of eptifibatide (36- to 180-μg/kg i.v. bolus followed by 0.2 to 0.75 μg/kg/min); or placebo. All patients were given front-loaded tPA, heparin [40-U/kg i.v. bolus (except two highest integrelin dose groups) and then 15 U/kg/hr], and aspirin, 325 mg/day and front-loaded tPA. The final 48 patients were randomized in 3:1 fashion to high-dose eptifibatide (180-μg/kg bolus and then 0.75 μg/kg/min); or placebo.

Results: Highest-dose group had better 90-minute TIMI grade 3 flow [66% vs. 39% (placebo); $p = 0.006$] and shorter time to ST-segment recovery (65 vs. 116 minutes; $p = 0.05$). However, no significant difference was observed in the in-hospital composite end points of death, reinfarction, stroke, revascularization, new CHF, and pulmonary edema (43% vs. 42%). Similar bleeding complication rates were observed (4% vs. 5%).

Comments: Study was weakly powered. Editorial points out that the open and double-blind data were inappropriately pooled. If only the double-blind data were analyzed, 90-minute TIMI grade 3 flow was actually better with placebo (77% vs. 64%).

44. **Brener SJ**, et al., on behalf of the Reopro And Primary PTCA Organization and Randomized Trial (**RAPPORT**) Investigators. Randomized, placebo-controlled trial of primary glycoprotein IIb/IIIa blockade with primary angioplasty for acute MI. *Circulation* 1998;98:734–741.

Design: Prospective, randomized, double-blind, placebo-controlled, multicenter study. Primary end point (at 6 months) was death, MI, and any TVR.

Purpose: To evaluate whether platelet IIb/IIIa–receptor blockade with abciximab reduces ischemic events in AMI patients undergoing primary angioplasty.

Population: 483 patients seen within 12 hours of onset of symptoms with ischemic chest pain lasting more than 20 minutes accompanied by significant ST elevation in at least two contiguous leads or new LBBB.

Exclusion Criteria: Included severe thrombocytopenia, baseline PTT greater than 1.2× control, previous stroke, severe uncontrolled hypertension, PTCA of IRA in prior 3 months, cardiogenic shock, prior abciximab or thrombolytic therapy.

Treatment: Abciximab, 0.25-mg/kg bolus, and then 0.125 μg/kg/min (maximum, 10 μg/min) for 12 hours. All patients received aspirin and heparin, 100-U/kg bolus before PTCA [with further boluses as needed to keep activated clotting time (ACT) longer than 300 seconds]. Stenting was discouraged but was allowed for residual dissection with more than 50% restenosis and for abrupt or threatened closure.

Results: No difference was observed between the two groups in incidence of 6-month primary end points (28.1% vs. 28.2%). However, the abciximab group had lower rates of death, MI, and urgent TVR at 7 days (3.3% vs. 9.9%; $p = 0.003$), 30 days (5.8% vs. 11.2%; $p = 0.03$), and 6 months (11.6% vs. 17.8%; $p = 0.05$). The abciximab group had 42% less bailout stenting (11.9% vs. 20.4%; $p = 0.008$). Abciximab was associated with increased major bleeding (defined as hematocrit decrease of more than 5; 16.6% vs. 9.5%; $p = 0.02$), mostly at the arterial access site. On-treatment analysis

showed that abciximab was associated with decreased death and MI at 7 days (1.4% vs. 4.7%; $p = 0.047$) with a trend at 6 months (6.9% vs. 12%; $p = 0.07$).
Comments: Increased bleeding with abciximab was likely due to double-blind design, as the investigators were unwilling to discontinue heparin immediately after procedure(s) for early sheath removal.

45. **van den Merkhof,** et al. Glycoprotein Receptor Antagonist Patency Evaluation (**GRAPE**) Pilot Study. Abciximab in the treatment of acute MI eligible for primary percutaneous transluminal coronary angioplasty. *J Am Coll Cardiol* 1999;33:1528–1532.

This study was composed of 60 patients seen within 6 hours of onset of symptoms who had abciximab (250-μg/kg bolus and then 10 μg/min for 12 hours) started before proceeding to the catheterization laboratory for possible primary angioplasty. Median time from initiation of abciximab to contrast injection of the IRA was 45 minutes. TIMI grade 3 flow was observed in 18%, and TIMI 2 flow, in 22%. These numbers are higher than those seen in primary angioplasty trials without abciximab pretreatment.

46. **Montalescot G,** et al., for the **ADMIRAL** Investigators. Platelet glycoprotein IIb/IIIa inhibition with coronary stenting for acute myocardial infarction. *N Engl J Med* 2001;344:1895–1903.

Design: Prospective, randomized, multicenter, double-blind, placebo-controlled trial. Primary composite end point at 30 days: death, reinfarction, or urgent TVR.
Purpose: To compare the combination of primary stenting and platelet glycoprotein IIb/IIIa receptor inhibition with primary stenting alone in AMI.
Population: 300 patients seen within 12 hours of onset of symptoms with 1 mm or more ST elevation in two or more contiguous leads.
Exclusion Criteria: Included bleeding diathesis, thrombolytic administration for current episode, recent stroke, uncontrolled hypertension, recent surgery, oral anticoagulant therapy, known contraindications to aspirin, ticlodipine, or heparin.
Treatment: Abciximab (0.25-mg/kg bolus and then 0.125 μg/kg/min for 12 hours) plus stent implantation or primary stenting alone. Therapy was initiated before sheath insertion and coronary angiography. Follow-up angiography at 24 hours and 6 months.
Results: Abciximab group had a significantly higher initial TIMI grade 3 flow compared with placebo (16.8% vs. 5.4%; $p = 0.01$; grade 2 or 3, 25.8% vs. 10.8%; $p = 0.006$). TIMI grade 3 flow after procedure and at 6 months also was higher in the abciximab group (95.1% vs. 86.7%; $p = 0.04$; 94.3% vs. 82.8%; $p = 0.04$). At 30 days, the abciximab group had a nearly 60% lower incidence of the primary end point (6.0% vs. 14.6%; $p = 0.01$; at 6 months, 7.4% vs. 15.9%). Much of this benefit was from a lower rate of urgent TVR with abciximab (at 30 days, 1.3% vs. 6.6%; $p = 0.02$), although mortality also trended lower (at 30 days, 3.4% vs. 6.6%; $p = 0.19$). The abciximab group had a significantly higher LV ejection fraction at 24 hours (57.0% vs. 53.9%; $p < 0.05$) and at 6 months (61.1% vs. 57.0%; $p = 0.05$).

47. **Stone GW,** et al., for The Controlled Abciximab and Device Investigation to Lower Late Angioplasty Complications (**CADILLAC**) Investigators. Comparison of angioplasty with stenting, with or without abciximab, in acute myocardial infarction. *N Engl J Med* 2002;346:957–966.

Design: Prospective, randomized, open, 2×2 factorial, multicenter trial. Primary end point at 6 months: death, reinfarction, disabling stroke, and ischemia-driven TVR.
Purpose: To determine whether used in combination with PTCA, coronary stenting and platelet glycoprotein IIb/IIIa inhibitors can further improve outcomes in AMI patients.
Population: 2,082 patients seen within 6 hours who underwent urgent cardiac catheterization and were eligible for stent placement.
Exclusion Criteria: Included cardiogenic shock, bleeding diathesis, cerebrovascular accident (CVA) in previous 2 years, history of leukopenia, thrombocytopenia, or hepatic or renal dysfunction.

Treatment: PTCA alone, PTCA plus abciximab, stenting alone (MultiLink stent), or stenting plus abciximab.

Results: TIMI grade 3 flow rates were similar in the four groups (95% to 97%). At 6 months, the primary composite end point occurred in 20.0% of the PTCA-alone group, 16.5% with PTCA plus abciximab, 11.5% with stenting, and 10.2% with stenting plus abciximab ($p < 0.001$). No significant differences were found in 6-month mortality between the four groups (PTCA alone, 4.5%; PTCA + abciximab, 2.5%; stenting, 3.0%; stenting + abciximab, 4.2%). Stroke and reinfarction rates also were similar. The difference in the incidence of the primary end point was owing to differences in the rates of TVR (15.7% with PTCA alone, 13.8% with PTCA + abciximab, 8.3% with stenting, and only 5.2% with stenting + abciximab; $p < 0.001$). Follow-up angiography demonstrated a lower restenosis rate with stenting compared with PTCA (22.2% vs. 40.8%; $p < 0.001$). Reocclusion rates of the IRA were 11.3% and 5.7% ($p = 0.01$), respectively, and both were independent of abciximab use.

Comments: Inclusion criteria were "soft" because patients with infarct suspicion and angiographic evidence were enrolled; as a result, fewer than 90% had ST elevation or new LBBB.

Glycoprotein IIb/IIIa Inhibitors and Reduced-dose Thrombolysis

48. **Antman EM,** et al., for the **TIMI-14** Investigators. Abciximab facilitates the rate and extent of thrombolysis. *Circulation* 1999;99:2720–2732 (editorial, 2714–2716).

Design: Prospective, randomized, dose-ranging, multicenter study. Primary end point was IRA TIMI grade 3 flow at 90 minutes (also see ASSENT-3, reference 82).

Purpose: To determine whether abciximab is an effective and safe addition to reduced-dose thrombolytic regimens for STEMI.

Population: 888 patients aged 18 to 75 years seen within 12 hours of symptom onset with 1 mm or greater ST elevation in at least two contiguous ECG leads.

Exclusion Criteria: LBBB, 6,000 U heparin in the hour before randomization, prior CABG surgery, PCI or thrombolytic therapy in prior 7 days, and history of stroke or transient ischemic attack (TIA).

Treatment: (a) 100 mg of accelerated-dose alteplase (control); (b) abciximab (0.25-mg/kg bolus, and then 0.125 μg/kg/min for 12 hours) plus reduced-dose SK (500,000 to 1.5 million U); (c) abciximab plus reduced-dose alteplase (20 to 65 mg); (d) abciximab alone. All patients received aspirin. Control patients received standard weight-based heparin (70-U/kg bolus; initial infusion, 15 U/kg/hr), whereas the abciximab groups received low-dose heparin (60-U/kg bolus, and then 7 U/kg/hr). Very low-dose heparin also was tested in the dose-confirmation phase (30-U/kg bolus, and then 4 U/kg/hr).

Results: Abciximab alone achieved TIMI grade 3 flow at 90 minutes in only 32%, and abciximab plus streptokinase, 500,000 to 1.25 million U in only 34% to 46%. Higher rates of TIMI grade 3 flow at 60 and 90 minutes were seen with increasing duration of alteplase infusion, progressing from bolus alone to bolus and 30- or 60-minute infusion ($p < 0.02$). Best regimen was abciximab and alteplase, 50 mg (15-mg bolus, 35 mg over 60 minutes), which produced TIMI 3 flow in 77% at 90 minutes (vs. 62% with alteplase alone; $p = 0.02$). TIMI 3 flow at 60 minutes also was significantly better with this regimen [72% vs. 43% (alteplase alone); $p = 0.0009$]. Major hemorrhage occurred in 3% receiving abciximab alone, 6% with alteplase alone, 10% with SK plus abciximab, 7% with 50 mg alteplase plus abciximab plus low-dose heparin, 1% with 50 mg alteplase plus abciximab plus very low-dose heparin.

49. Strategies for Patency Enhancement in the Emergency Department (**SPEED**) Group. Trial of abciximab with and without low-dose reteplase for acute myocardial infarction. *Circulation* 2000;101:2788–2794.

This prospective, randomized, open-label, multicenter, phase II study enrolled 528 patients with STEMI within 6 hours of chest-pain onset. Patients were randomized in a 4:1 fashion to abciximab alone ($n = 63$) or with 5 U, 7.5 U, 10 U, 5 U + 2.5 U, or 5 U + 5 U of reteplase ($N = 241$). Phase B tested the best phase A strategy (abciximab plus 5 U + 5 U reteplase, $n = 115$) against 10 U + 10 U reteplase alone ($n = 109$). Initial angiography was performed at a median of 63 minutes from the beginning of reperfusion therapy. In phase A, 62% of the abciximab-reteplase 5 + 5 U group had TIMI grade 3 flow (primary end point) versus 27% of the abciximab-only patients ($p = 0.001$). In phase B, 54% of the abciximab-reteplase 5 + 5 U group had grade 3 flow versus 47% of the reteplase-only patients ($p = 0.32$). TIMI grade 3 flow rates were 61% for a 60-U/kg heparin bolus and abciximab-reteplase 5 + 5 U, 51% for a 40-U/kg heparin bolus and abciximab-reteplase 5 + 5 U ($p = 0.22$), and 47% for reteplase alone ($p = 0.05$ vs. the 60-U/kg heparin group). Major bleeding rates in phase A were 3.3% for abciximab alone and 5.3% for abciximab-reteplase 5 + 5 U; rates in phase B were 9.8% for abciximab-reteplase 5 + 5 U and 3.7% for reteplase alone. Major bleeding rates were not significantly different with standard- or low-dose heparin (6.3% vs. 10.5%; $p = 0.30$). An analysis of the 323 (61%) patients who underwent early PCI found that it was used more frequently in patients with initial TIMI flow grade 0 or 1 versus flow grade 2 or 3 (83% vs. 60%; $p < 0.0001$) (see *J Am Coll Cardiol* 2000;36:1489). The early PCI group had a significantly lower incidence of reinfarction [1.2 vs. 4.9% (no early PCI); $p = 0.03$], urgent revascularization (1.6% vs. 9.3%; $p = 0.001$), transfusion requirement (9.0% vs. 16%; $p = 0.02$), and a significantly higher freedom from death, reinfarction, urgent revascularization, major bleeding, or transfusion at 30 days (85.4% vs. 70.4%; $p < 0.001$).

50. **Topol EJ.** The **GUSTO-V** Investigators. Reperfusion therapy for acute myocardial infarction with fibrinolytic therapy or combination reduced fibrinolytic therapy and platelet glycoprotein IIb/IIIa inhibition: the GUSTO-V randomised trial. *Lancet* 2001;357:1905–1914.

Design: Prospective, randomized, open, multicenter trial. Primary end point was 30-day mortality, and secondary end points included various complications of MI.
Purpose: To compare the effect of reteplase alone with reteplase plus abciximab in patients with AMI.
Population: 16,588 patients seen within 6 hours of symptom onset with ST elevation.
Exclusion Criteria: Included planned PCI, contraindications to thrombolysis.
Treatment: Standard-dose reteplase (two 10-U boluses, 30 minutes apart) or half-dose reteplase (two 5-U boluses) and full-dose abciximab.
Results: No significant differences were seen between the two groups in 30-day mortality [5.9% (reteplase) vs. 5.6% (OR, 0.95); $p = 0.43$]; the 0.3% absolute decrease with combination therapy fulfilled the criteria of noninferiority. At 1 year, mortality rates were identical (8.38% in both groups) (*JAMA* 2002;288:2130). The combination-therapy group had significantly lower rates of death and reinfarction (7.4% vs. 8.8%; $p = 0.0011$) and reinfarction (at 7 days: 2.3% vs. 3.5%). Reinfarction was associated with much higher 1-year mortality (22.6% vs. 8.0%). However, more nonintracranial bleeding complications were seen in the combination group (4.6% vs. 2.3%). The rates of intracranial hemorrhage and nonfatal disabling stroke were similar.

51. **Brenner SJ,** et al., for the **INTRO AMI** Investigators. Eptifibatide and low-dose tissue plasminogen activator in acute myocardial infarction: the Integrelin and Low-Dose Thrombolysis in Acute MI (INTRO AMI) Trial. *J Am Coll Cardiol* 2002;39:277–286.

This prospective, randomized, open-label, multicenter trial enrolled 649 patients with acute STEMI seen within 6 hours of symptom onset. In phase A, patients were randomized to eptifibatide, single or double bolus (30 minutes apart) of 180, 180/90, or 180/180 μg/kg, followed by infusion of 1.33 or 2.0 μg/kg/min (sequentially added to 25 mg or 50 mg of tPA). In phase B, patients were randomized to (a) double-bolus eptifibatide, 180/90 (30 minutes apart) and 1.33 μg/kg/min infusion with 50 mg tPA (group I); (b) 180/90 (10 minutes apart) and 2.0 g/kg/min with 50 mg tPA (group II); or (c) full-dose, weight-adjusted tPA (group III). In phase A, the highest rate of Thrombolysis In Myocardial Infarction (TIMI) flow grade 3 (primary end point) was seen with eptifibatide 180/90/1.33 and 50 mg tPA (65% and 78% at 60 and 90 minutes, respectively). In phase B, the incidence of TIMI grade 3 flow at 60 minutes was 42%, 56%, and 40%, for groups I through III, respectively ($p = 0.04$, group II vs. group III). The median corrected TIMI frame counts were 38, 33, and 50, respectively ($p = 0.02$). No differences were found between the three groups in TIMI major bleeding or intracranial hemorrhage. Mortality, reinfarction, and revascularization rates at 30 days also were similar.

52. **Giugliano RP,** et al., on behalf of the **INTEGRETI** Investigators. Combination reperfusion therapy with eptifibatide and reduced dose tenecteplase for ST-elevation myocardial infarction: results of the Integrelin and Tenecteplase in Acute Myocardial Infarction (INTEGRETI) Phase II angiographic trial. *J Am Coll Cardiol* 2003;41:1251–1260.

This prospective, randomized, open-label, multicenter trial enrolled 438 STEMI patients seen within 6 hours.

In the dose-finding phase, 189 patients were randomized to different combinations of double-bolus eptifibatide and reduced-dose TNK. In dose confirmation, 249 patients were randomized to eptifibatide, 180-μg/kg boluses, 2-μg/kg/min infusion, and a second bolus 10 minutes later (180/2/180) plus half-dose TNK (0.37 mg/kg), or standard dose (0.53 mg/kg) TNK monotherapy. All received aspirin and UFH [60-U/kg bolus and then 7 U/kg/hr (combination therapy) or 12 U/kg/hr (monotherapy)]. In dose finding, TIMI grade 3 flow rates at 60 minutes (primary end point) were similar across groups (64% to 68%). Arterial patency (TIMI grade 2 or 3 flow) was highest for eptifibatide, 180/2/180, plus TNK (96%; $p = 0.02$) vs. eptifibatide, 180/2/90, plus half-dose TNK. In dose confirmation, this combination, compared with TNK monotherapy, tended to achieve better TIMI 3 flow (59% vs. 49%; $p = 0.15$), arterial patency (85% vs. 77%; $p = 0.17$), and ST resolution (71% vs. 61%; $p = 0.08$). However, it was associated with increased rates of noncerebral major bleeding (7.6% vs. 2.5%; $p = 0.14$) and transfusion (13.4% vs. 4.2%; $p = 0.02$).

β-Blockers

53. **Norwegian Multicenter Group.** Timolol-induced reduction in mortality and re-infarction in patients surviving acute MI. *N Engl J Med* 1981;304:801–807.

Design: Prospective, randomized, double-blind, placebo-controlled, multicenter study. Mean follow-up period was 17 months. Primary end point was all-cause mortality.
Purpose: To evaluate the efficacy of long-term β-blockade after MI.
Population: 1,884 patients randomized at 7 to 28 days after AMI meeting at least two of the following criteria: (a) chest pain longer than 15 minutes, acute pulmonary edema, or cardiogenic shock; (b) pathologic Q waves and/or ST elevation followed by T-wave inversion in at least two leads; or (c) elevated serum markers.
Exclusion Criteria: HR, less than 50 beats/min; severe CHF; second- or third-degree AV block; SBP less than 100 mm Hg.
Treatment: Timolol, 10 mg twice daily, or placebo.
Results: Timolol group had a 39% lower mortality rate (13.3% vs. 21.9%; $p < 0.001$) and a 28% lower reinfarction rate (14.4% vs. 20.1%; $p < 0.001$).
Comments: Six-year follow-up showed a persistent mortality benefit of timolol (26.4% vs. 32.3%; $p = 0.003$).

54. β-Blocker Heart Attack Trial (**BHAT**) Research Group. A randomized trial of propranolol in patients with acute MI. *JAMA* 1982;247:1707–1714.

Design: Prospective, randomized, double-blind, placebo-controlled, multicenter study. Mean follow-up period was 25 months. Primary end point was all-cause mortality.
Purpose: To evaluate if long-term propranolol administration after MI reduces mortality.
Population: 3,837 patients younger than 70 years enrolled 5 to 21 days after an AMI.
Exclusion Criteria: Marked bradycardia, current β-blocker therapy, history of severe heart failure or asthma, and planned cardiac surgery.
Treatment: Propranolol, 60–80 mg, 3 times daily, or placebo.
Results: Propranolol group had 26.5% lower mortality (7.2% vs. 9.8%; $p < 0.005$), 28% fewer sudden cardiac deaths (3.3% vs. 4.6%; $p < 0.05$), and 23% fewer major

cardiac events (nonfatal MI plus fatal coronary disease). Serious side effects were infrequent.

Comments: Post hoc analysis showed that the benefit of propranolol was restricted to a high-risk group of 383 patients: 43% mortality reduction ($p < 0.01$).

55. The Metoprolol in Acute MI (**MIAMI**) Trial Research Group. Metoprolol in Acute MI (MIAMI): a randomised placebo-controlled international trial. *Eur Heart J* 1985;6:199–226.

Design: Prospective, randomized, double-blind, placebo-controlled, multicenter study. Primary end point was all-cause mortality.
Purpose: To evaluate whether metoprolol administration after MI reduces mortality.
Population: 5,728 patients younger than 75 years, seen within 24 hours of onset of symptoms (average, 7 hours).
Exclusion Criteria: Current treatment with β-blockers or calcium antagonists, and heart rate 65 beats/min or less.
Treatment: Metoprolol, 15 mg i.v., and then 200 mg/day orally, or placebo.
Results: Metoprolol group had a nonsignificant 13% mortality reduction at 15 days (4.3% vs. 4.9%). The high-risk subgroup (meeting at least three of the following criteria: older than 60 years, prior MI, ECG consistent with MI, previous angina, CHF, diabetes, taking digoxin or diuretics) had 29% lower mortality.

56. **ISIS-1** Collaborative Group. Randomised trial of intravenous atenolol among 16,107 cases of suspected acute MI. *Lancet* 1986;328:57–65.

Design: Prospective, randomized, open, parallel-group, multicenter study. Primary end point was vascular mortality at 7 days.
Purpose: To determine the effects of atenolol in MI patients on 7-day vascular mortality.
Population: 16,107 patients seen within 12 hours (average, 5 hours) of an AMI who were not taking a β-blocker or verapamil.
Exclusion Criteria: Heart rate less than 50 beats/min, SBP less than 100 mm Hg, second- or third-degree heart block, severe heart failure, and bronchospasm.
Treatment: Atenolol, 5 to 10 mg i.v., over a 5-minute period, followed by 100 mg/day orally for 7 days. No placebo was given to controls.
Results: Atenolol group had a 15% lower 7-day vascular mortality rate (3.89% vs. 4.57%; $p < 0.04$). Most of mortality difference occurred in the first 24 hours. At 1 year, the benefit persisted, with an 11% vascular mortality reduction (10.7% vs. 12.0%; $p < 0.01$). After year 1, nonsignificant excess of vascular deaths was found in the atenolol group (179 vs. 145; $p = 0.07$).
Comments: A later analysis showed that the benefit of atenolol in the first 24 hours was primarily owing to a lower rate of pulseless electrical activity, reflecting less cardiac rupture (see *Lancet* 1988;331:921).

57. **Roberts R,** et al., for the **TIMI-IIB** Investigators. Immediate vs. deferred beta-blockade following thrombolytic therapy in patients with acute MI: results of TIMI II-B. *Circulation* 1991;83:422–437.

Design: Prospective, randomized, open, parallel-group, multicenter study. Primary end point was predischarge left ventricular ejection fraction (LVEF).
Purpose: To compare immediate intravenous versus deferred (started on day 6) β-blocker in AMI patients treated with rtPA.
Population: 1,434 patients aged 75 years or younger seen within 4 hours of chest pain and with 1 mm or greater ST elevation in at least two contiguous ECG leads and having no contraindications to β-blockade. Low-risk subgroup is defined as an absence of all the following: history of MI, anterior ST elevation, rates greater than one-third up lung fields, SBP less than 100 mm Hg or cardiogenic shock, HR more than 100 beats/min, atrial fibrillation or flutter, and age 70 years or older.
Exclusion Criteria: HR less than 55 beats/min, SBP consistently less than 100 mm Hg, severe first-degree or advanced heart block, and wheezing or significant COPD.

Treatment: Immediate β-blockade group received metoprolol, 5 mg i.v., for three doses (given within 2 hours of rtPA), and then 50 to 100 mg twice daily. The deferred β-blockade group received metoprolol, 50 mg twice daily on day 6, followed by 100 mg twice daily. All patients received aspirin, heparin (intravenously for 5 days, and then subcutaneously every 12 hours), and lidocaine (1.0 to 1.5 mg/kg, and then 2.0 to 4.0 mg/min for 24 hours).

Results: No significant differences in mortality or LVEF were observed at discharge, but the subgroup of low-risk patients receiving β-blockade had a lower rate of death and nonfatal reinfarction (5.4% vs. 13. 7%; $p = 0.01$), as well as less recurrent chest pain (18.8% vs. 24.1%; $p < 0.02$).

58. **Gottlieb SS,** et al. Cooperative Cardiovascular Project. Effect of beta-blockade on mortality among high-risk and low-risk patients after MI. *N Engl J Med* 1998;339:489–497.

Design: Retrospective, observational study. Primary efficacy end point was 2-year mortality rate.

Purpose: To compare the mortality rates of patients in high- and low-risk subgroups who were treated with β-blockers with rates among those not receiving these agents.

Population: 201,752 patients from the Cooperative Cardiovascular Project data base (most discharges occurred between February 1994 and July 1995) with a principal diagnosis of AMI. Approximately two thirds of patients had relative contraindications to β-blocker administration (per ACC/AHA guidelines). Only 8,464 patients were not followed up for 24 months.

Treatment: Of patients, 34.3% received β-blockers (based on discharge prescription data).

Results: Patients with the following characteristics received β-blockers less frequently: very elderly, blacks, low EF, heart failure, COPD, elevated creatinine, or type 1 diabetes mellitus. However, mortality was lower in all of these subgroups of patients who were treated with β-blockers. Overall, 2-year mortality was 40% lower among patients without complications. Mortality also was 40% lower with β-blockers in patients with a non–Q-wave MI or COPD, whereas slightly smaller reductions (28% to 35%) were seen in those with an EF less than 20%, blacks, age older than 80 years, creatinine greater than 1.4 mg/dL, and diabetes. However, absolute mortality reduction in these latter groups was similar to or greater than that among patients with no risk factors.

59. **Dargie HJ.** Effect of carvedilol on outcome after myocardial infarction in patients with left-ventricular dysfunction: the **CAPRICORN** randomised trial. *Lancet* 2001;357:1385–1390.

Design: Prospective, randomized, placebo-controlled, multicenter trial. The primary end point was all-cause mortality or CV-related hospital admission.

Purpose: To investigate the long-term efficacy of carvedilol on morbidity and mortality in patients with LV dysfunction after AMI treated according to current evidence-based practice.

Population: 1,959 patients with AMI and a LVEF of 40% or less.

Treatment: Carvedilol (6.25 mg once daily titrated to 25 mg twice daily over 4 to 6 weeks), or placebo.

Results: No significant difference was observed between the carvedilol and placebo groups in the incidence of primary end point [35% vs. 37%; hazard ratio, 0.92 (95% CI, 0.80 to 1.07)]. However, all-cause mortality was significantly lower in the carvedilol group [12% vs. 15%; HR, 0.77 (CI, 0.60 to 0.98); $p = 0.03$]. The carvedilol group also had lower rates of cardiovascular mortality, nonfatal MI, and all-cause mortality or nonfatal MI.

60. **Hjalmarson A,** et al. Effect on mortality of metoprolol in acute MI. *Lancet* 1981;2:823–827.

A total of 1,395 patients with chest pain lasting 30 minutes or longer and ECG changes were randomized at an average of 11 hours from onset of symptoms to 15 mg i.v. and then 100 mg twice daily or placebo. MI was confirmed in 69.6% of patients. The metoprolol group had a 36% lower 90-day mortality rate (5.7% vs. 8.9%; $p < 0.03$).

61. **Ryden L,** et al. A double-blind trial of metoprolol in acute MI: effects on ventricular arrhythmias. *N Engl J Med* 1983;308:614–618.

A total of 1,395 patients with suspected MI were given metoprolol, 15 mg i.v., 50 mg every 6 hours for 2 days, and then 100 mg twice daily for 3 months. Antiarrhythmic drugs were given only for ventricular fibrillation and sustained VT. Only 58% of patients had a definite MI. The metoprolol group had less ventricular fibrillation (0.9% vs. 2.4%; $p < 0.05$) and less lidocaine use ($p < 0.01$).

62. **Soumerai SB,** et al. Adverse outcomes of underuse of β-blockers in elderly survivors of acute MI. *JAMA* 1997;227:115–121.

This large retrospective cohort study was composed of 5,332 patients; 1987 to 1992 Medicare and drug-claims data were used. Only 21% received treatment (no change in frequency from 1987 to 1991). A threefold greater likelihood of being started on calcium-channel blockers was observed. Underuse of β-blockers was predicted by use of calcium-channel blockers and increasing age. Overall, β-blocker use was associated with an adjusted 43% better survival, an effect seen in all age groups.

63. **Vantrimpoint P,** et al. Additive beneficial effects of beta-blockers to angiotensin converting enzyme inhibitors in the SAVE study. *J Am Coll Cardiol* 1997;29:229–236.

This retrospective analysis of SAVE data showed that β-blocker use was associated with a 30% lower rate of adjusted risk of cardiovascular mortality ($p = 0.002$), 21% less severe CHF ($p = 0.02$), and a nonsignificant 11% lower rate of recurrent MI. These lower rates were independent of captopril use.

Thrombolytic Therapy
Review Articles, Meta-Analyses, and Miscellaneous

64. **White HD.** Thrombolytic therapy for patients with MI presenting after six hours. *Lancet* 1992;340:221–222.

This analysis of trials with late thrombolytic administration showed a significant 12% reduction in 35-day mortality with treatment at 7 to 12 hours. A nonsignificant 6% reduction was seen with treatment at 13 to 24 hours.

65. Fibrinolytic Therapy Trialists (**FTT**) Collaborative Group. Indications for fibrinolytic therapy in suspected acute MI: collaborative overview of early mortality and major morbidity results from all randomised trials of >1000 patients. *Lancet* 1994;343:311–322.

This analysis focused on nine studies (GISSI-1, ISAM, AIMS, ISIS-2 and ISIS-3, ASSET, USIM, EMERAS, and LATE) with more than 1,000 patients (58,600 total). During days 0 and 1, the use of thrombolytics was associated with a higher mortality rate, especially in the elderly and those treated more than 12 hours after symptom onset. However, much greater benefit was seen on days 2 to 35. Thrombolytic-treated patients with ST-segment elevation or BBB had a 3% lower mortality rate when treated from 0 to 6 hours versus 2% lower at 7 to 12 hours and only 1% lower ($p = $ NS) at 13 to 18 hours.

66. **Boersma E,** et al. Early thrombolytic therapy in acute MI: reappraisal of the golden hour. *Lancet* 1996;348:771–775.

This analysis focused on 22 randomized trials enrolling 100 or more patients (total, 50,246 patients). Substantial mortality benefit (6.5% absolute reduction) was seen when a thrombolytic was given within 1 hour of onset of symptoms (vs. 2.6% at 1 to 2 hours, 2.6% at 2 to 3 hours, and 2.9% at 3 to 6 hours). Comparing those treated within 2 hours with those treated after 2 hours, the proportional mortality reduction was -44% versus -20% ($p = 0.001$). These data fit a nonlinear regression equation (i.e., most benefit early). In contrast, a similar prior analysis by the FTT Collaborative

Group (see *Lancet* 1994;343:311) had generated a linear model (1.6 additional lives per 1,000 treated patients for each hour of delay). However, their analysis included data from 4,250 patients who had unstable angina (USIM trial) and minimal or no ST elevation (ISIS-3).

67. **Krumholz HM,** et al. Thrombolytic therapy for eligible elderly patients with MI. *JAMA* 1997;277:1683–1688.

This retrospective, multicenter cohort study was composed of 753 of 3,093 MI patients aged 65 years or older with ST elevation of 1 mm or more, new LBBB, and no thrombolytic contraindications. Only 44% were administered a thrombolytic agent. Predictors of no thrombolysis were advanced age, no chest pain, seen more than 6 hours after onset of symptoms, LBBB, ST elevation less than 6 mm, presence of Q waves, ST elevation in only two leads, and altered mental status. Reasons for no thrombolysis were cited in the chart in only 19% of cases (top two reasons were delay and age). A 75% thrombolysis rate was observed if the patient had chest pain and was seen within 6 hours.

68. **Eagle KA,** et al. Practice variation and missed opportunities for reperfusion in ST-segment-elevation myocardial infarction: findings from the Global Registry of Acute Coronary Events (**GRACE**). *Lancet* 2002;359:373–377.

This study assessed current treatment practices of STEMI from prospectively collected data in the multinational (14 countries) Global Registry of Acute Coronary Events. Of 9,251 patients enrolled, 1,763 were seen within 12 hours of symptom onset with STEMI; of these, 30% did not receive reperfusion therapy. Patients less likely to receive reperfusion therapy were elderly patients (aged 75 years or older), those seen without chest pain, and those with a history of diabetes, CHF, MI, or coronary bypass surgery. A substantial percentage of eligible patients failed to receive reperfusion treatment. The United States had the highest rate of primary PCI. The rate at sites with a catheterization laboratory was only 19%.

Thrombolytic Comparative Studies
69. **TIMI-1,** The Thrombolysis in MI (TIMI) Trial. Phase I findings. *N Engl J Med* 1985;312:932–936.

Design: Prospective, randomized, double-blind, placebo-controlled, multicenter study. Primary end point was IRA patency at 90 minutes.
Purpose: To evaluate the efficacy of intravenously administered thrombolytic therapy and to compare the effects of tPA and SK.
Population: 316 patients younger than 76 years seen 7 hours or less from onset of symptoms with chest pain lasting 30 minutes or longer and ST-segment elevation in at least two ECG leads.
Treatment: Streptokinase, 1.5 million U over a 60-minute period and a 3-hour infusion of tPA placebo, or a 3-hour infusion of plasminogen activator [80 mg (40 mg in the first hour, then 20 mg for 2 hours)] and a 1-hour infusion of SK placebo.
Results: The 290 patients received treatment; 26 had a less than 50% reduction in the diameter of the IRA not treated. Among the 214 patients with total baseline occlusion, tPA achieved better reperfusion at 90 minutes: 60% versus 35% (TIMI grade 2 or 3 flow; $p < 0.001$). No significant differences in rates of bleeding events were observed.

70. Gruppo Italiano per lo Studio della Streptochinasi nell'Infarto Miocardico (**GISSI-2**). GISSI-2: a factorial randomised trial of alteplase vs. streptokinase and heparin vs. no heparin among 12,490 patients with acute MI. *Lancet* 1990;336:65–71.

Design: Prospective, randomized, open, parallel-group, 2 × 2 factorial, multicenter study. Primary end point was death, clinical heart failure, and EF 35% or less.
Purpose: To compare the efficacy of i.v. SK and tPA for the treatment of suspected acute STEMI and to study the effects of heparin on the incidence of recurrent ischemia.

Population: 12,490 patients seen within 6 hours of onset of symptoms with chest pain and 1 mm or more ST elevation in any limb lead or 2 mm or more in any precordial lead.

Treatment: (a) SK, 1.5 million U over a 30- to 60-minute period, and heparin, 12,500 U s.c. twice daily (starting 12 hours after initiation of the thrombolytic and continued through hospital discharge); (b) tPA, 10-mg bolus, and then 50 mg over 1 hour, and then 40 mg over 2 hours, and heparin, 12,500 U s.c. twice daily; (c) SK, 1.5 million U over 30 to 60 minutes without heparin; or (d) tPA, 10-mg bolus, and then 50 mg over 1 hour, and then 40 mg over 2 hours without heparin.

Results: No significant difference was observed in combined end points between SK and tPA [22.5% vs. 23.1% (mortality, 8.6% vs. 9.0%)]. No difference was observed in the rates of recurrent infarction, postinfarction angina, stroke, or bleeding. No differences were observed between heparin and no heparin, except for increased bleeding with heparin (1.0% vs. 0.6%; RR, 1.64; 95% CI, 1.09 to 2.45).

Comments: The International Study Group recruited an additional 8,401 patients (see *Lancet* 1990;336:71). Among these 20,891 patients, no difference was seen in in-hospital mortality rates (tPA, 8.9%; SK, 8.5%), but tPA was associated with a significantly higher stroke rate (1.33% vs. 0.94%).

71. **ISIS-3** Collaborative Group. A randomised comparison of streptokinase versus tissue plasminogen activator versus anistreplase and of aspirin and heparin versus aspirin alone among 41,299 cases of suspected acute MI. *Lancet* 1992;339:753–770.

Design: Prospective, randomized, double-blind (thrombolytic agents) and open-label (heparin), 3×2 factorial, multicenter study. Primary end point was 35-day mortality rate.

Purpose: To compare the effects on mortality of tPA, streptokinase, and acylated plasminogen-streptokinase activator complex (APSAC) and to compare aspirin alone with aspirin plus s.c. administered heparin.

Population: 41,299 patients with suspected MI seen within 24 hours of onset of symptoms (no ECG criteria).

Exclusion Criteria (suggested): Recent severe trauma, stroke, GI bleeding or ulcer, SK allergy.

Treatment: (a) SK, 1.5 million U over 60 minutes; (b) rtPA, 0.6 million U/kg over 4 hours (0.04 million U/kg as a bolus, 0.36 million U/kg over 1 hour, and then 0.067 million U/kg/hr for 3 hours); or (c) APSAC 30 U over 3 minutes. All patients received aspirin (162.5 mg daily), and half of the patients also received heparin, 12,500 U twice daily s.c. for 7 days (started 4 hours after initiation of thrombolytic therapy).

Results: No differences in 35-day mortality rate were seen between the three thrombolytic groups: SK, 10.6%; tPA, 10.3%; APSAC, 10.5%. The SK group did have fewer strokes (1.04% vs. 1.39% for tPA; $p < 0.01$), whereas tPA was associated with fewer reinfarctions [2.9% vs. 3.5% (SK)]. A trend toward a lower mortality difference was seen with heparin while it was being administered [7-day mortality rate, 7.4% vs. 7.9% (aspirin alone); $p = 0.06$], but this disappeared at 35-day and 6-month follow-ups. Heparin was associated with an excess of major noncerebral and cerebral hemorrhages (1.0% vs. 0.8%; $p < 0.01$; 0.56% vs. 0.40%; $p < 0.05$), but no difference was seen in the total stroke rate (1.28% vs. 1.18%).

Comments: No difference in mortality seen with tPA and SK, but questions remained because of the suboptimal heparin regimen (i.e., delayed and subcutaneous).

72. **GUSTO I.** The Global Utilization of Streptokinase and tPA for Occluded Coronary Arteries Study (GUSTO) Investigators. An international randomized trial comparing four thrombolytic strategies for acute MI. *N Engl J Med* 1993;329:673–682 (editorial, 723–724).

Design: Prospective, randomized, open label, multicenter study. Primary end point was 30-day all-cause mortality rate.

Purpose: To compare the effects of four thrombolytic regimens using SK and/or tPA.

Population: 41,021 patients seen less than 6 hours from onset of symptoms with chest pain lasting more than 20 minutes and ST elevation 1 mm or more in at least two limb leads or 2 mm or more in at least two precordial leads.

Exclusion Criteria: Prior stroke, active bleeding, prior treatment with SK or anistreplase, recent trauma or major surgery; relative contraindication was SBP 180 or greater unresponsive to therapy.

Treatment: (a) SK, 1.5 million U over 60 minutes, with s.c. heparin, 12,500 U twice daily; (b) SK, 1.5 million U over 60 minutes and i.v. heparin (5,000-U bolus and then 1,000 U/hr); (c) accelerated tPA [15-mg bolus, and then 0.75 mg/kg (maximum, 50 mg) over 30 minutes, and then 0.5 mg/kg (maximum, 35 mg) over 60 minutes] with i.v. heparin (5,000-U bolus and then 1,000 U/hr); or (d) tPA, 1.0 mg/kg over 60 minutes (10% given as a bolus; maximum dose, 90 mg), and SK, 1 million U over 60 minutes with i.v. heparin (5,000-U bolus and then 1,000 U/hr).

Results: Accelerated tPA with i.v. heparin (c) was associated with the lowest 30-day mortality rate: 6.3% (vs. 7.2%, 7.4%, and 7.0% for regimens a, b, and c), which corresponds to a 14% reduction compared with the SK-only regimens ($p = 0.001$). Despite an increased intracranial hemorrhage risk seen with tPA (0.72% vs. 0.49%, 0.54%, and 94%), tPA still was associated with a significant reduction in the combined end point of death or disabling stroke (6.9% vs. 7.8% in SK-only groups; $p = 0.006$). tPA appeared to confer a greater benefit in patients with anterior MI (8.6% vs. 10.5% mortality). A mortality benefit similar to that of tPA overall was seen in patients older than 75 years (1.3% vs. 1.1%), although limited numbers prevented the subgroup analysis from having the power to achieve statistical significance.

Comments: The mortality rate was only 4.3% in patients treated within 2 hours versus 5.5% at 2 to 4 hours and 8.9% at 4 to 6 hours. Thus time to therapy also is an important factor. A secondary analysis showed age to be a powerful mortality predictor: 3% if younger than 65 years old versus 9.5%, 19.6%, and 30.3% if 65 to 74, 75 to 85, and older than 85 years, respectively (see *Circulation* 1996;94:1826). One-year follow-up showed a persistent benefit of tPA with an increase in mortality of only 1.4% from 30 days to 1 year (see *Circulation* 1996;94:1233). Another secondary analysis showed the optimal PTT range to be 50 to 70 seconds (lowest 30-day mortality, stroke, and bleeding rates) with a clustering of reinfarctions in the first 10 hours after discontinuation of heparin (see *Circulation* 1996;93:870). Finally, a cost-effectiveness analysis (see *N Engl J Med* 1995;332:1418) showed that tPA costs $32,678 per year of life saved.

73. The **GUSTO Angiographic** Investigators. The effects of tissue plasminogen activator, streptokinase, or both on coronary artery patency, ventricular function and survival after acute MI. *N Engl J Med* 1993;329:1615–1622 (editorial, 1650–1652).

Design: Prospective, randomized, open-label, multicenter study. Primary end point was TIMI grade 2 or 3 flow at 90 minutes.

Purpose: To compare the patency rates and the effect on LV function of tPA and SK.

Population: 2,431 patients seen less than 6 hours from onset of symptoms with chest pain lasting more than 20 minutes and ST elevation 1 mm or more in at least two limb leads or 2 mm or more in at least two precordial leads.

Exclusion Criteria: See GUSTO-I trial summary.

Treatment: Four thrombolytic regimens (see GUSTO-I trial summary). Patients were then randomized to cardiac catheterization at 90 minutes, 180 minutes, 24 hours, or 5 to 7 days. The 90-minute group underwent repeated catheterization at 5 to 7 days.

Results: Highest patency (TIMI grade 2 or 3 flow) at 90 minutes was seen with tPA and intravenous heparin: 81% versus 54% with SK and s.c. heparin, 60% with SK and i.v. heparin, and 73% with combination therapy ($p < 0.001$ for tPA vs. SK groups). Normal flow (TIMI grade 3) was seen in 54% of the tPA patients versus 29%, 32%, and 38% in the other three groups. Surprisingly, the differences between the tPA and SK groups disappeared at 180 minutes. The reocclusion rate was low and similar in all four groups (4.9% to 6.4%). LV function paralleled patency at 90 minutes,

with the tPA group having better regional wall motion. Mortality also was strongly correlated with 90-minute patency: a low 4.4% with TIMI grade 3 flow versus 8.9% with grade 1 flow ($p = 0.009$).
Comments: Results support the open-artery theory asserting that early reperfusion of the IRA results in improved outcome (see accompanying editorial). A subsequent analysis of the 559 patients who underwent catheterization twice (at 90 minutes and 5 to 7 days) showed that early patency results were not predictive of reocclusion (see *J Am Coll Cardiol* 1994;24:1439). Another analysis showed that the mortality benefit of achieving 90-minute TIMI grade 3 flow was amplified beyond the initial 30 days: unadjusted mortality hazard ratio (TIMI grade 3 vs. 2 or less) from 30 days to 688 days was only 0.39 (vs. 0.57 at 30 days) (see *Circulation* 1998;97:1549).

74. **Cannon CP,** et al., **TIMI-4.** Comparison of front-loaded recombinant tissue plasminogen activator, anistreplase and combination thrombolytic therapy for acute MI. *J Am Coll Cardiol* 1994;24:1602–1610.

This prospective, double-blind, multicenter study randomized 382 patients seen within 6 hours of symptom onset to front-loaded rtPA [15-mg bolus, and then 0.75 mg/kg (maximum, 50 mg) over a 30-minute period, and then 0.50 mg/kg (max, 35 mg) over a 30-minute period]; or anistreplase, 30-U bolus over 2 to 5 minutes; or rtPA [15-mg bolus, and then 0.75 mg/kg (max, 50 mg) over 30 minutes] and anistreplase, 20-U bolus. All received i.v. heparin and aspirin. The rtPA group had higher patency (TIMI grade 2 or 3 flow) at 60 minutes: 78% versus 59% for two other groups ($p = 0.02$). Similar results were observed at 90 minutes [TIMI grade 3 flow in 60%, 43% (anistreplase only), and 44% (combination)]. No significant differences were seen in the composite primary end point, consisting of in-hospital death, severe CHF or cardiogenic shock, low EF, reinfarction, TIMI grade flow less than 2 at 90 minutes or 18 to 36 hours, reocclusion (on sestamibi imaging), major spontaneous hemorrhage, and severe anaphylaxis (rtPA, 41.3%; anistreplase, 49%; combination, 53.6%). However, the 6-week mortality rate was lowest in the rtPA group: 2.2% versus 8.8% with anistreplase ($p = 0.02$) and 7.2% with combination therapy ($p = 0.06$).

75. **Smalling RW,** et al., **RAPID.** More rapid, complete and stable coronary thrombolysis with bolus administration of reteplase compared with alteplase infusion in acute MI. *Circulation* 1995;91:2725–2732.

Design: Prospective, randomized, open-label, parallel-group, multicenter study. Primary end point was TIMI grade 2 or 3 flow at 90 minutes.
Purpose: To compare bolus administration of reteplase with a standard infusion of alteplase.
Population: 606 patients aged 18 to 75 years seen within 6 hours of onset of symptoms with chest pain lasting 30 minutes or longer and ST elevation 1 mm or more in inferior or lateral leads or 2 mm or more in precordial leads.
Treatment: (a) Reteplase, 15 million–U single bolus; (b) reteplase, 10 million–U bolus, and then 5 million–U bolus, 30 minutes later; (c) reteplase, 10 million–U bolus, and then 10 million–U bolus 30 minutes later; or (d) alteplase, given as a 6- to 10-mg bolus followed by an infusion over the first hour to a total dose of 60 mg, and then 20 mg/hr for 2 hours.
Results: Reteplase group receiving two 10 million–U boluses had better TIMI grade 3 flow than did the alteplase group at 90 minutes (63% vs. 49%) and at 5 to 14 days (88% vs. 71%). This group also had a better EF before hospital discharge (53% vs. 49%; $p = 0.034$). The incidence of bleeding complications was similar in all four treatment groups.
Comments: The results of this study demonstrate the efficacy of bolus reteplase administration, but the lack of a front-loaded alteplase regimen (used in RAPID II) was a major limitation of this trial.

76. International Joint Efficacy Comparison of Thrombolytics (**INJECT**). Randomized, double-blind comparison of reteplase double-bolus administration with streptokinase in acute MI: trial to investigate equivalence. *Lancet* 1995;346:329–336.

Design: Prospective, randomized, double-blind, double-dummy, multicenter study. Primary end point was 35-day mortality rate.

Purpose: To determine whether the effect of reteplase on 35-day mortality is at least equivalent to that of streptokinase.

Population: 6,010 patients seen within 12 hours of onset of symptoms with chest pain lasting 30 minutes or longer and ST elevation 1 mm or more in at least two of three inferior leads or leads I and aVL, 2 mm or more in at least two contiguous precordial leads, or new LBBB.

Treatment: SK, 1.5 million U over a 60-minute period, or reteplase, 10 million–U bolus, and repeated 30 minutes later. All patients received heparin for 24 hours.

Results: The 35-day mortality rates were similar: 9.0% (reteplase) and 9.5% (SK). Results show that reteplase is at least as effective as SK. Reinfarction and bleeding rates also were similar (5.0% vs. 5.4%; 0.7% vs. 1.0%), whereas the reteplase group had less atrial fibrillation (7.2% vs. 8.8%; $p < 0.05$), cardiogenic shock (4.7% vs. 6.0%; $p < 0.05$), heart failure (23.6% vs. 26.3%; $p < 0.05$), and hypotension (15.5% vs. 17.6%; $p < 0.05$).

Comments: No angiographic substudy has been conducted to confirm the high TIMI grade 3 patency achieved in the phase II study. The accompanying editorial suggests a probable lower TIMI grade 3 flow rate, especially because delay to treatment was longer in INJECT than in GUSTO.

77. **Bode C,** et al., for the **RAPID II** Investigators. Randomized comparison of coronary thrombolysis achieved with double-bolus reteplase (recombinant plasminogen activator) and front-loaded, accelerated alteplase (recombinant tissue plasminogen activator) in patients with acute MI. *Circulation* 1996;94:891–898.

Design: Prospective, randomized, open-label, parallel-group, multicenter study.

Purpose: To compare the bolus-administered thrombolytic reteplase with an accelerated infusion of alteplase on infarct-related patency and major events.

Population: 324 patients aged 18 to 75 years seen within 12 hours (from onset of symptoms to planned administration of treatment) with chest pain lasting 30 minutes or longer and ST elevation 1 mm or more in at least two of three inferior leads or lateral leads or 2 mm or more in at least two contiguous leads, or LBBB.

Treatment: Reteplase, 10 million U, over 2 to 3 minutes, and then 10 million U repeated 30 minutes later, or front-loaded alteplase. All patients received aspirin and i.v. heparin.

Results: The reteplase group had better TIMI grade 3 flow at 90 minutes (60% vs. 45%; $p = 0.01$) and 51% fewer coronary interventions (13.6% vs. 26.5%; $p < 0.01$); a greater than 50% statistically nonsignificant mortality reduction (4.1% vs. 8.4%) also was observed, as were similar rates of transfusion, hemorrhage, and stroke.

78. **GUSTO III** Investigators. A comparison of reteplase with alteplase for acute MI. *N Engl J Med* 1997;337:1118–1123 (editorial, 1159–1161).

Design: Prospective, randomized (2:1), open-label, parallel-group, multicenter study. Primary end point was 30-day mortality rate.

Purpose: To determine whether reteplase is superior to alteplase in reducing mortality in AMI.

Population: 15,059 patients seen with 30 minutes or more of continuous symptoms and within 6 hours of their onset and 1 mm or more ST elevation in at least two limb leads or 2 mm or more in precordial leads, or BBB.

Exclusion Criteria: Active bleeding, history of stroke, recent major surgery, SBP 200 mm Hg or higher or DBP 110 mm Hg or higher, and requirement for oral anticoagulation.

Treatment: Reteplase given as two 10 million–U boluses 30 minutes apart or an accelerated infusion of alteplase [15-mg bolus, and then 0.75 mg/kg (maximum, 50 mg) over a 30-minute period, and then 0.50 mg/kg (maximum, 35 mg) over 60 minutes].

Results: Reteplase and alteplase groups had similar 30-day mortality rates: 7.47% versus 7.24% ($p = 0.54$; 95% CI for absolute difference in mortality rates was -1.1%

to 0.66%). Stroke rate and combined end points of death or nonfatal, disabling stroke were both similar (1.64% vs. 1.79%; 7.89% vs. 7.91%).

Comments: Although this trial was designed as a superiority trial, the accompanying editorial points out that these results do not demonstrate equivalence according to the extremely strict COBALT trial criterion. Nonetheless, clinical equivalence of reteplase was observed in this large trial.

79. **Cannon CP,** et al., for the **TIMI-10B** Investigators. TNK-tissue plasminogen activator compared with front-loaded alteplase in acute MI. *Circulation* 1998;98: 2805–2814.

This prospective, randomized, multicenter trial was composed of 886 acute STEMI patients seen within 12 hours of onset of symptoms. Patients received TNK, 30 mg or 50 mg, or front-loaded tPA. All patients underwent immediate angiography. The 50-mg dose of TNK was discontinued early because of an increased rate of intracranial hemorrhage and was replaced by a 40-mg dose, and heparin doses were decreased. TNK, 40 mg, and tPA produced similar rates of TIMI grade 3 flow at 90 minutes (62.8% vs. 62.7%; p = NS; TNK, 30 mg, 54.3%, p = 0.035). TNK doses of 0.5 mg/kg resulted in higher TIMI grade 3 flow and lower median corrected TIMI frame counts (i.e., faster flow) than did lower doses. Lower rates of major bleeding and intracranial hemorrhage were observed after the heparin doses were lowered and titration of heparin was begun at 6 hours.

80. Assessment of the Safety and Efficacy of a New Thrombolytic: TNK-tPA (**ASSENT-2**). Single-bolus tenecteplase compared with front-loaded alteplase in acute MI: the ASSENT-2 double-blind randomized trial. *Lancet* 1999;354:716–722.

Design: Prospective, randomized, open-label, multicenter study. Primary end point was all-cause mortality at 30 days.

Purpose: To assess the efficacy and safety of TNK compared with alteplase (tPA).

Population: 16,949 patients seen within 6 hours of symptom onset with ST-segment elevations of 1 mm or more in two or more limb leads or 2 mm or more in two or more contiguous precordial leads; or new LBBB.

Treatment: TNK administered over 5 to 10 seconds (30 mg if greater than 60 kg; 35 mg if 60 to 60.9 kg; 40 mg if 70 to 79.9 kg; 45 mg if 80 to 89.9 kg; 50 mg if 90 kg or more) or accelerated infusion of tPA over a 90-minute period (100 mg or less).

Results: All-cause mortality rate at 30 days was nearly identical in the two groups: 6.18% (TNK) and 6.15% (tPA). Intracranial hemorrhage rates also were similar [0.43% (TNK), 0.44% (tPA), but fewer noncerebral bleeding complications (26.4% vs. 29.0%; p = 0.0003) and less need for blood transfusion (4.3% vs. 5.5%; p = 0.0002)] were observed with TNK. Subgroup analysis showed that the mortality rate among patients treated more than 4 hours after the onset of symptoms was significantly lower with TNK (7.1% vs. 9.2%; p = 0.018). This finding may be owing to the increased fibrin specificity of TNK.

81. The **InTIME-II** Investigators. Intravenous NPA for the treatment of infarcting myocardium early: InTIME-II, a double-blind comparison of single-bolus lanoteplase vs accelerated alteplase for the treatment of patients with acute myocardial infarction. *Eur Heart J* 2000;21:2005–2013.

This prospective, randomized, multicenter, double-blind, double-dummy trial was composed of 15,078 patients seen within 6 hours of pain and randomized in 2:1 fashion to lanoteplase, 120 IU/kg (single intravenous bolus), or tPA. The 30-day mortality rate between the two groups was statistically similar (and also met the FDA requirement for equivalence): 6.6% in the tPA group and 6.77% in the lanoteplase group. The incidence of intracranial hemorrhage was significantly higher in the nPA group (1.13% vs. 0.62; p = 0.003), whereas a trend toward a lower incidence of several secondary end points was seen, including death plus MI, recurrent MI, urgent revascularization, and severe heart failure.

82. The Assessment of the Safety and Efficacy of a New Thrombolytic Regimen (**ASSENT-3**) Investigators. Efficacy and safety of tenecteplase in combination

with enoxaparin, abciximab, or unfractionated heparin: the ASSENT-3 randomized trial in acute myocardial infarction. *Lancet* 2001;358:605–613.

Design: Prospective, randomized, open-label, multicenter trial. Primary composite end
   point at 30 days: death, in-hospital MI, or in-hospital refractory ischemia.
Purpose: To evaluate whether the combination of TNK plus enoxaparin or abciximab
   is safe and efficacious compared with tenecteplase and UFH in AMI patients.
Population: 6,095 AMI patients seen within 6 hours of symptom onset.
Treatment: Three groups: (a) full-dose TNK and enoxaparin for a maximum of 7 days;
   (b) half-dose TNK with weight-adjusted low-dose UFH and a 12-hour infusion of
   abciximab; or (c) full-dose TNK with weight-adjusted UFH for 48 hours
Results: The enoxaparin and abciximab groups had a lower incidence of the primary
   efficacy end point compared with the UFH group (11.4% and 11.1% vs. 15.4%, respectively; RR, 0.74 and 0.72; both $p < 0.001$). Similarly, the efficacy plus safety end
   point (in-hospital intracranial hemorrhage or in-hospital major bleeding complications) were significantly lower for the enoxaparin group [13.7% vs. 17.0% (UFH);
   $p = 0.0146$] and trended to be lower in the abciximab group (14.2% vs. 17.0%;
   $p = 0.057$). Among patients older than 75 years, the incidence of efficacy or safety
   events was *higher* in the abciximab group compared with the UFH group (36.9%
   vs. 28.0%; $p = 0.001$); a similar finding was seen among diabetic patients (22.3% vs.
   16.5%; $p = 0.0007$). Overall, the abciximab group had nearly twice the risk of major
   hemorrhage compared with the UFH group (4.3% vs. 2.2%; $p = 0.0002$; enoxaparin
   group, 3.0%; $p = $ NS vs. UFH).

Single-agent Studies

83. **GISSI-1.** Effectiveness of intravenous thrombolytic treatment in acute MI. *Lancet*
   1986;327:397–401.

Design: Prospective, randomized, open, parallel-group, multicenter study. Primary
   end point was 21-day mortality rate.
Purpose: To evaluate the safety and efficacy of i.v. SK in AMI and to determine whether
   any effect is dependent on the interval between onset of pain and treatment.
Population: 11,806 patients seen within 12 hours of onset of symptoms with chest pain
   and ST elevation or depression 1 mm or more in any limb lead or 2 mm or more in
   any precordial lead.
Treatment: SK, 1.5 million U over a 60-minute period.
Results: SK-treated patients had a 21-day mortality rate that was 18% lower than
   that of controls (10.7% vs. 13.0%; $p = 0.0002$). The largest mortality advantage [23%
   ($p = 0.0005$)] was associated with administration to those seen within 3 hours of
   onset of symptoms (RR, 0.74 vs. 1.19 for 9 to 12 hours). At 1 year, the mortality
   benefit persisted (17.2% vs. 19.0%; $p = 0.0008$).
Comments: The 10-year follow-up showed that the mortality benefit was still significant, with 19 lives saved/1,000 patients ($p = 0.02$) (see *Circulation* 1998;98:
   2659).

84. **ISIS-2** Collaborative Group. Randomised trial of intravenous streptokinase, oral,
   both, or neither among 17,187 cases of suspected acute MI. *Lancet* 1988;332:349–
   360.

Design: Prospective, randomized, double-blind, placebo-controlled, multicenter study.
   Primary end point was vascular mortality.
Purpose: To assess the separate and combined effects on mortality of i.v. SK and oral
   aspirin in patients with suspected AMI.
Population: 17,187 patients with suspected MI seen within 24 hours (median,
   5 hours) of onset of symptoms.
Exclusion Criteria: Any history of stroke, GI hemorrhage, or ulcer. Possible contraindications included recent trauma, severe persistent hypertension (not defined), and
   allergy to SK or aspirin.
Treatment: SK, 1.5 million U over a 60-minute period, and/or aspirin, 162.5 mg daily;
   or placebo.
Results: SK and aspirin-alone groups had 25% and 23% lower 5-week vascular mortality rates, respectively [9.2% vs. 12.0% (placebo), $p < 0.00001$; 9.4% vs. 11.8%,

$p < 0.00001$]. The SK-and-aspirin group had an even larger 42% mortality reduction (8% vs. 13.2%). Combination therapy also was effective in patients with LBBB (mortality, 14% vs. 27.7%). SK was associated with hypotension in 10% and more bleeds requiring transfusion (0.5% vs. 0.2%), but fewer strokes (0.6% vs. 0.8%). Aspirin reduced nonfatal reinfarction and stroke rates (1.0% vs. 2.0%; 0.3% vs. 0.6%).

85. Intravenous Streptokinase in Acute MI (**ISAM**) Study Group. A prospective trial of intravenous streptokinase in acute MI: mortality, morbidity and infarct size at 21 days. *N Engl J Med* 1986;314:1465–1471.

Design: Prospective, randomized, double-blind, placebo-controlled, multicenter study. Primary end point was 21-day mortality rate.

Purpose: To assess the effects of i.v. SK on 21-day mortality and to compare results in those treated within 3 hours with those treated at 3 to 6 hours.

Population: 1,741 patients aged 75 years or younger seen within 6 hours of onset of symptoms.

Treatment: SK, 1.5 million U over a 60-minute period, or placebo. All patients received heparin for 72 to 96 hours and coumadin for 3 weeks.

Results: The SK group had nonsignificant reduction in 21-day mortality (6.3% vs. 7.1%), significantly higher LVEF (56.8% vs. 53.9%), and an earlier CK-MB peak (13.9 vs. 19.2 hours). Among those treated within 3 hours, the mortality rates were lower [5.2% (SK) vs. 6.5%; $p = $ NS].

Comments: A subsequent report (see *Eur Heart J* 1990;11:885) determined that anterior MI patients treated with SK had higher EFs (50% vs. 42%; $p = 0.013$), especially those treated within 3 hours ($p = 0.004$). These differences persisted through 3-year follow-up (see *J Am Coll Cardiol* 1991;18:1610).

86. **Wilcox RG,** et al., Anglo-Scandinavian Study of Early Thrombolysis (**ASSET**). Trial of tissue plasminogen activator for mortality reduction in acute MI. *Lancet* 1988;332:525–530.

Design: Prospective, randomized, double-blind, placebo-controlled, multicenter study. Primary end point was mortality at 1 month.

Purpose: To evaluate the effects of tPA on mortality after AMI.

Population: 5,013 patients aged 18 to 75 years with suspected AMI who were treated within 5 hours of onset of symptoms.

Treatment: tPA, 10 mg bolus, followed by 50 mg over a 1-hour period, and then 20 mg/hr for 2 hours (100 mg total), or placebo.

Results: The tPA group had a 26% lower 1-month mortality rate: 7.2% vs. 9.8% [26% RRR (95% CI, 11% to 39%)]. This benefit persisted at 6 months: 10.4% vs. 13.1%. Among patients with proven MI, the mortality difference was more impressive: 12.6% versus 17.1%. The tPA group had more bleeding and more frequent bradycardia (27 vs. five patients).

87. **Topol EJ,** et al., and the Thrombolysis and Angioplasty in MI (**TAMI-6**) Study Group. A randomized trial of late reperfusion therapy for acute MI. *Circulation* 1992;85:2090–2099.

This prospective, randomized, double-blind, placebo-controlled, multicenter study enrolled 197 patients aged 75 years or younger seen 6 to 24 hours after onset of symptoms with 1 mm or more ST elevation in at least two contiguous leads. Patients received tPA over a 2-hour period [1 mg/kg over the first 60 minutes (10% as bolus; maximum, 80 mg), and then 20 mg over the second hour], or placebo. Angiography was performed within 24 hours; 71 patients had persistent IRA occlusion and met eligibility criteria for randomization to PTCA or no PTCA. Better early patency (TIMI grade 2 or 3 flow) was achieved with tPA [65% vs. 27% (placebo)], but similar rates were observed for late (6-month) patency (both 59%), in-hospital mortality, and LVEF. At 6 months, the tPA group had no increase in LV end-diastolic volume (vs. approximately 25% increase in the placebo group). PTCA patients had an 81% initial recanalization rate and improved ventricular function at 1 month, but no advantage was evident at late follow-up (no PTCA group had a 38% spontaneous recanalization rate).

88. The European MI Project (**EMIP**) Group. Prehospital thrombolytic therapy in patients with suspected MI. *N Engl J Med* 1993;329:383–389.

Prospective, randomized, double-blind, crossover, multicenter study of 5,469 patients seen within 6 hours with 1 mm or greater ST elevation in two or more limb leads or 2 mm or more in two or more precordial leads. Patients received anistreplase, 30 U, before hospitalization, followed by placebo in hospital or placebo followed by anistreplase. Trial was terminated early because of failure to reach target of 10,000 patients in a 2-year period. Patients in the prehospital group received anistreplase 55 minutes earlier on average than did those in the hospital group. Prehospital anistreplase was associated with a nonsignificant 13% overall mortality reduction (9.7% vs. 11.1%; $p = 0.08$) and a significant 16% cardiac mortality reduction (8.3% vs. 9.8%; $p = 0.049$). More adverse events [VF ($p = 0.02$), shock ($p < 0.001$), symptomatic hypotension ($p < 0.001$), bradycardia ($p = 0.001$)] occurred in the prehospital group before hospitalization, but this was offset by a higher incidence during the hospital period in the hospital group.

89. **Weaver WD,** et al., MI Triage and Intervention (**MITI**). Pre-hospital versus hospital-initiated thrombolytic therapy. *JAMA* 1993;270:1211–1216.

Design: Prospective, randomized, open, parallel-group study. Primary end point was a composite score that combined death, stroke, major bleeding, and infarct size.
Purpose: To compare prehospital and hospital initiation of thrombolytic therapy in patients with chest pain and ST-segment elevation.
Population: 360 patients aged 75 years or younger seen within 6 hours of onset of symptoms with ST elevation.
Exclusion Criteria: History of stroke, recent bleeding or surgery, SBP less than 180 mm Hg or DBP greater than 120 mm Hg.
Treatment: Prehospital or hospital administration of alteplase (100 mg over a 3-hour period) plus aspirin (325 mg).
Results: Despite earlier time to treatment in the prehospital-initiated group (77 vs. 110 minutes), no significant differences were seen in primary composite end point score ($p = 0.64$), mortality rate (5.7% vs. 8.1%; $p = 0.49$), EF, or infarct size. A secondary analysis showed that when treatment was initiated at sooner than 70 minutes, prehospital therapy was associated with a lower mortality rate (1.2% vs. 8.7%) and better EF (53% vs. 49%; $p = 0.03$). However, at 2-year follow-up (see *Am J Cardiol* 1996;78:497), the mortality benefit in this subgroup was no longer statistically significant [2% (less than 70 minutes) vs. 12%; $p = 0.12$].

90. Late Assessment of Thrombolytic Efficacy (**LATE**) Study Group. Late Assessment of Thrombolytic Efficacy study with alteplase 6–24 hours after onset of MI. *Lancet* 1993;342:759–766.

Design: Prospective, randomized, double-blind, placebo-controlled, multicenter study. Primary end point was 35-day mortality rate.
Purpose: To compare administration of alteplase with placebo in AMI patients seen at 6 to 24 hours.
Population: 5,711 patients seen 6 to 24 hours after onset of symptoms with 1 mm or more ST elevation in at least two limb leads, 2 mm or more ST elevation in at least two precordial leads, ST depression 2 mm or more in at least two leads, pathologic Q waves, or abnormal T-wave inversion in at least two leads thought to represent a non–Q-wave infarct.
Treatment: Alteplase, 100 mg over a 3-hour period (10-mg bolus, 50 mg for 1 hour, 20 mg/hr for 2 hours); or placebo.
Results: Intention-to-treat analysis showed a nonsignificant 14% 35-day mortality reduction in the alteplase group (8.9% vs. 10.3%). However, prespecified survival analysis according to treatment within 12 hours showed that the alteplase group had a 25.6% mortality reduction (8.9% vs. 11.9%; $p = 0.023$). Treatment for 12 to 24 hours was associated with a nonsignificant 5% mortality reduction (8.7% vs. 9.2%). Alteplase was not associated with a higher cardiac rupture rate, but rather earlier occurrence of rupture (within 24 hours after thrombolysis).

91. **Rawles J,** et al., on behalf of the Grampian Region Early Anistreplase Trial (**GREAT**) Group. Halving of mortality at one year by domiciliary thrombolysis in the GREAT. *J Am Coll Cardiol* 1994;23:1–5.

Design: Prospective, randomized, double-blind, parallel-group, multicenter study.

Purpose: To evaluate the feasibility, safety, and efficacy of home-administered thrombolysis by general practitioners compared with hospital thrombolysis.

Population: 311 patients with suspected MI seen by their general practitioners within 4 hours of symptom onset (ECG recordings required but not reported).

Treatment: Anistreplase, 30 U, at home or in hospital.

Results: Home-administered anistreplase was given more than 2 hours sooner, at a median 101 versus 240 minutes. The home-treated group had a 52% lower 1-year mortality rate (10.4% vs. 21.6%; $p = 0.007$).

Comments: Subsequent analysis showed the highest mortality rate in those randomized earliest. However, among patients at 2 hours, a 2.1% higher 30-day mortality per hour delay to thrombolytic therapy and a 6.9% higher 30-month mortality per hour delay were observed (see *BMJ* 1996;312:212).

92. The Continuous Infusion versus Double-Bolus Administration of Alteplase (**COBALT**) Investigators. A comparison of continuous infusion of alteplase with double-bolus administration for acute MI. *N Engl J Med* 1997;337:1124–1130 (editorial, 1159–1161).

Design: Prospective, randomized, open, multicenter study. Primary end point was 30-day mortality rate.

Purpose: To compare an accelerated infusion of alteplase over a 90-minute period with a two-bolus regimen in patients with AMI.

Population: 7,169 patients seen within 6 hours of symptom onset with 1 mm or more ST elevation in at least two limb leads and/or 2 mm or more in at least two contiguous precordial leads.

Treatment: Front-loaded alteplase [15-mg bolus, and then 0.75 mg/kg over a 30-minute period (maximum, 50 mg) and 0.50 mg/kg over final the 60 minutes (maximum, 35 mg)] or bolus regimen [50 mg over 1 to 3 minutes followed by 50 mg, 30 minutes later (or 40 mg if greater than 60 kg)]. Adjunctive therapy included aspirin and i.v. heparin (goal aPTT, 60 to 85 seconds).

Results: Double-bolus group had a 0.44% higher 30-day mortality rate (7.98% vs. 7.53%). The upper boundary of the 95% CI was +1.48%, which exceeded the prespecified upper limit of 0.40% to indicate equivalence. The double-bolus group also had statistically nonsignificant higher rates of stroke and hemorrhagic stroke (1.92% vs. 1.53%; $p = 0.24$; 1.12% vs. 0.81%).

Comments: Editorial points out that the definition of equivalence used was very strict because a sample size of 50,000 patients is required to rule out, with 80% power, an excess mortality of 0.4% when the true mortality rates are identical and in the 7.5% range.

93. **Morrow DA,** et al. Evaluation of the time saved by prehospital initiation of reteplase for ST-elevation myocardial infarction: results of The Early Retavase-Thrombolysis in Myocardial Infarction (**ER-TIMI 19**) trial. *J Am Coll Cardiol* 2002;40:71–77.

Design: Prospective, randomized, controlled, open, multicenter trial. Time from emergency medical service (EMS) arrival to fibrinolytic administration was compared between study patients receiving prehospital rPA and sequential control patients from 6 to 12 months before the study who received a fibrinolytic in the hospital.

Purpose: To test the feasibility of prehospital initiation of the bolus fibrinolytic reteplase and determine the time saved by prehospital rPA in the setting of contemporary emergency cardiac care.

Population: 315 patients with STEMI at 20 North American emergency medical systems; 630 controls were treated in-hospital with fibrinolytic therapy.

Treatment: Prehospital administration of reteplase (10 U over a 2-minute period followed by second bolus 30 minutes later, either in ambulance or in ED). All received aspirin and i.v. UFH [60-U/kg bolus (maximum, 4,000 U), and then 12 U/kg/hr (maximum, 800 U/hr)].

Results: AMI was verified in 98%. The median time from EMS arrival to initiation of reteplase was 31 minutes. The time from EMS arrival to in-hospital fibrinolytic for 630 control patients was 63 minutes, resulting in a time saved of 32 minutes ($p < 0.0001$). By 30 minutes after first medical contact, 49% of study patients had received the first bolus of fibrinolytic compared with only 5% of controls ($p < 0.0001$). In-hospital mortality was 4.7%. Intracranial hemorrhage occurred in 1.0%.

94. **Kennedy JW,** et al. Western Washington randomized trial of intracoronary streptokinase in acute MI. *N Engl J Med* 1985;312:1073–1078.

This early trial used intracoronary SK (4,000 U/min started at average 4.5 hours; average dose, 286,000 U). SK was beneficial in patients in whom reperfusion occurred (1-year mortality rate, 2.5% vs. 17%).

95. **White HD,** et al. Effect of intravenous streptokinase on left ventricular function and early survival after acute MI. *N Engl J Med* 1987;317:850–855.

This randomized, double-blind trial was composed of 219 patients with first MIs seen within 4 hours of onset of symptoms and treated with 1.5 million U of SK over a 30-minute period or placebo. All patients were given i.v. heparin for 48 hours, aspirin, and dipyridamole. At 3 weeks, the SK group had increased LVEF (primary end point): 59% vs. 53%; $p < 0.005$. The SK group also had a significantly lower mortality rate (2.5% vs. 12.9%; $p = 0.012$).

96. **Carney RJ,** et al. Randomized angiographic trial of recombinant tissue-type plasminogen activator (alteplase) in MI. *J Am Coll Cardiol* 1992;20:17–23.

This study demonstrated that the commonly used accelerated tPA regimen safely achieves more rapid reperfusion. The 281 patients were randomized in open fashion to a standard regimen (initial 10-mg bolus, and then 50 mg over a 1-hour period, and then 20 mg/hr for 2 hours) or an accelerated regimen (15-mg bolus, 50 mg over a 30-minute period, and then 35 mg over a 60-minute period). The accelerated tPA group had better patency at 60 minutes (76% vs. 63%; $p = 0.03$) but not at 90 minutes (81% vs. 77%; $p = 0.21$). Similar rates of recurrent ischemia, reinfarction, stroke, and bleeding were observed.

Percutaneous Coronary Intervention
Operator and Hospital Volume Studies

97. **Thiemann DR,** et al. The association between hospital volume and survival after acute myocardial infarction in elderly patients. *N Engl J Med* 1999;340:1640.

This retrospective cohort analysis focused on 98,898 Medicare patients aged 65 years or older with a principal discharge diagnosis of AMI. Patients admitted to hospitals in the lowest quartile of volume of invasive procedures had a 17% higher in-hospital mortality rate compared with patients at highest-volume-quartile hospitals (HR, 1.17; 95% CI, 1.09 to 1.26; $p < 0.001$).

98. **Magid DJ,** et al. Relation between hospital primary angioplasty volume and mortality for patients with acute MI treated with primary angioplasty vs thrombolytic therapy. *JAMA* 2000;284:3131–3138.

This retrospective cohort study analyzed 62,299 AMI patients at 446 acute care hospitals treated with primary angioplasty or thrombolytic therapy from June 1994 to July 1999. At hospitals with intermediate volume (17 to 48 procedures/year) and high volume (more than 49 procedures), mortality was significantly lower among patients undergoing angioplasty compared with thrombolysis (4.5% vs. 5.9%; $p < 0.001$; 3.4% vs. 5.4%; $p < 0.001$). At low-volume hospitals, no significant difference in mortality was found between the two treatment modalities (6.2% vs. 5.9%; $p = 0.58$).

99. **Vakili BA,** et al. Volume-outcome relation for physicians and hospitals performing angioplasty for acute myocardial infarction in New York state. *Circulation* 2001;104:2171–2176.

This analysis examined 1,342 patients who underwent angioplasty procedures within 23 hours of onset of AMI without preceding thrombolytic therapy. Primary PTCA performed by a high-volume operator (11 or more cases/year) was associated with a 57% lower in-hospital mortality compared with those treated by low-volume operators (one to ten cases/year; adjusted RR, 0.43; 95% CI, 0.21 to 0.83). Primary PTCA performed in high-volume hospitals (57 or more cases/year) resulted in a 44% in-hospital mortality reduction compared with that in low-volume hospitals (adjusted RR, 0.56; 95% CI, 0.29 to 1.1).

Meta-Analyses of Percutaneous Transluminal Coronary Angioplasty versus Thrombolysis

100. **Weaver WD,** et al. Comparison of primary coronary angioplasty and intravenous thrombolytic therapy for acute MI: a quantitative review. *JAMA* 1997;278:2093–2098.

Data analysis from 10 randomized trials with a total of 2,606 patients. Mortality at 30 days or less was significantly lower in patients treated with primary PTCA compared with thrombolysis (4.4% vs. 6.5%; OR, 0.66; 95% CI, 0.46 to 0.94; $p = 0.02$). Primary PTCA also was associated with lower rates of reinfarction [7.2% vs. 11.9%, or 0.58% (95% CI, 0.44 to 0.75); $p < 0.001$]. Authors point out that the primary angioplasty results were primarily achieved in specialized, high-volume centers.

101. **Keeley EC,** et al. Primary angioplasty versus intravenous thrombolytic therapy for acute myocardial infarction: a quantitative review of 23 randomised trials. *Lancet* 2003;361:13–20.

This analysis identified 23 studies with a total of 7,739 patients. Streptokinase was used in eight trials ($n = 1,837$), and fibrin-specific agents in 15 ($n = 5,902$). Stents were used in 12 trials. Primary PTCA had lower short-term mortality compared with thrombolytic therapy (7% vs. 9%; $p = 0.0002$), nonfatal MI (3% vs. 7%; $p < 0.0001$), and stroke (1% vs. 2%; $p = 0.0004$). Results with primary PTCA remained better during long-term follow-up.

Primary Angioplasty

102. **Grines CL,** et al. Primary Angioplasty in MI **(PAMI).** A comparison of immediate angioplasty with thrombolytic therapy for acute MI. *N Engl J Med* 1993;328:673–679 (editorial, 726–728).

Design: Prospective, randomized, open, multicenter study. End points included in-hospital death, reinfarction, and intracranial bleeding and EF at 6 weeks.
Purpose: To compare immediate PTCA with thrombolytic therapy in AMI.
Population: 395 patients seen within 12 hours of ischemic pain with 1 mm or more ST elevation in at least two contiguous ECG leads.
Exclusion Criteria: Complete LBBB, cardiogenic shock, and increased bleeding risk.
Treatment: tPA, 100 mg i.v. (or 1.25 mg/kg if patient weighed less than 65 kg) over a 3-hour period; or immediate PTCA. All patients received i.v. heparin for 3 to 5 days.
Results: A 97% PTCA success rate was observed. The PTCA group had a 60% lower in-hospital mortality rate (2.6% vs. 6.5%; $p = 0.06$) and a significant 58% reduction in in-hospital death or reinfarction (5.1% vs. 12.0%; $p = 0.02$). The PTCA group also had less intracranial bleeding (none vs. 2.0%; $p = 0.05$). No difference was seen between groups in EF at 6 weeks (both at rest and during exercise). The benefits of primary angioplasty were maintained at 2-year follow-up: lower incidence of death or MI (14.9% vs. 23%; $p = 0.034$), less recurrent ischemia (36.4% vs. 48%; $p = 0.026$), lower reintervention rates (27.2% vs. 46.5%; $p < 0.0001$), and lower rehospitalization rates (58.5% vs. 69.0%; $p = 0.035$) (see *Circulation* 1999;33:640).
Comments: A short randomization to balloon time was observed (average, 60 minutes vs. 42 minutes for door-to-thrombolysis time). Editorial asserts that high-risk

patients are most likely to benefit from immediate PTCA (e.g., older than 75 years, anterior MI, cardiogenic shock).

103. **Every NR,** et al., for the MI Triage and Intervention **(MITI)** Investigators. A comparison of thrombolytic therapy with primary coronary angioplasty for acute MI. *N Engl J Med* 1996;335:1253–1260.

Design: Retrospective cohort analysis of MITI Registry (19 Seattle-area hospitals, 10 with primary angioplasty capability).
Purpose: To compare outcomes in AMI patients receiving thrombolytic therapy and primary angioplasty.
Population: 3,145 MITI patients (thrombolytic group, $n = 2,095$; PTCA group, $n = 1,050$) treated between 1988 and 1994.
Exclusion Criteria: Lack of ECG data and angioplasty more than 6 hours after admission.
Treatment: Thrombolysis with alteplase (65%), SK (32%), or urokinase (3%; 8% were treated before hospitalization); or coronary angiography within 6 hours of admission followed by angioplasty if indicated.
Results: No significant differences were observed between thrombolysis and PTCA in the in-hospital [5.6% (thrombolytic) vs. 5.5%] or 3-year mortality rates. At 3-year follow-up, the thrombolysis group had 30% less coronary angiography, 15% fewer coronary angioplasties, and 13% lower costs. Thrombolysis patients were treated faster (1 vs. 1.7 hours after arrival) and sooner after chest pain than the PAMI thrombolysis group (198 vs. 230 minutes). Low-volume-PTCA hospitals did provide later treatment (2.3 vs. 1.5 hours) and had higher in-hospital mortality rates (8.1% vs. 4.5%).

104. **GUSTO IIb** Angioplasty Substudy. The Global Use of Strategies To Open occluded arteries in acute coronary syndromes: Angioplasty Substudy Investigators. *N Engl J Med* 1997;336:1621–1628.

Design: Prospective, randomized, open, multicenter substudy (57 sites; all performed 200 angioplasties/yr, with one operator doing 50/yr). Thirty-day primary end point was death, MI, and stroke.
Purpose: To compare thrombolytic therapy with primary angioplasty in patients with acute STEMI.
Population: 1,138 patients seen within 12 hours of STEMI.
Exclusion Criteria: Same as main GUSTO-IIb trial.
Treatment: Accelerated tPA [15-mg i.v. bolus, and then 0.75 mg/kg over a 30-minute period (maximum, 50 mg), 0.50 mg/kg over a 60-minute period (maximum, 35 mg)] or primary angioplasty (average door-to-balloon time, 1.9 hours).
Results: PTCA group had one-third lower rate of death, MI, and stroke (OR, 0.67; 9.6% vs. 13.7%; $p = 0.033$). Most of the observed benefit occurred from days 5 to 10. By 6 months, the difference was no longer significant (14% vs. 16%). Breakdown by end point (at 30 days): death, 5.7% versus 7% ($p = 0.37$); MI, 4.5% versus 6.5% ($p = 0.13$); stroke, 0.2% versus 0.9% ($p = 0.11$). PTCA was not associated with any extra benefit in high-risk groups. PTCA achieved TIMI grade 3 flow in a surprisingly low 73% of cases (technical success rate, 93%), which was associated with a 1.6% mortality rate (vs. 21.4%, 14.3%, 19.9% for TIMI flow grades 0 to 2).

105. **Brener SJ,** et al., on behalf of the Reopro and Primary PTCA Organization and Randomized Trial **(RAPPORT)** Investigators. Randomized, placebo-controlled trial of primary glycoprotein IIb/IIIa blockade with primary angioplasty for acute MI. *Circulation* 1998;98:734–741.

Design: Prospective, randomized, double-blind, placebo-controlled, multicenter study. Primary end point was death, MI, and any TVR at 6 months.
Purpose: To evaluate whether platelet IIb/IIIa receptor blockade with abciximab reduces ischemic events in AMI patients undergoing primary angioplasty.
Population: 483 patients seen within 12 hours of onset of symptoms with ischemic chest pain lasting more than 20 minutes accompanied by significant ST elevation in at least two contiguous leads or new LBBB.

Treatment: Abciximab, 0.25-mg/kg bolus, and then 0.125 μg/kg/min (maximum, 10 μg/min) for 12 hours. All patients received aspirin and heparin, 100-U/kg bolus before PTCA (with further boluses as needed to keep activated clotting time more than 300 seconds). Stenting was discouraged but was allowed for residual dissection with 50% restenosis and for abrupt or threatened closure.

Results: No difference was observed between the two groups in incidence of 6-month primary end point (28.1% vs. 28.2%). However, the abciximab group had less death, MI, and urgent TVR at 7 days (3.3% vs. 9.9%; $p = 0.003$), 30 days (5.8% vs. 11.2%; $p = 0.03$), and 6 months (11.6% vs. 17.8%; $p = 0.05$). The abciximab group had 42% less bailout stenting (11.9% vs. 20.4%; $p = 0.008$). Abciximab was associated with increased major bleeding (defined as a hematocrit decrease of more than 5%; 16.6% vs. 9.5%; $p = 0.02$), mostly at the arterial access site. On-treatment analysis showed that abciximab was associated with decreased death and MI at 7 days (1.4% vs. 4.7%; $p = 0.047$) with a trend at 6 months (6.9% vs. 12%; $p = 0.07$).

Comments: Low-risk population (30-day mortality rates, approximately 2%) may have attenuated the impact of abciximab. Increased bleeding with abciximab was likely due to the double-blind design because the investigators were unwilling to discontinue heparin immediately after the procedure(s) for early sheath removal.

106. **Grines CL,** et al. A randomized trial of transfer for primary angioplasty vs. on-site thrombolysis in patients with high risk myocardial infarction: the **Air PAMI** Study. *J Am Coll Cardiol* 2002;39:1713–1719.

Design: Prospective, randomized, open, multicenter study. Primary end point was a 30-day composite of death, recurrent MI, and disabling stroke.

Purpose: To evaluate whether early transfer for primary PTCA of AMI results in better outcomes than on-site thrombolysis.

Population: High-risk MI patients (older than 70 years, anterior MI, Killip class II/III, heart rate more than 100 beats/min, or SBP less than 100 mm Hg) who were eligible for thrombolytic therapy and seen in hospitals without on-site PCI.

Treatment: On-site thrombolysis or emergency transfer for primary PCI.

Results: Because of slow recruitment, the study was terminated after 138 patients enrolled (32% of the projected sample size). Median door-to-therapy time was 51 minutes in the thrombolytic group and 155 minutes in the transfer group. The long delay in the transfer group was mostly due to initiation of transfer (43 minutes) and transport time (26 minutes), as time from arrival in hospital to catheterization laboratory was 11 minutes, and catheterization laboratory arrival to treatment was only 14 minutes. No deaths occurred during transfer. In the transfer group, all patients underwent catheterization, and 89% had primary PCI. At 30-day follow-up, a nonsignificant 38% reduction in the primary composite end point in the transfer group was found compared with the thrombolytic group (8.4% vs. 13.6%; $p = 0.331$). Multivariate logistic regression analysis identified randomization to transfer as independent predictor of a reduction in the primary end point (OR, 0.159; 95% CI, 0.031 to 0.820; $p = 0.028$). The transfer group had a reduced hospital stay (6.1 vs. 7.5 days; $p = 0.015$) and less ischemia (12.7% vs. 31.8%; $p = 0.007$).

107. **Aversano T,** et al. Atlantic Cardiovascular Patient Outcomes Research Team **(C-PORT).** Thrombolytic therapy vs primary percutaneous coronary intervention for myocardial infarction in patients presenting to hospitals without on-site cardiac surgery: a randomized controlled trial. *JAMA* 2002;287:1943–1951.

Design: Prospective, randomized trial conducted from July 1996 through December 1999 at 11 community hospitals without on-site cardiac surgery or existing PCI programs. Primary end point at 6 months was death, recurrent MI, or stroke.

Purpose: To determine whether treatment of acute MI with primary PCI is superior to thrombolytic therapy at hospitals without on-site cardiac surgery.

Population: 451 thrombolytic-eligible patients with acute STEMI seen within 12 hours of symptom onset.

Exclusion Criteria: Included those ineligible for thrombolytic therapy.

Treatment: Primary PCI program was developed at all sites. Patients were randomized to receive primary PCI or accelerated tPA.

Results: The primary PCI group had a significantly lower incidence of the primary composite end point at 6 weeks (10.7% vs. 17.7%; $p = 0.03$) and 6 months (12.4% vs. 19.9%; $p = 0.03$). The benefit was primarily driven by a lower incidence of recurrent MI (at 6 months: 5.3% vs. 10.6%; $p = 0.04$). Mortality rates were similar (6.2% vs. 7.1%; $p = 0.72$), whereas stroke occurred in 2.2% and 4.0%, respectively ($p = 0.28$). The primary PCI group also had a shorter median length of stay (4.5 vs. 6.0 days; $p = 0.02$).

108. **DANAMI-2** (Danish Trial in Acute Myocardial Infarction-2). Preliminary results presented at the 51st ACC Annual Scientific Session, Atlanta, GA, March 2002.

Design: Prospective, randomized, open, multicenter trial. Primary end point at 30 days: death, clinical reinfarction, or significant disabling stroke.

Purpose: The invasive strategy is superior to the conservative, thrombolytic strategy in treatment of STEMI. The invasive strategy will be superior both in patients seen at on-site interventional facilities (no transfer of patient required) and without (transfer of patient required).

Population: 1,572 patients seen within 12 hours with a sum of greater than 4-mm ST elevation in all leads.

Exclusion Criteria: Included contraindications to thrombolytic therapy, expected time between randomization and arrival in catheterization laboratory longer than 3 hours for patients randomized in referral hospitals, and more than 2 hours in invasive-equipped hospitals.

Treatment: Primary PCI or front-loaded tPA. PCI patients were transferred to referring center if catheterization laboratory facilities were not available on-site. All received aspirin (300 mg, and then 75 to 150 mg daily) and heparin (5,000 U bolus + 1,000 U/hr infusion for at least 48 hours in patients randomized to tPA; 10,000-U initial bolus + additional heparin to keep the ACT between 350 and 450 seconds during the procedure in patients randomized to PCI).

Results: The trial was terminated early because of a clear benefit for PCI. The PCI group had 45% reduction in the primary composite end point compared with the fibrinolytic group (8.0% vs. 13.7%; $p = 0.0003$), primarily because of a lower incidence of recurrent MI (6.3% vs. 1.6%; $p < 0.0001$). The 30-day mortality was 7.6% in the fibrinolysis group versus 6.6% in the PCI group ($p = 0.35$), and disabling stroke occurred in 2.0% and 1.1% ($p = 0.15$), respectively. A similar benefit with PCI was seen in patients who were transferred and those who were not transferred (time difference to balloon inflation between the referred and on-site patients was only 10 minutes).

109. **PRAGUE-2, Widimsky P,** et al. Long distance transport for primary angioplasty vs immediate thrombolysis in acute myocardial infarction. *Eur Heart J* 2003;24:94–104.

This prospective, randomized trial enrolled 850 patients with acute STEMI seen within 12 hours in a community hospital and compared on-site thrombolysis (SK) with transfer for primary PCI. Exclusion criteria included contraindications to thrombolytic therapy and failure to initiate transfer within 30 minutes. Routine glycoprotein IIb/IIIa receptor antagonists before planned PCI was not used. At 30 days, mortality rates were not significantly different [10.4% (thrombolysis) vs. 6.0% (PCI); $p < 0.05$]. However, among those seen at 3 to 12 hours (vs. less than 3 hours), the PCI group had a stronger relative mortality reduction (6% vs. 15.3%; $p < 0.02$). The incidence of death, MI, and stroke also was significantly lower in the PCI group (8.4% vs. 15.2%; $p < 0.003$).

110. **O'Neill W,** et al. A prospective randomized clinical trial of intracoronary streptokinase versus coronary angioplasty for acute MI. *N Engl J Med* 1986;314:812–818.

In this first randomized trial of angioplasty versus thrombolysis (albeit intracoronary), only 56 patients were enrolled, all younger than 75 years and with symptoms for less than 12 hours. No differences were seen in the recanalization rate (83% vs. 85%), but the angioplasty group had decreased residual stenosis (43% vs. 83%) and significant EF improvement ($+8\%$ vs. $+1\%$; $p < 0.001$).

111. **Zijlstra F,** et al. A comparison of immediate angioplasty with intravenous streptokinase in acute MI. *N Engl J Med* 1993;328:680–684.

In this randomized trial of 142 patients seen within 6 hours of onset of pain, patients were randomized to balloon angioplasty or SK, 1.5 million U over a 60-minute period. The angioplasty group had a lower reinfarction rate (none vs. 12.5%) and higher EF by discharge (51% vs. 45%; $p = 0.004$).

112. **Gibbons RJ,** et al. Immediate angioplasty compared with the administration of a thrombolytic agent followed by conservative treatment for MI. *N Engl J Med* 1993;328:685–691.

In this small randomized trial of 108 patients seen within 12 hours of chest pain, the PTCA group did not have better myocardial salvage (by technetium 99 scan) nor were any differences in EF or mortality rate observed. However, PTCA patients did have a shorter stay (7.7 vs. 10.6 days; $p = 0.01$) and less rehospitalization (in first 6 months, 4% vs. 18%).

113. **Tiefenbrunn AJ,** et al. Clinical experience with primary percutaneous transluminal coronary angioplasty compared with alteplase (recombinant tissue-type plasminogen activator) in patients with acute MI: a report from the Second National Registry of MI (**NRMI-2**). *J Am Coll Cardiol* 1998;31:1240–1245.

This analysis showed that the outcomes of PTCA and rtPA are comparable in thrombolysis-eligible patients not in cardiogenic shock. Data were from 4,939 nontransfer primary PTCA patients treated within 12 hours of symptom onset and 24,705 rtPA-treated patients. Longer delay to treatment was seen in the PTCA group: 111 minutes (door to balloon) versus 42 minutes ($p < 0.0001$). Cardiogenic shock patients did better with PTCA: in-hospital mortality rate 32% versus 52% ($p < 0.0001$). A similar mortality rate was observed among thrombolytic-eligible patients not in cardiogenic shock [5.4% (rtPA) vs. 5.2%]. A higher stroke rate was observed in the thrombolytic group (1.6% vs. 0.7%; $p < 0.0001$), but no difference in combined incidence of death and nonfatal stroke (6.2% vs. 5.6%). No significant differences in reinfarction rates were found (2.9% vs. 2.5%).

Percutaneous Transluminal Coronary Angioplasty after Thrombolysis
114. **Topol EJ,** et al., and the Thrombolysis and Angioplasty in MI (**TAMI**) Study Group. A randomized trial of immediate versus delayed elective angioplasty after intravenous tissue plasminogen activator in acute MI. *N Engl J Med* 1987;317: 581–588 (editorial, 624–626).

Design: Prospective, randomized, multicenter study. Primary end point was infarct-related vessel patency and global LV function.
Purpose: To compare immediate with delayed elective angioplasty in patients undergoing thrombolysis for AMI.
Population: 386 patients met initial criteria (75 years or younger, within 6 hours of onset of symptoms, and 1 mm or more ST elevation in at least two contiguous leads); 197 patients had appropriate catheterization findings (i.e., lesions amenable to angioplasty) and were randomized to immediate or delayed angioplasty.
Exclusion Criteria: Contraindications related to angiographic findings included more than 50% left main stenosis, severe/diffuse disease, and infarct-related vessel unidentifiable.
Treatment: Predominantly single-chain tPA, 150 mg i.v. over a 6- to 8-hour period followed by angiography with either immediate angioplasty or deferred angioplasty (latter performed at 7 to 10 days and if indicated). The immediate group also had angiography at 7 to 10 days to assess for reocclusion and LV function.
Results: Immediate PTCA success rate was 86%. Similar reocclusion rates were observed [11% (immediate) vs. 13%]. Neither group had an improvement in global LV function. In the delayed group, 14% did not require angioplasty (residual stenosis

less than 50%), but a higher crossover rate was found to emergency angioplasty (16% vs. 5%). Immediate angioplasty had its own risks: Seven of nine patients with abrupt closure required emergency CABG surgery.

115. **Rogers WJ**, et al., for the **TIMI-IIA** Investigators. Comparison of immediate invasive, delayed invasive and conservative strategies after tissue-type plasminogen activator. *Circulation* 1990;81:1457–1476.

Design: Prospective, randomized, open, multicenter study. Primary end point was predischarge LVEF.
Purpose: To compare immediate versus delayed (at 18 to 48 hours) PTCA or CABG versus conservative treatment in AMI patients treated with tPA.
Population: 586 patients 75 years or younger seen within 4 hours of chest pain and with 1 mm or more ST elevation in at least two contiguous ECG leads.
Treatment: All patients received tPA [first 195 patients, 150 mg over a 6-hour period; next 391 patients, 100 mg over a 6-hour period (6-mg bolus, and then 54 mg over the first hour, 20 mg in the second hour, and 5 mg/hr for 4 hours)]; 195 underwent immediate invasive treatment, 194, delayed invasive treatment, and 197, conservative treatment [angiography ± angioplasty allowed with ischemic symptoms (spontaneous or provoked with testing)]. All patients received heparin for 5 days.
Results: All groups had similar predischarge LVEF (average, 49.3%) and IRA patency (TIMI grade 2 or 3 flow; mean, 83.7%). The immediate invasive group had a significantly higher CABG rate [7.7% vs. 2.1% (delayed invasive) vs. 2.5% (conservative); $p < 0.01$], and more transfusions were required among non-CABG patients (13.8% vs. 3.1% vs. 2.0%). Similar 1-year mortality rates were observed despite higher PTCA rates in immediate and delayed invasive groups (76% vs. 64% vs. 24%).

116. **Califf RM**, et al., for the **TAMI** Study Group. Evaluation of combination thrombolytic therapy and timing of cardiac catheterization in acute MI. *Circulation* 1991;83:1543–1556.

Design: Prospective, randomized, open, parallel-group, factorial (3×2), multicenter study. Primary end point was global LVEF.
Purpose: To evaluate combination thrombolytic therapy by comparison with monotherapy and to compare an aggressive with a deferred angiography strategy.
Population: 575 patients aged 75 years or younger seen within 6 hours of symptoms and with greater than 1 mm ST elevation in at least two contiguous ECG leads.
Treatment: Urokinase (1.5 million-U i.v. bolus, and then 1.5 million U over a 60-minute period), rtPA [100 mg over a 3-hour period (6-mg i.v. bolus, 60 mg over a 1-hour period, 20 mg/hr for 2 hours)], or combination therapy [urokinase, 1.5 million U over a 1-hour period and rtPA, 1 mg/kg, over a 1-hour period (10% as i.v. bolus; maximum dose, 90 mg)]. Aggressive strategy consisted of immediate angiography, whereas deferred strategy involved angiography before discharge (days 5 to 10).
Results: Global LVEF was well preserved and nearly identical at predischarge angiography (54%), regardless of thrombolytic or catheterization strategy. Combination thrombolysis resulted in higher 90-minute patency: TIMI grade 2 or 3 flow in 76% [tPA, 71% (p = NS); urokinase, 62% (p = 0.049)]. Less reocclusion [2% vs. 12% (p = 0.04) and 7% (p = NS)] and recurrent ischemia (25% vs. 31% vs. 35%) were observed. An aggressive strategy yielded better results with fewer adverse outcomes: death, stroke, reinfarction, heart failure, or recurrent ischemia in 55% versus 67% (p = 0.004), as well as a trend toward a higher predischarge patency rate (94% vs. 90%; p = 0.065).

117. Should We Intervene Following Thrombolysis **(SWIFT)** Trial Study Group. SWIFT trial of delayed elective intervention vs conservative treatment after thrombolysis with anistreplase in acute MI. *BMJ* 1991;302:555–560.

In this prospective, multicenter (n = 21) trial of 800 patients younger than 70 years, patients randomized to early angiography and appropriate intervention (PTCA, 43%; CABG, 15%) or conservative care [PTCA, 2.5%; CABG, 1.7% (initial admission)]. All patients were treated with anistreplase, 30 U over a 5-minute period. No differences in 1-year mortality (5.8% vs. 5%) and reinfarction rates (15% vs. 13%) were observed. Intervention group did have longer stay (11 days vs. 10 days).

118. **Madsen JK,** et al., Danish Trial in Acute MI **(DANAMI).** Danish multi-center randomized study of invasive vs. conservative treatment in patients with inducible ischemia after thrombolysis in acute MI (DANAMI). *Circulation* 1997;96:748–755 (editorial, 713–715).

Design: Prospective, randomized, open, multicenter study. Median follow-up period was 2.4 years. Primary end point was death, AMI, and admission with unstable angina.

Purpose: To compare an invasive strategy of PTCA or CABG with a conservative strategy in patients with inducible ischemia after thrombolysis for MI.

Population: 1,008 patients younger than 70 years with a first MI and inducible ischemia [spontaneous ischemia 36 hours or less after admission or positive bicycle exercise tolerance test result (0.1 mm or more ST depression, 0.2 mm or more ST elevation)].

Exclusion Criteria: Prior MI, PTCA, or CABG; incomplete thrombolysis; BP decrease during exercise; significant noncoronary disease; ECG abnormalities precluding ST-segment evaluation during exercise (e.g., LBBB).

Treatment: Invasive therapy group received angiography within 2 weeks, PTCA and CABG if significant disease (50% or greater stenosis). In the conservative arm, angiography was allowed if severe angina developed (e.g., Canadian Cardiovascular Society class 3 or 4).

Results: In the invasive group, PTCA was performed in 52.9%, and CABG, in 29.2% (at 2 to 10 weeks). In the conservative group, at 2 months, only 1.6% had undergone revascularization (at 1 year, 15%). At follow-up, no significant mortality difference was observed [3.6% (invasive) vs. 4.4%], but the invasive group had 47% fewer MIs (5.6% vs. 10.5%; $p = 0.0038$) and fewer unstable angina admissions (17.9% vs. 29.5%; $p < 0.00001$). Overall, the invasive group had 36% fewer primary end points (death, MI, and unstable angina) at 2 years (23.5% vs. 36.6%; $p < 0.0001$).

Comments: Editorial points out that few U.S. cardiologists follow ACC/AHA guidelines that recommend stress testing before invasive testing, and proposes performing angiography for medium or large MIs, and revascularization if evidence of an incomplete infarct is present (e.g., lower than expected CK peak, ECG evolution, preserved wall motion of infarct zone), and stress testing first those with only small MIs (e.g., leads II, III, aVF only).

119. **Ross AM,** et al. A randomized trial comparing primary angioplasty with a strategy of short-acting thrombolysis and immediate planned rescue angioplasty in acute myocardial infarction: the **PACT** trial. *J Am Coll Cardiol* 1999;34:1954–1962.

Design: Prospective, randomized, open, multicenter trial. Primary end point: predischarge EF. Follow-up, 1 year.

Purpose: To evaluate the effectiveness and safety of a "facilitated" PCI approach to AMI management.

Population: 606 patients seen 6 hours or less after symptom onset with ST 0.1 mV or more in two or more limb leads or 0.2 mV or more in two or more contiguous leads.

Treatment: Precatheterization thrombolysis (tPA, 50-mg bolus) or placebo followed by immediate angiography. If TIMI grade 3 flow present, second bolus of tPA, 50 mg, administered. If TIMI grade 0 to 2 flow, PCI performed.

Results: Initial angiography demonstrated that the tPA group had higher TIMI grade 3 flow (32.8% vs. 14.8%) and patency (TIMI grade 2 or 3; 61% vs. 34%; $p = 0.001$). After angioplasty, TIMI flow grade was similar between the two groups [TIMI grade 3 flow in 77% (rescue) and 79% (primary)], indicating that tPA administration did not adversely affect procedural outcomes. No significant difference was noted between the groups in predischarge EF (primary end point), but the EF was higher in those with TIMI 3 flow on catheterization laboratory arrival (62.4%). The small group of patients (12%) who had PTCA performed less than 1 hour after the tPA bolus also had better EFs (62.5% vs. 57.3%). No significant differences were found in bleeding rates, suggesting that immediate angioplasty could be performed safely after reduced-dose tPA.

120. **Bonnefoy E,** et al., on behalf of the Comparison of Angioplasty and prehospital Thrombolysis in Acute Myocardial infarction **(CAPTIM)** study group. Primary angioplasty versus prehospital fibrinolysis. *Lancet* 2002;360:825–829.

Design: Prospective, randomized, open, multicenter trial. Primary end point: death, nonfatal reinfarction, and nonfatal disabling stroke at 30 days.
Purpose: To determine whether primary angioplasty is better than prehospital fibrinolysis followed by transfer to an interventional facility for possible rescue PTCA.
Population: 840 patients seen within 6 hours of symptom onset with 2 mm or more ST elevation in at least two contiguous leads or LBBB.
Treatment: Prehospital fibrinolysis (accelerated alteplase) with angiography only for ongoing chest pain or ECG signs of continuing ischemia OR primary angioplasty. Each ambulance was staffed with a physician.
Results: The median delay between onset of symptoms and treatment was 130 minutes in the fibrinolysis group and 190 minutes (time to first balloon inflation) in the primary PTCA group. Rescue angioplasty was performed in 26% of fibrinolysis patients. No significant differences were seen between the groups in the incidence of the primary composite end point (primary PTCA, 6.2%; fibrinolysis, 8.2%; $p = 0.29$).
Comments: Study was underpowered: planned enrollment was 1,200 patients, which would have allowed a detection of a 40% relative reduction in incidence of primary end point.

121. **GRACIA.** Preliminary results presented at 24th Annual Meeting of the European Society of Cardiology, September 2002, Munich.

This prospective, randomized trial enrolled 500 acute STEMI patients and compared routine angiography within 24 hours of thrombolysis versus an ischemia-guided approach. In the routine invasive arm, 80% underwent stenting of the IRA; CABG was performed in 2%. In the ischemia-guided group arm, 30% underwent angiography, and 19% underwent PCI. At 30 days, the interventional group had a significantly lower incidence of death, reinfarction, or revascularization (0.8% vs. 3.7%; $p = 0.03$). This trial suggests that now routine coronary angiography and revascularization after thrombolytic administration is safe and associated with fewer adverse cardiac events at 30 days. These findings require validation in larger studies.

122. **Schweiger MJ,** et al., for the TIMI 10B and TIMI 14 Investigators. Early coronary intervention following pharmacologic therapy for acute myocardial infarction (the combined TIMI 10B-TIMI 14 experience). *Am J Cardiol* 2001;88:831–836.

This study analyzed 1,938 AMI patients from TIMI 10B (tPA vs. TNK) and TIMI 14 (thrombolytic therapy with or without abciximab). All patients underwent angiography at 90 minutes. Patients who underwent PCI were described as having a rescue procedure (TIMI 0 or 1 flow at 90 minutes), an adjunctive procedure (TIMI 2 or 3 flow at 90 minutes), or a delayed procedure [performed more than 150 minutes after symptom onset (median, 2.8 days)]. Among patients with TIMI 0 or 1 flow, a trend was found toward lower 30-day mortality with rescue PCI compared with no PCI (6% vs. 17%; $p = 0.01$, adjusted $p = 0.28$). Patients who underwent adjunctive PCI had 30-day mortality and/or reinfarction rates similar to those who underwent delayed PCI. In a multivariate model, adjunctive and delayed PCI patients had lower 30-day mortality and/or reinfarction rates ($p = 0.02$) than did patients with "successful thrombolysis" (i.e., TIMI 3 flow at 90 minutes) who did not undergo revascularization. Thus, early PCI after AMI is associated with favorable outcomes. Randomized trials of an early invasive strategy after thrombolysis are warranted.

Rescue Percutaneous Transluminal Coronary Angioplasty
123. **Abbottsmith CW,** et al. Fate of patients with acute MI with patency of the infarct-related vessel achieved with successful thrombolysis versus rescue angioplasty. *J Am Coll Cardiol* 1990;16:770–778.

This retrospective analysis focused on 776 TAMI patients with a patent IRA; 607 received only thrombolysis, and 169 had rescue angioplasty. The rescue success rate was 88%. However, at 7 to 10 days, the thrombolysis group had less reocclusion [11% vs. 21% (successful rescue); $p < 0.001$] and better EFs (52.3% vs. 48.1%; $p < 0.01$), whereas the in-hospital mortality rates were similar (4.6% vs. 5.9%). Failed rescue angioplasty was associated with a high mortality rate [39.1% vs. 5.9% (successful rescue)].

124. **Ellis SG,** et al. Present status of rescue coronary angioplasty: current polarization of opinion and randomized trials. *J Am Coll Cardiol* 1992;19:681–686.

This overview of 12 trials (only one randomized) included a total of 560 patients. The average success rate of rescue PTCA was 80%. Reocclusion occurred in 18%. The overall mortality rate was 10.6%, but it was much higher (up to 39%) in those for whom rescue failed.

125. **Ellis SG,** et al., **RESCUE.** Randomized comparison of rescue angioplasty with conservative management of patients with early failure of thrombolysis for acute anterior MI. *Circulation* 1994;90:2280–2284.

Design: Prospective, randomized, multicenter study. Primary end point was LVEF at 25 to 35 days.
Purpose: To assess the clinical benefit of rescue angioplasty in a relatively high-risk population.
Population: 151 patients aged 21 to 79 years seen with ST elevation 2 mm or more in at least two precordial leads.
Exclusion Criteria: Cardiogenic shock, prior MI, and left main stenosis 50% or more.
Treatment: Thrombolysis followed by PTCA or aspirin, heparin, and vasodilators.
Results: Rescue PTCA was successful in 92%. The rescue PTCA group had less death and severe heart failure (6% vs. 17%; $p = 0.05$) and better exercise (but not rest) EFs (43% vs. 38%; $p = 0.04$).

126. **Gibson CM,** et al. Rescue angioplasty in the thrombolysis in MI **(TIMI)** 4 trial. *Am J Cardiol* 1997;80:21–26.

This retrospective analysis focused on 402 TIMI-4 patients with either successful rescue angioplasty (PTCA) or successful thrombolysis. The successful PTCA group had better 90-minute TIMI grade 3 flow (87% vs. 65%; $p = 0.002$) and a lower TIMI frame count (27 vs. 39; $p < 0.001$). The successful versus failed rescue PTCA group had fewer in-hospital adverse end points, consisting of death, MI, severe CHF/shock, and EF 40% or less (29% vs. 83%; $p = 0.01$). The rescue PTCA (all) versus other groups had similar event rates (both with adverse outcomes in 35%).

127. **Ross AM,** et al. Rescue angioplasty after failed thrombolysis: technical and clinical outcomes in a large thrombolysis trial. *J Am Coll Cardiol* 1998;31:1511–1517.

This retrospective analysis focused on GUSTO-I angiographic substudy data. Rescue PTCA was performed in 198 patients; the artery was successfully opened in 88.4%, with 68% achieving TIMI grade 3 flow. Successful rescue PTCA resulted in better LV function and 30-day mortality than did failed rescue, comparable with outcomes in those with closed infarct arteries managed conservatively (266 patients), but less favorable than those with successful thrombolysis (1,058 patients). Failed rescue was associated with high 30.4% mortality (multivariate analysis predictor, severe heart failure).

Cardiogenic Shock
128. **Berger PB,** et al. Impact of an aggressive invasive catheterization and revascularization strategy on mortality in patients with cardiogenic shock in the GUSTO-I trial. *Circulation* 1997;96:122–127.

This analysis focused on 2,200 patients with SBP less than 90 mm Hg for 1 hour who survived 1 hour after onset of shock. The early angiography (24 hours or less) group had a lower 30-day mortality rate (38% vs. 62 %; $p = 0.0001$). After multiple logistic regression analysis, the early angiography group was found to be younger (63 vs. 68 years), to have had fewer prior MIs (19% vs. 27%), and to have been given thrombolysis earlier (2.9 vs. 3.2 hours). An aggressive strategy is still associated with a lower 30-day mortality rate (OR, 0.43; $p = 0.0001$). A subsequent GUSTO-I analysis showed that most patients (88%) with cardiogenic shock who were alive at 30 days survived at least 1 year, and that those who underwent revascularization within 30 days had better 1-year survival than did patients not revascularized (see *Circulation* 1999;99:873).

129. **Hochman JS,** et al. Should We Emergently Revascularize Occluded Coronaries for Cardiogenic Shock **(SHOCK)** Investigators. Early revascularization in acute MI complicated by cardiogenic shock. *N Engl J Med* 1999;341:625–634 (editorial, 686–688).

This prospective, randomized, multicenter trial was composed of 302 patients with STEMI (or new LBBB), pulmonary capillary wedge pressure, 15 mm Hg or more; cardiac index, 2.2 or less; SBP more than 90 mm Hg for 30 minutes before inotropes/vasopressors or IABP initiated; and heart rate, 60 beats/min. Patients underwent emergency revascularization (ERV) within 6 hours (PTCA or CABG) or medical management [thrombolysis recommended (given in 64%), delayed revascularization allowed at 54 hours]. The ERV group had a 97% angiography rate and 87% revascularization rate [PTCA, 49% (at average 0.9 hours); CABG, 38% (average 2.7 hours)]. Among initial medical stabilization (IMS) patients, 4% had revascularization performed before 54 hours, and 22% underwent late revascularization. No significant difference was found in 30-day all-cause mortality (primary end point) between the two groups (ERV, 46.7%, vs. IMS, 56.0%; $p = 0.11$); however, at 6 months, a significant mortality benefit was associated with early revascularization strategy (50.3% vs. 63.1%; $p = 0.027$). In the subgroup of patients aged 75 years or younger, ERV was significantly better than IMS (at 30 days, 41% vs. 57%; $p < 0.01$; 6 months, 48% vs. 69%; $p < 0.01$). The PTCA success rate was 76%, and the mortality rate was 100% if PTCA did not achieve TIMI grade 2 or 3 flow.

Stenting
130. **Antoniucci D,** et al. Florence Randomized Elective Stenting in Acute Coronary Occlusions **(FRESCO).** A clinical trial comparing primary stenting of the infarct-related artery with optimal primary angioplasty for acute MI. *J Am Coll Cardiol* 1998;31:1234–1239.

This prospective, randomized, multicenter study enrolled 150 patients seen within 6 hours of onset of symptoms with STEMI and who underwent successful primary PTCA. Patients were randomized to primary PTCA or primary PTCA followed by stenting. No PTCA was attempted if stenosis was less than 70% or the IRA could not be identified. No randomization to PTCA alone or stenting was performed if the reference diameter was less than 2.5 mm. Stenting success rate was 100%. At 6 months, the incidence of death, reinfarction, and repeated TVR due to recurrent ischemia at 6 months (primary end point) was only 9% in the stent group versus 28% in the PTCA group ($p = 0.003$). Repeated angiography was performed at 6 months, and the incidence of restenosis or reocclusion was 17% in the stent group and 43% in the PTCA group ($p = 0.001$).

131. **Suryapranata H,** et al. Randomized comparison of coronary stenting with balloon angioplasty in selected patients with acute MI. *Circulation* 1998;97:2502–2505.

This prospective, single-center study randomized 227 AMI patients seen within 6 hours of symptom onset (or after 6 to 24 hours if ongoing ischemia) to primary stenting (Palmaz-Schatz) or angioplasty (with bailout stenting only if prolonged inflation unsuccessful). Initial patients received warfarin for 3 months, but patients enrolled after January 1996 received ticlodipine, 250 mg/day for 2 weeks. Exclusion criteria were cardiogenic shock, prior bypass surgery or angioplasty, and prior MI. Angiographic exclusion criteria included unprotected left main, significant side branch jeopardy, excessive tortuosity, extensive thrombus, or inability to cross lesion with guide wire. Overall 6-month mortality rate was 2%. The stent group had fewer reinfarctions (1% vs. 7%; $p = 0.036$) and less need for subsequent TVR (4% vs. 17%; $p = 0.0016$). The stent group also had better cardiac event-free survival rate (95% vs. 80%; $p = 0.012$). The stent group had a larger reference vessel.

132. **Grines CL,** et al., for the **Stent PAMI** Study Group. Coronary angioplasty with or without stent implantation for acute myocardial infarction. *N Engl J Med* 1999;341:1949–1956 [also see *J Am Coll Cardiol* 1998;31:23 (pilot study)].

Design: Prospective, randomized, open, multicenter trial. The primary end point was the 6-month incidence of death, reinfarction, and disabling stroke, or ischemia-driven TVR.
Purpose: To compare stent implantation with primary angioplasty alone in AMI.
Population: 900 patients within 12 hours of symptom onset with ST elevation 1 mm or more in at least two contiguous leads or a nondiagnostic ECG with evidence of AMI in the catheterization laboratory and with lesions amenable to stenting.
Exclusion Criteria: Included prior administration of thrombolytic agents for index infarction, current use of warfarin, stroke in prior month, cardiogenic shock.
Treatment: Angioplasty alone or stenting (heparin-coated Palmaz-Schatz).
Results: Acute procedural success rates were greater than 99% in both groups. The postprocedural TIMI grade 3 flow rates were 89.4% in the angioplasty group and 92.7% in the stent group ($p = 0.10$). At 6 months, the stent group had a larger mean luminal diameter (2.56 mm vs. 2.12 mm; $p < 0.001$) and lower restenosis rate (20.3% vs. 33.5%; $p < 0.001$). Stenting was associated with a significant reduction in the 6-month composite primary end point (12.6% vs. 20.1%; $p < 0.01$). This difference was driven entirely by a decreased need for TVR because of ischemia (7.7% vs. 17%; $p < 0.001$). The 6-month mortality rate was 4.2% in the stent group and 2.7% in the angioplasty group ($p = 0.27$). Bleeding rates were similar.
Comments: Stenting of a closed artery was associated with a higher mortality rate at 30 days and 6 months compared with PTCA alone (*J Am Coll Cardiol* 1999;33 (suppl A):368A), but it should be noted that the use of glycoprotein IIb/IIIa inhibitors was infrequent (5%), rigid early-generation stents were used (increased thrombus embolization), and high-pressure deployment and oversizing of the stent were common. Many of these practice patterns have now changed, and this finding should be reevaluated in future studies.

133. **Le May MR,** et al. Stenting versus thrombolysis in acute myocardial infarction trial **(STAT).** *J Am Coll Cardiol* 2001;37:985–991.

A total of 123 patients with STEMI were randomized to primary stenting or accelerated tPA. Patients with cardiogenic shock, active bleeding, history of stroke, major surgery, severe hypertension, prolonged CPR, inadequate vascular access, PTCA within 6 months, prior stenting of culprit artery, and prior CABG were excluded. The primary end point was a 6-month composite of TVR. At 6-month follow-up, the primary end point (death, reinfarction, stroke or repeated TVR) had occurred in 24.2% of stent patients and 55.7% of TPA patients ($p < 0.001$); this difference was due to a significant reduction in TVR in the stent group (14.5% vs. 49.2%; $p < 0.001$).

134. **Kastrati A,** et al., for The Stent versus Thrombolysis for Occluded Coronary Arteries in Patients With Acute Myocardial Infarction **(STOPAMI-2)** Study. Myocardial salvage after coronary stenting plus abciximab versus fibrinolysis plus abciximab in patients with acute myocardial infarction: a randomised trial. *Lancet* 2002;359:920–925.

Design: Prospective, randomized, open, multicenter trial. The primary end point was the salvage index (the ratio of the degree of myocardial salvage to the initial perfusion defect).

Purpose: To determine whether AMI patients benefit from the addition of glycoprotein IIb/IIIa inhibitors to fibrinolytic or mechanical reperfusion strategies.

Population: 162 patients with AMI seen within 12 hours of onset of symptoms.

Treatment: Stenting or alteplase. All received abciximab. Technetium-99m sestamibi scintigraphy was done at admission and at a median of 11 days in 141 (87%) patients.

Results: Stenting was associated with greater myocardial salvage than was alteplase (median, 13.6% vs. 8.0% of the left ventricle; $p = 0.007$). The salvage index was greater in the stent group than in the alteplase group [median, 0.60 (0.37 to 0.82) vs. 0.41 (0.13 to 0.58); $p = 0.001$]. Six-month mortality rate was 5% in the stent group and 9% in the alteplase group [RR, 0.56 (95% CI, 0.17 to 1.88); $p = 0.35$].

135. **Stone GW,** et al., for The Controlled Abciximab and Device Investigation to Lower Late Angioplasty Complications **(CADILLAC)** Investigators. Comparison of angioplasty with stenting, with or without abciximab, in acute myocardial infarction. *N Engl J Med* 2002;346:957–966 (see reference 47, full summary).

This 2,082-patient trial found a significantly lower incidence of major events with stenting compared with angioplasty, regardless of abciximab use (see reference 47 for full summary).

Angiotensin-converting Enzyme Inhibitors with or without Nitrates
General Reviews and Meta-Analyses

136. **Ball SG,** et al. ACE inhibitors after MI: indications and timing. *J Am Coll Cardiol* 1995;25(suppl):42–46.

This review article emphasizes the significant benefit of ACE inhibition in patients with LV dysfunction. Early initiation and total length of therapy (e.g., 4 to 6 weeks vs. longer or indefinite) also are discussed.

137. ACE Inhibitor MI Collaborative Group. Indications for ACE inhibitors in the early treatment of acute MI: systematic overview of individual data from 100,000 patients in randomized trials. *Circulation* 1998;97:2202–2212.

This meta-analysis was composed of four randomized trials (CONSENSUS II, GISSI-3, ISIS-4, and CCS-1), 98,496 total patients, in which ACE inhibitors were started within 36 hours of AMI. ACE inhibition was associated with a 7% reduction in 30-day mortality (7.1% vs. 7.6%; $p < 0.004$). Most of the benefit was observed within the first week of treatment. The greatest mortality benefit was seen in high-risk groups (e.g., anterior MI; Killip class 2 to 3; heart rate, 100 beats/min at entry). ACE inhibition also was associated with a reduction in nonfatal cardiac failure (14.6% vs. 15.2%; $p = 0.01$) but led to more frequent hypotension (17.6% vs. 9.3%; $p < 0.01$) and renal dysfunction (1.3% vs. 0.6%; $p < 0.01$).

138. **Domanski MJ,** et al. Effect of angiotensin converting enzyme inhibition on sudden cardiac death in patients following acute MI. *J Am Coll Cardiol* 1999;33:598–604.

The results of this meta-analysis of 15 trials with 15,134 patients suggest that part of the benefit of ACE inhibition in AMI is related to a reduction in risk of sudden cardiac death. The majority of deaths (87%) were cardiovascular, of which 38.2% were deemed sudden cardiac deaths. Overall, ACE-inhibitor therapy was associated with significant reductions in overall mortality [OR, 0.83 (95% CI, 0.71 to 0.97)], cardiovascular death [OR, 0.82 (95% CI, 0.69 to 0.97)], and sudden cardiac death [OR, 0.80 (95% CI, 0.70 to 0.92)].

Studies

139. **Pfeffer MA,** et al., on behalf of the Survival and Ventricular Enlargement **(SAVE)** Investigators. Effect of captopril on mortality and morbidity in patients with left ventricular dysfunction after MI. *N Engl J Med* 1992;327:669–677.

Design: Prospective, randomized, double-blind, placebo-controlled, multicenter study. Mean follow-up period was 42 months. Primary end point was all-cause mortality.

Purpose: To determine the effect of captopril on mortality and morbidity when started 3 to 16 days after MI in patients with LV dysfunction.

Population: 2,231 patients aged 21 to 80 years with an EF 40% or less but no overt heart failure.

Exclusion Criteria: Requirement or contraindication to ACE inhibition, creatinine greater than 2.5 mg/dL, unstable post-MI course.

Treatment: Captopril initiated 3 to 16 days after MI and titrated from 12.5 mg, 3 times daily, to 25 mg, 3 times daily, by hospital discharge (and later 50 mg, 3 times daily if tolerated); or placebo.

Results: Captopril group had the following risk reductions: 19% lower all-cause mortality (20% vs. 25%; $p = 0.019$), 21% lower cardiovascular mortality ($p = 0.014$), 25% fewer recurrent MIs (11.9% vs. 15.2%; $p = 0.015$), and 22% less severe heart failure requiring hospitalization ($p = 0.019$). No difference was observed in deterioration of 9% in EF as measured by repeated radionuclide ventriculography at mean 36 months (13% vs. 16%; $p = 0.17$). Overall, captopril was associated with a 14% reduction in composite ischemic index of recurrent MI, revascularization, and unstable angina ($p = 0.047$) (see *Circulation* 1994;90:1731).

140. **Swedeberg K,** et al., on behalf of the Cooperative New Scandinavian Enalapril Survival Study **(CONSENSUS II)** Group. Effects of early administration of enalapril on mortality in patients with acute MI. *N Engl J Med* 1992;327:678–684.

Design: Prospective, randomized, double-blind, placebo-controlled, multicenter study. Average follow-up period was 188 days. Primary end point was all-cause mortality rate.

Purpose: To evaluate the effect on mortality of early i.v. administration of enalapril in AMI patients.

Population: 6,090 patients within 24 hours of symptom onset and one of the following: ST elevation in at least two contiguous leads, new Q waves, or elevated serum enzymes.

Exclusion Criteria: Included BP less than 105/65 mm Hg, history of adverse reaction to or requirement for ACE inhibition, severe valvular stenosis.

Treatment: Intravenous enalaprilat, 1 mg, over a 2-hour period (stopped if BP decreased below 90/60 mm Hg). Oral enalapril was begun at 6 hours (initial dose, 2.5 mg, and increased up to 20 mg/day); or placebo.

Results: Trial was terminated early by the safety committee. No significant mortality difference was observed at 180 days: 10.2% (placebo) vs. 11.0% (enalapril). Enalapril was associated with more frequent hypotension (BP less than 90/50 mm Hg): 12% vs. 3% ($p < 0.001$).

141. Acute Infarction Ramipril Efficacy **(AIRE)** Study Investigators. Effect of ramipril on mortality and morbidity of survivors of AMI with clinical evidence of heart failure. *Lancet* 1993;342:821–828.

Design: Prospective, randomized, double-blind, parallel-group, placebo-controlled, multicenter study. Average follow-up period was 15 months. Primary end point was all-cause mortality.

Purpose: To evaluate whether ramipril started 3 to 10 days after MI reduces mortality in patients whose course is complicated by heart failure.

Population: 2,006 patients with a definite AMI and clinical evidence of heart failure at any point after MI.

Exclusion Criteria: Heart failure due to valvular disease, unstable angina, contraindications to ACE inhibition, and severe and resistant heart failure.

Treatment: Ramipril, 2.5 mg twice daily for 2 days, and then 5 mg twice daily if tolerated.

Results: All-cause mortality was significantly lower in the ramipril group: 27% risk reduction (17% vs. 23%; $p = 0.002$). Ramipril patients also had a 30% lower risk of sudden death ($p = 0.011$) and a 19% risk reduction in combined end points consisting of death, severe heart failure, MI, and stroke ($p = 0.008$). No significant difference was observed in reinfarction or stroke rates.

142. **GISSI-3.** Effects of lisinopril and transdermal glyceryl trinitrate singly and together on 6-week mortality and ventricular function after acute MI. *Lancet* 1994;343:1115–1122.

Design: Prospective, randomized, open-label, 2 × 2 factorial, multicenter study. Primary outcomes were 6-week all-cause mortality and combination of death, heart failure at 5 days after MI, and EF 35% or less or 45% or more myocardial segments with abnormal motion.

Purpose: To evaluate the effect of lisinopril and nitrates, alone and in combination, on all-cause mortality and LV function after AMI.

Population: 18,895 patients seen within 24 hours with 1 mm or more ST elevation or depression in at least one limb lead or 2 mm or more in at least one precordial lead.

Exclusion Criteria: Severe heart failure, SBP less than 100 mm Hg, serum creatinine more than 177 μM, and severe comorbidity.

Treatment: (a) Lisinopril, 5 mg in first 24 hours, and then 10 mg once daily for 6 weeks or open control; (b) glyceryl nitrate (GTN), 5 μg/min i.v., and increased by 5 to 20 μg/min or until SBP was lowered by 10%. At 24 hours, transdermal GTN was started (10 mg/day, 14 hours each day) for 6 weeks. If not tolerated, isosorbide mononitrate (50 mg once daily) or open control. Overall, 72% of patients received a thrombolytic agent, 31% were taking a β-blocker, and 84%, aspirin.

Results: Overall, 6-week mortality rate was only 6.7%. Lisinopril was associated with significant mortality reduction (6.3% vs. 7.1%; OR, 0.88; $p = 0.03$), with survival curves beginning to diverge on the first day. Reduction also was seen in combined primary outcome (15.6% vs. 17.0%; OR, 0.90; $p = 0.009$). No difference between lisinopril and controls was observed in recurrent infarction, postinfarct angina, cardiogenic shock, and stroke. No difference in mortality was observed between patients with and without GTN (18.4% vs. 18.9%; $p = 0.39$). Of note, 13.3% of controls received nonstudy ACE inhibitors, and 57.1% received nonstudy nitrates.

Comments: At 6 months, the lisinopril group had fewer deaths and LV dysfunction (18.1% vs. 19.3%; $p = 0.03$) (see *J Am Coll Cardiol* 1996;27:337). A retrospective analysis showed that lisinopril was more beneficial in diabetic patients (6-week mortality, 8.7% vs. 12.4%; OR, 0.68) than in nondiabetic patients ($p < 0.025$) (see *Circulation* 1997;26:4245).

143. **Ambrosioni E,** et al., for the Survival of MI Long-term Evaluation **(SMILE)** Study Investigators. The effect of the angiotensin-converting-enzyme inhibitor zofenopril on mortality and morbidity after anterior MI. *N Engl J Med* 1995; 332:80–85.

Design: Prospective, randomized, double-blind, placebo-controlled, multicenter study. Follow-up was 1 year. Primary end point was death or severe heart failure (three or more of following: S_3, bilateral pulmonary rales, radiologic evidence, peripheral edema).

Purpose: To determine whether short-term ACE inhibition after MI reduces mortality and severe heart failure.

Population: 1,556 patients (of 20,261 cardiac care unit patients) at less than 24 hours from symptom onset and not administered thrombolytic therapy.

Exclusion Criteria: Cardiogenic shock, SBP less than 100 mm Hg, creatinine greater than 2.5 mg/dL, and history of CHF or ACE inhibitor use.

Treatment: Zofenopril, 7.5 to 30 mg twice daily, or placebo.

Results: At 6 weeks, the zofenopril group had a significant 34% reduction in the incidence of death and severe heart failure (7.1% vs. 10.6%; $p = 0.018$). A significant 46% reduction in severe heart failure and a statistically nonsignificant 25% reduction in death was found (7.1% vs. 10.6%; $p = 0.19$). At 1 year, the zofenopril group had 29% lower mortality (10.0% vs. 14.1%; $p = 0.011$).

144. **ISIS-4** Collaborative Group. ISIS-4: a randomised factorial assessing early oral captopril, oral mononitrate and intravenous magnesium sulfate in 58,050 patients with suspected acute MI. *Lancet* 1995;345:669–685.

Design: Prospective, randomized, double-blind, partially placebo-controlled (including captopril arm), multicenter study. Primary end point was 5-week mortality rate.
Purpose: To assess the effects of early initiation of captopril, oral nitrate, and intravenous magnesium on mortality and morbidity in AMI patients.
Population: 58,050 patients with suspected AMI (confirmed in 92%) seen within 24 hours (median, 8 hours) of symptom onset.
Exclusion Criteria (recommended): Cardiogenic shock, persistent severe hypotension, severe fluid depletion, and negligibly low risk of cardiac death.
Treatment: Captopril arm received 6.25 mg, 12.5 mg 2 hours later, 25 mg at 10 to 12 hours, and then 50 mg twice daily for 28 days; or placebo. The isosorbide mononitrate (Imdur) arm received 30 mg, 30 mg 10 to 12 hours later, 60 mg once daily for 28 days; 70% received thrombolytic therapy, and 94%, antiplatelet therapy.
Results: Captopril was associated with a 7% reduction in mortality: 7.19% versus 7.69% ($p^2 = 0.02$). The benefit doubled in high-risk groups (prior MI, CHF, anterior ST elevation). More hypotension was seen with captopril, but no increased deaths were seen among patients with low BP (90 to 100 mm Hg). Imdur administration did not have a significant effect on mortality (7.34% vs. 7.54%).

145. Chinese Cardiac Study **(CCS-1).** Oral captopril versus placebo among 13,634 patients with suspected acute MI: interim report from the Chinese Cardiac Study (CCS-1). *Lancet* 1995;345:686–687.

Design: Prospective, randomized, placebo-controlled, multicenter study. Primary end point was 4-week all-cause mortality.
Purpose: To assess the effect of ACE inhibition in a broad group of MI patients.
Population: 13,634 patients with or without ST elevation seen within 36 hours of symptom onset.
Exclusion Criteria: Persistent hypotension (SBP less than 90 mm Hg), long-term use of large doses of diuretics, and contraindications to ACE inhibitors.
Treatment: Captopril, 6.25 mg initial dose, 12.5 mg 2 hours later, and then 12.5 mg 3 times daily; or placebo.
Results: Captopril group had a nonsignificant mortality reduction at 4 weeks: 9.05% vs. 9.59% ($p = 0.03$). Captopril was associated with a significant excess of hypotension, resulting in discontinuation of therapy (8.4% vs. 4.9%) and higher incidence of persistent hypotension (16.3% vs. 10.8%). In patients with an admission SBP less than 100 mm Hg, mortality was slightly higher in the captopril group (11.0% vs. 10.0%; $p = $ NS).
Comments: The additive results of CCS-1, ISIS-4, CONSENSUS-II, GISSI-3, and 11 smaller trials show a clear benefit of ACE inhibitors: 6.5% odds reduction (7.27% vs 7.73%; total of 100,963 patients).

146. **Kober L,** et al., for the Trandolapril Cardiac Evaluation (**TRACE**) Study Group. A clinical trial of the angiotensin-converting-enzyme inhibitor trandolapril in patients with left ventricular dysfunction after MI. *N Engl J Med* 1995;333:1670–1676.

Design: Prospective, randomized, double-blind, placebo-controlled, multicenter study. Follow-up period was 24 to 50 months. Primary end point was all-cause mortality rate.
Purpose: To evaluate the effect of long-term ACE inhibition with trandolapril on mortality in AMI complicated by LV dysfunction.
Population: 1,749 of 2,606 eligible patients with an EF of 35% or less and an AMI 3 to 7 days before enrollment.
Exclusion Criteria: Contraindications to or need for ACE inhibition, severe diabetes, hyponatremia (less than 125 mM), unstable angina requiring immediate intervention, and severe comorbidity.
Treatment: Trandolapril, 1 mg/day, and titrated up to 4 mg/day; or placebo.

Results: Trandolapril group had a 22% reduction in the relative risk of death (34.7% vs. 42.3%; $p = 0.001$), as well as significantly fewer cardiovascular and sudden cardiac deaths (RRs, 0.75 vs. 0.76) and less frequent progression to severe heart failure (RR, 0.71). A nonsignificant reduction in recurrent MI was seen (RR, 0.86; $p = 0.29$).

147. **Pfeffer MA,** et al., for the Healing and Early Afterload Reducing Therapy **(HEART)** Trial Investigators. Early versus delayed angiotensin-converting-enzyme inhibition therapy in acute MI. *Circulation* 1997;95:2643–2651.

Design: Prospective, randomized, double-blind, placebo-controlled, multicenter study. Follow-up period was 90 days.

Purpose: To compare the safety and efficacy of immediate versus delayed ACE inhibition on echocardiographic evidence of ventricular dilatation in patients with anterior MI.

Population: 352 patients seen within 24 hours of symptom onset.

Exclusion Criteria: Contraindications to or need for ACE inhibitor; creatinine, 2.5 mg/dL; cardiogenic shock; SBP less than 100 mm Hg; and persistent ischemia.

Treatment: Three groups: (a) early (days 1 to 14) placebo, and then full-dose ramipril (10 mg/day); (b) early and late low-dose ramipril (0.625 mg); and (c) early and late full-dose ramipril.

Results: Trial was terminated early (600 patients planned) based on GISSI-3 and ISIS-4 results showing benefit of early initiation of ACE inhibition. Early full-dose ramipril (group c) showed the largest increase in ejection fraction at 90 days [+4.9 vs. 3.9 (low dose) vs. 2.4 (delayed full dose); p trend < 0.05]. No significant differences were observed in LV diastolic area. Groups had similar event rates and incidence of low BP (90 mm Hg or less).

148. **OPTIMAAL.** Effects of losartan and captopril on mortality and morbidity in high-risk patients after acute myocardial infarction: presented at the 24th Annual Meeting of the European Society of Cardiology, September 2002. Published online in *Lancet* September 1, 2002.

Design: Prospective, randomized, double-blind, parallel, multicenter study. Primary end point: all-cause mortality. Mean follow-up, 2.7 years.

Purpose: To determine whether losartan is superior or noninferior to captopril at decreasing all-cause mortality in high-risk patients after AMI.

Population: 5,477 patients enrolled within 10 days of presentation AND with. (a) AMI and signs or symptoms of heart failure (rales, S_3, treatment with diuretics or vasodilators, persistent sinus tachycardia, or radiographic evidence of heart failure); OR (b) AMI, EF, less than 35%, or LV end-diastolic diameter (LVEDD) greater than 65 mm; OR (c) new Q-wave anterior wall MI; OR (d) reinfarction with previous pathologic Q-waves in the anterior wall.

Exclusion Criteria: Included SBP less than 100 mm Hg, current ACE inhibitor or ARB therapy, unstable angina, stenotic valvular heart disease, planned coronary revascularization.

Treatment: Losartan (target dose, 50 mg orally once daily) or captopril (target dose, 50 mg orally 3 times each day).

Results: At follow-up, no significant difference in all-cause mortality was found between the two groups (losartan, 18.2%; captopril, 16.4%; $p = 0.069$). The confidence interval boundary (less than 1.10) showed that losartan did not fulfill criteria for noninferiority. No significant increase in mortality was found in either group when stratified by β-blocker use. The losartan group had a significantly lower CV mortality than did the captopril group (15.3% vs. 13.3%; $p = 0.032$). Losartan was better tolerated than captopril, with 17% discontinuing losartan for any reason compared with 23% with captopril ($p < 0.0001$).

Comments: These results confirm that ACE inhibitors should remain first-line therapy in high-risk AMI patients. Data from the RENAAL and LIFE trials suggest that higher doses of losartan may be more beneficial. The large ongoing VALIANT study is examining higher doses of ARB and combination ARB-ACE inhibitor therapy in post-MI patients.

Nitrates
General Reviews
149. **Yusuf S,** et al. Effect of intravenous nitrates on mortality in acute MI: an overview of the randomized trials. *Lancet* 1988;1:1088–1092.

Analysis of data from seven small i.v. NTG trials enrolling 851 patients found that use of i.v. NTG was associated with a significant 41% mortality reduction (12.0% vs. 20.5%; $p < 0.001$). Analysis of three trials studying i.v. nitroprusside found that its use was associated with a nonsignificant mortality reduction (14.3% vs. 17.8%).

Studies
150. **Cohn JN,** et al. Effect of short-time infusion of sodium nitroprusside on mortality rate in acute MI complications by left ventricular failure. *N Engl J Med* 1982;306:1129–1135.

This prospective, double-blind, placebo-controlled trial was composed of 812 men with LV filling pressures of 12 mm Hg or more randomized to nitroprusside (10 to 200 μg/min) or placebo for 48 hours. The goal of therapy was to reduce LV filling pressures by 40%. Overall, no differences were seen in 13-week mortality [19% vs. 17% (placebo)]. However, nitroprusside appeared beneficial if given late (more than 9 hours; 13-week mortality rates, 14.4% vs. 22.3%, $p = 0.04$) and harmful if given early (24.2% vs. 12.7%; $p = 0.025$).

151. **Flaherty JT,** et al. A randomized prospective trial of intravenous nitroglycerin in patients with acute MI. *Circulation* 1983;68:576–588.

In this prospective, blinded study, 104 patients were randomized to NTG (initially 5 μg/min, goal SBP decrease of 10%) or placebo for 48 hours. Early NTG [started within 10 hours of symptoms (*post hoc* definition)] was associated with less cardiac death, new CHF, and infarct extension at 10 days [15% vs. 39% (other three groups); $p = 0.003$]. More early-treated patients had an EF improvement of 10% at 7 to 14 days [35% vs. 6% (late NTG) vs. 11% and 0%; $p = 0.004$]. No significant differences were observed in 3-month mortality (15% vs. 25%) or peak CK or infarct size.

152. **Jugdutt BI,** et al. Intravenous nitroglycerin therapy to limit myocardial infarct size, expansion and complications: effect of timing, dosage, and infarct location. *Circulation* 1988;78:906–919.

This small randomized study showed that mortality benefit was associated with i.v. NTG. A total of 310 patients were randomized to i.v. NTG (infusion titrated to lower mean BP: 10% if normotensive, 30% if hypertensive) or control. The i.v. NTG group had a smaller CK infarct size ($p < 0.0001$), less cardiogenic shock (5% vs. 15%; $p < 0.005$), and decreased LV thrombi (5% vs. 22%; $p < 0.0005$). At 10-day follow-up, a 22% higher EF, 40% less LV asynergy, 41% lower Killip class, and no difference in expansion index (vs. +31%) were observed. The i.v. NTG group had lower 30-day and 1-year mortality rates (14% vs. 26%; $p < 0.005$; 21% vs. 31%; $p < 0.05$). Subgroup analysis showed that this benefit was limited to those with anterior infarcts.

153. **ISIS-4** Collaborative Group. ISIS-4: a randomised factorial assessing early oral captopril, oral mononitrate and intravenous magnesium sulfate in 58,050 patients with suspected acute MI. *Lancet* 1995;345:669–685.

This megatrial that enrolled 58,050 patients with suspected AMI admitted within 24 hours of symptom onset included a randomization to oral mononitrate (30 mg, 30 mg 10 to 12 hours later, and then 60 mg/day for 28 days), or placebo. In the nitrate arm, a nonsignificant reduction was seen in 35-day mortality (7.34% vs. 7.54%). Nearly half the placebo group received i.v. nitrate therapy, which could have diluted the results. See reference 144 for a full summary.

Calcium-channel Blockers
154. **The Danish Study Group on Verapamil in MI (DAVIT I).** Verapamil in acute MI. *Eur Heart J* 1984;5:516–528.

This randomized trial was composed of 3,498 patients younger than 75 years with suspected MI. Patients received verapamil, 0.1 mg/kg i.v., followed by 120 mg orally 3 times daily; or matched placebo. Treatment continued for 6 months in the 1,436 (41%) patients with confirmed MI. Verapamil use was associated with a nonsignificant 9% mortality reduction at 6 months (12.8% vs. 13.9%; OR, 0.91; 95% CI, 0.67 to 1.24).

155. **Wilcox RG,** et al. Trial of Early Nifedipine in Acute MI **(TRENT)**. Trial of early nifedipine in acute MI: the TRENT study. *BMJ* 1986;293:1204–1208.

Design: Prospective, randomized, double-blind, placebo-controlled, multicenter study. Primary end point was all-cause mortality rate.
Purpose: To evaluate the effects of early nifedipine on mortality in acute MI patients.
Population: 4,491 patients 70 years or younger seen within 24 hours of onset of chest pain.
Exclusion Criteria: SBP less than 100 mm Hg or DBP less than 50 mm Hg; HR, more than 120 beats/min; and current treatment with calcium-channel blocker.
Treatment: Nifedipine, 10 mg 4 times daily, or placebo.
Results: Of the patients, 64% had confirmed MI. Nifedipine was associated with a nonsignificant 7% increase in mortality at 1 month (6.7% vs. 6.3%).

156. The Multicenter Diltiazem Post-Infarction Trial **(MDPIT)** Research Group. The effect of diltiazem on mortality and reinfarction after MI. *N Engl J Med* 1988;319: 385–392.

Design: Prospective, randomized, double-blind, placebo-controlled, multicenter study. Mean follow-up period was 25 months. Primary end point was total mortality, cardiac death, and nonfatal MI.
Purpose: To evaluate the effects of long-term diltiazem on mortality or reinfarction rates after documented MI.
Population: 2,466 patients aged 25 to 75 years with a documented MI (enzyme confirmation required).
Exclusion Criteria: Included cardiogenic shock; second- or third-degree heart block; HR, less than 50 beats/min; and requirement for calcium antagonist.
Treatment: Diltiazem, 60 mg twice or 4 times daily, or placebo.
Results: No difference was observed in total mortality between the diltiazem and placebo groups (166 and 167 patients, respectively). However, among patients without pulmonary congestion (1,909 patients), diltiazem was associated with fewer cardiac events (hazard ratio, 0.77; 95% CI, 0.61 to 0.98), whereas diltiazem-treated patients with pulmonary congestion had more cardiac events (hazard ratio, 1.41; 95% CI, 1.01 to 1.96).

157. The Danish Study Group on Verapamil in MI **(DAVIT II)**. Effect of verapamil on mortality and major events after acute MI (DAVIT II). *Am J Cardiol* 1990;66:779–785.

Design: Prospective, randomized, double-blind, placebo-controlled, multicenter study. Average follow-up period was 16 months. Primary end point was death and reinfarction.
Purpose: To evaluate the effect on total mortality and major cardiac events of verapamil started in the second week after MI.
Population: 1,975 patients younger than 75 years enrolled 7 to 15 days after proven MI.
Exclusion Criteria: Included BP less than 90 mm Hg, second- or third-degree heart block at 3 days.
Treatment: Verapamil, 120 mg 3 times daily (once- or twice-daily dosing allowed in cases of adverse drug reactions), or placebo.
Results: Verapamil group had 17% fewer major events (18.0% vs. 21. 6%; $p = 0.03$) and 20% lower mortality (11.1% vs. 13.8%; $p = 0.11$). A significant mortality reduction was seen in patients with CHF (7.7% vs. 11.8%; $p = 0.02$), whereas no benefit was seen in those without CHF (17.9% vs. 17.5%).

158. **Goldbourt U,** et al. Secondary Prevention Reinfarction Israel Nifedipine Trial **(SPRINT 2).** Early administration of nifedipine in suspected acute MI. *Arch Intern Med* 1993;153:345–353.

Design: Prospective, randomized, double-blind, placebo-controlled study. Primary end point was 6-month all-cause mortality rate.

Purpose: To evaluate the effect on mortality of nifedipine started early after AMI in high-risk patients.

Population: 1,006 patients aged 50 to 79 years meeting at least one of the following criteria: prior MI, angina in preceding month, hypertension, NYHA class II or higher, anterior MI, and lactate dehydrogenase 3 times the upper limit of normal.

Treatment: Nifedipine, 20 mg 3 times daily (6-day titration period), or placebo.

Results: Trial was terminated early. The nifedipine group had a 20% higher 6-month mortality rate (18.7% vs. 15.6%; 95% CI, 0.94 to 1.84). The majority of the mortality difference was owing to excessive mortality during the first 6 days (7.8% vs. 5.5%; CI, 0.86 to 3.0). No differences were observed in reinfarction rates (5.1% vs. 4.2%) or in outcomes based on CHF status.

159. **Rengo F,** et al., Calcium Antagonist Reinfarction Italian Study **(CRIS).** A controlled trial of verapamil in patients after acute MI: results of the CRIS. *Am J Cardiol* 1996;77:365–369 (editorial, 421–422).

Design: Prospective, randomized, double-blind, placebo-controlled study. Mean follow-up period was 2 years. Primary end point was all-cause mortality rate.

Purpose: To evaluate the effects of verapamil on mortality and major cardiac end points in AMI patients.

Population: 1,073 patients aged 30 to 75 years who survived 5 days after an AMI.

Exclusion Criteria: NYHA class III/IV heart failure; HR, less than 50 beats/min; SBP less than 90 mm Hg or greater than 190 mm Hg; DBP greater than 110 mm Hg; long-term therapy with calcium antagonists or β-blockers.

Treatment: Verapamil, 120 mg orally every 8 hours, or placebo started 7 to 21 days (mean, 13.8 days) after admission.

Results: No differences were observed between the verapamil and placebo groups in all-cause mortality (30 and 29 deaths, respectively). The verapamil group had 20% fewer reinfarctions and 20% less angina.

Comments: Editorial reports that pooled data from nine trials shows that verapamil is associated with a favorable effect on reinfarction (OR, 0.81; 95% CI, 0.67 to 0.98) but no overall mortality benefit (OR, 0.93; 95% CI, 0.78 to 1.10).

160. Incomplete Infarction Trial of European Research Collaborators Evaluating Progressing Post-Thrombolysis **(INTERCEPT).** Preliminary results presented at the 71st AHA Scientific Session in Dallas, TX, November 1999.

A total of 874 patients at 63 European sites who received thrombolytic therapy for AMI were randomized at 36 to 96 hours to long-acting diltiazem, 300 mg once daily, or placebo for 6 months. All patients received aspirin. At 6 months, the diltiazem group had a nonsignificant 23% relative reduction in death, MI, and refractory ischemia (22.6% vs. 29.5%). The diltiazem group had a significant reduction in the incidence of repeated revascularization (7% vs. 12%) and a strong trend toward fewer episodes of refractory ischemia (17.2% vs. 23.2%).

Magnesium

161. **Woods KL,** et al., Second Leicester Intravenous Magnesium Intervention Trial **(LIMIT-2).** Intravenous magnesium sulfate in suspected acute MI: results of LIMIT-2. *Lancet* 1992;339:1553–1558.

This prospective, randomized, double-blind, placebo-controlled, single-center study randomized 2,316 patients with suspected AMI (no ECG criteria specified) seen within 24 hours. Patients received magnesium sulfate, 8 mmol over a 5-minute period, followed by 65 mmol over a 24-hour period; or saline. AMI was confirmed in 65%. The magnesium group had a 24% lower 28-day mortality rate (7.8% vs. 10.3%; $p = 0.04$).

Long-term follow-up (mean, 2.7 years) showed persistent significant mortality benefit (16%) associated with magnesium (see *Lancet* 1994;343:816).

162. **ISIS-4** Collaborative Group. ISIS-4: a randomised factorial assessing early oral captopril, oral mononitrate and intravenous magnesium sulfate in 58,050 patients with suspected acute MI. *Lancet* 1995;345:669–685.

This megatrial of 58,050 patients with suspected AMI included a randomization to magnesium (8-mmol bolus over a 15-minute period, and then 72 mmol over a 24-hour period) or no magnesium. Magnesium group had a nonsignificant 6% increase in mortality (7.64% vs. 7.24%) and a higher incidence of CHF (+12/1,000), hypotension (+11/1,000), and cardiogenic shock (+5/1,000). No benefit of magnesium was seen in any subgroup.

163. **The Magnesium in Coronaries (MAGIC)** Trial Investigators. Early administration of intravenous magnesium to high-risk patients with acute myocardial infarction in the Magnesium in Coronaries (MAGIC) trial: a randomized controlled trial. *Lancet* 2002;360:1189–1196.

This prospective, randomized, placebo-controlled, multicenter trial enrolled 6,213 high-risk AMI patients aged 65 years or older seen within 6 hours of symptom onset who were ineligible for reperfusion or eligible for reperfusion. Exclusion criteria included high-grade AV block, cardiogenic shock, and renal failure. Patient received i.v. magnesium (2-g i.v. bolus over a 15-minute period, and then 17 g over a 24-hour period) or placebo. Of patients who underwent reperfusion (primarily thrombolysis), 96% received the magnesium at the time of reperfusion. At 30 days, no difference was found between the two groups in all-cause mortality (15% in both groups). No differences occurred when the patients were stratified by sex, geography, EF, concomitant medications, and other variables.

Antiarrhythmics

164. **Burkart F,** et al., Basel Antiarrhythmic Study of Infarct Survival **(BASIS).** Effect of antiarrhythmic therapy on mortality in survivors of MI with asymptomatic complex ventricular arrhythmias: BASIS. *J Am Coll Cardiol* 1990;16:1711–1718.

Design: Prospective, randomized, three-center study. Follow-up period was 1 year.
Purpose: To compare individualized antiarrhythmic therapy with low-dose amiodarone and no therapy.
Population: 312 of 1,220 consecutively screened MI survivors younger than 71 years with asymptomatic, complex ventricular arrhythmias (Lown class 3 or 4b) on 24-hour ECG before hospital discharge.
Treatment: (a) Individualized: initially quinidine or mexiletine (if both failed, others tried: ajmaline, disopyramide, flecainide, propafenone, sotalol); (b) amiodarone, 1 g/day for 5 days, and then 200 mg/day for 1 year; or (c) no therapy: drugs allowed if arrhythmias developed.
Results: Amiodarone group had a lower overall 1-year mortality rate compared with controls: 5.1% vs. 13.2% ($p < 0.05$); mortality for individually treated patients was 10% ($p =$ NS vs. amiodarone).
Comments: Post hoc analysis showed that the benefit of amiodarone was restricted to those with an EF of 40% (1.5% vs. 8.9% 1-year mortality; $p < 0.03$) (see *Am J Cardiol* 1992;69:1399). Late follow-up showed persistent benefit of amiodarone (after discontinuation at 1 year) compared with placebo: at 7 years, 30% versus 45% mortality ($p = 0.03$) (see *Circulation* 1993;87:309).

165. The Cardiac Arrhythmia Suppression Trial **(CAST)** Investigators. Preliminary report: effect of encainide and flecainide on mortality in a randomized trial of arrhythmia suppression after myocardial infarction. *N Engl J Med* 1989;321:406–412.

Design: Prospective, randomized, open-label (initial phase), double-blind (main phase), placebo-controlled, multicenter study. Follow-up period was 10 months.

Purpose: To evaluate whether suppression of asymptomatic or mildly asymptomatic ventricular arrhythmias after MI reduces death due to arrhythmia.

Population: 1,727 patients with MI in prior 6 days to 2 years, at least six ventricular premature contractions per hour on 24-hour Holter monitoring, EF 0.55 or less if 90 days or less after MI or 0.40 or less if more than 90 days after MI (if EF 30%, patients not eligible to receive flecainide), and suppressibility during open-label phase (at 4 to 10 days, 80% reduction of ventricular premature contractions and 90% reduction of unsustained runs of VT).

Exclusion Criteria: Ventricular arrhythmias associated with severe symptoms; unsustained VT with 15 beats at 120 beats/min; contraindications to drugs; and ECG abnormalities making rhythm interpretation difficult.

Treatment: Encainide, 35 or 50 mg orally 3 times daily; flecainide, 100 or 150 mg twice daily; or moricizine, 200 or 250 mg 3 times daily.

Results: Encainide and flecainide arms were discontinued early. Encainide and flecainide patients had more arrhythmic deaths [4.5% vs. 1.2% (placebo); RR, 3.6; 95% CI, 1.7 to 8.5], as well as higher overall mortality (7.7% vs. 3.0%; RR, 2.5; 95% CI, 1.6 to 4.5).

Comments: The moricizine arm of the trial continued. Later analysis showed that those patients with easily suppressible arrhythmias ($n = 1,778$) had fewer arrhythmic deaths than the 1,173 patients with difficult-to-suppress arrhythmias (RR, 0.59; $p = 0.003$). This likely explains the low placebo mortality rate (1.2%) (see *Circulation* 1995;91:79).

166. **CAST II** Investigators. Effect of the antiarrhythmic agent moricizine on survival after MI. *N Engl J Med* 1992;327:227–233.

Design: Prospective, randomized, open-label (titration phase), double-blind (main phase), placebo-controlled, multicenter study. Mean follow-up period was 18 months. Primary end point was death due to arrhythmia or cardiac arrest due to arrhythmia requiring resuscitation.

Purpose: To evaluate whether suppression of asymptomatic or mildly symptomatic ventricular arrhythmias after MI by moricizine reduces arrhythmia deaths.

Population: 1,325 patients in the initial 14-day phase, 1,155 patients in the long-term phase; inclusion criteria similar to those of CAST I (169).

Exclusion Criteria: Included ventricular arrhythmias associated with severe symptoms; unsustained VT with 15 beats at 120 beats/min; contraindications to drugs.

Treatment: Moricizine, 200 mg 3 times daily (initial trial), 200 to 300 mg 3 times daily (long-term trial), or placebo (both trials).

Results: In the initial 14-day trial, the moricizine group had higher mortality (2.3% vs. 0.3%; RR, 5.6; 95% CI, 1.7 to 19.1). In the long-term phase, the moricizine group had a nonsignificant excess of deaths (15% vs. 12%).

Comments: Trial stopped early because of a less than 8% chance of observing a significant benefit if it was continued to completion.

167. **Waldo AL,** et al., for the Survival with Oral D-sotalol **(SWORD)** Investigators. Effect of D-sotalol on mortality in patients with left ventricular dysfunction after recent and remote MI. *Lancet* 1996;348:7–12.

Design: Prospective, randomized, double-blind, placebo-controlled, multicenter study. Mean follow-up period was 148 days. Primary end point was all-cause mortality rate.

Purpose: To determine if the NYHA class III antiarrhythmic agent D-sotalol can decrease all-cause mortality in high-risk MI survivors.

Population: 3,121 patients with EF 40% or less and recent MI (6 to 42 days) or symptomatic heart failure (class II or III) with remote (longer than 42 days) MI.

Exclusion Criteria: Unstable angina, class IV heart failure, history of life-threatening arrhythmia, PTCA or CABG in previous 14 days, creatinine clearance 50 mL/min or less.

Treatment: D-Sotalol, 200 mg orally twice daily, or placebo.

Results: Trial was terminated early because of 65% higher overall mortality in the sotalol group: 5.0% vs. 3.1% ($p = 0.006$). Increased arrhythmic deaths (RR, 1.77; $p = 0.008$) accounted for the excess mortality. The effect was greatest in those with EF 30% or less (RR, 4.0 vs. 1.2; EF, 31% to 40%; $p = 0.007$).

168. **Julian DG,** et al., for the European MI Amiodarone Trial **(EMIAT)** Investigators. Randomised trial of effect of amiodarone on mortality in patients with left-ventricular dysfunction after recent MI: EMIAT. *Lancet* 1997;349:667–674.

Design: Prospective, randomized, double-blind, placebo-controlled, multicenter study. Mean follow-up period was 21 months. Primary end point was all-cause mortality rate.

Purpose: To evaluate the effect of amiodarone on mortality in post-MI patients with LV dysfunction.

Population: 1,486 patients aged 18 to 75 years with MI in the prior 5 to 21 days and EF of 40% or less by multiple-gated nuclear angiography (approximately 45% with EF 30% or less).

Exclusion Criteria: Amiodarone in previous 6 months; HR, less than 50 beats/min; second- or third-degree AV block; significant hepatic or thyroid dysfunction; need for antiarrhythmic(s) other than β-blockers or digoxin.

Treatment: Amiodarone, 800 mg/day for 14 days, 400 mg/day for 14 weeks, and then 200 mg/day; or placebo.

Results: Among all patients, total mortality was 13.4%, with no difference between amiodarone and placebo (RR, 0.99). No difference was observed in cardiac mortality (RR, 0.94; $p = 0.67$). The amiodarone group had fewer arrhythmic deaths (RR, 0.35; $p = 0.04$).

169. **Cairns JA,** et al., for the Canadian Amiodarone MI Arrhythmia Trial **(CAMIAT)** Investigators. Randomised trial of outcome after MI in patients with frequent or repetitive ventricular premature depolarisations: CAMIAT. *Lancet* 1997; 349:675–682.

Design: Prospective, randomized, double-blind, placebo-controlled, multicenter study. Median follow-up period was 1.8 years. Primary end point was resuscitated VF or arrhythmic death.

Purpose: To determine the effect of amiodarone on overall mortality in post-MI patients with frequent or repetitive ventricular premature depolarizations.

Population: 1,202 patients with MI in the prior 6 to 45 days, EF 40% or less, and 24-hour ECG monitoring showing 10 ventricular premature depolarizations per hour or one run of three beats of VT at 100 to 120 beats/min.

Exclusion Criteria: Contraindications to amiodarone (prior intolerance; HR, less than 50 beats/min; heart block (any degree); QT interval greater than 480 milliseconds; VT at more than 120 beats/min.

Treatment: Amiodarone, 10 mg/kg/day for 2 weeks, 300 to 400 mg/day for 3 to 5 months, 200 to 300 mg/day for 4 months, and 200 mg for 5 to 7 days/week for 16 months; or placebo.

Results: Amiodarone group with nearly 50% fewer arrhythmic deaths plus resuscitated VF [3.3% vs. 6.0%; $p = 0.016$ (intention-to-treat analysis, $p = 0.029$)]. Total mortality was not different.

Comments: Primary analysis was not based on intention-to-treat analysis. The trial also had many dropouts (221 amiodarone and 152 placebo patients; more than 70% and more than 50%, respectively, stopped because of adverse effects).

170. **Ceremuzynski L,** et al. Effect of amiodarone on mortality after MI: a double-blind, placebo-controlled pilot study. *J Am Coll Cardiol* 1992;20:1056–1062.

A total of 613 MI patients not eligible to receive β-blockers were randomized to placebo or amiodarone, 800 mg/day, and then 400 mg 6 times per week. The amiodarone group had a 45% lower 1-year mortality rate (6.2% vs. 10.7%; $p = 0.048$). The amiodarone group also had fewer class 4 ventricular arrhythmias (7.5% vs. 19.7%). Mild pulmonary toxicity was seen in only one patient.

171. **Teo KK,** et al. Effects of prophylactic antiarrhythmic drug therapy in acute MI. *JAMA* 1993;270:1589–1595.

This analysis focused on 138 randomized trials with approximately 98,000 enrolled patients. Lower mortality was seen with β-blockers (26,973 patients; OR, 0.81; $p^2 = 0.00001$) and amiodarone (778 patients; OR, 0.71; $p = 0.03$). Higher mortality was seen with class I agents (11,712 patients; OR, 1.14; $p = 0.03$). A statistically nonsignificant impact of calcium-channel blockers was observed (10,154 patients; OR, 1.04; $p = 0.41$).

172. **Sadowski ZP,** et al. Multicenter randomized trial and a systematic overview of lidocaine in acute myocardial infarction. *Am Heart J* 1999;137:792–798.

A total of 903 patients seen within 6 hours of symptom onset with ST elevation were randomized to lidocaine (four boluses of 50 mg each every 2 minutes, and then 3 mg/min for 12 hours, and then 2 mg/min for 36 hours) or no lidocaine. The lidocaine group had significantly less VF (2.0% vs. 5.7%; $p = 0.004$) but tended toward increased mortality (9.7% vs. 7.0%; $p = 0.145$). A meta-analysis of these results and those from 20 other randomized studies with more than 11,000 patients revealed nonsignificant trends toward reduced VF (OR, 0.71; 95% CI, 0.47 to 1.09) and increased mortality rates (OR, 1.12; 95% CI, 0.91 to 1.36) with lidocaine.

Intraaortic Balloon Pump

173. **Ohman EM,** et al., **IABP** Trial. Use of aortic counterpulsation to improve sustained coronary artery patency during acute MI. *Circulation* 1994;90:792–799.

Design: Prospective, randomized, multicenter study. Primary end point was angiographically detected reocclusion of IRA during initial hospitalization.
Purpose: To determine whether 48 hours of aortic counterpulsation therapy after reperfusion established during emergency catheterization would reduce the rate of reocclusion of the IRA.
Population: 182 AMI patients who underwent catheterization within 24 hours with successful restoration of IRA patency.
Exclusion Criteria: Included cardiogenic shock, pulmonary edema requiring aortic counterpulsation, severe PVD, more than 75% restenosis in one or two major epicardial arteries and TIMI grade 2 or 3 flow achieved in IRA with thrombolytic therapy, contraindication(s) to heparin.
Treatment: IABP for 48 hours or standard care.
Results: Primary angioplasty was performed in 106 patients, rescue angioplasty in 51 patients, and other methods (e.g., intracoronary thrombolysis) in the remaining 25 patients. Both groups had a similar incidence of severe bleeding complications and transfusions. Catheterization performed at a median of 5 days demonstrated that the aortic counterpulsation group had a lower IRA reocclusion rate (8% vs. 21%) and nearly 50% fewer clinical events (death, stroke, reinfarction, ERV, and recurrent ischemia; 13% vs. 24%; $p < 0.04$).

174. **Stone GW,** et al. A prospective, randomized evaluation of prophylactic intraaortic balloon pump (IABP) counterpulsation in high risk patients with acute MI treated with primary angioplasty. *J Am Coll Cardiol* 1997;29:1459–1467.

Design: Prospective, randomized, multicenter study. Primary end points were death, MI, IRA occlusion, stroke, new heart failure, and sustained hypotension.
Purpose: To determine whether AMI patients stratified as high risk benefit from a routine IABP strategy after PTCA.
Population: 437 PAMI II patients classified as high risk (meeting at least one of the following criteria: age older than 70 years, three-vessel disease, ejection fraction 45% or less, saphenous vein graft occlusion, persistent malignant ventricular arrhythmia, or suboptimal angioplasty result).
Exclusion Criteria: Cardiogenic shock, bleeding diathesis, and thrombolytic therapy before catheterization.
Treatment: IABP for 36 to 48 hours or standard care.

Results: The two groups had similar outcomes [composite end point incidence 28.9% (IABP) vs. 29.2%]. The IABP group had fewer unscheduled repeated catheterizations (7.6% vs. 13.3%; $p = 0.05$), but had more strokes (2.4% vs. 0%; $p = 0.03$). The authors suggest that the IABP effect may not have been detected because of low control group mortality (3.1%) and IRA occlusion rate (5.5%).

175. **Ohman EM,** et al. The use of intraaortic balloon pumping as an adjunct to reperfusion therapy in acute MI. *Am Heart J* 1991;121:895–901.

This retrospective analysis focused on 810 consecutive patients given thrombolysis within 6 hours of onset of symptoms. The balloon pump was inserted in 85 patients. This group had a higher frequency of three-vessel disease, left anterior descending (LAD) artery disease, and other risk factors, as well as a high in-hospital mortality rate of 32%. Reocclusion occurred in only two of 85 patients (after discharge), and no reinfarctions occurred while the balloon was inserted.

176. **Anderson RD,** et al. Use of intraaortic balloon bump counterpulsation in patients presenting with cardiogenic shock: observations from the GUSTO-I study. *J Am Coll Cardiol* 1997;30:708–715.

This analysis focused on 68 GUSTO-I patients with cardiogenic shock who had an IABP placed (91% within 1 day). Early IABP use was associated with increased bleeding (moderate, 47% vs. 12%; $p = 0.0001$; severe, 10% vs. 5%; $p = 0.16$). IABP use also was associated with increased arrhythmias, procedures, and bypass surgery. However, these increases were owing longer time to death (2.8 days vs. 7.2 hours). However, in part, a trend toward lower 30-day mortality was seen with IABP use [57% vs. 67%; adjusted $p = 0.11$ (if revascularization patients were excluded, 47% vs. 64%; $p = 0.07$)].

Other Treatments

177. **Malmberg K,** et al., Diabetic Insulin-Glucose Infusion in Acute MI **(DIGAMI).** Randomized trial of insulin-glucose infusion followed by subcutaneous insulin treatment in diabetic patients with acute MI: effects on mortality at 1 year. *J Am Coll Cardiol* 1995;26:57–65.

Design: Prospective, randomized, open, multicenter study. Primary end point was all-cause mortality.

Purpose: To evaluate whether rapid improvement of metabolic control in diabetic patients with an insulin/glucose infusion decreases early mortality and subsequent morbidity.

Population: 620 patients with suspected MI and blood glucose 11 mM on admission (with or without prior diagnosis of diabetes).

Treatment: Continuous i.v. insulin infusion for 24 hours (started at 5 U/h) or until normoglycemia was achieved (goal of 7 to 10 mM), and then s.c. insulin for 3 months; or conventional therapy.

Results: At 24 hours, the insulin/glucose-treated patients had lower glucose (9.6 vs. 11.7 mM) and 29% lower mortality at 1 year (18.6% vs. 26.1%; $p = 0.027$). Mortality reduction was most marked (52%) in patients with a low cardiovascular risk profile or no previous insulin therapy. Only 10% stopped insulin because of hypoglycemia with no associated morbidity.

Comments: Intense insulin may restore impaired platelet function, decrease plasminogen activator inhibitor (PAI)-1 activity, and possibly improve metabolism of noninfarcted areas. Long-term follow-up (see *BMJ* 1997;314:1512) showed that lower mortality was maintained at a mean 3.4 years: 33% vs. 44% (RR, 0.72; $p = 0.011$), with the largest benefit seen in patients with no prior insulin therapy (RR, 0.49).

178. **Fath-Ordoubadi F,** et al. Glucose-insulin-potassium therapy for treatment of acute MI. *Circulation* 1997;96:1152–1156.

This analysis focused on nine well-designed randomized, placebo-controlled trials with 1,932 patients (all prethrombolytic era). GIK was associated with lower hospital mortality (16.1% vs. 21%; OR, 0.72; $p = 0.004$). A 48% reduction was seen in the four trials using high-dose GIK (to suppress free fatty acid levels maximally).

179. **Diaz R,** et al., on behalf of the Estudios Cardiologicos Latinoamerica **(ECLA)** Glucose-Insulin-Potassium Pilot Trial Collaborative Group. Metabolic modulation of acute MI. *Circulation* 1998;98:2227–2234.

Design: Prospective, randomized, open, multicenter study.
Purpose: To evaluate the feasibility of GIK administration in contemporary practice and to assess its effect on clinical end points in patients with AMI.
Population: 407 patients with suspected AMI seen within 24 hours of symptom onset.
Exclusion Criteria: Severe renal impairment or hyperkalemia.
Treatment: High-dose GIK (25% glucose, 50 IU insulin/L, and 80 mM KCl at 1.5 mL/kg/hr for 24 hours), low-dose GIK (10% glucose, 20 IU insulin/L, and 40 mM KCl at 1.0 mL/kg/hr for 24 hours), or control. GIK was started an average 10 to 11 hours after onset of symptoms.
Results: GIK-treated patients had nonsignificant reductions in several in-hospital events, including severe heart failure, cardiogenic shock, VF, and reinfarction. Among the 252 (61.9%) patients treated with reperfusion strategies (thrombolysis, 95%; PTCA, 5%), GIK-treated patients had a significant 66% reduction in in-hospital mortality (5.2% vs. 15.2%; RR, 0.34; $p = 0.008$). At 1-year follow-up, only the high-dose GIK patients undergoing reperfusion had a significant mortality benefit (RR, 0.37; log rank test, 0.046). The GIK group had a higher frequency of phlebitis (severe in only 2%) and serum changes in plasma concentration of glucose or potassium.
Comments: High-dose regimen achieves maximal suppression of free fatty acid levels (see *Am J Cardiol* 1975;36:929). A meta-analysis of 1,932 patients showed no interaction between GIK and reperfusion.

180. **Mahaffey KW,** et al. Adenosine as an adjunct to thrombolytic therapy for acute myocardial infarction: results of a multicenter, randomized, placebo-controlled trial: the Acute Myocardial Infarction STudy of ADenosine **(AMISTAD)** trial. *J Am Coll Cardiol* 1999;34:1711–1720.

Design: Prospective, randomized, placebo-controlled, multicenter study. Primary end point was infarct size.
Purpose: To assess whether adenosine as an adjunct to thrombolysis would reduce MI size.
Population: 236 patients seen within 6 hours of onset of chest pain lasting 20 minutes or longer and with ST elevation 0.1 mV or more in two contiguous leads. Clinical decision made to treat with thrombolytic therapy.
Exclusion Criteria: Included dipyridamole within past 24 hours, bronchospastic lung disease or prior bronchodilator therapy, advanced AV block, LBBB, sustained bradycardia (less than 60 beats/min for more than 20 minutes).
Treatment: Adenosine (70 mg/kg/min i.v. for 3 hours) or placebo (normal saline) begun before thrombolytic therapy. Tc-99m sestamibi was injected before thrombolytic therapy began, and single-photon emission computed tomography (SPECT) imaging was performed within 6 hours.
Results: Infarct size was assessed in 83% of patients and was significantly reduced in adenosine-treated patients (adjusted $p = 0.03$). A 67% relative reduction in infarct size with adenosine was found in patients with anterior MI (15% in the adenosine group vs. 45.5% in the placebo group; $p = 0.014$) but no reduction in patients with nonanterior infarcts (11.5% for both groups; $p = 0.96$). A trend was seen toward more major clinical events in the adenosine group compared with placebo (22% vs. 16%; OR, 1.43; 95% CI, 0.71 to 2.89).

181. **AMISTAD II.** Preliminary results presented at the 51st ACC Scientific Session, Atlanta, GA. March 2002.

This prospective, randomized, placebo-controlled trial enrolled 2,118 patient with anterior AMI seen within 6 hours of symptom onset. Patients were randomized to low-dose i.v. adenosine (50 μg/kg/min), high-dose adenosine (70 μg/kg/min), or placebo for 3 hours. Patients underwent reperfusion therapy (thrombolysis or mechanical reperfusion) within 15 minutes of initiation of study drug infusion. At 6 months, a nonsignificant reduction in death or CHF was seen in the pooled adenosine groups (16%) and with the high-dose group (15%) versus placebo (18%). In the prespecified subgroup analysis of patients with reperfusion success, a significant reduction in death or CHF was seen in the pooled adenosine group versus placebo (11% vs. 15%; $p = 0.043$). Among patients treated within 2 hours, adenosine had a greater RRR than did placebo (9% vs. 13%). Infarct size trended toward being smaller in pooled adenosine groups compared with placebo (17% vs. 26%; $p = 0.078$) and reached statistical significance in the high-dose adenosine group (11% vs. 26%; $p = 0.028$).

182. **GIPS.** Preliminary results presented at 24th Annual Meeting of the European Society of Cardiology, September 2002, Munich.

This prospective, randomized, placebo-controlled, open trial enrolled 940 patients with AMI treated with primary angioplasty. Patients received potassium, 80 mmol in 500 mL, and 20% glucose at a rate of 3 mL/kg body weight/hr over 8 to 12 hours and continuous i.v. insulin titrated with dose adjustment every hour, or placebo. At 30 days, a nonsignificant trend was observed toward a reduction in the combined end point of death, reinfarction, and repeated revascularization in the GIK group (8.0% vs. 9.9%; $p = 0.08$). In a subgroup analysis, a significant reduction was found in the primary end point among those without heart failure symptoms (Killip class 1) (4.2% vs. 8.4%; $p = 0.01$).

Specific Cases

Anterior Myocardial Infarction

183. **Stone PH,** et al. Prognostic significance of location and type of MI: independent adverse outcome associated with anterior location. *J Am Coll Cardiol* 1988;11:453–463.

This retrospective analysis focused on 471 Multicenter Investigation of the Limitation of Infarct Size (MILIS) patients with a first MI showing an anterior location associated with poor outcome. Anterior versus inferior patients: larger infarcts (higher CK-MB fraction; $p < 0.001$), approximately 3 times more heart failure (40.7% vs. 14.7%), more than 4 times more in-hospital deaths (11.9% vs. 2.8%; $p < 0.001$), and higher cumulative cardiac mortality (27% vs. 11%; $p < 0.001$). Q wave versus non-Q wave: worse in-hospital course [higher CK-MB, lower EF, more heart failure and deaths (9.3% vs. 4.1%; $p < 0.05$)], but no significant difference in long-term cardiac mortality (21% vs. 16%). After adjustment for infarct size, anterior patients still had higher mortality rates. If location and type were considered, anterior patients still had worse outcomes (whether Q wave or non–Q wave).

Inferior Myocardial Infarction

184. **Berger PB,** et al. Incidence and prognostic implications of heart block complicating inferior MI treated with thrombolytic therapy: results from TIMI II. *J Am Coll Cardiol* 1992;20:533–540.

This retrospective analysis focused on 1,786 patients. Complete heart block occurred in 12% (6.3% at presentation). The complete heart block group had a higher unadjusted 21-day mortality rate (7.1% vs. 2.7%; $p = 0.007$), but adjusted RR was not statistically significant. Mortality was nearly 5 times higher in those with complete heart block after thrombolysis (9.9% vs. 2.2%; $p < 0.001$). Increased deaths were attributable to more severe cardiac dysfunction.

185. **Behar S,** et al. Complete atrioventricular block complicating inferior acute wall MI: short and long-term prognosis. *Am Heart J* 1993;125:1622–1627.

This analysis focused on 2,273 SPRINT Registry patients with inferior Q-wave MIs. An 11% incidence of complete heart block was observed (women, 14%; age 70 years, 15%). The complete heart block group had more than a threefold higher in-hospital mortality rate (37% vs. 11%; $p < 0.0001$; adjusted OR, 2.0; 95% CI, 1.12 to 3.57).

However, no difference in 5-year mortality was observed among hospital survivors (28% vs. 23%).

186. **Peterson ED,** et al. Prognostic significance of precordial ST segment depression during inferior MI in the thrombolytic era: results in 16,521 patients. *J Am Coll Cardiol* 1996;28:305–312.

This *post hoc* GUSTO-I analysis focused on 6,422 patients without any precordial depression. The ST-depression group had a 47% higher 30-day mortality rate (4.7% vs. 3.2%; at 1 year, 5% vs. 3.4%; $p < 0.001$). Magnitude of depression (sum of V_1 through V_6) added significant prognostic information after risk factor adjustment: 36% higher mortality per 0.5 mm.

187. **Matetzky S,** et al. Significance of ST segment elevations in posterior chest leads (V_7 to V_9) in patients with acute inferior MI: application for thrombolytic therapy. *J Am Coll Cardiol* 1998;31:506–511.

This analysis showed that ST elevation in V_7 to V_9 correlates with posterolateral involvement, and such patients benefit more from thrombolysis. Eighty-seven patients who had a first inferior MI and were treated with rtPA were stratified according to the presence (46 patients) or absence (41 patients) of ST elevation in V_7 to V_9. The ST-elevation group had a higher incidence of posterolateral wall-motion abnormalities ($p < 0.001$) on radionuclide ventriculography, a larger infarct area (higher peak CK, $p < 0.02$), lower predischarge EF ($p < 0.008$), and higher incidence of death, reinfarction, or heart failure ($p < 0.05$). Patency of the IRA in the V_7 to V_9 elevation group resulted in an improved EF at discharge ($p < 0.012$), whereas EF in the nonelevation patients was unchanged, regardless of IRA patency.

Right Ventricular Infarction

188. **Zehender M,** et al. Right ventricular infarction as an independent predictor of prognosis after acute MI. *N Engl J Med* 1993;328:981–988.

This analysis of 200 consecutive patients showed that ST elevation in lead V_4R was highly predictive of RV infarction: sensitivity, 88%; specificity, 78%. ST elevation in V_4R also was associated with higher mortality (31% vs. 19% overall) and more in-hospital complications (64% vs. 28%).

189. **Kinch JW, Ryan TJ.** Right ventricular infarction. *N Engl J Med* 1994;330:1211–1217.

This excellent overview discusses the pathophysiology, diagnosis, complications, treatment, and prognosis of patients with RV infarction.

190. **Zehender M,** et al. Eligibility for and benefit of thrombolytic therapy in inferior MI: focus on the prognostic importance of right ventricular infarction. *J Am Coll Cardiol* 1994;24:362–369.

This prospective analysis focused on 200 patients with an inferior MI. Thrombolytic therapy (accelerated tPA regimen) was received by 36%; this group of patients had a lower mortality than did patients ineligible for tPA (8% vs. 25%; $p < 0.001$). However, benefit of tPA was restricted to patients with RV infarction (RVI) complicating acute inferior MI: 76% lower mortality (10% vs. 42%; $p < 0.005$) and fewer overall complications (34% vs. 54%; $p < 0.05$). In the absence of RVI, no difference was observed in mortality (7% vs. 6%), whether or not patients received tPA.

191. **Bowers TR,** et al. Effect of reperfusion on biventricular function and survival after right ventricular infarction. *N Engl J Med* 1998;338:933–940.

This prospective study was composed of 53 inferior MI patients with echocardiographic evidence of RVI (RV free-wall dysfunction, dilatation, and depressed global performance). Complete reperfusion was achieved by balloon angioplasty in 77% of patients (i.e., normal flow in right coronary artery and its major RV branches) and led to recovery of RV function [mean score for free-wall motion, 1.4 (at 3 days) vs. 3.0 (baseline); $p < 0.001$]. In contrast, unsuccessful reperfusion (no RV branch flow) was associated with a lack of RV recovery, as well as persistent hypotension and low cardiac output (83% vs. 12%; $p = 0.002$) and markedly higher mortality (58% vs. 2%; $p = 0.001$).

192. **Zeymer U,** et al. Effects of thrombolytic therapy in acute inferior MI with or without right ventricular involvement. *J Am Coll Cardiol* 1998;32:876–881.

This analysis of 522 inferior MI patients from the HIT-4 trial showed that RV involvement is not an independent predictor of survival. RV involvement was associated with higher 30-day cardiac mortality rates (5.9% vs. 2.5%), but this was related to larger infarct size rather than to RVI. Among large inferior MI patients (sum ST elevation greater than 0.8 mV or precordial depression), a proximal right coronary artery lesion was seen in 52% with and 23% without RVI. Among small-MI patients, lesions were mostly distal in location, and cardiac mortality was less than 1% irrespective of the presence of RVI.

193. **Shiraki H,** et al. Association between preinfarction angina and a lower risk of right ventricular infarction. *N Engl J Med* 1998;338:941–947.

This retrospective analysis focused on 113 patients with a first MI due to occlusion of the right coronary artery. Absence of preinfarction angina (defined as chest pain less than 30 minutes 7 or fewer days before MI) was a strong predictor of RVI (OR, 6.3; $p < 0.001$), complete AV block (OR, 3.6; $p = 0.01$), and combined hypotension and shock (OR, 12.4; $p < 0.001$). Angina in the preceding 24 to 72 hours was associated with a lower incidence of RVI (OR, 0.2; $p = 0.02$) and hypotension/shock (OR, 0.1; $p = 0.02$).

Posterior Myocardial Infarction

194. **Boden WE,** et al. Electrocardiographic evolution of posterior acute MI: importance of early precordial ST-segment depression. *Am J Cardiol* 1987;59:782–787.

This analysis focused on 50 patients from the Diltiazem Reinfarction Study who had isolated precordial ST-segment elevation of 1 mm or more in at least two precordial leads (V_1 to V_4). Serial ECGs showed that 46% developed evidence of posterior MI, defined as R-wave 0.04 seconds or more in lead V_1 and R:S 1 or more in V_2. The posterior group had a higher peak CK than the anterior group (1,051 vs. 663 IU; $p < 0.009$). All 23 posterior MI patients had horizontal ST depression and upright precordial T waves versus downsloping ST depression and T-wave inversion in 27 patients with an anterior non–Q-wave MI.

195. **Casas RE,** et al. Value of leads V_7–V_9 in diagnosing posterior wall acute MI and other causes of tall R waves in V_1–V_2. *Am J Cardiol* 1997;80:508–509 (see reference 8 for summary).

Cocaine-associated Myocardial Infarction

196. **Hollander JE,** et al. Prospective multicenter evaluation of cocaine-associated chest pain. *Acad Emerg Med* 1994;1:330–339.

This prospective cohort study was composed of 246 patients with cocaine-associated chest pain. Pain began at a median 60 minutes after cocaine use and persisted for 120 minutes. Fourteen (5.7%) patients had a confirmed MI (elevated CK-MB). ECG showed a low sensitivity (35.7%) and high specificity (89.9%). No clinical differences were seen between those with and without MI.

197. **Hollander JE.** The management of cocaine-associated myocardial ischemia. *N Engl J Med* 1995;333:1267–1272.

This review covers pathophysiology, initial evaluation, treatment, complications, diagnostic evaluation, long-term prognosis, and secondary prevention of cocaine-associated ischemia.

198. **Hollander JE,** et al. Predictors of coronary artery disease in patients with cocaine-associated MI. *Am J Med* 1997;102:158–163.

This retrospective analysis of 70 patients from 29 centers found CAD, defined as 50% or more stenosis or positive stress test result, demonstrated in 70%. The patient with CAD was older (42 vs. 31 years) and had more cardiac risk factors (2.3 vs. 1.5), hypertension (OR, 5.3), and bradyarrhythmias (OR, 8.0). A greater percentage also had inferior location (p = 0.04).

Non–Q-wave/Non–ST Elevation Myocardial Infarction
See Chapter 3.

Assessment and Prognosis

General Review Articles/Miscellaneous
199. **Shaw LJ,** et al. A meta-analysis of pre-discharge risk stratification after acute MI with stress electrocardiography myocardial perfusion and ventricular function imaging. *Am J Cardiol* 1996;78:1327–1337.

This analysis of 54 studies (76% retrospective) with 19,874 patients shows the low positive predictive value of predischarge noninvasive testing.

200. **Morrow DA,** et al. TIMI risk score for ST-elevation myocardial infarction: a convenient, bedside, clinical score for risk assessment at presentation: an intravenous nPA for treatment of infarcting myocardium early II trial substudy. *Circulation* 2000;102:2031–2037.

The TIMI risk score for STEMI was created as the arithmetic sum of independent mortality predictors based on a logistic regression analysis of the 14,114-patient Intravenous nPA for Treatment of Infarcting Myocardium Early II (InTIME II) trial. The ten baseline variables constituting the TIMI risk score accounted for 97% of the predictive capacity of the multivariate model. These included age 65 to 74 years (2 points); age older than 75 years (3 points); diabetes, hypertension or angina (1 point); SBP less than 100 mm Hg (3 points); heart rate more than 100 beats/min (2 points); Killip class II to IV (2 points); weight less than 67 kg (1 point); anterior STEMI or LBBB (1 point); and time to treatment more than 4 hours (1 point). The risk score showed a more than 40-fold graded increase in mortality (less than 1% with a score of 0 vs. 35.9% for a score greater than 8). The prognostic capacity of the TIMI risk score was similar to the full multivariable model (c statistic, 0. 779 vs. 0.784). External validation in the TIMI 9 trial showed similar prognostic capacity (c statistic, 0.746).

201. **Morrow DA,** et al. Application of the TIMI risk score for ST-elevation MI in the National Registry of Myocardial Infarction 3. *JAMA* 2001;286:1356–1359.

The TIMI risk score was evaluated in 84,029 STEMI patients treated from 1998 to 2000 and data recorded in the National Registry of MI 3 (NRMI 3) registry. Only 48% received reperfusion therapy. NRMI 3 patients were older and more often female and with a history of CAD than were those in the derivation set. A significant graded increase in mortality was found with increasing TIMI risk score (range, 1.1% to 30.0%; $p < 0.001$ for trend). The risk score showed strong prognostic capacity overall (c = 0.74 vs 0.78 in derivation set). The risk score was equally predictive in those treated with fibrinolysis (c = 0.79) and primary PCI (c = 0.80). Among patients not receiving fibrinolytic therapy, absolute mortality rates were much higher for a given risk score, but the same pattern (higher score, higher risk) was seen, although with lower discriminatory capacity (c = 0.65).

Electrocardiography, Arrhythmias, and Conduction System
202. **Volpi A,** et al. In-hospital prognosis of patients with acute MI complicated by primary ventricular fibrillation. *N Engl J Med* 1987;317:257–261.

This analysis focused on 11,112 GISSI patients. Primary VF (defined as not due to shock or MI) occurred in 2.8% and was associated with a nearly twofold higher in-hospital mortality rate (10.8% vs. 5.9%; RR, 1.94; 95% CI, 1.35 to 2.78).

203. Multicenter Investigation of the Limitation of Infarct Size **(MILIS).** Prognosis after cardiac arrest due to ventricular tachycardia or ventricular fibrillation associated with acute MI. *Am J Cardiol* 1987;60:755–761.

This analysis focused on 849 MILIS study patients aged 75 years or younger with a confirmed MI. Mean follow-up period was 32 months. VT and VF patients had a fourfold higher in-hospital mortality rate (27% vs. 7%; $p < 0.001$). This difference was attributable to a sevenfold higher risk in patients with secondary causes of VT and VF (e.g., presence of heart failure, hypotension). A worse outcome was attained if the episode occurred after 72 hours (57% vs. 20%; $p < 0.05$). No cases of primary VT and VF occurred after 72 hours. No difference in mortality at follow-up was seen among hospital survivors.

204. **Berger PB,** et al. Incidence and significance of ventricular tachycardia and fibrillation in the absence of hypotension or heart failure in acute MI treated with recombinant tissue-type plasminogen activator: results from the Thrombolysis in Myocardial Infarction (TIMI) phase II trial. *J Am Coll Cardiol* 1993;22:1773–1779.

This analysis focused on 2,456 TIMI II patients without CHF or hypotension during the first 24 hours after study entry. Sustained VT or VF developed in 1.9% within 24 hours. Among patients undergoing angiography at 18 to 48 hours (per protocol), the VT and VF group had lower IRA patency (68% vs. 87%; $p = 0.01$). Mortality at 21 days was more than 10 times higher in the VT and VF patients (20.4% vs. 1.6%; $p < 0.001$). Survival from 21 days to 1 year was similar in both groups.

205. **Schroder R,** et al. Extent of early ST segment elevation resolution: a strong predictor of outcome in patients with acute MI and a sensitive measure to compare thrombolytic regimens. *J Am Coll Cardiol* 1995;26:1657–1664.

This prospective study was composed of 1,398 INJECT patients seen within 6 hours of symptom onset. ST resolution at 3 hours was classified into three groups: complete (more than 70%), partial (30% to 70%), and no (less than 30%) resolution. The 35-day mortality rates in these groups were 2.5%, 4.3%, and 17.5% ($p < 0.0001$). Even after baseline characteristics were included, ST resolution was the most powerful predictor of 35-day mortality.

206. **Mont L,** et al. Predisposing factors and prognostic value of sustained monomorphic ventricular tachycardia in early phase of acute MI. *J Am Coll Cardiol* 1996;28:1670–1676.

This retrospective analysis focused on 1,120 consecutive cardiac care unit patients. The incidence of monomorphic VT was 1.9%. This group had larger infarcts (peak CK-MB, 435 vs. 168 IU/L) and 4 times higher mortality (43% vs. 11%; $p < 0.001$). VT was an independent mortality predictor, whereas independent predictors of VT were CK-MB (OR, 11.8), Killip class (OR, 4, 0), and bifascicular block (OR, 3.1).

207. **Hathaway WR,** et al. Prognostic significance of the initial electrocardiogram in patients with acute MI. *JAMA* 1998;279:387–391.

This retrospective analysis focused on 34,166 GUSTO-I patients without paced or ventricular rhythms or LBBB. In multivariate analysis, 30-day mortality predictors were found to be the sum of ST deviation (depression and elevation; OR, 1.53), heart rate (OR, 1.49), and QRS duration.

208. **Volpi A,** et al. Incidence and prognosis of early primary ventricular fibrillation in acute MI: results of the GISSI-2 database. *Am J Cardiol* 1998;82:265–271.

This retrospective analysis focused on 9,720 patients with a first MI. Early (4 hours or less) and late (more than 4 to 48 hours) primary VF occurred in 3.1% and 0.6%, respectively. Recurrence rates were 11% and 15%. Early primary VF occurred more frequently if SBP was less than 120 mm Hg and in the presence of hypokalemia. In-hospital mortality was higher in patients with both early and late primary VF [ORs, 2.47 (95% CI, 1.48 to 4.13) and 3.97 (95% CI, 1.51 to 10.48)]. Mortality from hospital discharge to 6 months was similar for both primary VF subgroups and controls.

209. **Go AS,** et al. Bundle-branch block and in-hospital mortality in acute MI. *Ann Intern Med* 1998;129:690–697.

This large retrospective cohort study of 297,832 patients from 1,571 hospitals showed that the prevalences of RBBB and LBBB are similar (6.2% and 6.7%, respectively) and that RBBB is a stronger independent predictor of in-hospital death [adjusted OR, 1.64 vs. 1.34 (LBBB)].

210. **Cheema AN,** et al. Nonsustained ventricular tachycardia in the setting of acute MI. *Circulation* 1998;98:2030–2036.

This prospective database analysis showed that contrary to prevailing opinion, nonsustained VT (NSVT) that occurs beyond several hours after AMI is associated with adverse outcomes. NSVT was identified in 118 patients within 72 hours of AMI. The control group was matched for age, sex, type of MI, and thrombolytic therapy. The NSVT group had more frequent in-hospital VF (9% vs. none; $p < 0.001$), but in-hospital mortality (10% vs. 4%) and follow-up mortality (10% vs. 17%) were not significantly different. However, a multivariate analysis showed that time from presentation to NSVT was the strongest mortality predictor (risk became significant at 13 hours and peaked at 24 hours; RR, 7.5).

211. **Savonitto S,** et al. Prognostic value of the admission electrocardiogram in acute coronary syndromes. *JAMA* 1999;281:707–713.

This retrospective analysis focused on 12,142 GUSTO-IIb patients. Presenting ECG characteristics included T-wave inversion in 22%, ST elevation in 28%, ST depression in 35%, and 15% with a combination of ST elevation and depression. The 30-day incidence of death or MI was 5.5% in patients with T-wave inversion, 9.4% in those with ST elevation, 10.5% in those with ST depression, and 12.4% in those with both ST elevation and depression. After adjusting for factors associated with increased death or MI at 30 days, compared with those with T-wave inversion only, patients with ST-segment changes were at significantly increased risk (ORs, 1.68, 1.62, and 2.27 for ST elevation, ST depression, and both, respectively). Admission CK levels were associated with increased risk of death (OR, 2.36) and death or MI (OR, 1.56). In a multivariate analysis, ECG category and CK levels at admission remained highly predictive of death and MI.

Exercise Testing

212. **Hamm LF,** et al. Safety and efficacy of exercise testing early after acute MI. *Am J Cardiol* 1989;63:1193–1197.

This analysis focused on 151,949 tests performed at 570 institutions; 42% were symptom-limited tests. Overall, only 41 fatal (0.03%) and 141 major cardiac complications (0.09%) were noted. Symptom-limited testing was associated with a similar mortality rate, but with 1.9 times more major cardiac complications.

213. **Chaitman BR,** et al. Impact of treatment strategy on predischarge exercise test in TIMI-II. *Am J Cardiol* 1993;71:131–138.

This analysis focused on 3,339 patients showing a fourfold higher 1-year mortality rate if no predischarge exercise test was done (7.7% vs. 1.8%; $p < 0.001$). No predictive value of ST depression or chest pain was observed: conservative RR, 0.6 (95% CI, 0.1 to 2.9); invasive RR, 2.1 (95% CI, 0.5 to 9.4). However, catheterization and revascularization are recommended if ETT is positive.

214. **Jain A,** et al. Comparison of symptom-limited and low level exercise tolerance tests early after MI. *J Am Coll Cardiol* 1993;22:1816–1820.

This analysis focused on 150 consecutive patients [44 others were excluded (death, ischemia at rest or with minimal ambulation, complications, physician/patient preference)]. Bruce protocol was performed at 6.4 ± 3.1 days. Low-level test results were positive in only 23% versus 40% with symptom-limited tests ($p < 0.001$). At follow-up (15 ± 5 months), only five patients with a negative maximal test result versus 14 patients with a nondiagnostic symptom-limited test had cardiac events.

215. **Zaret BL,** et al. Value of radionuclide rest and exercise left ventricular ejection fraction in assessing survival of patients after thrombolytic therapy for acute MI: results of TIMI II Study. *J Am Coll Cardiol* 1995;26:73–79.

The 2,567 patients were studied at average 9 hours after onset of symptoms. Rest EF was strongly associated with 1-year mortality (overall, 9.9%). The RR for EF of 30% to 39% was 3.1; 40% to 49%, 2.2; and 50% to 59%, 1.2. The differential between rest and exercise EF was not helpful.

216. **Villella A,** et al. Prognostic significance of maximal exercise testing after MI treated with thrombolytic agents: the GISSI-2 data base. *Lancet* 1995;346:523–529.

This *post hoc* analysis focused on 6,295 GISSI-2 patients tested an average of 28 days after AMI. The same mortality rate (7.1%) was observed among those with a positive ETT result as in those who did not undergo testing; lower rates were associated with nondiagnostic and negative tests (1.3% and 0.9%, respectively). Independent predictors of mortality were symptomatic ischemia and low work capacity (RRs, 2.1 and 1.8).

217. **Vanhees L,** et al. Comparison of maximum vs. submaximal exercise testing in providing prognostic information after acute MI and/or coronary artery bypass grafting. *Am J Cardiol* 1997;80:257–262.

This retrospective analysis focused on 527 patients (MI, $n = 297$; bypass surgery, $n = 119$; both, $n = 111$) with a maximal test result at 12.9 ± 2.7 weeks after the event. After adjustments, peak oxygen uptake significantly related to all-cause and total mortality [HRs, 0.43 ($p < 0.05$) and 0.31 ($p < 0.01$)]. Five METS and anaerobic threshold were not predictive of mortality. In contrast, 7 METS (reached by 37%, encompasses 94% of events) was a strong predictor: HRs 0.16 and 0.15 (both $p < 0.01$) and had excellent diagnostic accuracy (loss of specificity with a cutoff of 8 METS).

Echocardiography and Other Noninvasive Tests

218. **Sutton MSJ,** et al. Quantitative two-dimensional echocardiography measurements are major predictors of adverse cardiovascular events after acute MI. *Circulation* 1994;89:68–75.

A total of 521 SAVE trial patients had echocardiograms at 11.1 ± 3.2 days. At 1 year, LVED and LV end-systolic areas were smaller in the captopril group ($p = 0.038$, 0.015). The captopril group had 35% fewer cardiovascular events. In these patients with cardiovascular events, a more than threefold increase in LV cavity areas was observed.

219. **Picano E,** et al. Stress echocardiography results predict risk of reinfarction early after uncomplicated acute MI: large-scale multicenter study. *J Am Coll Cardiol* 1995;26:908–913.

The 1,080 patients underwent a dipyridamole echocardiography study at 10 ± 5 days. Follow-up period was 14 months. A positive test result (44%) was associated with a higher reinfarction rate (6.3% vs. 3.3%; $p < 0.01$).

220. **Sicari R,** et al., ECHO Dobutamine International Cooperative **(EDIC)** Study. Prognostic value of dobutamine-atropine stress echocardiography early after acute MI. *J Am Coll Cardiol* 1997;29:254–260.

In this prospective, observational, multicenter trial, 778 patients with first MI were tested at an average of 12 days, with follow-up testing at 9 ± 7 months. Positive test results were attained in 56%. No difference in event rates (death, MI, unstable angina, angioplasty, bypass surgery) was observed regardless of positive or negative test results: 14% versus 12% ($p = 0.3$). However, when only spontaneously occurring events were considered, myocardial viability was the best predictor (HR, 2.0; $p < 0.002$). Wall-motion stroke index is a very strong predictor of cardiac deaths only (HR, 9.2; $p < 0.0001$).

221. **Migrino RQ,** et al. End-systolic volume index at 90 to 180 minutes into reperfusion therapy for acute MI is a strong predictor of early and late mortality. *Circulation* 1997;96:116–121.

The 1,300 patients underwent left ventriculography. End-systolic volume index of 40 mL/m^2 or less was independently associated with increased 30-day and 1-year mortality rates [adjusted ORs, 3.4 (95% CI, 2.0 to 5.9), 4.1 (95% CI, 2.6 to 6.2); $p < 0.001$]. Independent predictors of high end-systolic volume index of 40 or less were SBP less than 110 mm Hg, anterior MI, male, prior angina or MI, weight less than 70 kg, and heart rate 80 beats/min or less.

Flow and Vessel Patency

222. **Dewood MA,** et al. Prevalence of total coronary occlusion during the early hours of transmural MI. *N Engl J Med* 1980;303:897–902.

This classic angiography study demonstrated the central role of thrombotic occlusion in the pathogenesis of transmural MI. A total of 322 patients underwent catheterization at less than 24 hours. Total occlusion of the IRA was seen in 87% at less than 4 hours versus 65% at 12 to 24 hours.

223. **Karagounis L,** et al. Does TIMI perfusion grade 2 represent a mostly patent artery or a mostly occluded artery? Enzymatic and electrocardiographic evidence from the TEAM-2 study (Trial of Eminase in Acute MI). *J Am Coll Cardiol* 1992;19:1–10.

This analysis focused on 359 TEAM II patients treated with APSAC or SK. Angiography was performed at 90 to 240 minutes. TIMI grade 3 flow was associated with earlier enzymatic peaks and better ECG indexes of MI than TIMI grade flows 0 to 2 ($p = 0.02$ to 0.0001). No differences were found between TIMI flow grades 0, 1, and 2.

224. **Gibson CM,** et al. Angiographic predictors of reocclusion after thrombolysis: results from TIMI-4. *J Am Coll Cardiol* 1995;25:582–589.

The 278 patients were randomized to APSAC, rtPA, or combination therapy. Higher reocclusion (at 18 to 36 hours) was associated with TIMI grade 2 versus 3 flow (10% vs. 2%; $p = 0.003$), ulcerated lesions (10% vs. 3%; $p = 0.009$), and positive collateral vessels (18% vs. 5.6%; $p = 0.03$). Similar trends were seen for eccentric (7% vs. 2%; $p = 0.06$) and thrombotic lesions (8% vs. 3%; $p = 0.06$). Reocclusion also was associated with more severe mean stenosis at 90 minutes (78% vs. 74%; $p = 0.04$).

225. **Simes RJ,** et al. Link between the angiographic substudy and mortality outcomes in a large randomized trial of myocardial reperfusion: importance of early and complete infarct artery reperfusion. *Circulation* 1995;91:1923–1928.

This GUSTO-I substudy of 1,210 patients showed that TIMI grade 3 flow at 90 minutes was associated with decreased mortality. A model was developed that assumed any difference in treatment effects on 30-day mortality were mediated through differences in 90-minute IRA patency. The model showed a strong correlation ($r = 0.97$) between actual and predicted mortality rates. These data provide support for the idea that improved survival is due to achievement of early and complete reperfusion.

226. **Lenderink T,** et al. Benefit of thrombolytic therapy is sustained throughout 5 years and is related to TIMI perfusion grade 3 but not grade 2 flow at discharge. *Circulation* 1995;92:1110–1116.

This study showed the benefits of achieving TIMI grade 3 flow. Five-year follow-up data were analyzed on 923 hospital survivors enrolled in the European Cooperative Study Group (ECSG) studies. Patients with TIMI grade 3 flow had a 91% 5-year survival rate compared with 84% for the TIMI grade 0 to 1 and TIMI grade 2 groups ($p^2 = 0.01$).

227. **Anderson JL,** et al. Meta-analysis of five reported studies on the relation of early coronary patency grades with mortality and outcomes after acute MI. *Am J Cardiol* 1996;78:1–8.

This meta-analysis focused on five studies with 3,969 patients. The mortality rate was 8.8% for TIMI grade 0/1, 7% for grade 2, and only 3.7% for grade 2 patients (grade 3 vs. 2; $p = 0.001$). TIMI grade 3 flow also was associated with better EFs and less time to CK peak.

228. **Reiner JS,** et al. Evolution of early TIMI 2 flow after thrombolysis for acute MI. *Circulation* 1996;94:2441–2446.

This analysis of the GUSTO Angiography Study showed the benefit of progressing from early TIMI grade 2 flow to grade 3 at follow-up. Of 914 patients with TIMI grade 2 flow, 278 underwent angiography at both 90 minutes and 5 to 7 days. In the group that improved to grade 3 flow by the second catheterization (67%), a higher mean EF (57.5% vs. 52.8%; $p = 0.02$), better infarct zone wall motion ($p = 0.01$) and less visible thrombus (26% vs. 38%; $p = 0.04$) were found. However, TIMI grade 3 flow at 90 minutes remained the best, with less thrombus (42% vs. 58%; $p < 0.0001$) and highest 5- to 7-day EF (61.7% vs. 57.5%; $p = 0.002$).

229. **Pilote L,** et al. Determinants of the use of angiography and revascularization after thrombolysis for acute MI. *N Engl J Med* 1996;335:1198–1205.

This *post hoc* analysis focused on 21,772 GUSTO-I patients; 71% had predischarge angiography, of whom 58% underwent revascularization (PTCA, 73%). Overall, the best predictor of angiography use was age [if younger than 73 years, 76% (vs. 53%)]. Among young patients, PTCA availability was the most important predictor [83% vs. 67% (no PTCA)]. The number two predictor was recurrent ischemia. Reassuringly, coronary anatomy was the top predictor of the use and type of revascularization. However, the study yielded several unexpected findings: (a) similar revascularization rate in those with three-vessel disease and LV dysfunction as those with an EF less than 50% and one- or two-vessel disease and LAD stenosis of 50% or less; (b) many without symptoms had revascularization for one- or two-vessel disease; and (c) patients younger than 80 years with CHF or cardiogenic shock had similar angiography rates to those without these findings.

230. **Selby JV,** et al. Variation among hospitals in coronary angiography practices and outcomes after MI in a large health maintenance organization. *N Engl J Med* 1996;335:1888–1896.

This retrospective cohort study was composed of 6,851 patients treated from 1990 to 1992 at 16 hospitals. By 3 months, 30% to 77% had undergone angiography. After multivariate analysis, angiography rates in all hospitals were found to be inversely related to the risk of death from heart disease and heart disease events ($p = 0.03$; $p < 0.001$). However, at higher-angiography-rate hospitals, angiography was associated with lower risks of death and any heart disease event (HRs, 0.67 and 0.72). In patients without indications for angiography, less benefit was seen at high-volume centers (HRs, 0.85 and 0.90).

231. **Barbagelata NA,** et al. TIMI grade 3 flow and reocclusion after intravenous thrombolytic therapy: a pooled analysis. *Am Heart J* 1997;133:273–282.

Analysis of 15 TIMI flow studies with 5,475 angiograms and 27 reocclusion studies with 3,147 angiograms. TIMI grade 3 flow rates at 60 minutes and 90 minutes were as follows: with accelerated tPA, 57.1%/63.2%; standard tPA, 39.5%/50.2%; APSAC, 40.2%/50.1%; and SK, 31.5% (90 minutes). Reocclusion rates were as follows: with accelerated tPA, 6.0%; standard tPA, 11.8%; APSAC, 3.0%; and SK, 4.2%.

232. **Puma JA,** et al. Support for the open-artery hypothesis in survivors of acute MI: analysis of 11,228 patients treated with thrombolytic therapy. *Am J Cardiol* 1999;83:482–487.

This analysis focused on 11,228 GUSTO-I patients with available IRA patency data. Both univariable and multivariable analyses showed that an open artery was associated with a significantly lower 30-day mortality rate ($p < 0.001$). This benefit appears to extend beyond that provided by myocardial salvage because the effect remained after adjustment for LVEF.

233. **Gibson CM,** et al. Relationship between TIMI frame count and clinical outcomes after thrombolytic administration. *Circulation* 1999;99:1945–1950.

Corrected TIMI frame count (CTFC) was measured in 1,248 patients in TIMI 4, 10A, and 10B trials. Patients who died in the hospital and by 30 to 42 days had higher CTFCs (69.6 vs. 49.5, $p = 0.0003$; 66.2 vs. 49.9, $p = 0.006$). In a multivariate model, CTFC was an independent predictor of in-hospital mortality (OR, 1.21 per 10-frame increase). The risk of in-hospital mortality increased in a graded fashion from none in patients with the fastest flow (0 to 13 frames, hyperemia, TIMI grade 4 flow), to 2.7% in patients with CTFC of 14 to 40 (CTFC 40 is the cutoff for TIMI grade 3 flow), to 6.4% in patients with CTFC greater than 40 ($p = 0.003$).

Microvascular Perfusion

234. **Gibson CM,** et al. for the TIMI Study Group. Relationship of TIMI myocardial perfusion grade to mortality after administration of thrombolytic drugs. *Circulation* 2000;101:125–130.

The TIMI myocardial perfusion (TMP) grade system was developed to assess the filling and clearance of contrast in the myocardium. TMP grade 0 was defined as no apparent tissue-level perfusion (no ground-glass appearance of blush or opacification of the myocardium) in culprit artery distribution; TMP grade 1 indicates presence of myocardial blush but no clearance from the microvasculature (blush or a stain was present on the next injection); TMP grade 2 blush clears slowly (blush is strongly persistent and diminishes minimally or not at all during three cardiac cycles of the washout phase); and TMP grade 3 indicates that blush begins to clear during washout (blush is minimally persistent after three cardiac cycles of washout). Among 762 patients enrolled in the TIMI 10B trial, a significant mortality gradient was found across TMP grades, with mortality lowest in those patients with TMP grade 3 (2.0%), intermediate in TMP grade 2 (4.4%), and highest in TMP grades 0 and 1 (6.0%; three-way $p = 0.05$). Even among patients with TIMI grade 3 flow in the epicardial artery, the TMP grades allowed further risk stratification of 30-day mortality: 0.73% for TMP grade 3; 2.9% for TMP grade 2; 5.0% for TMP grade 0 or 1 ($p = 0.03$ for TMP grade 3 vs. grades 0, 1, and 2; three-way $p = 0.066$). TMP grade 3 flow was a multivariate correlate of 30-day mortality (OR, 0.35; 95% CI, 0.12 to 1.02; $p = 0.054$) in a multivariate model that adjusted for the presence of TIMI 3 flow ($p = $ NS), the corrected TIMI frame count (OR, 1.02; $p = 0.06$), the presence of an anterior MI (OR, 2.3; $p = 0.03$), admission heart rate ($p = $ NS), female sex ($p = $ NS), and age (OR, 1.1, $p < 0.001$).

235. **Gibson CM,** et al. Relationship of the TIMI myocardial perfusion grades, flow grades, frame count, and percutaneous coronary intervention to long-term outcomes after thrombolytic administration in acute myocardial infarction. *Circulation* 2002;105:1909–1913.

This analysis examined 848 patients from the TIMI 10B trial (compared tPA with TNK) who had 2-year follow-up. Improved survival was associated with TIMI grade 2/3 flow (Cox HR, 0.41; $p = 0.001$), reduced CTFCs ($p = 0.02$), and an open microvasculature (TMPG, 2/3; HR, 0.51; $p = 0.038$). Rescue PCI of closed arteries (TFG, 0/1) at 90 minutes was associated with lower mortality ($p = 0.03$), and mortality trended lower with adjunctive PCI of open (TFG, 2/3) arteries ($p = 0.11$). In a multivariate model correcting for previously identified correlates of mortality (age, sex, pulse, LAD as culprit vessel, and any PCI during initial hospitalization), patency (TFG, 2/3; HR, 0.32; $p < 0.001$), CTFC ($p = 0.01$), and TMPG 2/3 remained associated with reduced mortality (HR, 0.46; $p = 0.02$).

Pre- or Postinfarct Angina

236. **Ruocco NA Jr,** et al. Invasive vs. conservative strategy after thrombolytic therapy for acute MI in patients with antecedent angina. *J Am Coll Cardiol* 1992;20: 1445–1451.

This retrospective analysis focused on 3,534 TIMI-2 patients. The antecedent angina group was characterized by more multivessel disease [37.9% vs. 26.4% (invasive group)] and a higher 1-year reinfarction rate (11.2% vs. 7.9%; $p = 0.001$). However, as in the rest of the trial, a similar rate of death and MI between conservative and invasive strategies was observed in those with or without antecedent angina.

237. **Anzai T,** et al. Preinfarction angina as a major predictor of left ventricular function and long-term prognosis after a first Q wave MI. *J Am Coll Cardiol* 1995;26: 319–327.

This analysis of 291 patients showed that preinfarction angina was associated with lower peak CK, a decreased incidence of in-hospital VT and VF (anterior, 8% vs. 24%; inferior, 3% vs. 13%), and decreased cardiac mortality (anterior, 8% vs. 27%; inferior, 3% vs. 13%). In multiple regression analysis, preinfarction angina was the most powerful predictor of cardiac mortality [RR, 1.85 (vs. 1.83 for anterior location and 1.76 for absence of successful revascularization)].

238. **Andreotti F,** et al. Preinfarction angina as a predictor of more rapid coronary thrombolysis in patients with MI. *N Engl J Med* 1996;334:7–12 (editorial, 51–52).

This small study was composed of 14 (of 23) MI patients with preceding unstable angina. Angiography was performed at 15 minutes, 35 minutes, 55 minutes, and 24 hours. The preinfarction angina group had higher TIMI grade 3 flow at 35 minutes (64% vs. 0%; $p = 0.006$) and lower peak CK-MB ($p < 0.01$). The time to reperfusion correlated with the indices of infarct size ($r = 0.53$; $p^2 = 0.02$). The preinfarction angina group had a faster time (by 27%) to initiation of thrombolytic therapy. These patients also had an increased incidence of prior coronary disease (43% vs. 22%) and thus were more likely to have a good collateral network. The accompanying editorial by Braunwald offers four possible explanations for this phenomenon: (a) coronary collaterals are closed in the absence of ischemia; (b) ischemic preconditioning (adenosine release) occurs; (c) patients taking aspirin and heparin are more amenable to thrombolysis; and (d) more rapid reperfusion occurs (this study).

239. **Galli M,** et al. GISSI-3 Angina Precoce Post-Infarto **(APPI).** Early and 6 month outcome in patients with angina pectoris early after acute MI. *Am J Cardiol* 1996;78:1191–1197.

This prospective study was composed of 2,363 patients (at 31 of 200 GISSI-3 centers lacking revascularization capability); 74% were thrombolyzed. Multivariate predictors of postinfarction angina with ECG changes (14% incidence) were preinfarction angina, age 70 years, female gender, and history of MI. Early angina was associated with increased in-hospital and 6-month reinfarction [RRs, 3.1 (7% vs. 2%) and 2.9 (12% vs. 5%); both $p < 0.001$] and 6-month mortality [RR, 2.3 (13% vs. 7%); $p < 0.001$]. Unfortunately, no factors predicted reinfarction after angina.

240. **Kobayashi Y,** et al. Previous angina reduces in-hospital death in patients with acute myocardial infarction. *Am J Cardiol* 1998;81:117–122.

This retrospective analysis focused on 2,262 consecutive AMI patients. In-hospital mortality was lower in those with previous angina than without (first MI, 6.9% vs. 11.4%; $p < 0.01$; prior MI, 17.7% vs. 25.3%; $p < 0.05$). In multivariate analysis, previous angina was an independent predictor of in-hospital death. In patients with a first MI, death due to cardiac rupture was less common in those with previous angina (1.4% vs. 5.0%; $p < 0.01$). Among those with a prior MI, a trend toward fewer deaths due to cardiogenic shock or CHF was found in patients with previous angina (12.8% vs. 19.0%; $p = 0.05$).

Thrombolysis-specific Studies
241. **Hillis LD,** et al. Risk stratification before thrombolytic therapy in patients with acute MI. *J Am Coll Cardiol* 1990;16:313–315.

This analysis focused on 3,339 TIMI II patients (78 excluded with shock or pulmonary edema). The low-risk group (26%; zero of eight risk factors) had a low 6-week mortality rate of 1.5%. The group with one risk factor (age 70 years, female gender, diabetes, prior MI, anterior MI, atrial fibrillation, SBP less than 100 mm Hg, or heart rate more than 100 beats/min) had a 6-week mortality rate of 5.3% ($p < 0.001$). If four risk factors, 17.2% mortality rate.

242. **Cragg DR,** et al. Outcome of patients with acute MI who are ineligible for thrombolytic therapy. *Ann Intern Med* 1991;115:173–177.

This retrospective analysis focused on 1,471 patients; 16% were given thrombolysis on protocols (88% TIMI IIB), and 7% had nonprotocol lysis, primary balloon angioplasty, or both. The nonthrombolyzed group was older, more likely to be female, and more frequently had hypertension and prior MIs. Ineligible patients had a fivefold higher mortality rate (19% vs. 4%; $p < 0.001$). Independent mortality predictors were age older than 76 years, stroke or other bleeding risk, ineligible ECG, or two exclusion criteria.

243. **Barbash GI,** et al. Significance of smoking in patients receiving thrombolytic therapy for acute MI: experience gleaned from the International tPA/Streptokinase Mortality Trial. *Circulation* 1993;87:53–58.

This analysis of 8,259 International tPA/Streptokinase Trial patients found a protective effect of smoking in patients with acute MI (see also *Am J Cardiol* 1995;75:232). Both nonsmokers (more diabetes, higher Killip class, and older) and ex-smokers had more in-hospital reinfarctions (4.7% and 5% vs. 2.7%; $p < 0.001$) and decreased in-hospital and 6-month mortality rates (13%/18%, 8%/12%, 5%/8%).

244. **Grines CL,** et al. Effect of cigarette smoking on outcome after thrombolytic therapy for MI. *Circulation* 1995;91:298–303.

This study showed that better outcomes in smokers with MI may be due to a low-risk profile. Analysis of 1,619 patients treated with tPA, urokinase, or both in six MI trials showed that smokers had similar 90-minute patency (but higher grade 3 flow: 41.1% vs. 34.6%; $p = 0.03$) but lower in-hospital mortality rates (4% vs. 8.9%; $p = 0.0001$). However, after adjustments [lower age (54 vs. 60 years), more inferior MIs (60% vs. 53%), less three-vessel disease (16% vs. 22%), and higher baseline EF (53% vs. 50%)], no independent prognostic significance was associated with smoking.

245. **Lee KL,** et al. Predictors of 30-day mortality in the era of reperfusion for acute MI: results from an international trial of 41,021 patients. *Circulation* 1995;91: 1659–1668.

Multivariate analysis showed the strong influence of age on mortality rate (only 1.1% if younger than 45 years, 20.5% if older than 75 years). Other factors associated with mortality included lower SBP, higher Killip class, elevated HR, and anterior infarct. These five factors contribute approximately 90% of prognostic information.

246. **Woodfield SL,** et al. Gender and acute MI: is there a different response to thrombolysis? *J Am Coll Cardiol* 1997;29:35–42.

This GUSTO Angiography Substudy analysis showed female gender to be an independent risk factor for mortality. The women had some high-risk features (e.g., older, and more hypertension, diabetes, and heart failure) and some low-risk features (e.g., fewer prior MIs and bypass surgery, less smoking). The unadjusted 30-day mortality rate was nearly 3 times higher (13.1% vs. 4.8%; $p < 0.001$), and after multivariate analysis, female gender remained an independent mortality predictor.

Other
247. **Case RB,** et al. Living alone after MI. *JAMA* 1992;267:515–519.

This analysis of 1,234 MI patients with an average follow-up of 2.1 years showed that living alone was associated with 54% more end points (nonfatal MI plus cardiac death).

248. **Frasure-Smith N,** et al. Depression following MI. *JAMA* 1993;270:1819–1825 (editorial, 1860–1861).

This small study was composed of 222 MI patients who survived to hospital discharge. Patients were interviewed at average 7 days (major depression, 2 weeks). Depression was associated with a 4.3-fold higher mortality rate ($p = 0.013$). The impact was at least equivalent to that of LV dysfunction (Killip class) and prior MI. Editorial points out that typically 15% to 20% of post-MI patients have major depression.

249. **Jollis JG,** et al. Outcome of acute MI according to the specialty of the admitting physician. *N Engl J Med* 1996;335:1880–1887.

This retrospective analysis of 8,241 Medicare patients showed that cardiologists provide optimal care for MI patients. All-cause 1-year mortality HRs (based on admitting physician) were as follows: cardiologists, 0.88; family medicine, 0.98; general practitioner, 1.06; and other, 1.16. Cardiologist-treated patients were younger and healthier and had less diabetes, more Killip class I, lower predicted 30-day mortality rates (GUSTO-I model; 18 vs. 20%), and longer hospital stay (9.3 vs. 7.3 to 8.6 days). Cardiologists used thrombolysis about twice as often; used angiography, revascularization, treadmill tests, nuclear imaging, Holter monitoring, and echocardiography more frequently; and gave more patients aspirin, β-blockers, and heparin. In an analysis of all 1992 Medicare claims (approximately 220,000 patients), the same mortality pattern emerged: with cardiologists, 30%; internists, 37%; family medicine, 39%; and general practitioners, 40%. Although 82% of the attending physicians were the same as the admitting physician, the roles of consultants and transfers were not assessed.

250. **Chen J,** et al. Do America's best hospitals perform better for acute MI? *N Engl J Med* 1999;340:286–292.

Analysis of more than 149,000 Medicare beneficiaries with AMI in 1994 or 1995. Hospitals were classified as one of three types: (a) top-ranked, (b) similarly equipped (not in top rank but with on-site facilities for catheterization, PCI, and bypass surgery), and (c) nonsimilarly equipped. Patients admitted to a top-ranked hospital had a lower adjusted 30-day mortality rate [OR, 0.87 (vs. other two types); 95% CI, 0.76 to 1.00; $p = 0.05$]. Top-ranked hospitals were more likely to prescribe aspirin and β-blockers to those without contraindications (96.2% vs. 88.6% and 83.4%; 75.0% vs. 61.8% and 58.7%). Not surprisingly, after adjusting for the increased appropriate use of these medications, the mortality benefit associated with admission to a top-ranked hospital was attenuated (OR, 0.94; $p = 0.38$).

Complications of Myocardial Infarction

Arrhythmias, Bundle Branch Block

251. **Antman EM, Berlin JA.** Declining incidence of ventricular fibrillation in MI: implications for prophylactic use of lidocaine. *Circulation* 1992;86:764–773.

This analysis focused on 18 randomized trials with 4,754 patients. Earlier year of publication (range, 1969 to 1988) was a significant predictor of VF ($p = 0.002$), even after adjusting for other variables. The incidence of VF in controls decreased from 4.5% in 1970 to only 0.35% in 1990.

252. **Solomon SD,** et al. Ventricular arrhythmias in trials of thrombolytic therapy for acute MI: a meta-analysis. *Circulation* 1993;88:2575–2581.

This analysis focused on 15 randomized trials with 39,606 patients. Thrombolytic administration was associated with lower risk of VF during the entire hospitalization (OR, 0.83; 95% CI, 0.76 to 0.90; $p < 0.0001$) but not in the first 6 or 24 hours after thrombolysis (ORs, 0.98 and 1.00). Thrombolytic use also was associated with a higher incidence of VT during hospitalization (OR, 1.34; 95% CI, 1.15 to 1.55; $p < 0.0001$).

253. **Newby KH,** et al. Incidence and clinical relevance of the occurrence of bundle branch block in patients treated with thrombolytic therapy. *Circulation* 1996;94:2424–2428.

This study was composed of 681 TAMI-9 and GUSTO-I patients who underwent continuous 12-lead ECG monitoring for 36 to 72 hours. BBB occurred in 23.6% (RBBB, 13%; LBBB, 7%; alternating, 3.5%). Mortality was 2.5 times higher in BBB patients compared with those without BBB (8.7% vs. 3.5%; $p = 0.007$). The highest mortality rate was observed in those with persistent BBB [19.4% vs. 5.6 (transient) and 3.5% (none); $p < 0.001$]. BBB patients also had decreased EF, increased peak CK, and more diseased vessels.

254. **Crenshaw BS,** et al. Atrial fibrillation in the setting of acute MI: the GUSTO-I experience. *J Am Coll Cardiol* 1997;30:406–413.

AF on admission ECG in 2.5%, increasing to 7.9% after study enrollment. The group with early *and* late AF had more three-vessel disease, less TIMI grade 3 flow, more in-hospital strokes (3.1% vs. 1.3%; $p = 0.0001$), and more than twofold higher unadjusted 30-day *and* 1-year mortality rates (14.3% vs. 6.2%; $p = 0.0001$; 21.5% vs. 8.6%, $p < 0.0001$). In multivariate analysis, late AF predictors were age, peak CK, Killip class, and heart rate. Adjusted ORs of mortality were 1.1 for baseline AF (85% CI, 0.88 to 1.3) and 1.4 for late AF (95% CI, 1.3 to 1.5).

Cardiac Rupture

255. **Becker RC,** et al. Cardiac rupture associated with thrombolytic therapy: impact of time to treatment in the LATE (Late Assessment of Thrombolytic Efficacy) study. *J Am Coll Cardiol* 1995;25:1063–1068.

This analysis of 5,711 LATE patients found that cardiac rupture was the listed cause of death in 53 (9.7%) of 547 patients who died in the first 35 days. No increased risk of rupture was found in the group receiving rtPA at 6 to 24 hours compared with the placebo group. However, rupture events did occur earlier in the thrombolytic group (Treatment × Time to death interaction; $p = 0.03$).

256. **Becker RC,** et al. A composite view of cardiac rupture in the U.S. National Registry of MI. *J Am Coll Cardiol* 1996;27:1321–1326.

In this analysis of 350,755 patients, thrombolytic administration (approximately 12,000 patients) was associated with 5.9% mortality (no thrombolytic therapy, 12.9%). Cardiac rupture was reported as the cause of death in 12% of patients who received thrombolysis [vs. 6% (no thrombolysis)] and occurred more frequently within the first 24 hours.

257. **Anzai T,** et al. C-reactive protein as a predictor of infarct expansion and cardiac rupture after a first Q-wave acute MI. *Circulation* 1997;96:778–784.

Elevated C-reactive protein (CRP) was shown to be a risk factor for cardiac rupture. CRP was measured every 24 hours in 220 patients. Among the rupture patients, CRP levels were twice as high (23.7 vs. 12.2 mg/dL; $p = 0.001$). In a multivariate analysis, a CRP of 2 mg/L or more was an independent risk factor for rupture (RR, 4.72; $p = 0.004$), as well as LV aneurysm (RR, 2.11; $p = 0.03$), and 1-year cardiac death (RR, 3.44; $p < 0.0001$).

258. **Becker RC,** et al. Fatal cardiac rupture among patients treated with thrombolytic agents and adjunctive thrombin antagonists. *J Am Coll Cardiol* 1999;33: 479–487.

This analysis of 3,759 patients enrolled in the TIMI 9A and 9B trials showed a 1.7% incidence of cardiac rupture. By multivariate analysis, independent predictors of rupture were age older than 70 years (OR, 3.77; 95% CI, 2.06 to 6.91), female gender (OR, 2.87; 95% CI, 1.44 to 5.73), and prior angina (OR, 1.82; 95% CI, 1.05 to 3.16). No association was found between the intensity of anticoagulation or type of thrombin inhibition (e.g., heparin or hirudin) and cardiac rupture.

259. **Moreno R,** et al. Primary angioplasty reduces the risk of left ventricular free wall rupture compared with thrombolysis in patients with acute myocardial infarction. *J Am Coll Cardiol* 2002;39:598–603.

This analysis consisted of 1,375 patients with AMI seen within 12 hours of symptom onset; 55.4% underwent primary angioplasty, and 44.6% were treated with thrombolytic therapy. Free-wall rupture (FWR) was diagnosed when sudden death occurred because of pulseless electrical activity (PEA) with large pericardial effusion on an echocardiogram or when demonstrated postmortem or at surgery. The overall incidence of FWR was 2.5% (angioplasty, 1.8%; thrombolysis, 3.3%; $p = 0.69$). In the univariate analysis, the following were risk factors for FWR: age older than 70 years (5.2% vs. 1.2%; $p < 0.001$), female gender (5.1% vs. 1.8%, $p = 0.006$), anterior location (3.3% vs. 1.4%; $p = 0.02$) and treatment more than 2 hours after symptom onset (3.6% vs. 1.7%, $p = 0.043$). In the multivariate analysis, independent risk factors were age older than 70 (OR, 4.12; 95% CI, 2.04 to 8.62; $p < 0.001$) and anterior location (OR, 2.91; 95% CI, 1.36 to 6.63; $p = 0.008$), whereas treatment with primary angioplasty was an independent protective factor (OR, 0.46; 95% CI, 0.22 to 0.96; $p = 0.037$).

Cardiogenic Shock and Congestive Heart Failure

260. **Goldberg RJ,** et al. Cardiogenic shock after acute MI: incidence and mortality from a community-wide perspective, 1975–88. *N Engl J Med* 1991;325:1117–1122.

This retrospective analysis focused on 4,762 AMI patients. Cardiogenic shock (incidence, 7.5%) patients had a high rate of mortality: 77% vs. 13.5%. No significant changes were noted between 1975 and 1988.

261. **Holmes DR Jr,** et al. Contemporary reperfusion therapy for cardiogenic shock: the GUSTO-I experience. *J Am Coll Cardiol* 1995;26:668–674.

Cardiogenic shock occurred in 2,972 (7.2%) patients, with 89% of cases developing after hospital admission. These shock patients had a higher reinfarction rate (11% vs. 3%) and much higher mortality rate [57% (shock on presentation) and 55% (shock after admission) versus 3%; $p < 0.001$]. Shock developed less frequently in patients treated with rtPA (6.3% vs. 7.7% and 8.1% in SK groups). The 30-day mortality was lower among the 19% who underwent angioplasty (31% vs. 61%).

262. **Holmes DR Jr,** et al. Difference in countries' use of resources and clinical outcome for patients with cardiogenic shock after MI: results from the GUSTO trial. *Lancet* 1997;349:75–78.

Analysis of GUSTO data showed that the following features were evident among U.S. patients: younger ($p < 0.001$), more anterior MIs (49% vs. 53%), and treated earlier (3.1 vs. 3.3 hours; $p < 0.01$). They underwent procedures much more often: catheterization, 58% vs. 23%; PTCA, 26% vs. 8%; IABP, 35% vs. 7%; pulmonary artery use, 57% vs. 22%. Revascularization was associated with decreased mortality in all nations; however, the United States had a 24% lower 30-day mortality rate [50% vs. 66% (other nations); $p < 0.001$ (adjusted for revascularization rates)]. Authors suggest better U.S. outcomes are owing to earlier identification of patients as a result of closer monitoring.

263. **Goldberg RJ,** et al. Temporal trends in cardiogenic shock complicating acute MI. *N Engl J Med* 1999;340:1162–1168.

This observational study was composed of 9,076 patients admitted to all local hospitals of a metropolitan area (Worcester, MA) during eleven 1-year periods between 1975 and 1997. The incidence of cardiogenic shock was relatively stable during this period (average, 7.1%). Cardiogenic shock was associated with a 71.7% in-hospital mortality rate (vs. 12.0%; $p < 0.001$). A significant trend toward better in-hospital survival was seen among patients treated in the mid-to-late 1990s compared with mid-to-late 1970s [ORs, 0.49 (1993 and 1995) and 0.46 (1997)].

Stroke

264. **Maggioni AP,** et al. Risk of stroke in patients with acute MI after thrombolytic and antithrombotic therapy. *N Engl J Med* 1992;327:1–6.

This analysis focused on GISSI-2 and International Study patients; complete data were available on 20,768 patients. The in-hospital stroke rate was 1.14% (hemorrhagic, 0.36%; ischemic, 0.48%; undefined cause, 0.30%). Patients treated with tPA had a small but significant excess of stroke versus SK-treated patients (1.33% vs. 0.94%; adjusted OR, 1.42; 95% CI, 1.09 to 1.84). Factors associated with increased risk of stroke were older age, higher Killip class, and anterior infarction.

265. **Simoons ML,** et al. Individual risk assessment for intracranial hemorrhage during thrombolytic therapy. *Lancet* 1993;342:1523–1528.

This analysis focused on data from the Netherlands registry, European Cooperative Study Group, GISSI-2 and International Study Group trials, TIMI II trials, TAMI trials, and ISAM study. By multivariate analysis, independent predictors of intracranial hemorrhage were age older than 65 years (OR, 2.2; 95% CI, 1.4 to 3.5), body weight less than 70 kg (OR, 2.1; CI, 1.3 to 3.2), hypertension on hospital admission (OR, 2.0; CI, 1.2 to 3.2), and administration of alteplase (OR, 1.6; 95% CI, 1.0 to 2.5).

266. **Loh E,** et al. Ventricular dysfunction and the risk of stroke after MI. *N Engl J Med* 1997;336:251–257.

This analysis focused on 2,231 SAVE patients (all with EF 0.4 or less), with a 5-year stroke rate of 8.1%. Independent stroke risk factors were lower EF (28% or less vs. more than 35%; RR, 1.86), age (18% higher risk per 5 years), no aspirin or anticoagulation (with aspirin, RR 0.44; with anticoagulation, RR only 0.19). Limitations of the analysis were (a) aspirin and anticoagulation not randomly assigned, (b) no data on anticoagulation intensity, and (c) role of atrial dysfunction not assessable.

267. **Gurwitz JH,** et al. Risk for intracranial hemorrhage after tissue plasminogen activator for acute MI. *Ann Intern Med* 1998;129:597–604.

This analysis focused on 71,073 patients from the National Registry of MI 2 treated with tPA between June 1994 and September 1996. The in-hospitalization intracranial hemorrhage rate was 0.95% [0.88% confirmed (CT or MRI)]. In multivariate models, the following were intracranial hemorrhage predictors: older age, female sex, black ethnicity, SBP more than 140 mm Hg, DBP greater than 100 mm Hg, history of stroke, tPA dose more than 1.5 mg/kg, and lower body weight.

Reocclusion, Recurrent Ischemia, and Reinfarction

268. **Benhorin J,** et al. Prognostic significance of nonfatal myocardial reinfarction. *J Am Coll Cardiol* 1990;15:253–258.

This analysis focused on 1,234 placebo patients in the Multicenter Diltiazem Trial. At follow-up (1 to 4 years), nonfatal MI had occurred in 9.4%, with a higher frequency in women and those with prior cardiac symptoms. Nonfatal MI was associated with a threefold higher risk of subsequent cardiac mortality (5.4 times higher if the index event was a first MI).

269. **Ohman EM,** et al. Consequences of reocclusion after successful reperfusion therapy in acute MI. *Circulation* 1990;82:781–791.

This analysis focused on 810 TAMI patients with repeated angiography at average 7 days that showed a reoccluded IRA in 12.4% (58% with symptoms). At follow-up, occluded patients had a similar EF, but worse infarct-zone function and increased in-hospital mortality (11% vs. 4.5%; $p = 0.01$).

270. **Kornowski R,** et al. Predictors and long-term prognostic significance of recurrent infarction in the year after a first MI. *Am J Cardiol* 1993;72:883–888.

This retrospective analysis focused on 3,695 SPRINT patients, with a 1-year reinfarction rate of 6% (associated in-hospital mortality, 30%). Reinfarction predictors were peripheral vascular disease (adjusted RR, 2.12), anterior MI (RR, 1.62), angina before MI (RR, 1.53), CHF on admission (RR, 1.34), diabetes (RR, 1.33), hypertension (RR, 1.28), and age increment (RR, 1.13). Reinfarction rates were as follows: zero or one risk factor, 4.0%; five or six risk factors, 23.3%. Recurrent MI is the strongest long-term mortality predictor (adjusted RR, 4.76).

271. **Mueller HS,** et al. Prognostic significance of nonfatal reinfarction during 3 year follow-up of the TIMI II clinical trial. *J Am Coll Cardiol* 1995;26:900–907.

The incidence of reinfarction was 10.1% (43 of 339 died). Relative risks of death were 1.9 if reinfarction occurred at less than 42 days, 6.2 at 43 to 365 days, and 2.9 at 1 to 3 years.

272. **Verheught FWA,** et al. Reocclusion: the flip of coronary thrombolysis. *J Am Coll Cardiol* 1996;27:766–773.

This analysis focused on 61 studies with 6,061 patients undergoing angiography twice. Reocclusion usually occurs within weeks. Overall, an 11% reocclusion rate was observed, but a 16% incidence was seen in true occlusion studies; thus initial occlusion is a risk factor. Aspirin and heparin were not associated with benefit in prevention (APRICOT, HART trials). Hirudin and hirulog appear beneficial (see TIMI-5 and *Circulation* 1994;89:1567). Half of reocclusions are clinically silent. Revascularization is helpful, especially if symptoms are present (see *N Engl J Med* 1992;27:1825).

273. **Bauters, C** et al. Angiographically documented late reocclusion after successful coronary angioplasty of an infarct-related lesion is a powerful predictor of long-term mortality. *Circulation* 1999;99:2243–2250.

Retrospective analysis of 528 patients who had a patent IRA after balloon angioplasty procedure 10 ± 6 days after MI. At 6-month follow-up angiography, IRA reocclusion occurred in 17% (TIMI flow grade 0 or 1). At long-term follow-up (median, 6.4 years), the reocclusion group had a 2.5-fold higher mortality rate (20% vs. 8%; $p = 0.002$). The actuarial 8-year total mortality rates were 28% and 10% ($p = 0.0003$), and the CV mortality rates were 25% and 7% ($p < 0.0001$). The mortality differences between reoccluded and patent IRA patients were greater in patients with an anterior MI.

Left Ventricular Thrombi

274. **Gueret P,** et al. Effects of full-dose heparin anticoagulation on the development of left ventricular thrombosis in acute transmural MI. *J Am Coll Cardiol* 1986;8:419–426.

This small prospective study showed that thrombi occur frequently in anterior MIs. Ninety patients (46 anterior, 44 inferior) seen an average 5.2 hours after onset of symptoms were randomized to heparin or no heparin. No thrombi were detected on first echocardiograms (done at 10.3 ± 8 hours). In the anterior MI group, 46% had thrombi at 4.3 ± 3.0 days [38% (heparin) vs. 52% (no heparin); $p = 0.76$]. No thrombi formed in the inferior group.

275. **Vecchio C,** et al. Left ventricular thrombus in anterior acute MI after thrombolysis. *Circulation* 1991;84:512–519.

This GISSI-2 ancillary echocardiography study was composed of 180 consecutive patients with first MI. Echocardiography was performed within 48 hours and before discharge. Left ventricular thrombi were found in 28% (no difference between the four treatment groups). Mural shape was more common, especially in heparinized patients. Only one in-hospital embolic event was documented.

276. **Vaitkus PT, Barnathan ES.** Embolic potential, prevention and management of mural thrombus complicating anterior MI: a meta-analysis. *J Am Coll Cardiol* 1993;22:1004–1009.

This analysis focused on 11 studies with 856 patients. Thrombus by echocardiography was associated with an odds ratio of embolization of 5.45 (11% vs. 2%). In anterior MI patients, the odds ratio was 8.0. Anticoagulation was associated with 86% less embolization. Primary anticoagulation led to 68% less embolization, whereas thrombolytic therapy was associated with 52% less embolization (16% vs. 32%).

277. **Greaves SC,** et al. Incidence and natural history of left ventricular thrombus following anterior wall acute MI. *Am J Cardiol* 1997;80:442–448.

This analysis focused on 309 Healing and Early Afterload Reducing Treatment (HEART) substudy patients, 78% with Q-wave anterior MIs. Echocardiography was performed on days 1, 14, and 90. LV thrombus rates were low: day 1, 0.6%; day 14, 3.7%; day 90, 2.5%. Only one thrombus was detected on two echocardiograms. Thrombus patients had a greater LV size increase and wall-motion abnormalities.

Valvular Damage and Septal Defects

278. **Lehmann KG,** et al. Mitral regurgitation in early MI: incidence, clinical detection and prognostic implications. *Ann Intern Med* 1992;117:10–17.

This analysis focused on 206 TIMI I patients with contrast left ventriculography within 7 hours of symptom onset. Mitral regurgitation was present in 27 (13%) patients and associated with a markedly increased 1-year mortality rate (RRs, 12.2 and 7.5 by univariate and multivariate analyses, respectively).

279. **Tcheng JE,** et al. Outcome of patients sustaining acute ischemic mitral regurgitation during MI. *Ann Intern Med* 1992;117:18–24.

This inception cohort case study was composed of 1,480 consecutive patients who underwent catheterization within 6 hours of infarction. Acute ischemic moderately severe to severe (3+ to 4+) mitral regurgitation was associated with a mortality rate of 24% at 30 days and 52% at 1 year. Physical examination did not identify 50% of these patients. Acute reperfusion by thrombolysis or angioplasty did not reliably reverse valvular incompetence.

280. **Lamas GA,** et al. Clinical significance of mitral regurgitation after acute MI. *Circulation* 1997;96:827–833.

This study was composed of 727 SAVE patients with catheterization and left ventriculography data (done within 16 days of MI). Mitral regurgitation (19.4%) patients were more likely to have a persistently occluded IRA (27.2% vs. 15.2%; $p = 0.001$). At follow-up (median, 3.5 years), mitral regurgitation patients had a more than twofold higher CV mortality rate (29% vs. 12%; $p < 0.001$), more severe CHF (24% vs. 16%; $p = 0.015$), and a higher rate of CV mortality, severe CHF, and reinfarction (47% vs. 29%; $p < 0.001$). In multivariate analysis, mitral regurgitation was an independent CV mortality predictor [RR, 2.0; 95% CI, 1.28 to 3.04].

281. **Birnbaum Y,** et al. Ventricular septal rupture after acute myocardial infarction. *N Engl J Med* 2002;347:1426–1432.

This review article discusses numerous topics, including the incidence, risk factors, pathogenesis, hemodynamics, time course, clinical manifestations, angiographic findings, medical and surgical therapy, and prognosis of ventricular septal rupture after acute MI.

5. CONGESTIVE HEART FAILURE

EPIDEMIOLOGY

Congestive heart failure (CHF) is now responsible for more than 1 million hospital admissions each year in the United States, at a cost of nearly $40 billion.

The aging of the population and improved survival after myocardial infarction (MI) has resulted in an increasing prevalence of CHF, which now affects nearly 5 million Americans. Data from the Framingham Heart Study suggest that the incidence of CHF over the past 50-year period has declined among women but not among men, whereas survival has continued to improve in both sexes (by 12% per decade), which accounts for the increasing prevalence (12). Most studies show women surviving longer than men (7,9,10,12; see also *Arch Intern Med* 1999;159:1816), whereas the Studies of Left Ventricular Dysfunction (SOLVD) trial found the opposite (11). The likely explanation for this discrepancy is that the SOLVD trial enrolled a higher percentage of women with coronary artery disease (CAD), and CHF due to an ischemic etiology is associated with increased mortality.

Factors associated with an increased risk of CHF are advanced age, male gender, black race, diabetes, obesity, smoking, and hypertension (8,9). Among women, those with hypertension and diabetes are more likely than men to develop CHF (11). Echocardiographic findings associated with increased risk include low left and/or right ventricular ejection fraction (EF), left ventricular (LV) dilatation, and valvular disease (21,22; also see *N Engl J Med* 1997;336:1350).

Among those diagnosed with HF, progression of disease is predicted by functional class. The New York Heart Association (NYHA) classification is as follows:

Class I: no limitation
Class II: slight HF; comfortable at rest but ordinary activity causes fatigue, dyspnea, or angina
Class III: marked failure; less than ordinary activity causes symptoms
Class IV: severe failure; symptoms of CHF at rest

The mortality rate in NYHA class III patients with peak oxygen consumption of 10 to 15 mL/kg/min is 15% to 20% per year, and it increases to 50%/yr or more in class IV patients with oxygen consumption of less than 10 mL/kg/min.

HISTORY AND PHYSICAL EXAMINATION

Symptoms include dyspnea, fatigue, paroxysmal nocturnal dyspnea, orthopnea, and nocturia. Orthopnea appears to be the most sensitive symptom for predicting elevated pulmonary capillary wedge pressure (PCWP) (13). Impaired concentration may occur in individuals with decreased cardiac output at rest.

The physical examination may be notable for rales (often not present if chronic or gradual in onset), elevated jugular venous pressure, presence of third heart sound, peripheral edema, cool extremities, narrowed pulse pressure, and tachycardia (see **Table 5.1**). Hepatomegaly and ascites are often seen with right HF. Most of these signs have limited sensitivity at predicting elevated PCWP. In one study, jugular venous distention, at rest or inducible by an abdominojugular test, had a sensitivity of 80% for predicting elevated PCWP (14). In another study, low pulse pressure was an excellent predictor of poor cardiac output, with a pulse pressure of less than 25% having a 91% sensitivity and 83% specificity for a cardiac index of 2.2 L/min/m^2 or less (13).

ETIOLOGY

Systolic dysfunction is due to pump failure, typically from ischemic cardiomyopathy, dilated cardiomyopathy (DCM), or valvular disease. Nonischemic dilated cardiomyopathy is also relatively common; alcohol and viral illnesses are responsible for some cases but many are idiopathic. High-output causes of CHF are less common, and include anemia, hyperthyroidism, and pregnancy. Rare causes include Paget disease,

TABLE 5.1. FINDINGS OF PHYSICAL EXAMINATION

	Systolic Dysfunction	Diastolic Dysfunction
Third heart sound	Frequent	Rare
Fourth heart sound	Rare	Frequent
Rales	Occasional	Occasional
Peripheral edema	Frequent	Rare
Jugular venous distention	Frequent	Rare
Cardiomegaly	Usual	Rare

Modified from Braunwald E. *Heart disease.* Philadelphia: W.B. Saunders, 1997.

arteriovenous fistula, pheochromocytoma, and beriberi. Diastolic dysfunction is a component in approximately one third of CHF cases; it is typically associated with hypertension, hypertrophic cardiomyopathy, and infiltrative disease.

An important precipitating factor of CHF is noncompliance with a prescribed drug regimen and poor diet (e.g., high salt). In one study of patients hospitalized for HF, more than 60% were found to be noncompliant with drugs and/or diet (1). Abrupt/acute precipitating causes of CHF include acute MI, acute pulmonary embolism, acute mitral regurgitation and aortic insufficiency, acute ventricular septal defect, and infection. (Tachycardia results in higher cardiac output.) More chronic precipitating causes of CHF include drugs [nonsteroidal antiinflammatory drugs; verapamil, diltiazem, and procainamide (negative inotropy); estrogens, androgens and minoxidil (water retention); doxorubicin (Adriamycin). Sleep apnea often co-exists with heart failure and has an adverse effect on prognosis.

TESTS

1. Laboratory tests. Low serum sodium is common (dilutional hyponatremia from expansion of extracellular fluid volume) and predictive of poor outcome (16); elevated creatinine and liver function tests also are predictors of poor outcome. The use of brain natriuretic peptide has been found to be beneficial in the evaluation and triage of patients with acute dyspnea in the emergency department (18; also see *J Am Coll Cardiol* 2001;37:379). Finally, inflammatory markers (e.g. c-reactive protein IL-6) appear to be elevated in CHF patients (see Circulation 2003;107:1486). Their prognostic role requires further study.
2. Chest radiograph. Findings of increased pulmonary capillary pressure are seen in approximately 50% of patients; bilateral pleural effusions and cardiomegaly also may be present (see *JAMA* 1997;277:1712).
3. Electrocardiography (ECG). Q waves and left bundle branch block are good predictors of systolic dysfunction. A wide QRS (more than 220 milliseconds) is predictive of increased mortality.
4. Echocardiogram (22). A simple and useful tool, echocardiography can help determine systolic versus diastolic dysfunction and left and/or right ventricular impairment.
5. Six-minute walk test. Short distance correlates with higher mortality and increased HF-related hospitalizations (21; see also *Chest* 1996;110:325 and *Am Heart J* 1998;136:449).
6. Metabolic stress testing. Used to measure oxygen consumption; a peak oxygen consumption of less than 12 to 14 mL/kg/min portends a poor prognosis (20).
7. Endomyocardial biopsy. Biopsy may be useful in selected cases, such as suspected amyloidosis, sarcoidosis, and giant cell myocarditis.

TREATMENT

Acute

1. Nitrates. Nitrates are given sublingually or intravenously in cases in which preload reduction is necessary. In the case of severe HF, nitroprusside administration

should be considered if both PCWP and systemic vascular resistance (SVR) are elevated.

2. Nesiritide. This form of human B-type natriuretic peptide causes vasodilation and increased renal blood flow and urine output and has resulted in rapid symptomatic and hemodynamic improvement in patients with acutely decompensated HF (44). In the Vasodilation in The Management of Acute CHF (VMAC) study, nesiritide also was compared with nitroglycerin in the management of acutely decompensated CHF. Although no significant difference was noted in outcomes at 24 hours, hemodynamic benefit was somewhat improved at 3 hours (45). Subgroup analysis of patients receiving dobutamine in a study comparing nesiritide with standard CHF management showed that compared with dobutamine, nesiritide was used for a shorter total duration ($p < 0.001$), and the total duration of all intravenous vasoactive therapy also was shorter ($p < 0.012$). No difference was found in length of stay between the groups, but a trend toward decreased readmissions in the nesiritide groups was noted (see *J Am Coll Cardiol* 2002;39:798). Another study which randomized 255 patients to nesiritide or dobutamine found nesiritide reduced or had a neutral impact on ventricular ectopy, while dobutamine was associated with increased arrhythmias and higher heart rate (PRECEDENT; see *Am Heart J* 2003;144:1102).

3. Diuretics. Furosemide, 20 to 200 mg, is administered intravenously to alleviate lung edema due to volume overload, again by reducing preload. (Initial dose should be based on prior diuretic history.) Addition of a thiazide (e.g., metolazone or chlorothiazide) may help potentiate diuresis. In cases of massive fluid overload that respond poorly to diuretics, ultrafiltration may be effective (see *J Am Coll Cardiol* 1993;21:424).

4. Inotropic agents. No single agent has been found to be clinically superior, but adrenergic agents (such as dobutamine and dopamine and the phosphodiesterase inhibitor, milrinone) each may have a role in certain hemodynamic states. Dopamine may be preferable in those with low blood pressure because dobutamine reduces SVR to a greater extent. Milrinone has greater vasodilating-unloading properties. This agent was evaluated for short-term use in acute exacerbations of CHF in the OPTIME-CHF trial and was not shown to be beneficial (69).

Data from small clinical trials and anecdotal case experience suggest that inotropic agents reduce hospitalization, lead to hemodynamic and clinical improvement, and may serve as a bridge to transplantation. Some reports have suggested that intermittent infusion therapy in outpatients also may be effective in attenuating CHF symptoms in the long term (see *J Heart Lung Transplant* 2000;19:S49). The safety of prolonged outpatient use of these agents has been questioned. Data from more than 1,000 patients with chronic CHF randomized to milrinone or placebo showed an increase in mortality (30% vs. 24%) with more adverse reactions, including syncope and hypotension (PROMISE; 63). The increase in mortality has led some to suggest that inotropic drugs used in this fashion may exacerbate arrhythmias with subsequent sudden cardiac death. In severely symptomatic HF patients, the trade-off between symptomatic amelioration and the chance of sudden cardiac death must be considered.

Long-term Therapies

Angiotensin-converting Enzyme Inhibitors

Clearly indicated if LV dysfunction is present (see Table 5.2), angiotensin-converting enzyme (ACE) inhibitors should be initiated before aggressively performing diuresis in CHF patients. The Cooperative North Scandinavian Enalapril Survival Study (CONSENSUS I) showed that enalapril reduced 1-year mortality by 31% in NYHA class IV patients (24), whereas the larger SOLVD trial enrolled NYHA class II and III patients and showed that enalapril reduced mortality by 16% (average follow-up, 41 months) (25). Subsequent trials have shown similar benefits with other ACE inhibitors [e.g., Acute Infarction Ramipril Efficacy Study (AIRE) (27)].

The beneficial effect of administering larger doses of ACE inhibition has been demonstrated. A study of 248 CHF patients randomized to 20 mg of enalapril or up to

TABLE 5.2. DIFFERENTIAL DIAGNOSIS

	Acute Heart Failure	Decompensated Chronic Heart Failure	Chronic Heart Failure
Severity of symptoms	Severe	Severe	Mild to moderate
Pulmonary edema	Rare	Common	Rare
Peripheral edema	Rare	Common	Common
Weight gain	None to minimal	Moderate to severe	Mild to moderate

Modified from Braunwald E. *Heart disease.* Philadelphia: W.B. Saunders, 1997.

60 mg of enalapril showed no beneficial effect of larger doses (see *J Am Coll Cardiol* 2000;36:2090). The ATLAS trial randomized more than 3,000 patients and demonstrated 8% lower mortality and 24% fewer hospitalizations in patients treated with 35 mg/day of lisinopril (29). A meta-analysis of 32 studies found ACE inhibitor therapy to be associated with significant reductions in total mortality [odds ratio, 0.77; 95% confidence interval (CI), 0.67 to 0.88; $p < 0.001$] and mortality or hospitalization for CHF (odds ratio, 0.65; 95% CI, 0.57 to 0.74; $p < 0.001$) (23). The use of ACE inhibition in diastolic heart failure is being evaluated. In the ongoing PEP-CHF trial, patients older than 70 years with preserved EF but symptoms of CHF are being randomized to perindopril or placebo.

Angiotensin II–receptor Antagonists

Current trial data comparing angiotensin II–receptor antagonists with ACE inhibitors confirm that ACE inhibitors should remain first-line therapy for patients with CHF, and angiotensin II–receptor blockers should be reserved for those who are intolerant because of cough. In the ELITE trial, losartan was reported to have a lower mortality rate compared with captopril in patients with CHF. Mortality was not the primary end point, and the trial enrolled only 722 patients (28). Furthermore, these findings were not confirmed in the larger ELITE II study that again compared captopril with losartan in 3,152 patients. After a median follow-up of 1.5 years, losartan was not superior to captopril in reducing mortality, but was better tolerated (30).

Other angiotensin II blockers also have been evaluated in patients with CHF. In the Val-HeFT trial, valsartan was compared with placebo in more than 5,000 CHF patients with NYHA class II to IV symptoms (31). Whereas no difference in mortality was noted, patients had improved quality of life and fewer hospitalizations. In

TABLE 5.3. MAJOR ACE INHIBITOR TRIALS

	Number of Patients	Patient Characteristics	Placebo Mortality	Hazard Ratio
V-HeFT II (40)	804	NYHA I–III	25% at 2 yr[a]	0.72
CONSENSUS I (24)	253	NYHA IV	52% at 1 yr	0.69
SOLVD (25)	2,569	NYHA II, III	40% at 3.4 yr	0.84
SOLVD Prevention (26)	4,228	NYHA I	16% at 3.1 yr	0.91
AIRE (27)	2,006	Post-MI, clinical HF	23% at 1.3 yr	0.73
SAVE (Chapter 4)	2,231	Post-MI, EF ≤ 40%	25% at 3.5 yr	0.81
ISIS-4 (Chapter 4)	58,050	24 hr post-MI[b]	7.7% at 5 wk	0.93

This table demonstrates that studies that enrolled higher-risk patients showed a strong benefit (15%–30% lower mortality) from ACE inhibitor therapy, whereas a modest benefit was seen in the lower-risk populations (SOLVD Prevention, ISIS-4).
EF, ejection fraction; HF, heart failure; NYHA, New York Heart Association; MI, myocardial infarction; ACE, angiotensin-converting enzyme.
[a]Hydralazine and isosorbide.
[b]No HF required for enrollment.

addition, subgroup analysis showed a trend toward increased mortality in patients receiving valsartan, ACE inhibition, and β-blockers. The benefit or danger of combining valsartan with ACE inhibition and/or β-blockers in patients with CHF after MI will be more fully studied in the ongoing VALIANT trial.

Candesartan was evaluated in a study of 844 patients with CHF randomized to placebo or candesartan, and significant improvements in exercise tolerance, cardiothoracic ratio, and symptoms and signs of CHF were noted (STRETCH; see *Circulation* 1999;100:2224). The CHARM trial will evaluate the use of candesartan in various groups of patients in NYHA class II to IV. Several groups will be evaluated, including patients with (a) LVEF less than or equal to 40% treated with an ACE inhibitor ($n = 2,300$); (b) LVEF of 40% or less, ACE-inhibitor intolerant ($n = 1,700$); and (c) LVEF greater than 40%, not treated with ACE inhibitors ($n = 2,500$). The three studies will be combined to evaluate the effect of candesartan on all-cause mortality in the broad spectrum of symptomatic HF.

Diuretics

Diuretics are used to control and reduce fluid retention. In most cases, they should be used in conjunction with an ACE inhibitor with or without a β-blocker. A few small studies have found that a continuous intravenous infusion of furosemide in patients hospitalized with severe CHF may provide improved diuresis and natriuresis (32).

Aldosterone Blockers

The Randomized Aldactone Evaluation Study (RALES), which evaluated the potassium-sparing diuretic spironolactone in patients receiving optimal therapy (including a loop diuretic), showed a significantly lower mortality rate among spironolactone-treated patients compared with those treated with a loop diuretic (33). When spironolactone therapy is initiated, hyperkalemia occurs frequently, so careful monitoring of serum potassium levels is necessary.

Eplerenone is a selective aldosterone blocker which has a favorable side effect profile compared to aldosterone, especially a lower incidence of gynecomastia. The Eplerenone Post-Acute MI Heart Failure Efficacy and Survival Study (EPHESUS) compared eplerenone with placebo in 6,632 MI patients with an ejection fraction ≤40%. The Eplerenone group had a significant reduction in all-cause mortality compared to placebo (relative risk 0.85, $p = 0.008$).

Digoxin

Two digoxin-withdrawal trials [the Randomized Assessment of Effect of Digoxin on Inhibitors of ACE (RADIANCE) and Prospective Randomized Study of Ventricular Failure and Efficacy of Digoxin (PROVED) (36,37)] showed that fewer hospitalizations for worsening CHF occurred in those who continued taking digoxin. Although the large Digoxin Investigation Group (DIG) mortality trial (38) found that digoxin had no significant effect on total mortality (positive or negative), it also found that digoxin-treated patients had fewer hospitalizations than placebo patients.

Vasodilators

Hydralazine and Isosorbide Dinitrate

This combination was associated with a higher mortality rate than was enalapril in the Second VA Cooperative Heart Failure Trial (V-HeFT II; 25% vs. 18% at 2 years) (40), but yielded better results than placebo in V-HeFT I (39). Short-term use of high-dose transdermal nitrates appears to result in significant improvement in exercise tolerance and hemodynamics.

Calcium-Channel Blockers

Negative inotropic effects are not desirable in systolic dysfunction. However, in the Prospective Randomized Amlodipine Survival Evaluation (PRAISE) trial (41), amlodipine showed a trend toward lower mortality (-16%; $p = 0.07$), with a 46% lower mortality rate among patients with nonischemic cardiomyopathy. PRAISE-2 compared amlodipine with placebo in a group of patients without ischemic heart disease (42). Patients with CHF with LVEF less than 30% were randomized to receive placebo or amlodipine. No significant difference was found in this cohort with regard to all-cause or cardiac mortality.

β-Blockers

β-Blockers are safe when given carefully in controlled fashion; recent Consensus Recommendations advocate the use of β-blockers in patients in NYHA functional classes II or III. However, they should not be used in those with congested, decompensated HF. All β-blocker trials of more than 1 month duration have shown improved LV function, and a meta-analysis of 17 randomized trials with approximately 3,000 patients showed an approximately 30% mortality reduction, mostly due to fewer sudden deaths (46). The Cardiac Insufficiency Bisoprolol Study (CIBIS II) enrolled more than 2,600 NYHA class III or IV patients with an EF of less than 35% and found that bisoprolol-treated patients had a mortality rate approximately one third lower than that of placebo-treated patients (57), whereas the recently completed Metoprolol CR/XL Randomized Intervention Trial in HF (MERIT-HF) trial enrolled nearly 4,000 patients with an EF of less than 40% and found that metoprolol-XL reduced mortality by 35% compared with placebo (58).

The largest published experience to date of the nonselective β-blocker and α_1-antagonist carvedilol pooled data from different small studies (49–51), and found an impressive 65% mortality reduction at 6 months in carvedilol-treated patients (52). Carvedilol also was shown to be beneficial in improving EF and NYHA functional class, and reducing LV volumes (see *J Am Coll Cardiol* 2001;37:407). The recent Carvedilol Prospective Randomized Cumulative Survival (COPERNICUS) trial extended these results to a more advanced patient population with NYHA class IV symptoms (54). Patients with far advanced heart failure symptoms and those who could not reach compensation were not enrolled nor were significant number of black patients. Future studies focusing on these patients and patients with asymptomatic LV dysfunction are needed.

The Carvedilol or Metoprolol European Trial (COMET) directly compared these two agents in 3029 patients. At a mean follow-up of more than 3 years, carvedilol was associated with a significantly lower mortality than metoprolol therapy (preliminary results presented at ESC Heart Failure meeting, Strasburg, France, June 2003.

β-Blockade has, in general, been added to background therapy with digoxin, diuretics, and ACE inhibition. A study presented at the 24th Annual Meeting of the European Society of Cardiology (September 2002), CARMEN, compared carvedilol monotherapy, enalapril monotherapy, and combination therapy in 572 patients with mild CHF and found no significant differences between the groups. Whereas this study suggests that β-adrenergic blockade may be shown to be efficacious as initial monotherapy, the neutral finding in this trial also may be due to extended use of ACE inhibition by patients in both arms before enrollment. The results of this trial are enticing, but ACE inhibition remains first-line therapy in patients with symptomatic CHF.

Not all trials of β-adrenergic blockade have shown positive results. The BEST trial compared bucindolol with placebo in patients with NYHA class III or IV symptoms and found no difference in overall mortality rates. These findings called into question the concept of beneficial class effects for β-blockade in CHF (54).

Amiodarone

One South American study of the Grupo de Estudio de la Sobrevida en la Insuficiencia Cardiaca en Argentina (GESICA) (60) showed a mortality benefit, whereas the more recent and better designed Survival Trial of Antiarrhythmic Therapy in CHF (CHF-STAT) (61) found no mortality advantage in the amiodarone group. In the CHF-STAT, a trend was seen toward a lower mortality rate with amiodarone in the subgroup of patients with nonischemic cardiomyopathy.

Other Agents

1. Oral milrinone. A higher mortality rate was found in the Prospective Randomized Milrinone Survival Evaluation (PROMISE) trial, with more adverse reactions including syncope and hypotension (63).

2. Vesnarinone. Despite one study that suggested a benefit with 60 mg/day (64), a subsequent larger study showed increased mortality with 60 mg/daily compared with placebo (67).

3. Intravenous inotropic agents. Data from small clinical trials and anecdotal case experience suggest that inotropic agents reduce hospitalization, lead to hemodynamic and clinical improvement, and may serve as a bridge to transplantation. Some reports have suggested that intermittent infusion therapy in outpatients also may be effective in attenuating CHF symptoms in the long term (see *J Heart Lung Transplant* 2000;19:S49). The safety of prolonged outpatient use of these agents has been questioned, and an increase in mortality has led some to suggest that inotropic drugs used in this fashion may exacerbate of arrhythmias with subsequent sudden cardiac death. In severely symptomatic heart failure patients, the trade-off between symptomatic amelioration and the chance of sudden cardiac death may be worthwhile.

4. L-type calcium channel blockade. Mibefradil was compared with placebo in 2,590 NYHA class II to IV patients in the MACH-1 study (see *Circulation* 2000;101:758). A trend was noted toward increased mortality with mibefradil (14% higher at 3 months; $p = 0.09$). Patients co-medicated with mibefradil and antiarrhythmics (class I or III), including amiodarone, had a significantly increased risk of death.

Investigational Agents

1. Vasopeptidase inhibitor. Ompatrilat was compared with enalapril in the OVERTURE study, but no mortality advantage was found (68).

2. Endothelin-receptor antagonism. Preliminary results have been reported with two agents. Bosentan was compared with placebo in the Endothelin Antagonist Bosentan for Lowering Cardiac Events in Heart Failure (ENABLE) trial. No significant difference was seen in the primary end point of death or rehospitalization for heart failure in 1,613 patients with NYHA class IIIB or IV symptoms. Treatment with this drug led to fluid retention in some patients and further adverse cardiac events (see *J Am Coll Cardiol* 2002;40:1). The EARTH trial randomized 642 patients with NYHA class II to IV symptoms and LVEF 35% or less to darusentan or placebo for at least 1 month. At 6 months, darusentan was associated with a nonsignificant trend toward reduced LV end-systolic dimension (primary end point). Finally, tezosentan was compared with placebo in the randomized intravenous tezosentan study (RITZ-4) (see *J Am Coll Cardiol* 2003;41:1452). No significant difference was seen in the primary composite end point of death, worsening HF, recent ischemia, and recurrent or new MI within 72 hours.

Biventricular Pacing

Among those with chronic CHF due to systolic dysfunction, 30% or more have electrical conduction defects (bundle branch block or intraventricular conduction delay) that cause delayed activation of portions of the ventricular myocardium. Please see Chapter 6 for a discussion of biventricular (BiV) pacing, also known as "resynchronization" therapy.

Surgical Options

Left Ventricular Assist Device

Useful as a bridging device to transplantation, the left ventricular assist device (LVAD) significantly improves peak oxygen consumption (73). Failure of long-term therapy is predicted by several preoperative variables, including poor urine output, elevated central venous pressure, mechanical ventilation, prolonged prothrombin time, and reoperation (70). The use of the LVAD as destination therapy was evaluated in the REMATCH trial. A significant survival advantage was noted in patients with end-stage heart failure who received an LVAD, but this therapy was limited by device malfunction, the high incidence of infection, and the fact that only 25% of patients receiving LVAD were alive at 2 years (75).

Coronary Artery Bypass Graft Surgery
In CHF patients with CAD and moderate to severe LV dysfunction (EF less than 40%), coronary artery bypass graft (CABG) improves 3-year survival by 30% to 50% (3). It is not clear whether this magnitude of benefit is obtained in patients with primarily heart failure symptoms and little or no angina.

Cardiac Transplantation
Heart transplantation should be considered if peak oxygen consumption is below 10 to 12 mL/kg/min on optimal therapy. Other eligibility criteria also must be met [typically, age 65 years or younger, no active infection, and no malignancy; see American Heart Association (AHA)/American College of Cardiology (ACC) guidelines in *Circulation* 1995;92:3593].

Experimental or Controversial Treatment
1. Partial ventriculectomy (Batista procedure). A wedge of the LV muscle is removed from apex to base, and the mitral valve apparatus is often repaired or replaced. Various centers have reported perioperative mortality in excess of 20%. The largest series reported a surgical mortality of 3.2%, but 16% required LVADs. Long-term results were disappointing, with an incidence of death, return to NYHA class IV symptoms, or need for transplant or LVAD of 50% at 1 year and 67% at 2 years. Mortality rates have ranged from 15% to 30%, and LVAD rescue is often necessary (see *Ann Thorac Surg* 1997;64:634, *Eur J Cardiothorac Surg* 1998;13:337).
2. Mitral valve repair. This option has been used in patients with CHF due to DCM, which is complicated by severe, refractory mitral regurgitation. In one study, mitral valve reconstruction resulted in significant NYHA class improvement and a 2-year survival rate of more than 70% (71).

Miscellaneous
Tailored Therapy
Right heart catheterization is performed in patients with severe CHF, and intravenous and ultimately oral vasodilators are used to achieve optimal hemodynamics (see *Am J Cardiol* 1990;66:1348, and *J Heart Lung Transplant* 1991;10:468).

Continuous Positive Airway Pressure (CPAP)
In heart failure patients with depressed LV function and obstructive sleep apnea treatment of the latter with CPAP has been shown to reduce SBP and improve LV systolic function (see *N Eng J Med* 2003;348:1233).

Exercise Training and Rehabilitation
Numerous studies have shown tolerability and benefits of exercise in most patients. Regular exercise typically results in increased peak oxygen uptake and increased peak workload. Patients with circulatory failure in addition to deconditioning may not respond to exercise training (74–77).

Multidisciplinary Approach
One study found that a comprehensive, nurse-directed management approach, consisting of patient and family education, prescribed diet, social service consult, medication review, and intensive follow-up, led to more than 50% fewer CHF-related hospitalizations, improved quality of life, and significant cost savings (2). Preliminary results of the TEN-HMS study were presented at the 24th Annual Meeting of the European Society of Cardiology, September 2002. This trial randomized 427 patients with CHF home telemonitoring, nurse phone follow-up, or usual care. Patients receiving nurse follow-up or in-home telemonitoring had fewer days in the hospital than did those treated with standard measures.

COMPLICATIONS

Sudden Cardiac Death

CAD is the major substrate of sudden cardiac death, and cardiomyopathies, valvular heart disease, and abnormalities of the conduction system also are implicated, and the baseline EF is a significant predictor of sudden cardiac risk. Sudden cardiac death is responsible for 30% to 70% of deaths among those with CHF. The incidence is 2% to 3% per year in those with asymptomatic LV dysfunction and up to 20%/yr in those with severe CHF. Patients with advanced CHF who have a syncopal episode have a high incidence of subsequent sudden death [in one study, 45% at 1 year (81)]. The incidence of sudden cardiac death appears lower in patients receiving ACE inhibitors.

Whereas predictors of sudden cardiac death have been established in patients with prior MI and reduced EF (see Chapter 6, MADIT and MUSTT), risk stratification is difficult because few clinical predictors are specific for sudden cardiac death in those with nonischemic CHF. The relative utility of implantable cardioverter defibrillators (ICDs) versus antiarrhythmic drug therapy in this patient population is unknown. Ongoing trials including SCD-HeFT, which is comparing amiodarone with ICD implantation, will address this question in patients with nonischemic cardiomyopathy, NYHA class II to III symptoms, and LVEF less than 35%.

Atrial Fibrillation

The prevalence of atrial fibrillation is approximately 20%, and it is associated with an increased risk of stroke (15%/yr if LV dysfunction is present) and higher total mortality (80).

Embolism

Incidence is 1% to 2% per year in NYHA class II or III patients who are in normal sinus rhythm and 3% to 4% per year in patients awaiting transplantation. Oral anticoagulation should be considered if mural thrombus is present (embolic risk much higher).

REFERENCES

Guidelines, Miscellaneous

1. **Ghali JK,** et al. Precipitating factors leading to decompensation of heart failure: traits among urban blacks. *Arch Intern Med* 1988;148:2013.

This study of 101 patients admitted to an inner city hospital with a diagnosis of heart failure established precipitating factor(s) in 93%. The most common causes were noncompliance with diet and/or drugs (63%), uncontrolled hypertension (44%), arrhythmias (29%; mostly atrial fibrillation), environmental factors (19%), inadequate therapy (17%), pulmonary infection (12%), emotional stress (7%), and MI (6%).

2. **Rich MW,** et al. A multidisciplinary intervention to prevent the readmission of elderly patients with congestive heart failure. *N Engl J Med* 1995;333:1190–1195.

This prospective, randomized trial was composed of 282 high-risk patients aged 70 years or older hospitalized with CHF. Patients were assigned to standard care (control group) or nurse-directed, multidisciplinary care, consisting of comprehensive education of the patient and family, a prescribed diet, social service consultation, medication review, and intensive follow-up. A trend was noted toward improved survival without readmission (primary end point) in the multidisciplinary intervention group (64.1% vs. 53.6%; $p = 0.09$). The total number of hospital admissions was significantly lower in the multidisciplinary intervention group (53 vs. 94; $p = 0.02$), including 56% fewer CHF-related admissions (24 vs. 54; $p = 0.04$). The intervention group had an overall lower cost of care ($460 less per patient). Finally, in a subgroup of 126 patients, quality-of-life scores at 90 days improved significantly more in the intervention patients ($p = 0.001$).

3. **Frazier OH,** Myers TJ. Surgical therapy for severe failure. *Curr Probl Cardiol* 1998;23:726–764.

This review covers heart transplantation, mechanical circulatory support measures, cardiomyoplasty, and myocardial revascularization (bypass surgery, transmyocardial laser).

4. **Feenstra J,** et al. Drug-induced heart failure. *J Am Coll Cardiol* 1999;33:1152–1162.

This review discusses the anthracyclines, cyclophosphamide, paclitaxel, mitoxantrone, other chemotherapeutic agents, nonsteroidal antiinflammatory drugs, immunomodulating agents (e.g., interferons, interleukin-2), and antidepressants. The contributory roles of three major cardiac drug classes in causing heart failure also are reviewed: antiarrhythmics, β-blockers, and calcium-channel blockers.

5. **Hunt SA,** et al. **ACC/AHA guidelines** for the evaluation and management of chronic heart failure in the adult: executive summary. *J Am Coll Cardiol* 2001;38:2101–2113. Available at: http://www.acc.org/clinical/guidelines/failure/hf_index.htm.

This consensus document outlines the assessment and therapy of patients with CHF. The report outlines management of patients with symptomatic and asymptomatic LV dysfunction as well as patients with refractory end-stage heart failure. Interventions that are of proven value are discussed in detail, as are end-of-life issues and the treatment of special populations such as women, racial minorities, and elderly patients.

6. **Jessup M, Brozena S.** Heart failure. *N Eng J Med* 2003;348:2007–2018.

This recent article reviews the epidemiology, pathophysiology, and etiologies of heart failure. Treatment modalities are then discussed for patients in various stages (A to D) of heart failure. Two final sections briefly review nonpharmacologic therapies.

Epidemiology

7. **Schocken DD,** et al. Prevalence and mortality rate of congestive heart failure in the United States. *J Am Coll Cardiol* 1992;20:301–306.

This analysis focused on prevalence data obtained from the National Health and Nutritional Examination Survey (NHANES I; 1971 to 1975) and mortality data from the NHANES-I Epidemiologic Follow-up Study (1982 to 1986). Prevalence based on clinical criteria was 2% for the noninstitutionalized U.S. population. Mortality increased with advancing age and was higher in men than in women (15-year rates in patients older than 55 years: men, 71.8%; women, 39.1%).

8. **Levy D,** et al. The progression from hypertension to congestive heart failure. *JAMA* 1996;275:1557–1562.

This analysis focused on 5,143 Framingham Study subjects with a mean follow-up period of 14.1 years. Hypertension antedated 91% of new heart failure cases. After risk-factor adjustment, hypertension was associated with relative risks of developing heart failure of approximately 2.0 (men) and 3.0 (women). Poor 5-year survival was observed among hypertensive CHF subjects: 24% in men and 31% in women.

9. **Adams KF Jr,** et al. Relation between gender, etiology and survival in patients with symptomatic heart failure. *J Am Coll Cardiol* 1996;28:1781–1788.

This prospective, observational study was composed of 557 patients (177 women; nonischemic etiology in 68%). At a mean follow-up of 2.4 years, the all-cause mortality rate was 36%. Women with better survival ($p < 0.001$), primarily due to the lower mortality associated with a nonischemic etiology (men vs. women, relative risk 2.36; $p < 0.001$).

10. **Adams KF,** et al. Gender differences in survival in advanced heart failure. *Circulation* 1999;99:1816–1821.

This analysis focused on 471 Flolan International Randomized Survival Trial (FIRST) patients, of whom 112 were women; 60% were NYHA class IV, and average EF was 18%. A Cox proportional-hazards model, which included adjustments for age, gender, and 6-minute walk results, showed a significant association between female gender and better survival. (Relative risk of death for men vs. women was 2.18; $p < 0.001$.)

11. **Petrie MC.** Failure of women's hearts. *Circulation* 1999;99:2334–2341.

This review discusses epidemiologic data on CHF in women, including the higher risk among those with diabetes, hypertension, and obesity. The prevalence of CHF in the United States is higher in women because it is more common in elderly individuals. Conflicting data exist on the median survival of CHF patients. Framingham Heart Study data showed that women had a longer survival than men, whereas the SOLVD trial found the opposite (the latter enrolled more women with CAD).

12. **Levy D,** et al. Long-term trends in the incidence of and survival with heart failure. *N Engl J Med* 2002;347:1397–1402 (editorial, 1442–1444).

This analysis consisted of 1,075 Framingham Heart Study participants who developed heart failure (HF) from 1950 to 1999. As compared with the period from 1950 to 1969, the incidence of HF remained virtually unchanged among men in the three subsequent periods (1970 to 1979, 1980 to 1989, 1990 to 1999) but declined by 31% to 40% among women (rate ratio for 1990 to 1999, 0.69; 95% CI, 0.51 to 0.93). Survival after onset of HF improved in both sexes. The 30-day, 1-year, and 5-year age-adjusted mortality rates among men declined from 12%, 30%, and 70% in the period from 1950 to 1969 to 11% to 28%, and 59% from 1990 to 1999. Corresponding rates among women were 18%, 28%, and 57% (1950 to 1969) and 10%, 24%, and 45% (1990 to 1999). Overall, the survival after HF onset improved by 12% per decade ($p = 0.01$ for men, $p = 0.02$ for women).

Assessment and Prognosis

Physical Examination

13. **Stevenson LW,** Perloff JK. The limited reliability of physical signs for estimating hemodynamics in chronic heart failure. *JAMA* 1989;261:884–888.

This prospective study was composed of 50 patients with known chronic HF. Orthopnea within the preceding week was the most sensitive (91%) symptom for predicting elevated PCWP (22 mm Hg or more). Physical signs were not sensitive at predicting elevated PCWP because rales, edema, and elevated mean jugular venous pressure were absent in 18 (41.9%) of 43 patients. A measured pulse pressure of less than 25% had a 91% sensitivity and 83% specificity for a cardiac index less than 2.2 L/min/m^2.

14. **Butman SM,** et al. Bedside cardiovascular exam with severe chronic heart failure: importance of rest or inducible jugular venous distention. *J Am Coll Cardiol* 1993;22:968–974.

This prospective study was composed of 52 patients with chronic CHF who underwent right heart catheterization. The presence of jugular venous distention had a 57% sensitivity and 93% specificity for a PCWP of 18 mm Hg. The combination of jugular venous distension at rest or inducible by an abdominojugular test had a sensitivity of 81%, specificity of 80%, and 81% predictive accuracy.

15. **Badgett RG,** et al. Can the clinical examination diagnose left-sided heart failure in adults? *JAMA* 1997;277:1712–1719.

This review of the literature asserts that the best findings for detecting increased filling pressure are jugular venous distention and radiographic redistribution. The best findings for detecting systolic dysfunction are abnormal apical impulse, cardiomegaly (by radiograph), and Q waves or left bundle branch block on ECG.

Laboratory, Other

16. **Lee WH,** et al. Prognostic importance of serum sodium concentration and its modification by converting enzyme inhibition in patients with severe chronic heart failure. *Circulation* 1986;73:257–267.

This analysis focused on 30 clinical, hemodynamic, and biochemical variables in 203 consecutive severe HF patients. At follow-up (6 to 94 months), a regression analysis showed that pretreatment with a serum sodium concentration was the most powerful predictor of cardiovascular mortality [median survival, 99 (serum Na, 30 mEq/L or less) vs. 337 days; $p < 0.001$]. The poor outcomes in hyponatremic patients appeared to be related to high plasma renin levels because hyponatremic patients did better if treated with ACE inhibitors [median survival, 108 (serum Na, 137 mEq/L or less) vs. 232 days; $p = 0.003$].

17. **Cohn JN,** et al. Plasma norepinephrine as a guide to prognosis in patients with chronic congestive heart failure. *N Engl J Med* 1984;311:819–823.

The 106 patients with moderate to severe CHF had hemodynamics, plasma norepinephrine, and plasma renin activity measured at supine rest; follow-up lasted 1 to 62 months. Multivariate analysis found only plasma norepinephrine to be an independent predictor of mortality ($p = 0.002$).

18. **McCullough PA,** et al. B-type natriuretic peptide and clinical judgment in emergency diagnosis of heart failure: analysis from Breathing Not Properly **(BNP)** Multinational Study. *Circulation* 2002;106:416–422.

Design: Prospective, blinded, multicenter study. Primary end point was diagnostic accuracy at the optimum cutoff of B-type natriuretic peptide (BNP) and at 80% or more emergency department (ED) physician estimate of clinical probability of CHF.
Purpose: To assess the correlation of serum BNP levels with the clinical diagnosis of CHF.
Population: 1,538 patients with clinical suspicion for CHF determined by the ED attending physician.
Exclusion Criteria: Advanced renal failure (creatinine clearance, less than 15 mL/min), acute MI, and overt cause of dyspnea (e.g., chest-wall trauma).
Treatment: Standard evaluation and management for CHF.
Results: The final diagnosis, as determined by two blinded independent cardiologists, was CHF in 47%. At an 80% cutoff level of certainty of CHF, clinical judgment had a sensitivity of 49% and specificity of 96%. At 100 pg/mL, BNP had a sensitivity of 90% and specificity of 73%. In determining the correct diagnosis (CHF vs. no CHF), adding BNP to clinical judgment would have enhanced diagnostic accuracy from 74% to 81%. In those participants with an intermediate (21% to 79%) probability of CHF, BNP at a cutoff of 100 pg/mL accurately classified 74% of the cases. The areas under the receiver-operating-characteristic curve were 0.86 (95% CI, 0.84 to 0.88), 0.90 (95% CI, 0.88 to 0.91), and 0.93 (95% CI, 0.92 to 0.94) for clinical judgment, for BNP at a cutoff of 100 pg/mL, and for the two in combination, respectively ($p < 0.0001$ for all pair-wise comparisons).

Noninvasive Testing
19. **Gradman A,** et al. Predictors of total mortality and sudden death in mild to moderate heart failure. *J Am Coll Cardiol* 1989;14:546–570.

This analysis focused on 295 patients with LVEF 40% or less, 81% in NYHA class II. The mean follow-up period was 16 months. In multiple regression analysis, LVEF was the strongest mortality predictor ($p = 0.006$): 27% with LVEF 20% or less died versus 7% with LVEF 30%. Ventricular tachycardia also was associated with increased mortality: 34% among those with more than 0.088 events/hr vs. 12% in those with no events.

20. **Mancini DM,** et al. Value of peak exercise oxygen consumption for optimal timing of cardiac transplantation in ambulatory patients with heart failure. *Circulation* 1991;83:778–786.

This study of 114 patients found a peak oxygen consumption of 14 mL/kg/min or less in 62 patients (35 were transplantation candidates, and 27 had noncardiac issues) and more than 14 mL/kg/min in 52 patients. All three groups had similar NYHA functional class, LVEF, and cardiac index. Patients with an oxygen consumption of more than 14 mL/kg/min had a lower PCWP and significantly better 1-year survival [94% vs. 70% (transplant candidates) and 47%]. A multivariate analysis found peak oxygen consumption to be the best survival predictor, whereas PCWP added further prognostic information.

21. **Bitner V,** et al. Prediction of mortality and morbidity with a 6-minute walk test in patients with left ventricular dysfunction. *JAMA* 1993;270:1702–1707.

This analysis focused on 898 SOLVD patients with radiologic evidence of CHF and/or EF less than 45%; mean follow-up period was 8 months. No significant test-related complications were found. Highest versus lowest performance level (distance walked, 450 m or more vs. less than 300 m): 71% lower mortality (3% vs. 10.2%), 51% fewer hospitalizations (19.9% vs. 40.9%), and 91% fewer HF hospitalizations (2% vs. 22.2%). Logistic regression analysis showed that EF and walk time were equally strong and independent predictors of mortality and hospitalization due to acute HF.

22. **de Groote P,** et al. Right ventricular ejection fraction is an independent predictor of survival in patients with moderate heart failure. *J Am Coll Cardiol* 1998;32:948–954.

This analysis focused on 205 consecutive NYHA class II or III patients who underwent exercise testing and radionuclide angiography. At follow-up (median, 2 years), 44 cardiac-related deaths (21.5%) occurred. Multivariate analysis showed three variables to be independent predictors of both survival and event-free cardiac survival: NYHA classification, percentage of maximal predicted Vo_2, and right ventricular EF.

Treatment

Angiotensin-converting Enzyme Inhibitors and Angiotensin II Inhibitors
Meta-Analysis
23. **Garg R,** Yusuf S. Overview of randomized trials of angiotensin-converting enzyme inhibitors on mortality and morbidity in patients with heart failure. *JAMA* 1995;273:1450–1456.

This analysis focused on 32 studies with 7,105 patients. All studies were placebo controlled, 8 weeks in duration, and assessed all-cause mortality by intention to treat. ACE-inhibitor therapy was associated with significant reductions in total mortality (odds ratio, 0.77; 95% CI, 0.67 to 0.88; $p < 0.001$) and mortality or hospitalization for CHF (odds ratio, 0.65; 95% CI, 0.57 to 0.74; $p < 0.001$). Patients with the lowest EF had the greatest benefit. The mortality reduction was mainly due to fewer deaths from progressive HF (odds ratio, 0.69; 95% CI, 0.58 to 0.83). Nonsignificant reductions were noted in the incidence of arrhythmic deaths (odds ratio, 0.91; 95% CI, 0.73 to 1.12) and fatal MI (odds ratio, 0.82; 95% CI, 0.60 to 1.12). No significant differences were found between several different agents (see Tables 5.1 and 5.2).

Studies
24. The Cooperative North Scandinavian Enalapril Survival Study **(CONSENSUS)** Group. Effects of enalapril on mortality in severe CHF. *N Engl J Med* 1987;316: 1429–1435.

Design: Prospective, randomized, double-blind, placebo-controlled, multicenter study. Average follow-up period was 6 months. Primary end point was all-cause mortality rate.
Purpose: To evaluate the effect of enalapril, in addition to conventional therapy, on mortality in patients with severe CHF.
Population: 253 NYHA class IV patients with heart size larger than 600 mL/m^2 body surface area in men and more than 550 mL/m^2 in women.
Exclusion Criteria: Acute pulmonary edema, MI in prior 2 months, unstable angina, planned cardiac surgery, and serum creatinine more than 300 μM.
Treatment: Enalapril, 2.5 mg/day orally, up to 20 mg twice daily. All patients were taking diuretics, 94% taking digoxin, and 50% taking vasodilators (mostly isosorbide dinitrate).

Results: Trial was terminated early because of significant mortality benefit in the enalapril group: 40% relative risk reduction (RRR) in mortality at 6 months (26% vs. 44%; $p = 0.0002$), 31% RRR at 1 year (36% vs. 52%; $p = 0.001$), and 27% RRR at end of the study (39% vs. 54%; $p = 0.003$). The entire mortality reduction was seen in patients with progressive heart failure (approximately 50% lower mortality). No difference in sudden death rates was observed. A significant mortality benefit was maintained at 2-year follow-up (see *Am J Cardiol* 1992;60:103).

25. The Studies of Left Ventricular Dysfunction (**SOLVD**) Investigators. Effect of enalapril on survival in patients with reduced ventricular ejection fraction and congestive heart failure. *N Engl J Med* 1991;325:293–302.

Design: Prospective, randomized, double-blind, placebo-controlled, multicenter study. Average follow-up period was 41 months. Primary end point was all-cause mortality rate.
Purpose: To evaluate the effect of enalapril on mortality in patients with LV dysfunction and HF symptoms.
Population: 2,569 NYHA class II and III patients aged 21 to 80 years with an EF of 35% or less.
Exclusion Criteria: Active angina requiring surgery, unstable angina, or MI within the preceding month; renal failure; pulmonary disease; and current ACE-inhibitor therapy.
Treatment: Enalapril, 2.5 to 5 mg twice daily initially, and then increased at 2 weeks to 5 to 10 mg twice daily; or placebo. Other drugs were not restricted (e.g., diuretics, digoxin, vasodilators).
Results: Enalapril group had 16% lower mortality (35.2% vs. 39.7%, 16% risk reduction; $p = 0.0036$). The majority of this effect was owing to fewer deaths from progressive heart failure (16.3% vs. 19.5%; $p = 0.0045$). The enalapril group also had a lower rate of death and rehospitalization due to worsening heart failure (47.7% vs. 57.3%, 26% risk reduction; $p < 0.0001$). Sudden-death rates were similar.

26. The SOLVD Investigators. Effect of enalapril on mortality and the development of heart failure in asymptomatic patients with reduced left ventricular ejection fractions. *N Engl J Med* 1992;327:685–691.

Design: Prospective, randomized, double-blind, placebo-controlled, multicenter study. Follow-up period was 37 months. Primary end point was all-cause mortality rate.
Purpose: To evaluate effect of enalapril on mortality in patients with LV dysfunction without overt HF.
Population: 4,228 patients aged 21 to 80 years with an EF of 35% or less and taking no medications for HF (diuretics allowed for hypertension, and digoxin, for atrial fibrillation).
Exclusion Criteria: See SOLVD trial earlier.
Treatment: Enalapril, 2.5 to 20 mg orally per day, or placebo.
Results: Total mortality rates were 14.8% and 15.8% in the enalapril and placebo groups, respectively ($p = 0.30$). Most of this nonsignificant difference was due to 12% fewer cardiovascular deaths in the enalapril group (12.5% vs. 14.1%; $p = 0.12$). Fewer enalapril patients developed HF (20.7% vs. 30.2%; $p < 0.001$), and fewer required hospitalization due to HF (8.7% vs. 12.9%; $p < 0.001$).

27. The Acute Infarction Ramipril Efficacy Study (**AIRE**) Investigators. Effect of ramipril on mortality and morbidity of survivors of acute MI with clinical evidence of heart failure. *Lancet* 1993;342:821–828.

Design: Prospective, randomized, double-blind, placebo-controlled, multicenter study. Mean follow-up period was 15 months. Primary end point was all-cause mortality.
Purpose: To compare the effects of ramipril with placebo on overall mortality in acute MI survivors with early evidence of CHF.
Population: 2,006 patients with an MI 2 to 9 days before study enrollment and clinical evidence of HF at any time since acute MI.
Exclusion Criteria: Severe CHF (usually NYHA class IV), unstable angina, and heart failure of primary valvular or congenital etiology.

Treatment: Ramipril, 2.5 mg orally twice daily for 2 days, and then 5 mg twice daily; or placebo.

Results: Ramipril group had a 27% risk reduction in mortality (17% vs. 23%; $p = 0.002$). This benefit was already apparent at 30 days. Sudden cardiac deaths were reduced by 30% ($p = 0.011$).

Comments: AIREX follow-up study analyzed 603 patients at a mean 59 months, and the ramipril group still had a significantly lower mortality rate (RR, 0.64; 27.5% vs. 38.9%; $p = 0.002$) (see *Lancet* 1997;349:1493).

28. **Pitt B,** et al. Evaluation of Losartan in the Elderly **(ELITE).** Randomized trial of losartan vs. captopril in patients over 65 with heart failure. *Lancet* 1997;349:747–752.

Design: Prospective, randomized, double-blind, placebo-controlled, multicenter study. Primary end point was increase in creatinine clearance of 0.3 mg/dL.

Purpose: To compare the effects of angiotensin II–receptor inhibitor losartan with captopril on creatinine clearance and major cardiac events in elderly HF patients.

Population: 722 ACE inhibitor–naive patients in NYHA class II to IV and with EF of 40% or less.

Exclusion Criteria: Included SBP less than 90 mm Hg, acute MI or coronary angioplasty in the prior 72 hours, bypass surgery in the prior 2 weeks, unstable angina in the prior 3 months, and stroke or transient ischemic attack in the prior 3 months.

Treatment: Losartan, 12.5 to 50 mg daily, or captopril, 6.25 to 50 mg 3 times daily for 48 weeks.

Results: Similar incidence of increased creatinine was observed in both groups (10.5%). Fewer losartan patients discontinued therapy: 12.2% vs. 20.8%; $p = 0.002$ (cough, 0 vs. 14 patients). The losartan group showed a trend toward lower rates of death and hospitalization (9.4% vs. 13.2%; $p = 0.075$) and a significant 45% lower overall mortality rate (4.8% vs. 8.7%, $p = 0.035$; sudden cardiac death: five vs. 14 patients). This mortality benefit was seen in all subgroups except women (240 patients, 7.6% vs. 6.6%).

Comments: Study was not designed to examine mortality.

29. **Packer M,** et al. Comparative effects of low and high doses of the angiotensin-converting enzyme inhibitor, lisinopril, on morbidity and mortality in chronic heart failure **(ATLAS).** *Circulation* 1999;100:2312–2318.

Design: Prospective, randomized, double-blind, placebo-controlled, multicenter study. Primary end point was all-cause mortality. Follow-up period was 4 years.

Purpose: To evaluate the comparative efficacy of lisinopril on mortality in patients with LV dysfunction and HF symptoms.

Population: 3,164 patients with NYHA class II to IV HF and an EF of 30% or less.

Exclusion Criteria: Included acute coronary ischemic event or revascularization procedure in the prior 2 months, history of sustained or symptomatic ventricular tachycardia (VT), intolerance to ACE inhibitors, and serum creatinine greater than 2.5 mg/dL.

Treatment: Low-dose lisinopril (2.5 to 5.0 mg daily) or high-dose lisinopril (32.5 to 35 mg daily). Before randomization, all patients received lisinopril for 4 weeks to assess their ability to tolerate the drug. Digitalis, ACE inhibitors, or vasodilators were allowed but not mandated.

Results: Patients in the high-dose group had a nonsignificant 8% lower risk of death ($p = 0.13$) but a significant 12% lower risk of death or hospitalization for any reason ($p = 0.002$) and 24% fewer hospitalizations for HF ($p = 0.002$). Dizziness and renal insufficiency was observed more frequently in the high-dose group, but the two groups were similar in the number of patients requiring cessation of the study medication.

30. **Pitt B,** et al. Effect of losartan compared with captopril on mortality in patients with symptomatic heart failure: randomised trial—the Losartan Heart Failure Survival Study **(ELITE II).** *Lancet* 2000;355:1582–1587.

Design: Prospective, randomized, double-blind, placebo-controlled, multicenter study. Primary end point was all-cause mortality.

Purpose: To compare the mortality benefit of the angiotensin II–receptor inhibitor losartan with captopril in elderly HF patients.

Population: 3,152 ACE inhibitor–naive patients in NYHA class II through IV and with EF 40% or less.

Exclusion Criteria: Included ACE inhibitor or angiotensin II–receptor antagonist intolerance, SBP less than 90 mm Hg, DBP greater than 95 mm Hg, hemodynamically important stenotic valvular heart disease, active myocarditis or pericarditis, ICD implantation, serum creatinine more than 220 mM, PTCA in previous week, cerebrovascular accident (CVA) or transient ischemic attack (TIA) in previous 6 weeks; CABG surgery, acute MI, or unstable angina in previous 2 weeks.

Treatment: Losartan, 12.5 to 50 mg daily, or captopril, 6.25 to 50 mg 3 times daily.

Results: No significant differences were found between the two groups in all-cause mortality (11.7% vs. 10.4% average annual mortality rate) or sudden death or resuscitated arrests (9.0% vs. 7.3%; $p = 0.08$). Fewer losartan patients had adverse effects (9.7% vs. 14.7%; $p < 0.001$), especially cough (0.3% vs. 2.7%).

Comments: These results demonstrate the problem of drawing conclusions from trials enrolling small numbers of patients (i.e., ELITE I). The trial was not designed to address equivalence between the two treatments, so these findings do not provide evidence regarding the efficacy of losartan compared with placebo.

31. **Cohn JN,** et al. A randomized trial of the angiotensin-receptor blocker valsartan in chronic heart failure **(Val-HeFT).** *N Engl J Med* 2001;345:1667–1675.

Design: Prospective, randomized, double-blind, placebo-controlled, multicenter study. Primary end point was all-cause mortality.

Purpose: To determine the mortality benefit of adding valsartan to usual therapy for CHF in patients with HF.

Population: 5,010 patients with NYHA class II to IV symptoms with EF 40% or less. Patients required to be on stable medical regimens, which could include diuretics, digoxin, ACE inhibition, and β-blockers.

Treatment: Valsartan, 40 to 50 mg daily, or captopril, 6.25 to 50 mg 3 times daily.

Results: No significant difference in overall mortality was found between the valsartan and captopril groups (19.7% vs. 19.4%). The incidence of the secondary combined end point of death or cardiac arrest with resuscitation, hospitalized for CHF, or intravenous inotropic or vasodilator for 4 hours or more, was significantly lower with valsartan (RR, 0.87; $p = 0.009$). This benefit was mainly owing to a lower incidence of hospitalization for HF (13.8% vs. 18.2%; $p < 0.001$). Treatment with valsartan also was associated with improvements in NYHA class, EF, signs and symptoms of HF, and quality of life.

Diuretics

32. **Dormans TPJ,** et al. Diuretic efficacy of high dose furosemide in severe heart failure: bolus injection vs. continuous infusion. *J Am Coll Cardiol* 1996;28:376–382.

In this crossover study, 20 patients were randomized to an equal dosage by intravenous bolus or an 8-hour continuous infusion after a loading dose (20% total). Doses used ranged from 250 to 2,000 mg/24 hr. The continuous-infusion group had an increased urinary volume (2.9 vs. 2.3 L; $p < 0.001$) and better sodium excretion. Reversible hearing loss was seen in five intravenous-bolus patients [maximal plasma concentration, 95 vs. 24 μg/mL (see *Chest* 1992;102:725); only nine patients, and the bolus plus 48-hour infusion yielded better results than intravenous boluses 3 times daily].

33. **Pitt B,** et al., Randomized Aldactone Evaluation Study **(RALES)** Investigators. The effect of spironolactone on morbidity and mortality in patients with severe heart failure. *N Engl J Med* 1999;341:709–719 (editorial, 753–755).

Design: Prospective, randomized, double-blind, placebo-controlled, multicenter study. Mean follow-up was 24 months. Primary end point was all-cause mortality.

Purpose: To evaluate whether spironolactone would significantly reduce mortality in patients with severe HF.

Population: 1,663 NYHA class III (69%) or IV (31%) patients with an EF of 35% or less. Ischemic etiology of HF in 54%.

Exclusion Criteria: Included valvular heart disease; unstable angina; hepatic failure; potassium, 5 mM or greater; creatinine, greater than 2.5 mg/dL.

Treatment: Spironolactone, 25 mg, or placebo once daily. Dose could be increased to 50 mg if worsening HF with normal potassium. All patients were taking loop diuretics, 95% were taking ACE inhibitors, and 74% were receiving digoxin.

Results: Spironolactone group had a significant (30%) reduction in mortality compared with placebo (35% vs. 46%; $p < 0.001$). This benefit was attributable to a lower risk of sudden death from cardiac causes (29% RRR) and death from progressive HF (36% RRR). Spironolactone was associated with a higher incidence of gynecomastia (10% vs. 1%; $p < 0.001$); whereas the incidence of serious hyperkalemia was similar (2% vs. 1%).

34. **EPHESUS (Eplerenone Post-Acute MI Heart Failure Efficacy and Survival Study). Pitt B,** et al. for the EPHESUS Investigators. Eplerenone, a selective aldosterone blocker in patients with left ventricular dysfunction after myocardial infarction. *N Engl J Med* 2003;348:1309–1321 (editorial pp. 1380–1382).

Design: Prospective, randomized, placebo-controlled, double-blind, multicenter study. Primary endpoints were all cause mortality and cardiovascular death or hospitalization for cardiovascular causes. Mean followup was 16 months.

Purpose: To evaluate the effect of eplerenone on morbidity and mortality among patients with acute MI complicated by left ventricular dysfunction.

Population: 6632 patients with an acute MI 3 to 14 days prior to randomization and LVEF = 40% by echocardiography.

Exclusion Criteria: Included use of potassium-sparing divretics, creatinine >2.5 mg/dL, potassium >5.0 mmol/L.

Treatment: Eplerenone, 25 to 50 mg twice daily, or placebo. Nearly all were on ACE inhibitors (94%) and 75% were on beta-blockers.

Results: Eplerenone group had a significant reduction in all-cause mortality compared to placebo (14.4% vs. 16.7%, relative risk 0.85, $p = 0.008$). It was also associated with a lower rate of cardiovascular death or CV-related hospitalization (RR 0.87, $p = 0.002$). Eplerenone also had a 21% relative reduction in sudden cardiac death ($p = 0.03$). Serious hyperkalemia occurred more frequently with eplerenone (5.5% vs. 3.9%, $p = 0.002$), while hypokalemia was less common (8.4% vs. 13.1%, $p < 0.001$).

Digoxin
Review Article
35. **Hauptman PJ,** Kelly RA. Digitalis *Circulation* 1999;99:1265–1270.

This review discusses the molecular and clinical pharmacology of cardiac glycosides, describes the clinical manifestations and treatment of digitalis toxicity, and examines recent trial data, with a focus on the DIG trial results.

Studies
36. **Packer M,** et al., Randomized Assessment of Effect of Digoxin on Inhibitors of ACE **(RADIANCE)** study. Withdrawal of digoxin from patients with chronic HF treated with ACE inhibitor. *N Engl J Med* 1993;329:1–7.

Design: Prospective, randomized, double-blind, placebo-controlled, multicenter study. Primary end point was study withdrawal due to worsening HF, time to withdrawal, and changes in exercise tolerance.

Purpose: To evaluate the effect of the withdrawal of digoxin from patients with chronic HF who were clinically stable while receiving digoxin, diuretics, and an ACE inhibitor.

Population: 178 NYHA class II or III patients taking digoxin, diuretics, and ACE inhibitors (captopril or enalapril).

Exclusion Criteria: SBP, 160 mm Hg or more or less than 90 mm Hg; DBP, greater than 95 mm Hg; history of supraventricular arrhythmias or sustained ventricular arrhythmias; MI in the prior 3 months; and stroke in the prior 12 months.

Treatment: Patients were randomized to continue digoxin or to placebo for 12 weeks.

Results: Cessation/placebo group had a markedly higher rate of worsening CHF requiring withdrawal from the study (24.7% vs. 4.7; RR, 5.9; $p < 0.001$), lower EF ($p < 0.001$), decreased functional capacity (maximal exercise tolerance; $p = 0.033$; submaximal exercise endurance; $p = 0.01$; NYHA class, $p = 0.019$), and poorer quality of life scores ($p = 0.04$).

37. **Uretsky BF,** et al., Prospective Randomized Study of Ventricular Failure and Efficacy of Digoxin **(PROVED).** Randomized study assessing effect of digoxin withdrawal in patients with mild-moderate chronic CHF. *J Am Coll Cardiol* 1993;22:955–962.

Design: Prospective, randomized, double-blind, placebo-controlled, multicenter study. Primary end point was incidence of treatment failure, time to treatment failure, treadmill time, and 6-minute walk distance.

Purpose: To evaluate the effects of digoxin withdrawal in patients with mild to moderate HF.

Population: 88 NYHA class II or III patients in normal sinus rhythm and taking digoxin and diuretics.

Exclusion Criteria: SBP less than 90 mm Hg, acute MI or coronary angioplasty in the prior 72 hours, bypass surgery in the prior 2 weeks, unstable angina in the prior 3 months, and stroke or TIA in the prior 3 months.

Treatment: Patients were randomized to continue digoxin or to placebo for 12 weeks.

Results: Cessation/placebo group had lower exercise tolerance (-96 vs. -4.5 seconds; $p = 0.003$), twice as many treatment failures (39% vs. 19%; $p = 0.039$), decreased time to treatment failure ($p = 0.037$), lower EF ($p = 0.016$), and higher heart rate ($p = 0.003$).

38. Digoxin Investigation Group **(DIG).** The effect of digoxin on mortality and morbidity in patients with heart failure. *N Engl J Med* 1997;336:525–533.

Design: Prospective, randomized, double-blind, placebo-controlled, multicenter study. Follow-up period was 37 months. Primary end point was all-cause mortality rate.

Purpose: To evaluate the effects of digoxin on mortality from any cause in HF patients.

Population: 6,800 patients with an EF of 45% or less and in normal sinus rhythm. Most patients were taking ACE inhibitors (94%) and diuretics (82%).

Treatment: Digoxin (average dose, 0.25 mg/day) or placebo.

Results: No significant difference in mortality rates (34.8% vs. 35.1%) was observed. The digoxin group had fewer CHF hospitalizations (26.8% vs. 34.7%; RR, 0.72; $p < 0.001$) and showed a trend toward fewer CHF deaths (RR, 0.88; $p = 0.06$), but this was offset by increased mortality due to other cardiac causes (not a prespecified outcome; 15% vs. 13%; $p = 0.04$). Subgroup analysis showed that greater reductions in death and hospitalization were due to worsening HF if EF less than 25% (-23% vs. -16%) or NYHA class III/IV (-22% vs. -18%). An overall decrease in hospital stays of only nine per 1,000 patient years was observed. An ancillary trial of 988 patients with EF greater than 45% also showed no difference in mortality (both 23.4%).

Comments: Subsequent *post hoc* subgroup analysis (see *N Engl J Med* 2002;347:1403) showed that among women, a significantly higher mortality was seen in those assigned to digoxin therapy [33.1% vs. 28.9% (no digoxin)]; in contrast, mortality rates were similar in men. This finding among women persisted after a multivariate analysis was performed. Another postnoc analysis of 3782 men with LVEF $\leq$ 45% found that the optimal serum digoxin concentration was 0.5 to 0.8 mg/ml (higher mortality if $\geq$ 0.9 mg/ml; see *JAMA* 2003;289:871).

Vasodilator Studies

39. **Cohn JN,** et al. VA Cooperative Heart Failure Trial **(V-HeFT I).** Effect of vasodilator therapy on mortality in chronic congestive heart failure. *N Engl J Med* 1986;314:1547–1552.

Design: Prospective, randomized, double-blind, placebo-controlled, multicenter study. Mean follow-up period was 2.3 years. Primary end point was all-cause mortality rate.

Purpose: To determine whether two widely used vasodilator regimens could alter life expectancy in men with stable chronic CHF.

Population: 642 men aged 18 to 75 years with chronic HF (defined as cardiac dilatation by chest radiography or echocardiography) or EF less than 45% in association with reduced exercise tolerance.

Exclusion Criteria: Exercise tolerance limited by chest pain, MI in prior 3 months, and requirement for long-acting nitrates, calcium-channel antagonists, and/or β-blockers.

Treatment: Prazosin, 20 mg once daily; hydralazine, 300 mg/day; and isosorbide dinitrate, 160 mg/day; or placebo. Digoxin and diuretics were permitted.

Results: Hydralazine-isosorbide dinitrate group had 38% lower mortality at 1 year [12.1% vs. 19.5% (placebo)], 25% reduction at 2 years [25.6% vs. 34.3% (placebo); $p < 0.028$], and 23% reduction at 3 years (36.2% vs. 46.9%). LVEF increased significantly at 8 weeks and at 1 year in the hydralazine-isosorbide dinitrate group (+2.9%, +4.2%; both $p < 0.001$). No significant benefits were seen with prazosin.

40. **Cohn JN,** et al., **V-HeFT II.** A comparison of enalapril with hydralazine-isosorbide dinitrate in the treatment of chronic CHF. *N Engl J Med* 1991;325:303–310.

Design: Prospective, randomized, double-blind, placebo-controlled, multicenter study. Average follow-up period was 2.5 years. Primary end point was 2-year all-cause mortality rate.

Purpose: To compare the efficacy of enalapril with hydralazine plus isosorbide dinitrate in HF patients.

Population: 804 men aged 18 to 75 years in mostly NYHA class II/III and taking digoxin and diuretics.

Exclusion Criteria: MI or cardiac surgery in the prior 3 months and angina limiting exercise or requiring long-term medical therapy.

Treatment: Enalapril, 20 mg/day, or hydralazine, 300 mg/day, plus isosorbide dinitrate, 160 mg/day.

Results: Enalapril group had a 28% lower 2-year mortality rate (18% vs. 25%; $p = 0.016$) and a 14% lower overall mortality rate (32.8% vs. 38.2%; $p = 0.08$). This mortality difference was owing to fewer sudden cardiac deaths (57 vs. 92 patients), mostly in NYHA class I or II patients. At 13 weeks, the enalapril group had a greater reduction in BP, whereas the hydralazine-isosorbide dinitrate group had a greater increase in EF and exercise tolerance.

41. **Packer M,** et al., Prospective Randomized Amlodipine Survival Evaluation **(PRAISE).** Effect of amlodipine on morbidity and mortality in severe chronic heart failure. *N Engl J Med* 1996;335:1107–1114.

Design: Prospective, randomized, double-blind, placebo-controlled, multicenter study. Average follow-up period was 14 months. Primary end point was mortality and CV morbidity [hospitalization for 24 hours for MI, pulmonary edema, severe hypoperfusion, VT, or ventricular fibrillation (VF)].

Purpose: To assess the safety and efficacy of the calcium-channel antagonist amlodipine in patients with severe chronic HF.

Population: 1,153 patients with an EF less than 30%. HF was associated with ischemic disease in 732 (63.5%) patients.

Exclusion Criteria: Unstable angina or MI in the prior month, cardiac arrest or sustained ventricular tachycardia or ventricular fibrillation in the prior year, stroke or cardiac revascularization in the prior 3 months, SBP less than 85 mm Hg or 160 mm Hg or more, active myocarditis, constrictive pericarditis, primary valvular disease.

Treatment: Amlodipine, 10 mg/day (5 mg/day for first 2 weeks), or placebo.

Results: Amlodipine group had a nonsignificant 9% lower incidence in the primary end point (39% vs. 42%; $p = 0.31$). Amlodipine group also had a nonsignificant 16% mortality reduction (33% vs. 38%; $p = 0.07$). Among nonischemic patients, amlodipine was associated with a 46% lower mortality rate ($p < 0.001$) and 31% fewer overall events ($p = 0.04$).

Comments: An interesting ancillary study of cytokines showed that high interleukin-6 levels correlated with increased CHF and death ($p = 0.048$) and were reduced by amlodipine ($p = 0.006$) but to values still more than 5 times normal (see *J Am Coll Cardiol* 1997;30:35).

42. **PRAISE-2** (Prospective Randomized Amlodipine Survival Evaluation–2). Effect of amlodipine on morbidity and mortality in severe nonischemic chronic heart failure: preliminary results presented at the 49th Annual American College of Cardiology Scientific Sessions, Anaheim, CA, November 2000.

Design: Prospective, randomized, double-blind, placebo-controlled, multicenter study. Primary end point was all-cause mortality and CV morbidity (hospitalization for 24 hours for MI, pulmonary edema, severe hypoperfusion, ventricular tachycardia, or ventricular fibrillation). Average follow-up was 4 years.

Purpose: To assess the safety and efficacy of the calcium-channel antagonist amlodipine in patients with severe nonischemic chronic HF.

Population: 1,652 patients with an EF less than 30% and NYHA class IIIb or IV symptoms despite therapy with diuretics, ACE inhibitors, and digoxin.

Exclusion Criteria: Included therapy with calcium channel blockers, β-blockers, or cardiodepressant antiarrhythmic drugs; unstable angina or MI in the prior month; cardiac arrest or sustained VT or VF in the prior year; stroke or cardiac revascularization in the prior 3 months; SBP less than 85 mm Hg or 160 mm Hg or greater; primary valvular disease.

Treatment: Amlodipine, 10 mg/day (5 mg/day for first 2 weeks), or placebo.

Results: No significant difference was found between the groups in all-cause mortality [31.7% (placebo), 33.7% (amlodipine); hazard ratio, 1.09; 95% CI, 0.92 to 1.29; $p = 0.32$].No subgroup was found to receive a mortality benefit with amlodipine.

Comments: Further analysis using the combined population of PRAISE-1 and PRAISE-2 showed no significant differences in all-cause mortality.

43. **Fonarow GC,** et al., **Hydralazine-Captopril study (Hy-C).** Effect of direct vasodilation with hydralazine versus ACE inhibition with captopril on mortality in advanced heart failure. *J Am Coll Cardiol* 1992;19:842–850.

This study was composed of 117 heart transplant evaluees with a mean EF of 20%. Patients were randomized to captopril (initial dose, 6.25 mg, titrated to maximum 100 mg every 6 hours) or hydralazine (initial dose, 25 mg, titrated up to 150 mg every 6 hours) with or without isosorbide dinitrate (discontinued if intolerable side effects occurred). Doses were titrated to achieve a PCWP of 15 mm Hg and SVR of 1,200 dynes sec/cm^5. The captopril group had a better 1-year survival rate (81% vs. 51%; $p = 0.05$). As seen in V-HeFT II, this benefit was owing to fewer sudden deaths ($p = 0.01$).

44. **Colucci WS,** et al., for **Nesiritide Study Group.** Intravenous nesiritide, a natriuretic peptide, in the treatment of decompensated congestive heart failure. *N Engl J Med* 2000;343:246–253.

Design: Prospective, randomized, partially blinded, partially open, multicenter trial. Primary end point: Change in pulmonary capillary pressure from baseline to 6 hrs (efficacy trial); global clinical status and clinical symptoms (comparative trial).

Purpose: To evaluate an intravenous infusion of nesiritide, a brain (B-type) natriuretic peptide, in patients with decompensated CHF.

Population: Efficacy study: 127 patients with a PCWP of 18 mm Hg or more and cardiac index of 2.7 L/min/m^2; comparative trial, 305 patients.

Exclusion Criteria: Included dopamine, dobutamine, or intravenous vasodilator infusion for more than 4 hours; MI or unstable angina in the previous 48 hours; clinically significant valvular stenosis; hypertrophic or restrictive cardiomyopathy; constrictive pericarditis; or active myocarditis.

Treatment: Efficacy trial: Swan-Ganz catheter placed and randomization to double-blind treatment with intravenous placebo or nesiritide (0.015 or 0.030 μg/kg/min) for 6 hours. Comparative trial: hemodynamic monitoring not required and open-label therapy with standard agents or nesiritide for up to 7 days.

Results: In the efficacy trial, at 6 hours, nesiritide was associated significant reductions in PCWP (6.0 and 9.6 mm Hg for 0.015 and 0.030 μg/kg/min, respectively, versus +2.0 mm Hg with placebo; $p < 0.001$). Nesiritide was also associated with improved global clinical status in 60% and 67% of patients (vs. 14% in placebo group; $p < 0.001$), less dyspnea [57% and 53% vs. 12% (placebo); $p < 0.001$], and less fatigue [32% and 38% vs. 5% (placebo); $p < 0.001$]. In the comparative trial, the improvements in global clinical status, dyspnea, and fatigue were sustained with nesiritide therapy for up to 7 days and were similar to those seen with standard intravenous therapy for HF. The most common side effect was dose-related hypotension [symptomatic: 11% and 17% vs. 4%; $p = 0.008$ (comparative); 2% and 5% vs. none; $p = 0.55$ (efficacy)].

45. Publication Committee for the **VMAC** Investigators (Vasodilatation in the Management of Acute CHF). Intravenous nesiritide vs nitroglycerin for treatment of decompensated congestive heart failure: a randomized controlled trial. *JAMA* 2002;287:1531–1540.

Design: Prospective, randomized, double-blind trial. Primary end points were change in PCWP in catheterized patients and self-evaluation of dyspnea at 3 hours after initiation of study drug.
Population: 489 inpatients with dyspnea at rest from decompensated CHF, including 246 who received pulmonary artery catheterization.
Treatment: Intravenous nesiritide, intravenous nitroglycerin, or placebo added to standard medications for 3 hours, followed by nesiritide or nitroglycerin added to standard medication for 24 hours.
Results: At 3 hours, the mean decrease in PCWP from baseline was greater with nesiritide compared with placebo ($p < 0.001$) and nitroglycerin ($p = 0.03$). At 3 hours, nesiritide resulted in improvement in dyspnea compared with placebo ($p = 0.03$), but no significant difference was found between nesiritide and nitroglycerin in dyspnea or global clinical status. At 24 hours, the reduction in PCWP was greater in the nesiritide group (8.2 mm Hg) than in the nitroglycerin group (6.3 mm Hg), but no significant difference was noted in dyspnea and only modest improvement in global clinical status.

β-Blockers
Review Articles and Meta-Analyses
46. **Heidenreich PA,** et al. Effect of β-blockade on mortality in patients with heart failure: a meta-analysis of randomized clinical trials. *J Am Coll Cardiol* 1997;30:27–34.

This analysis focused on 17 randomized trials enrolling a total of 3,039 patients with mortality data through at least 3 months. β-Blocker use was associated with significantly lower mortality (odds ratio, 0.69; 95% CI, 0.54 to 0.88), mostly because of fewer nonsudden cardiac deaths (odds ratio, 0.58; 95% CI, 0.4 to 0.83). For sudden cardiac death, the odds ratio was 0.84 (95% CI, 0.59 to 1.2). Similar mortality reductions were observed for ischemic and nonischemic cardiomyopathy patients.

47. **Lechat P,** et al. Clinical effects of β-adrenergic blockade in chronic heart failure. *Circulation* 1998;98:1184–1191.

This meta-analysis focused on 18 double-blind, placebo-controlled, parallel-group studies with a total of 3,023 patients. β-Blocker use was associated with a 29% increase in EF ($p < 0.0001$) and 37% reduction in the risk of death or hospitalization for HF ($p < 0.001$). All-cause mortality was decreased by 32% ($p = 0.003$). A greater reduction for nonselective β-blockers compared with β_1-selective agents was seen (49% vs. 18%; $p = 0.049$). The effect of β-blocker use on NYHA functional class was of only borderline significance ($p = 0.04$).

Carvedilol Studies
48. Australian-New Zealand **(ANZ)** Heart Failure Research Collaborative Group. Effects of carvedilol, a vasodilator–β-blocker, in patients with congestive heart failure due to ischemic heart disease. *Circulation* 1995;92:212–218.

Design: Prospective, randomized, double-blind, placebo-controlled, multicenter study. Primary end points were changes in LVEF and treadmill exercise duration from baseline to 6 months.

Purpose: To evaluate the effects of carvedilol on symptoms, exercise performance, and LV function in patients with CHF due to CAD.

Population: 415 NYHA class II or III patients with an EF less than 45% and ischemic etiology of HF.

Exclusion Criteria: SBP less than 90 mm Hg; HR, less than 50 beats/min; heart block, coronary event, or procedure within previous 4 weeks; primary myocardial or valvular disease; and verapamil and/or β-blocker therapy.

Treatment: After a 2- to 3-week run-in period (3.125 to 6.25 mg twice daily; only 4% withdrawal rate), patients were randomized to carvedilol (target dose, 25 mg twice daily), or placebo; 86% were taking ACE inhibitors.

Results: At 6 months, the carvedilol group had a 5.2% higher EF (by radionuclide ventriculography; $p < 0.0001$) and decreased LV end-systolic and LV end-diastolic dimensions [-2.6 mm ($p < 0.0001$) and -1.3 mm ($p = 0.048$)]. No changes were seen in exercise tolerance (6-minute walk test). NYHA class improvement was seen in 28% and 23% (placebo; $p = $ NS), whereas worsening symptoms occurred in 5% versus 12% ($p = 0.05$).

49. **Packer M,** et al., Prospective Randomized Evaluation of Carvedilol on Symptoms and Exercise **(PRECISE).** Double-blind, placebo-controlled study of the effects of carvedilol in patients with moderate to severe heart failure. *Circulation* 1996;94:2793–2799.

Design: Prospective, randomized, double-blind, placebo-controlled, multicenter study. Primary end point was exercise tolerance.

Purpose: To evaluate the clinical effects of carvedilol in patients with moderate to severe CHF.

Population: 278 patients with moderate to severe CHF (dyspnea or fatigue at rest or on exertion for 3 months), an EF 35% or less, and receiving digoxin, diuretics, and an ACE inhibitor.

Exclusion Criteria: MI, unstable angina, CABG surgery, or stroke in the prior 3 months; uncorrected primary valvular disease; SBP less than 85 mm Hg or more than 160 mm Hg or DBP more than 100 mm Hg; heart rate, less than 68 beats/min; and use of calcium-channel blockers or antiarrhythmic drugs.

Treatment: During the open-label run-in period, carvedilol, 6.25 mg twice daily for 2 weeks. If tolerated, the patient was randomized to carvedilol, 12.5 twice daily initially, with titration over a 2- to 6-week period to 25 to 50 mg twice daily for 6 months, or placebo.

Results: Carvedilol patients had more frequent improvement in symptoms, as evaluated by changes in NYHA functional class ($p = 0.014$) and global assessments by the patient ($p = 0.002$) and the physician ($p < 0.001$). Carvedilol patients also had a significant increase in EF ($+8\%$ vs. $+3\%$; $p < 0.001$) and a significant decrease in morbidity and mortality (19.6% vs. 31.0%; $p = 0.029$). However, no significant effect was seen on exercise tolerance or quality-of-life scores.

50. **Colucci WS,** et al. Carvedilol inhibits clinical progression in patients with mild symptoms of heart failure. *Circulation* 1996;94:2800–2806.

Design: Prospective, randomized, double-blind, placebo-controlled, multicenter study. Primary end point was progression of HF (defined as death or hospitalization due to HF or need for sustained increase in HF medications).

Purpose: To determine whether long-term treatment with carvedilol inhibits clinical progression in patients with mild symptoms of HF and receiving optimal therapy.

Population: 278 patients aged 18 to 85 years with an EF of 35% or less.

Exclusion Criteria: MI, unstable angina, or CABG surgery in the prior 3 months; SBP less than 85 mm Hg or more than 160 mm Hg or DBP more than 100 mm Hg; uncorrected primary valvular disease; and use of calcium-channel blockers or antiarrhythmic drugs.

Treatment: After the open-label run-in phase with carvedilol, 6.25 mg twice daily, patients were randomized to carvedilol, 12.5 to 50 mg twice daily, or placebo for 6 months.

Results: Carvedilol group had a 48% reduction in clinical progression of HF (11% vs. 21%; *p* = 0.008). The carvedilol group also had a significant reduction in all-cause mortality (0.9% vs. 4.0%; RR, 0.23; *p* = 0.048) and improved EF (+10% vs. +3%; *p* < 0.001) and NYHA functional class (*p* < 0.003). However, no differences in exercise tolerance or quality of life were noted, and no difference between idiopathic DCM and ischemic heart disease patients.

51. **Bristow MR,** et al., Multicenter Oral Carvedilol Heart Failure Assessment **(MOCHA).** Carvedilol produces dose-related improvements in left ventricular function and survival in subjects with chronic heart failure. *Circulation* 1996;94: 2807–2816.

Design: Prospective, randomized, double-blind, placebo-controlled, multicenter study. Follow-up period was 6 months. Primary end point was change in walk test distances (6-minute corridor test and 9-minute self-powered treadmill test).
Purpose: To evaluate the effects of carvedilol in addition to standard therapy on clinical events and quality of life in chronic HF patients.
Population: 345 patients aged 18 to 85 years with symptomatic, stable HF capable of walking 150 to 450 meters in 6 minutes.
Exclusion Criteria: MI or stroke in the prior 3 months, uncorrected primary valvular disease, planned bypass surgery or balloon angioplasty, SBP less than 85 or more than 160 mm Hg, and use of calcium-channel blockers or antiarrhythmic drugs.
Treatment: Carvedilol, 6.25 to 25 mg/day, or placebo. Concomitant therapy included diuretics, digoxin, and ACE inhibitors.
Results: No differences were seen in submaximal exercise performance (as assessed by two walk tests) or HF symptoms. Carvedilol was associated with dose-dependent improvements in LV function (+5%, +6%, and +8% in low-, medium-, and high-dose groups versus +2% with placebo; *p* < 0.001) and mortality (6.0%, 6.7%, and 1.1% vs. 15.5%; *p* < 0.001). When the three carvedilol groups were combined, the all-cause actuarial mortality risk was 73% lower (*p* < 0.001). Carvedilol patients also were hospitalized less frequently (by 58% to 64%; *p* = 0.01).

52. **Packer M,** et al., U.S. Carvedilol Heart Failure Study Group. The effect of carvedilol on morbidity and mortality in patients with chronic heart failure. *N Engl J Med* 1996;334:1349–1355 (editorial, 1396–1397).

Design: Prospective, randomized, double-blind, placebo-controlled, multicenter study. Primary end point was mortality.
Purpose: To evaluate the safety and efficacy of carvedilol in patients with chronic HF.
Population: 1,094 chronic HF patients with an EF 35% or less and taking digoxin, diuretics, and an ACE inhibitor.
Exclusion Criteria: SBP less than 90 mm Hg, acute MI or coronary angioplasty in the prior 72 hours, bypass surgery in the prior 2 weeks, unstable angina in the prior 3 months, and stroke or TIA in the prior 3 months.
Treatment: After the 2-week open-label phase (5.6% failed to complete this period because of adverse events), patients were assigned to one of four treatment groups based on exercise capacity [6-minute walk: mild, 426 to 550 m; moderate, 150 to 425 m; severe, less than 150 m (fourth group dose-ranging protocol)] and randomized to carvedilol, 6.25 to 50 mg twice daily (titrated over a 2- to 10-week period), or placebo.
Results: At 6 months, carvedilol-treated patients had 65% lower mortality (3.2% vs. 7.8%; *p* < 0.001), 27% fewer CV-related hospitalizations (14.1% vs. 19.6%; *p* = 0.036), and a 38% reduction in death and hospitalization (15.8% vs. 24.6%; *p* < 0.001). Patients with an initial HR of more than 82 beats/min had the most benefit. More placebo patients had worsening HF.
Comments: Analysis combined patients from three different studies [PRECISE, MOCHA, Colucci WS, et al. (52)]. This study had limited follow-up and only 53 total deaths; seven carvedilol deaths occurred in the run-in period, and 17 (1.4%) patients were excluded because of worsening HF [more problematic in severe HF patients (only 3% of this study population)].

53. Heart Failure Research Collaborative Group, **ANZ** (Australia/ New Zealand). Randomized, placebo-controlled trial of carvedilol in patients with congestive heart failure due to ischaemic heart disease. *Lancet* 1997;349:375–380.

Design: Prospective, randomized, double-blind, placebo-controlled, multicenter study. Average follow-up period was 19 months. Primary end point was changes in LVEF and treadmill exercise duration.

Purpose: To evaluate the longer-term effects on death and other serious clinical events of carvedilol in patients with chronic stable HF.

Population: 415 NYHA class II or III patients with chronic stable HF.

Exclusion Criteria: Current NYHA class IV; primary valvular disease; SBP less than 90 mm Hg or more than 160 mm Hg or DBP more than 100 mm Hg; and MI, unstable angina, bypass surgery, or coronary angioplasty in the prior 4 weeks.

Treatment: Twenty-seven patients were withdrawn during the 2- to 3-week open-label phase of carvedilol therapy (3.125 mg daily to 6.25 mg twice daily). Carvedilol was then given at 6.25 to 25 mg twice daily, or placebo.

Results: At 1 year, the carvedilol group had an increased EF (+5.3%; $p < 0.0001$) and decreased end-diastolic and end-systolic dimensions [−1.7 mm ($p = 0.06$) and −3.2 mm ($p = 0.001$)]. However, no differences were noted in exercise treadmill time, 6-minute walk distance, NYHA class, or specific activity score. At 19 months, no difference was seen in the number of HF episodes, but the carvedilol group had a lower incidence of death and hospitalization (50% vs. 63%; RR, 0.74; 95% CI, 0.57 to 0.95).

Comments: ANZ echocardiographic substudy of 123 patients (echocardiograms at baseline and 6 and 12 months) showed that the carvedilol group had a LV end-diastolic volume index 14 mL/m^2 lower than placebo ($p = 0.0015$), LV end-systolic volume index 15.3 mL/m^2 lower than placebo ($p = 0.0001$), and EF 5.8% higher ($p = 0.0015$) (see *J Am Coll Cardiol* 1997;29:1060).

54. **Packer M,** et al., for the Carvedilol Prospective Randomized Cumulative Survival Study **(COPERNICUS)** Group. Effect of carvedilol on survival in severe chronic heart failure. *N Engl J Med* 2001;344:1651–1658.

Design: Prospective, randomized, double-blind, placebo-controlled, multicenter study. Primary end point was changed in LVEF and treadmill exercise duration. Average follow-up period was 10 months.

Purpose: To evaluate the longer-term effects on death and other serious clinical events of carvedilol in patients with chronic stable HF.

Population: 2,289 NYHA class III or IV patients with chronic stable HF.

Exclusion Criteria: Included CHF due to uncorrected primary valvular disease or a reversible cardiomyopathy; eligibility for cardiac transplantation; contraindication to β-blocker therapy or use in the previous 2 months; coronary revascularization, acute myocardial or cerebral ischemic event in the previous 2 months; use of α-adrenergic blocker, calcium-channel blocker, or class I antiarrhythmic drug in the previous 4 weeks; SBP less than 85 mm Hg, creatinine more than 2.8 mg/dL.

Treatment: Patients received an initial dose of 3.125 mg of carvedilol or placebo twice daily for 2 weeks, which was then increased at 2-week intervals (if tolerated), first to 6.25 mg, then to 12.5 mg, and finally to a target dose of 25 mg twice daily.

Results: A 35% decrease was seen in the risk of death with carvedilol (95% CI, 19% to 48%; $p = 0.0014$). A 24% decrease in the combined risk of death or hospitalization with carvedilol was found ($p < 0.001$). Fewer patients in the carvedilol group than in the placebo group withdrew because of adverse effects or for other reasons ($p = 0.02$). A subsequent report showed that more patients felt improved and fewer patients felt worse in the carvedilol group than in the placebo group after 6 months of maintenance therapy ($p = 0.0009$; see *Circulation* 2002;106:2194).

Comments: Patients not included were those with far-advanced HF symptoms and those who could not reach compensation. A small proportion of black patients were included.

55. **Eichhorn E,** et al. A trial of the beta-blocker bucindolol in patients with advanced chronic heart failure (**BEST**). *N Engl J Med* 2001;344:1659–1667.

Design: Prospective, randomized, double-blind, placebo-controlled, multicenter trial. Primary end point was all-cause mortality. Average follow-up, 2.0 years.

Purpose: To evaluate the effect on survival of the β-blocker bucindolol in patients with advanced HF.

Population: 2,708 patients with NYHA III (92%) or IV (8%) heart failure and LVEF 35% or lower.

Exclusion Criteria: Included decompensated CHF, eligibility for heart transplantation, reversible causes of HF, uncorrected primary valvular disease, hypertrophic cardiomyopathy, MI within the previous 6 months, PCI or CABG within 60 days, calcium-channel–blocking or β-agonists within 1 week, β-blocking agents within 30 days, amiodarone within 8 weeks.

Treatment: Bucindolol, 3 to 100 mg orally, or placebo.

Results: Trial terminated after seventh interim analysis. Mortality rates were similar between the two groups [411 deaths (bucindolol) vs. 449 deaths; unadjusted $p = 0.16$]. The bucindolol group had a significantly lower incidence of CV death and heart transplantation or death.

Comments: The neutral results of this study are surprising and challenge the concept of a beneficial class effect with β-adrenergic blockade.

Other Studies

56. **Waagstein F,** et al., Metoprolol in Dilated Cardiomyopathy **(MDC).** Beneficial effects of metoprolol in idiopathic dilated cardiomyopathy (DCM). *Lancet* 1993;342:1441–1446.

Design: Prospective, randomized, double-blind, placebo-controlled, parallel-group, multicenter study. Follow-up period was 12 to 18 months. Primary end point was death and need for cardiac transplantation.

Purpose: To evaluate the effects of metoprolol versus placebo in patients with HF due to idiopathic DCM.

Population: 383 patients aged 16 to 75 years with LVEF less than 0.40; 94% were in NYHA functional class II or III.

Exclusion Criteria: Use of β-blockers or calcium-channel blockers, CAD (more than 50% stenosis), SBP less than 90 mm Hg, heart rate less than 45 beats/min, obstructive lung disease requiring β-agonists, and insulin-dependent diabetes.

Treatment: If the test dose was tolerated (metoprolol, 5 mg twice daily for 2 to 7 days), then patients were randomized to metoprolol [10 mg/day titrated up to 100 to 150 mg/day (mean, 108 mg/day)], or placebo.

Results: Metoprolol group had 34% risk reduction in death or need for heart transplantation (22.5% vs. 36.5%; $p = 0.058$). At follow-up, the metoprolol group had a significantly better improvement in LVEF ($+0.12$ vs. $+0.06$ at 12 months; $p < 0.0001$), increased exercise duration ($+76$ vs. $+15$ seconds at 12 months; $p = 0.046$), and showed a trend toward lower PCWP (-5 vs. -2 mm Hg; $p = 0.06$). The metoprolol group had better quality of life (based on patient assessment at 12 and 18 months; $p = 0.01$), and a significant correlation was found between the NYHA classification made by the physician and the quality-of-life assessment. A subsequent report showed that the metoprolol group had a significantly improved exercise oxygen consumption index ($p = 0.045$) (see *J Am Coll Cardiol* 1994;23:1397).

57. **Lechat P,** et al., Cardiac Insufficiency Bisoprolol Study **(CIBIS).** A randomized trial of β-blockade in heart failure. *Circulation* 1994;90:1765–1773.

Design: Prospective, randomized, double-blind, placebo-controlled, multicenter study. Mean follow-up period was 1.9 years. Primary end point was total mortality rate.

Purpose: To evaluate the effects of bisoprolol on all-cause mortality in HF patients.

Population: 641 patients aged 18 to 75 years with an EF less than 40%; 95% were NYHA class III and 5% class IV.

Exclusion Criteria: MI in the prior 3 months, planned bypass surgery, HF secondary to mitral or aortic valve disease, insulin-dependent diabetes, SBP less than 100 or more than 160 mm Hg, and resting heart rate, less than 65 beats/min.

Treatment: Bisoprolol, 1.25 to 5.0 mg/day, or placebo. All patients were taking diuretics and vasodilator therapy, and 90% were taking ACE inhibitors.

Results: Bisoprolol group had a nonsignificant 20% mortality reduction (16.6% vs. 20.8%; $p = 0.22$). Bisoprolol significantly improved the functional status of patients: fewer hospitalizations for cardiac decompensation (19% vs. 28%; $p < 0.01$) and more with an improvement of one NYHA class (21% vs. 15%; $p = 0.04$).

Comments: Study was underpowered and only half of the patients were titrated to the target dose. In the subgroup of patients with no history of MI, a clear survival benefit was noted ($p = 0.034$).

58. Cardiac Insufficiency Bisoprolol Study II **(CIBIS-II)** Investigators. The Cardiac Insufficiency Bisoprolol Study II (CIBIS II): A randomized trial. *Lancet* 1999;353: 9–12.

Design: Prospective, randomized, double-blind, placebo-controlled, multicenter study. Mean follow-up period was 1.3 years. Primary end point was all-cause mortality rate.

Purpose: To evaluate the efficacy of bisoprolol in decreasing all-cause mortality in patients with symptomatic chronic HF.

Population: 2,647 NYHA class III or IV patients with LVEF less than 35%.

Exclusion Criteria: Uncontrolled hypertension, MI, or unstable angina in the prior 3 months, PTCA or CABG in the prior 6 months, heart rate less than 60 beats/min, or preexisting or planned therapy with β-blockers.

Treatment: Bisoprolol, 1.25 to 10.0 mg/day, or placebo. All patients were taking diuretics and ACE inhibitors.

Results: Study was terminated because bisoprolol showed a significant mortality benefit: 11.8% versus 17.3% (hazard ratio, 0.66; $p < 0.0001$). The bisoprolol group also had a lower incidence of sudden death (3.6% vs. 6.3%; hazard ratio, 0.56; $p = 0.0011$) and 20% fewer hospital admissions; treatment effects were independent of severity or cause of HF.

Comments: No run-in period provided a better estimate of clinical effectiveness of bisoprolol. The low mortality rates suggest that not all patients were NYHA class III and IV patients.

59. **MERIT-HF** Study Group. Effect of metoprolol CR/XL in chronic heart failure: metoprolol CR/XL randomized intervention trial in congestive heart failure (MERIT-HF). *Lancet* 1999;353:2001–2007.

Design: Prospective, randomized, double-blind, placebo-controlled multicenter study. Mean follow-up period was 1 year. Primary end point was all-cause mortality.

Purpose: To evaluate whether metoprolol CR/XL, once daily, in addition to standard therapy, could lower mortality in symptomatic HF patients with impaired EF.

Population: 3,991 NYHA class II to IV (II, 41%; III, 55%) patients with an EF of 40% or less. Two thirds of patients that had an ischemic etiology of HF; 89% were taking an ACE inhibitor; 90% were taking a diuretic; and 63% were receiving digoxin.

Treatment: Metoprolol CR/XL, 12.5 mg (NYHA III or IV) or 25 mg (NYHA II) once daily; or placebo. Target dose was 200 mg/day with up-titration over an 8-week period. Randomization was preceded by a 2-week single-blind placebo run-in period.

Results: All-cause mortality was significantly lower in the metoprolol group (7.2% vs. 11.0%; RR, 0.66; $p < 0.001$). The metoprolol group also had a 38% reduction in CV mortality ($p < 0.001$), a 41% reduction in sudden death ($p < 0.001$), and a 49% reduction in death due to progressive HF ($p = 0.002$). The incidence of side effects was similar in both groups.

Amiodarone

60. **Doval HC,** et al., Grupo de Estudio de la Sobrevida en la Insuficiencia Cardiaca en Argentina **(GESICA).** Randomized trial of low-dose amiodarone in severe CHF. *Lancet* 1994;344:493–498.

Design: Prospective, randomized, open, parallel-group, multicenter study. Follow-up period was 2 years. Primary end point was total mortality.

Purpose: To evaluate the effect of low-dose amiodarone on mortality in patients with severe HF without symptomatic ventricular arrhythmias.

Population: 516 NYHA class II to IV patients with stable functional capacity and not requiring antiarrhythmic therapy.

Exclusion Criteria: Amiodarone treatment during the prior 3 months; MI, HF onset, or syncope in the prior 3 months; and history of sustained VT or VF.

Treatment: Amiodarone, 500 mg/day for 14 days, and then 300 mg once daily for 2 years; or standard therapy (diuretics, digoxin, ACE inhibitors).

Results: Amiodarone group had 28% RR in mortality at 2 years (33.5% vs. 41.4%; $p = 0.024$) and 31% RR in hospitalization due to worsening HF (45.8% vs. 58.2%; $p = 0.0024$). Reductions were seen in both sudden death (27% RR; $p = 0.16$) and death due to progressive HF (23% risk reduction; $p = 0.16$). These benefits were present in all examined subgroups and were independent of the presence of non-sustained VT. Side effects were reported in 17 (6.1%) amiodarone patients, of whom 12 discontinued therapy.

Comments: The study was blinded only to coordination center personnel, had a unique population (10% with Chagas disease), and was terminated at the two-thirds point.

61. **Singh SN,** et al., Survival Trial of Antiarrhythmic Therapy in CHF **(CHF-STAT).** Amiodarone in patients with congestive heart failure and asymptomatic ventricular arrhythmia. *N Engl J Med* 1995;333:77–82 (editorial, 121–122).

Design: Prospective, randomized, double-blind, placebo-controlled, multicenter study. Primary end point was overall mortality and sudden death from cardiac causes. Follow-up period was 45 months.

Purpose: To evaluate the effect of antiarrhythmic therapy on mortality in patients with CHF and asymptomatic ventricular arrhythmia.

Population: 674 patients with symptoms of CHF, cardiac enlargement, fewer than 10 premature ventricular contractions, and EF of 40% or less.

Exclusion Criteria: MI in the prior 3 months, history of cardiac arrest or sustained VT, need for antiarrhythmic therapy, and SBP less than 90 mm Hg.

Treatment: Amiodarone, 800 mg/day for 14 days, 400 mg/day for 50 weeks, and then 300 mg/day; or placebo. Other therapy consisted of vasodilators (all patients), with or without digoxin or diuretics.

Results: No significant differences were found in mortality or sudden death [30.6% (amiodarone) vs. 29.2%; 15% vs. 19%; $p = 0.43$]. However, amiodarone was associated with a trend toward lower mortality in the subgroup of patients with nonischemic cardiomyopathy ($p = 0.07$). The amiodarone group also had better suppression of ventricular arrhythmias and a greater increase in EF at 2 years (+10.5% vs. +4.1%).

Comments: This VA-based trial had notable differences compared with GESICA: older patients (+6 years), more men (GESICA, 48% lower mortality in females vs. 26% in men), and healthier patients with higher EFs. However, subgroup analysis showed that the greatest benefits in CHF-STAT occurred in NYHA class II patients.

Inotropic and Other Agents

62. **Dibianco,** et al. A comparison of oral milrinone, digoxin and their combination in the treatment of patients with chronic heart failure. *N Engl J Med* 1989;320:677–683.

This prospective, randomized trial was composed of 230 patients comparing 12 weeks of digoxin, milrinone, and their combination. Both agents alone improved exercise tolerance (+64 vs. +82 seconds) and lowered frequency of decompensation [15% and 34% vs. 47% (placebo)]. Overall, no significant difference was found between the effects of the two drugs. Milrinone and digoxin were no better than digoxin alone.

63. **Packer M,** et al., Prospective Randomized Milrinone Survival Evaluation **(PROMISE).** Effect of oral milrinone on mortality in severe chronic heart failure. *N Engl J Med* 1991;325:1468–1475.

Design: Prospective, randomized, double-blind, placebo-controlled, multicenter study. Mean follow-up period was 6.1 months. Primary end point was all-cause mortality.

Purpose: To evaluate the effect of oral administration of the phosphodiesterase milrinone on mortality in patients with severe CHF.

Population: 1,088 NYHA class III or IV patients and EF less than 35%.

Exclusion Criteria: Obstructive valvular disease; history of serious ventricular arrhythmia; MI in prior 3 months; SBP less than 85 mm Hg; and requirement for β-blockers, calcium-channel blockers, and antiarrhythmic drugs.

Treatment: Milrinone, 40 mg/day orally, or placebo. All patients were on digoxin, diuretics, and ACE inhibitors.

Results: Study was terminated early. Milrinone was associated with significantly higher all-cause mortality (30% vs. 24%; $p = 0.038$) and CV mortality rates (29.4% vs. 22.6%; $p = 0.016$). The milrinone group had a 69% increased risk of sudden cardiac deaths ($p = 0.005$), whereas no increased risk of death was found because of progressive HF. Adverse effects were worst among class IV patients (53% higher mortality; $p = 0.006$).

64. **Feldman AM,** et al. Effects of vesnarinone on morbidity and mortality in patients with heart failure. *N Engl J Med* 1993;329:149–155.

This prospective study randomized 477 patients to vesnarinone, 60 mg/day, or placebo. The vesnarinone group had 48% lower mortality at 6 months. However, the drug demonstrated a narrow therapeutic range, with a higher mortality rate associated with 120 mg/day. Neutropenia was seen in 2.5% of patients taking vesnarinone.

65. **Hampton JR,** et al. Prospective Randomised Study of Ibopamine on Mortality and Efficacy **(PRIME II).** Randomised study of effect of ibopamine on survival in patients with advanced severe HF. *Lancet* 1997;349:971–977.

This prospective, randomized, multicenter trial was composed of 1,906 NYHA II to IV patients. The average follow-up period was 1 year. The trial was terminated early because the ibopamine group had increased mortality (25% vs. 20%; $p = 0.017$). In multivariate analysis, antiarrhythmic use was associated with increased mortality in ibopamine patients.

66. **Califf RM,** et al., Flolan International Randomized Survival Trial **(FIRST).** A randomized controlled trial of epoprostenol therapy. *Am Heart J* 1997;134:44–54.

This prospective, randomized trial was composed of 471 patients with an EF less than 25% (less than 30% if taking inotropes); NYHA class IIIB or IV symptoms for 1 month with digoxin, diuretic, and ACE inhibitor; cardiac index, 2.2 mL/kg/m^2 or less; and PCWP, 15 mm Hg. Patients were randomized to epoprostenol (initial dose, 2 ng/kg/min; median, 4.0) or standard care. The epoprostenol group had an increased cardiac index (1.81 to 2.61) and decreased PCWP (24.5 to 20.0 mm Hg), but showed a trend toward increased mortality ($p = 0.055$), prompting early termination of the trial.

67. **Cohn JN,** et al., for the Vesnarinone Trial Investigators. A dose-dependent increase in mortality with vesnarinone among patients with severe heart failure. *N Engl J Med* 1998;339:1801–1806.

This prospective, randomized, double-blind, placebo-controlled, multicenter study enrolled 3,833 patients with NYHA class III or IV heart failure and an LVEF 30% or less despite optimal treatment (any regimen of diuretics, vasodilators, ACE inhibitor, and digitalis). Patients received vesnarinone (30 or 60 mg) or placebo once daily. At follow-up (mean, 286 days), the placebo group had significantly fewer deaths than the 60-mg vesnarinone group (18.9% vs. 22.9%; $p = 0.02$). Increased mortality with vesnarinone was mostly owing to increased sudden death rate (12.3% vs. 9.1%). Quality of life (assessed by Minnesota Living with Heart Failure Questionnaire) improved significantly more in the 60-mg vesnarinone group than in the placebo group at 8 weeks ($p < 0.001$) and 16 weeks ($p = 0.003$), but by 26 weeks, the differences were no longer significant. Agranulocytosis occurred in 1.2% and 0.2% of those given vesnarinone, 60 mg/day and 30 mg/day, respectively.

68. **Packer M,** et al. Comparison of ompatrilat and enalapril in patients with chronic heart failure: the Ompatrilat Versus Enalapril Randomized Trial of Utility in Reducing Events **(OVERTURE).** *Circulation* 2002;106:920–926.

Design: Prospective, randomized, placebo-controlled, blinded, parallel-group, multicenter trial. Primary end point was all-cause mortality or hospitalization for HF. Average follow-up, 15 months.

Purpose: To prove superiority or noninferiority of the vasopeptidase inhibitor ompatrilat compared to enalapril in patients with CHF.

Population: 5,770 patients with NYHA class II to IV CHF for more than 2 months due to ischemic or nonischemic heart disease, EF less than 30%, hospitalized for HF in the past year, and receiving diuretics at the time of enrollment.

Exclusion Criteria: Included reversible cause(s) of HF, no HF admission in the previous 48 hours, probable cardiac transplant or LVAD candidate, acute coronary syndrome in the previous month, coronary revascularization or an acute cerebral ischemic event in the previous 3 months, and history of VT, VF, or sudden death (unless ICD had been placed and had not fired in the previous 2 months).

Treatment: Ompatrilat, 40 mg/day, or enalapril, 20 mg/day.

Results: A nonsignificant trend was found toward a lower incidence of death or hospitalization for CHF in the ompatrilat group compared with the enalapril group (32% vs. 34%; $p = 0.19$). All-cause mortality rates were not significantly different (17% vs. 18%). The trend was strong enough to show that ompatrilat was not inferior to enalapril.

69. **Cuffe MS,** et al., for The Outcomes of a Prospective Trial of Intravenous Milrinone for Exacerbations of Chronic Heart Failure **(OPTIME-CHF)** Investigators. Short-term intravenous milrinone for acute exacerbation of chronic heart failure: a randomized controlled trial. *JAMA* 2002;287:1541–1547.

This trial randomized 951 patients with exacerbation of chronic HF not requiring intravenous inotropic support to 48 hours of milrinone or placebo. A total of the median number of days hospitalized for CV causes within 60 days after randomization did not differ significantly between patients given milrinone (6 days) compared with placebo (7 days; $p = 0.71$). Sustained hypotension requiring intervention (10.7% vs. 3.2%; $p < 0.001$) and new atrial arrhythmias (4.6% vs. 1.5%; $p = 0.004$) occurred more frequently in patients who received milrinone. The milrinone and placebo groups did not differ significantly in in-hospital mortality (3.8% vs. 2.3%; $p = 0.19$) or 60-day mortality (10.3% vs. 8.9%).

Mechanical Assist Devices and Surgical Options

70. **Oz MC,** et al. Screening scale predicts patients successfully receiving long-term implantable left ventricular assist devices. *Circulation* 1995;92(suppl II):II-169–173.

A risk-factor selection scale (range, 0 to 10) was developed based on an analysis of easily obtainable preoperative risk factors in 56 patients undergoing LVAD insertion. Points were assigned as follows: urine output less than 30 mL/hr (weight, 3); central venous pressure more than 16 mm Hg (weight, 2); mechanical ventilation (weight, 2); prothrombin time more than 16 seconds (weight, 2); and reoperation (weight, 1). The mortality rate among those with a score of 5 was 67%. The average score of nonsurvivors was 5.43 versus 2.45 among survivors ($p < 0.0001$).

71. **Bolling SF,** et al. Intermediate-term outcome of mitral construction in cardiomyopathy. *J Thorac Cardiovasc Surg* 1998;115:381–386.

The 48 NYHA class III or IV patients with severe DCM and 4+ mitral regurgitation underwent surgery; all had annuloplasty rings inserted, seven had CABGs for incidental disease, and 11 had tricuspid valve repair. Postoperative transesophageal echocardiography (TEE) showed no mitral regurgitation in 41 patients and mild mitral regurgitation in seven patients. One- and 2-year actuarial survival rates were 82% and 71%. At a median follow-up of 22 months, NYHA class had improved significantly from 3.9 to 2.0.

72. **Hunt SA,** et al. Mechanical circulatory support and cardiac transplantation. *Circulation* 1998;97:2079–2090.

This review article discusses several mechanical circulatory support devices and the complications associated with their use. The transplantation section discusses recipient selection and survival rates and provides a brief overview of immunosuppression and rejection surveillance.

73. **Mancini D,** et al. Comparison of exercise performance in patients with chronic severe heart failure versus left ventricular assist devices. *Circulation* 1998;98:1178–1183.

Metabolic exercise testing was performed in 65 CHF and 20 LVAD patients. Peak oxygen consumption was significantly higher in the LVAD group (15.9 vs. 12.0 mL/kg/min; $p < 0.001$). At peak exercise, the LVAD group also had a significantly higher HR, BP, and cardiac output, whereas PCWP was lower (14 vs. 31 mm Hg; $p < 0.001$). LVAD patients also had better hemodynamic measurements at rest, including higher cardiac output and lower PCWP.

74. **Mancini DM,** et al. Low incidence of myocardial recovery after left ventricular assist device implantation in patients with chronic heart failure. *Circulation* 1998;98:2383–2389.

A retrospective chart review of 111 LVAD recipients identified only five successfully explanted patients. A prospective attempt to identify explantable patients by using exercise testing was then undertaken on 39 consecutive patients, of whom 15 were able to exercise with maximal device support. Peak average oxygen consumption was 14.5 mL/kg/min, and Fick cardiac output, 11.4 L/min. Seven patients remained normotensive while exercising at 20 cycles/min, and their peak oxygen consumption decreased from 17.3 to 13.0 mL/kg/min. In one of these patients, the LVAD was successfully explanted.

75. **Rose EA,** et al. Randomized Evaluation of Mechanical Assistance for the Treatment of Congestive Heart Failure final results: **(REMATCH)** Study Group. *N Engl J Med* 2001;345:1435–1443.

Design: Prospective, randomized, multicenter trial. Primary end point was all-cause mortality or hospitalization for HF. Average follow-up, 14.5 months.
Purpose: To prove superiority of the implantable LVAD compared with standard therapy in patients with end-stage CHF.
Population: 129 patients with end-stage CHF who were ineligible for cardiac transplantation.
Exclusion Criteria: Included eligibility for cardiac transplantation, absence of symptoms of NYHA class IV symptoms in the previous 90 days, EF 25% or less, or a peak oxygen consumption of more than 14 mL/kg/min.
Treatment: A vented electric LVAD or optimal medical therapy. Patients could continue β-blockers if they had been administered for at least 60 of the 90 days before randomization.
Results: The LVAD group had a 48% reduction in mortality compared with the medical-therapy group ($p = 0.001$). At 1 year, survival rates were 52% in the LVAD group and 25% in the medical-therapy group ($p = 0.002$), whereas the rates at 2 years were 23% and 8% ($p = 0.09$), respectively. The frequency of serious adverse events in the LVAD was 2.35 times that in the medical-therapy group (95% CI, 1.86 to 2.95), with a predominance of infection, bleeding, and malfunction of the device. The quality of life was significantly improved at 1 year in the LVAD group.
Comment: Because fewer than 25% of LVAD patients were alive at 2 years, these results may not be of sufficient magnitude to convince the medical community and insurance companies that this technology (or at least this particular device) can be considered a good alternative to transplantation.

Exercise/Training

76. **Hambrecht R,** et al. Physical training in patients with stable chronic heart failure: effects of cardiorespiratory fitness and ultrastructural abnormalities of leg muscles. *J Am Coll Cardiol* 1995;25:1239–1249.

This small study showed the benefits of exercise and described accompanying physiologic changes. Twenty-two patients were randomized to training or inactivity. Average EF was 26%. At 6 months, trained patients had a 31% increase in oxygen uptake, a 19% increase in volume density of mitochondria, and a 41% increase in volume density of cytochrome-*c* oxidase–positive mitochondria (i.e., training delays anaerobic metabolism).

77. **Keteyiajn SJ,** et al. Exercise training in patients with heart failure. *Ann Intern Med* 1996;124:1051–1057.

This small randomized controlled trial was composed of 40 men with an EF of 35% or less. The treatment regimen was composed of three sets of three exercises, each performed for 11 minutes (target heart rate, 60% maximum) for 2 weeks, and then up to 80% as tolerated. At 24 weeks, the exercise group had increased exercise duration (+2.8 minutes), 16% higher peak oxygen consumption, and increased power output (+20 watts).

78. **Wilson JR,** et al. Circulatory status and response to cardiac rehabilitation in patients with heart failure. *Circulation* 1996;94:1567–1572.

This study showed that only some patients respond well to exercise and offered insights into the pathophysiology of nonresponders. Thirty-two patients underwent maximal exercise treadmill testing and then rehabilitation for 3 months. Twenty-one had a normal cardiac-output response to exercise, of whom 43% responded to the rehabilitation regimen (more than 10% increase in peak oxygen consumption and anaerobic threshold). Of the other 11 patients, three stopped rehabilitation (because of exhaustion), and one responded (9%; $p < 0.04$). The former group was likely limited by deconditioning, whereas the latter group was impaired by circulatory failures.

79. **Hambrecht R,** et al. Regular physical exercise corrects endothelial dysfunction and improves exercise capacity in patients with chronic heart failure. *Circulation* 1998;98:2709–2715.

This small prospective randomized study of 20 patients showed that exercise training resulted in increased peak oxygen uptake (+26% at 6 weeks; $p < 0.01$). This increase correlated with endothelium-dependent changes in peripheral blood flow ($r = 0.64$; $p < 0.005$), suggesting that improved endothelial function contributes modestly to increased exercise capacity.

Complications

80. **Middlekauff HR,** et al. Prognostic significance of atrial fibrillation in advanced heart failure: a study of 390 patients. *Circulation* 1991;84:40–48.

This retrospective analysis focused on 390 consecutive NYHA class III or IV patients with a mean EF of 19%. Actuarial survival and sudden death–free survival was significantly worse in the atrial fibrillation patients compared with those in normal sinus rhythm (52% vs. 71%; 69% vs. 82%, both $p = 0.0013$).

81. **Middlekauff HR,** et al. Syncope in advanced heart failure: high sudden death regardless of etiology. *J Am Coll Cardiol* 1993;21:110–116.

This retrospective analysis focused on 491 NYHA class III or IV HF patients with no history of cardiac arrest and a mean EF of 20%. Sixty (12%) patients had a history of syncope. At follow-up (mean, 1 year), sudden death had occurred in 14%, and 13% had died of progressive HF. The 1-year actuarial incidence of sudden death was more than threefold higher in patients with a history of syncope than in those without syncope (45% vs. 12%; $p < 0.00001$). The incidence of sudden death was similar in patients with either cardiac syncope or syncope from other causes (49% vs. 39%; $p = $ NS).

82. **Natterson PD,** et al. Risk of arterial embolization in 224 patients awaiting cardiac transplantation. *Am Heart J* 1995;129:564–570.

This analysis focused on 224 consecutive outpatients awaiting cardiac transplantation. Mean EF was 20%, and mean LV end-diastolic diameter was 7.6 cm. During follow-up (301 ± 371 days), arterial embolization only occurred in six (2.7%) patients. The risk of embolization was not significantly different between patients taking warfarin, those with LV thrombus on transthoracic echocardiography, or those with a history of embolization.

6. ARRYTHMIAS

EPIDEMIOLOGY

Atrial fibrillation (AF) is the most common sustained arrhythmia in the United States population (lifetime risk, approximately 7%) and leads to more hospitalizations than does any other arrhythmia. AF prevalence is highest in those with clinical cardiovascular disease and occurs most commonly among older age groups. The average age at onset is 70 to 74 years (age 65 years for lone AF); as with other cardiac illnesses, women tend to be first seen at an older age than do men. AF is causally related to a substantial proportion of ischemic strokes, and AF patients appear to have higher adjusted mortality rates than do those without AF. Atrial flutter, a related but more organized rhythm, also is associated with a modestly higher stroke risk than that for individuals in normal sinus rhythm (SR) (5,7). The current consensus is that atrial flutter should be treated the same as AF, in terms of thromboembolic risk and prophylaxis.

NATURAL HISTORY

The clinical course of AF is heterogeneous: some patients have only self-terminating paroxysms that occur with variable frequency, whereas others always require intervention to terminate episodes. Spontaneous conversion rates are variable (less than 15% to as high as 78%) and depend on the population studied. Higher rates of spontaneous conversion are associated with shorter AF duration (less than 12 hours), younger age, and lack of associated heart disease. In general, patients who are older, have more structural heart disease, and have a longer history of symptoms tend to progress toward more persistent and chronic AF, sometimes despite aggressive management. Among patients with persistent (non–self-terminating) AF, normal SR can be restored in most, but 50% or more will have recurrences within 1 year.

ETIOLOGIES AND RISK FACTORS

Many new cases of AF do not have a single clear etiology. From 3% to 11% of AF patients have structurally normal hearts (see *JAMA* 1985;254:3449 and *N Engl J Med* 1987;317:669). Conversely, new-onset AF often occurs in the setting of acute cardiac or noncardiac illness. Common examples include pneumonia, pulmonary embolism, and other acute pulmonary conditions; sepsis; acute myocardial infarction (MI); and major surgery. In these cases, treatment of the underlying illness is of primary importance. Cardiac surgery is associated with a distinctly high risk of postoperative AF, which occurs in 30% to 40% of patients undergoing coronary artery bypass graft (CABG; see *Circulation* 1996;94:390–397) or valve surgery. Other acute precipitants of AF include alcohol intoxication ("holiday heart syndrome"), pericarditis, myocarditis, and thyroid disease. AF also may be triggered by other primary arrhythmias that are curable by radiofrequency catheter ablation.

A variety of chronic cardiac conditions are associated with the development of AF; most common among these are hypertension and congestive heart failure (CHF). In a multivariable model based on subjects followed up for 38 years in the Framingham Heart Study (see *JAMA* 1994;271:840–844), odds ratios (ORs) for the development of AF were highest for CHF (men, 4.5; women, 5.9), and also were significant for valve disease (1.8, 3.4), hypertension (1.5, 1.4) and diabetes mellitus (1.4, 1.6). Prior MI was an independent risk factor for men (OR, 1.4) but not women. Rheumatic heart disease has a strong association with AF, but because of its declining prevalence in developed nations, the valvular lesion now most frequently associated with AF is mitral regurgitation. Other cardiopulmonary conditions associated with AF include hypertrophic, dilated, and restrictive cardiomyopathies; atrial septal defect and other congenital abnormalities; and the sleep-apnea syndrome. In addition, many older patients with AF have concomitant sinus node dysfunction, known as the tachycardia-bradycardia syndrome. In those patients, both arrhythmias appear related to underlying degeneration of normal atrial tissue.

The following is a list of causes of AF classified by prevalence:

Major causes: Hypertension, CHF, ischemic heart disease, postcardiac surgery
Common causes: Alcohol intoxication, pulmonary disease, valvular heart disease, rheumatic heart disease, cardiomyopathy, thyrotoxicosis
Uncommon to rare causes: Pericarditis, infiltrative disease, atrial myxoma, autonomic dysfunction, ventricular/atrial septal defect, pulmonary embolism

STROKE RISK FACTORS

Data from the Framingham Heart Study initially documented the roughly fivefold increased incidence of stroke among AF patients compared with age, sex, and hypertensive matched contemporaries without AF, and highlighted the remarkably high rates of stroke in patients with AF due to rheumatic heart disease (relative risk, 17.6; also see *Neurology* 1978;28:973). Predictors of stroke were further evaluated in a meta-analysis of pooled control-group patients from five major anticoagulation trials (3). Among clinical variables, independent risk factors for stroke (with associated ORs) included previous stroke or transient ischemic attack (TIA) (2.5), hypertension (1.6), CHF (1.4), age (1.4 per decade), and diabetes mellitus (1.7). One of the trials also assessed echocardiographic variables and found impaired left ventricular (LV) systolic function and increased left atrial size to be significant predictors, independent of clinical variables (see *Ann Intern Med* 1992;116:6). In patients with nonvalvular AF, transesophageal echocardiography (TEE) has identified additional markers of stroke risk, including the presence of thrombus, spontaneous echo contrast or reduced flow velocity in the left atrial appendage, and complex atherosclerotic plaque in the aorta (see *J Am Coll Cardiol* 1998;31:1622).

TREATMENT

The American College of Cardiology (ACC), American Heart Association (AHA), and European Society of Cardiology (ESC) recently published comprehensive guidelines on the management of AF (1). The following will briefly cover key aspects of management; the reader is referred to the guidelines for a more detailed review of these topics.

Atrial Fibrillation Prevention after Cardiac Surgery

Postoperative AF is especially common after cardiac operations, occurring in approximately 25% of patients. Postoperative AF occurs most frequently on postoperative days 2 to 3. Several studies have shown that its occurrence is associated with higher morbidity. Among cardiac surgery patients, one study found that postoperative AF was associated with increased mortality at 1 month and 6 months (see *Ann Surg* 1997;226:501). Postoperative AF also results in an extended length of hospital stay.

The use of β-blockers after surgery has been consistently shown to reduce the incidence of AF and has become standard practice (8; also see *Am J Cardiol* 1992;69:963). In one meta-analysis of 24 randomized studies, β-blocker therapy reduced post-CABG AF by 77% (8). Preoperative initiation of β-blockers also was found to be more effective than postoperative initiation.

Several randomized, controlled studies have evaluated the prophylactic use of intravenous (i.v.) or oral amiodarone (9; also see *J Am Coll Cardiol* 1999;34:343). Although amiodarone typically reduced the incidence of in-hospital AF, these reductions translated into a significantly shorter hospital stay in only one trial, when oral amiodarone was started 7 days preoperatively (9). Only one randomized study has compared amiodarone with a β-blocker (propranolol; see *Am Heart J* 2001;142:811). Amiodarone was associated with a lower incidence of postoperative AF, but no difference in length of hospital stay was found. Amiodarone has pulmonary toxicity, and an increased incidence of bradyarrhythmias has been seen in those receiving β-blocker therapy; therefore β-blockers remain first-line therapy for AF prophylaxis, whereas amiodarone should be considered in those who cannot take β-blockers and who are at high risk (i.e., history of AF, age older than 75 years, valve operations). Other trials have evaluated agents such as oral sotalol (no advantage over other β-blockers with increased risk of torsades de pointes; see *J Am Coll Cardiol* 1999;34:334), procainamide (not effective), and verapamil (not effective).

Two randomized studies have compared single-site with dual-site atrial pacing for prevention of postoperative AF (see Cardiac Pacing section later). Atrial overdrive pacing was superior to no pacing for AF prevention in both trials, but the studies were discrepant regarding which site of pacing is better and whether this approach reduced hospital length of stay.

Rate versus Rhythm Control

Some patients are unstable or severely symptomatic with AF due to hypotension, CHF, and/or angina. In such cases, cardioversion must be performed promptly, and in some occasions as an emergency. Often, however, the symptoms due to AF can be eliminated or at least minimized by controlling the rate of ventricular response. When AF becomes persistent, practitioners and patients then face a choice between rate control and rhythm control as alternative long-term strategies. Beyond the elimination of AF-related symptoms, advocates of rhythm control have hypothesized (if not assumed) that maintenance of SR will reduce the rates of stroke and potentially death, compared with a rate-control approach. These hypotheses have recently been tested in the North American AFFIRM and European RACE randomized trials (10,11). In both trials, rhythm control failed to lower the incidence of stroke or death, although questions remain regarding how optimally patients in the rhythm-control arms were treated. Clearly, symptoms will continue to drive many patients and their physicians to pursue rhythm-control measures, but these trials suggest that the simple approach of rate control and anticoagulation is acceptable for the majority of patients.

Pharmacologic Agents for Control of the Ventricular Rate

1. β-Blockers: metoprolol, 5 to 15 mg i.v.; esmolol, 500 μg/kg over a 1-minute period, and then 50 mg/min. β-Blockers should not be used in patients with severe bronchospasm and should be used with caution in the presence of severe LV dysfunction. Commonly used oral β-blockers include metoprolol and atenolol, 25 to 100 mg daily.
2. Calcium-channel blockers: diltiazem (half-life, 1 to 2 hours), 15 to 20 mg i.v. over a 2-minute period, and then 5 to 15 mg/hr; verapamil (half-life, less than 30 minutes), 2.5 to 10 mg i.v. over a 2-minute period or 40 to 120 mg orally every 8 hours.
3. Digoxin (0.5 mg i.v., and then 0.25 mg i.v. every 4 hours for two to four doses, and then 0.125 to 0.375 mg orally once daily). Digoxin is most effective for chronic AF, not paroxysmal AF. It takes hours to achieve effect and works poorly if high sympathetic tone is present. It should not be used in patients with LV diastolic dysfunction.

Pharmacologic Agents for the Acute Conversion of Atrial Fibrillation

Antiarrhythmic drugs have complex pharmacologic and physiologic actions, and all carry some potential for side effects, noncardiac toxicity, and proarrhythmia, that is, the induction of potentially dangerous rhythms other than the one being treated. These risks are modified by a number of factors, including renal function, gender, LV systolic function, LV hypertrophy, and the presence of coronary disease and prior infarction. Understanding of these risks is essential to maximize the therapeutic index of any treatment decision.

Intravenous Agents
1. Amiodarone (150 mg i.v. over a 10-minute period *or* 5 to 7 mg/kg over a 30-60 minute period, followed by 1.2 to 1.8 g per day continuously or in divided oral doses). Adverse effects may include hypotension, sinus bradycardia, phlebitis, and rarely,

torsades de pointes. Considered modestly effective for conversion of recent-onset AF (15) and of limited efficacy for AF of longer than 7 days duration.

2. Ibutilide (1 to 2 mg i.v. over a 10-minute period; can repeat once). Initial studies of this class III agent showed high conversion rates, but an approximate 2% risk of sustained polymorphic ventricular tachycardia (VT; highest incidence in women) [(16); see also *Am Heart J* 1998;136:642]. Ibutilide is slightly more effective at converting atrial flutter than AF.

3. Procainamide (loading dose of 15 to 17 mg/kg at 20 mg/min, and then 2 to 6 mg/min i.v.). Hypotension occurs in 10% to 15% of patients, and QT prolongation and torsades de pointes are known risks. Despite its long track record, procainamide was classified as a IIb recommendation for acute conversion in the AHA/ACC/ESC guidelines because of limited data on safety and efficacy (1).

4. Intravenous versions of flecainide and propafenone are available outside but not within the United States. Both are considered class I recommendations for conversion of AF 7 days or less in duration, and a class IIb recommendation for conversion of AF of more than 7 days in duration. Intravenous sotalol also is available outside the United States, but is not recommended for acute conversion of AF.

Oral Agents

1. Amiodarone (600 to 1,200 mg daily in divided doses for 10 to 14 days, and then 200 to 400 mg orally once daily). Because of its large volume of distribution, oral amiodarone is slower to take effect than other agents when used for acute conversion, but has a very low incidence of proarrhythmia and is considered effective in enhancing conversion by DC shock and preventing immediate recurrence of AF (IRAF) after cardioversion.

2. Flecainide [200 to 300 mg orally (p.o.)]: a single oral loading dose of flecainide has been shown to be more effective than placebo at converting AF of less than 7 days duration (see *Am J Cardiol* 1992;70:69–72). Transient hypotension, QRS widening, and conversion to atrial flutter with rapid ventricular response have occurred. This agent is contraindicated in patients with ischemia or LV dysfunction.

3. Propafenone (450 to 600 mg p.o.): a meta-analysis of oral propafenone loading— usually 600 mg given in a single dose—for recent-onset AF estimated success rates between 56% and 83%, depending on the duration of AF and the duration of follow-up after drug administration (see *J Am Coll Cardiol* 2001;37:542). These rates are superior to those of placebo, oral amiodarone, and oral quinidine, and comparable to those of oral flecainide. As with flecainide, transient arrhythmias around the time of cardioversion can occur, and the drug should be avoided in patients with impaired LV function or coronary disease.

4. Quinidine (0.75 to 1.5 g in divided doses over a 6- to 12-hour period). Considered moderately effective. Can cause QT prolongation and torsades de pointes. Its vagolytic properties can increase the ventricular response; thus coadministration of a rate-controlling agent is recommended (12).

5. Dofetilide (125 to 500 μg p.o., b.i.d.): short-term conversion rates of 10% to 30% for this newer class III agent are significantly better than those of placebo (17,18). QT prolongation and torsades de pointes can occur, and have led to requirements for inpatient drug initiation. Unlike that of most other agents, however, the safety of dofetilide has been established in patients with LV dysfunction and coronary disease.

6. Other: sotalol, digoxin, calcium-channel blockers, and disopyramide either have not been adequately studied or appear ineffective for the acute conversion of AF (14).

Pharmacologic Agents for Long-term Maintenance of Sinus Rhythm

With exceptions, the same oral agents reviewed earlier for immediate conversion also are used for maintenance of SR. Because of findings of increased mortality in specific clinical trials (CAST, SWORD), the class IA and IC drugs are generally recommended only for patients without structural heart disease. Brief additional comments follow.

1. Amiodarone (200 mg/day). In addition to its well-documented safety in the presence of coronary artery disease (CAD) and LV dysfunction, amiodarone appears to be the most effective agent for long-term maintenance of SR. Its superiority to alternative antiarrhythmic drugs in terms of efficacy has been shown in nonrandomized (13) and randomized trials (19), but the potential for noncardiac toxicity (liver, lung, thyroid) and other side effects (neurologic, skin discoloration) requires consideration, particularly in younger patients.
2. Dofetilide (125 to 500 μg p.o., b.i.d.). Dofetilide is the only antiarrhythmic drug other than amiodarone with good safety data in CHF and CAD (17,18). It is more effective than placebo in conversion of AF, maintenance of SR, and prevention of new AF in such patients. Dofetilide should be avoided in patients with renal impairment and has a number of important drug-to-drug interactions.
3. Sotalol (80 to 160 mg p.o., b.i.d.). For maintenance of SR, sotalol is better than placebo (see *Am J Cardiol* 1999;84:270) and probably similar in efficacy to quinidine and possibly propafenone. It has clinically relevant β-blocking as well as type III effects. Sotalol is renally excreted and prolongs the QT interval. It is not recommended for use in HF or in patients with marked LV hypertrophy.
4. Flecainide (100 to 150 mg p.o., b.i.d.). Flecainide is better than placebo for maintenance of SR, and also was superior to long-acting quinidine in one randomized trial (see *Am J Cardiol* 1989;64:1317). Its use should be targeted to patients with no structural heart disease.
5. Propafenone (150 to 300 mg p.o., b.i.d. to t.i.d.). Propafenone is probably similar in efficacy to flecainide, and carries the same adverse effects and warnings (see *Circulation* 1995;92:2550).
6. Class IA agents (disopyramide, quinidine, procainamide). As a group, the IA agents have less data supporting their efficacy than do either the IC or class III agents, although quinidine has been studied more than the others (12). Each of these agents is associated with QT prolongation and potentially important noncardiac adverse effects. Their use for maintenance of SR has been steadily declining, relative to other agents.

Electrical Cardioversion

Electrical cardioversion is favored for immediate management of unstable patients, and appears to have greater efficacy (in the 70% to 90% range) than drugs for the elective conversion of AF of short- to medium-term duration, although recurrence soon or late after cardioversion is common and often requires avoidance of certain drugs. Aside from minor skin irritation, adverse events are relatively rare and may include the unmasking of significant sinus bradycardia. The most significant potential risk related to cardioversion is thromboembolism, and specific guidelines regarding pericardioversion anticoagulation exist and are reviewed later.

Type and Amount of Energy
Although traditional teaching dictates starting cardioversion attempts at low energies (50 to 100 J), a recent randomized study using monophasic waveform devices found a significantly higher success rate at higher energies (see *Am J Cardiol* 2000;86:348). Success rates were 14%, 39%, and 95%, respectively, with initial energies of 100 J, 200 J, and 360 J. Patients treated with higher initial energies received fewer shocks and lower cumulative energy, and no patients had detectable myocardial injury by troponin testing. Recently, external defibrillators with biphasic waveforms have been introduced into clinical practice. These defibrillators, compared with older monophasic devices, achieve greater success at relatively lower energies (21) and have been used successfully in patients for whom previous attempts with monophasic defibrillators failed (see *Am J Cardiol* 2002;90:331).

Anticoagulation Before and After Cardioversion
Cardioversion, whether electrical or pharmacologic, is associated with a transient increase above the already elevated baseline risk of thromboembolism in AF, related

in part to the delayed recovery of atrial mechanical function. For that reason, specific recommendations regarding pericardioversion anticoagulation have been developed. The following summarizes the class I recommendations for antithrombotic therapy in patients undergoing cardioversion (see AHA/ACC/ESC Guidelines for further details):

a. Patients with AF less than 48 hours in duration may be cardioverted without prior anticoagulation. This empiric time point is not supported by prospective data, but retrospective data suggest that embolic complications with this approach are rare (see *Am J Cardiol* 1997;126:615 and *J Am Coll Cardiol* 2002;40:934).

b. Patients with AF hemodynamically unstable AF of recent onset should be cardioverted as an emergency without preceding anticoagulation, but should be given heparin concurrently if possible, and treated afterward with warfarin [international normalized ratio (INR), 2 to 3] for 3 to 4 weeks.

c. Patients with AF of longer than 48 hours or unknown duration should be given anticoagulation with warfarin (target INR, 2 to 3) for at least 3 to 4 weeks before and after cardioversion.

d. Documenting the absence of thrombus in the left atrial appendage by TEE is an acceptable alternative to the 3 to 4 weeks of anticoagulation preceding cardioversion. The safety of this approach has been established through both nonrandomized and randomized studies (20–22).

The potential role of low-molecular-weight heparin compounds as a substitute for i.v. heparin or warfarin around the time of cardioversion is under investigation. One randomized study recently reported preliminary data suggesting the noninferiority of enoxaparin for this indication (34), but this is difficult to prove, given the generally low rate of embolic events during this short time.

Long-term Anticoagulation

In meta-analyses of AF studies (3,25), anticoagulation with warfarin reduced stroke risk by 50% to 68% versus placebo, compared with approximately 25% to 35% reduction with aspirin. No difference in stroke rate was found between paroxysmal AF and chronic AF. When anticoagulation is used, a target INR of 2.0 to 3.0 should be targeted (25–35), as the SPAF III trial (34) showed an increased rate of ischemic stroke and embolic complications with lower INR (**Table 6.1**).

Recommendations for long-term anticoagulation are listed as follows:

1. If the patient has lone AF (i.e., no stroke risk factors) and is younger than 65 years, aspirin alone is considered by most experts to be adequate, as the baseline stroke risk of this cohort is low (approximately 0.5%/year) (2).

2. If the patient is older than 75 years or younger than 75 years with risk factors (e.g., history of stroke or TIA, hypertension, CHF, diabetes mellitus), anticoagulation with warfarin is recommended (target INR, 2.0 to 3.0).

3. The optimal duration of warfarin treatment after cardioversion is not known, although "at least" 3 to 4 weeks is recommended. Thus far, no study has clearly demonstrated that a strategy of SR maintenance reduces the risk of stroke if warfarin is discontinued.

Investigational Anticoagulants

The oral direct thrombin inhibitor ximelagratan does not require coagulation monitoring or dosage titrations. The third Stroke Prevention Using Oral Direct Thrombin Inhibitor Ximelagratan in Patients with Nonvalvular AF (SPORTIF III) trial enrolled 3,407 patients in an open-label fashion to ximelagratan, 36 mg twice daily, or warfarin. At follow up (mean 21 months), The ximelagratan group had a trend toward a lower annualized rate of stroke or systemic embolic events. An on-treatment analysis showed a 41% relative risk reduction with Ximelagratan (1.3% / yr. vs. 2.2% / yr, $p = 0.018$). Some ximelagratan patients developed liver enzyme elevations. The nearly 4,000 patient double-blind SPORTIF V trial is ongoing and will provide further data on the efficacy and side effect profile of this promising agent.

TABLE 6.1. MAJOR RANDOMIZED TRIALS OF WARFARIN FOR PREVENTION OF THROMBOEMBOLISM IN NONVALVULAR ATRIAL FIBRILLATION

Annual Event Rate (%) Study	Primary End Point(s)	Target INR	Warfarin	Control	Value
AFASAK (26)	Stroke, TIA, embolic complications to viscera and extremities	2.8–4.2	2.0	5.5[a]	<0.05
BAATAF (27)	Ischemic stroke	1.5–2.7	0.4	3.0[b]	0.002
SPAF I (28)	Ischemic stroke, systemic emboli	2.0–3.5	2.3	7.4[a]	0.01
CAFA (29)	Nonlacunar stroke, non-CNS embolic event, ICH, other fatal hemorrhage	2.0–3.0	3.5	5.2[a]	NS
SPINAF (30)	Cerebral infarction	1.4–2.8	0.9	4.3	0.001
EAFT (31)	Vascular death, any stroke, MI, recent stroke/TIA, systemic embolism	2.5–4.0	8.0	15.0[a]	0.001
SPAF II (32)	Ischemic stroke, systemic emboli	2.0–4.5	1.9	2.7[c]	0.15
SPAF III (34)	Ischemic stroke, systemic emboli	2.0–3.0	1.9	7.9[d]	<0.0001
AFASAK II (35)	Stroke, systemic emboli	2.0–3.0	2.8	3.6[e]	NS

CAF, chronic atrial fibrillation; PAF, paroxysmal atrial fibrillation; INR, international normalized ratio; ICH, intracranial hemorrhage; MI, myocardial infarction; TIA, transient ischemic attack; CNS, central nervous system; NS, not significant.
[a]Placebo group.
[b]No treatment but aspirin allowed.
[c]Aspirin.
[d]Aspirin and fixed low-dose warfarin (mean INR, 1.3).
[e]Low-dose warfarin.

Other Treatment Measures

1. *Focal ablation.* Promising early reports have led to growing enthusiasm for catheter-based ablation approaches targeting ectopic atrial foci that trigger AF, the great majority of which appear to arise in or near the ostia of the pulmonary veins. This approach has been studied mainly in relatively young patients with structurally normal hearts, and appears to improve or eliminate AF episodes in 70% or more of subjects, but is clearly more successful when AF is paroxysmal rather than persistent (see *N Engl J Med* 1998;339:659 and *Circulation* 2002;105:1077). As noted previously, sometimes catheter ablation of a primary arrhythmia—notably atrial flutter—serves to suppress AF episodes as well.
2. *Surgical maze procedure.* Cox and other investigators developed surgical approaches to compartmentalizing the atria to alter the underlying substrate for AF (see *J Thorac Cardiovasc Surg* 1995;110:473). A number of similar methods using ablative energy sources rather than incisions are now under investigation. These interventions are typically combined adjunctively with mitral valve or other cardiac surgery.
3. *Implantable atrial defibrillator.* Some patients with frequent, symptomatic episodes of AF for whom other modalities have failed may be candidates for sophisticated ICD devices that provide antitachycardia pacing as well as automated or

patient-activated shocks to terminate atrial arrhythmias (see *Circulation* 1998;98: 1651).

4. *Atrial pacemakers.* Pacing the right atrium from two sites and implanting pacemakers with automated atrial overdrive algorithms are two novel pacemaker-based interventions for reducing the "burden" of AF. These are reviewed in a separate chapter (see Cardiac Pacing section later).

5. *Atrioventricular junction (AVJ) ablation with permanent pacemaker implantation.* In patients for whom maintenance of SR is no longer feasible or desired, but who still have significant symptoms with AF, benefits have been demonstrated with the combination of AVJ ablation and implantation of a ventricular pacemaker. This provides the ultimate form of rate control and eliminates the irregular ventricular response that in some patients contributes to symptoms, even at moderate rates (see *Circulation* 1997;96:2617 and *Circulation* 1998;98:953).

VENTRICULAR ARRHYTHMIAS

Sudden cardiac death (SCD) accounts for more than 250,000 annual fatalities in the United States, and roughly half of all cardiac deaths are due to out-of-hospital cardiac arrest. The majority of these events are attributable to unstable ventricular arrhythmias.

Immediate Therapy: Automated External Defibrillators

Because most patients with witnessed cardiac arrest have "shockable" ventricular tachyarrhythmias just after collapse (see *Am Heart J* 1989;117:151), and survival rates are critically related to the rapidity of defibrillation (see *Circulation* 1978;57:20), substantial effort has been expended in developing and deploying automated external defibrillators (AEDs) in public areas. These devices, which require little to no training to operate, were originally shown to improve survival to hospital discharge among cardiac arrest victims when supplied by first-responder firefighters, as compared with waiting slightly longer for paramedics (37). More recently, pilot studies of AED use in casinos (38) and commercial airplanes (39) have demonstrated excellent performance of both AED rhythm diagnostics and shocking efficacy, leading to rates of survival to hospital discharge of 40% to 50% for victims of ventricular fibrillation (VF). The use of AEDs in other settings is under investigation, even as many public venues (e.g., sports stadiums) are investing in these life-saving devices for use by laypeople.

Immediate Therapy: Intravenous Amiodarone

Two recent important trials, ARREST and ALIVE, have provided more robust data than smaller prior studies on the immediate resuscitation of cardiac arrest (40,41). These trials demonstrated that a bolus of i.v. amiodarone, when given for patients with pulseless ventricular tachycardia (VT) or VF refractory to initial attempts at defibrillation, results in improved survival to hospital admission compared with either placebo or i.v. lidocaine. The ARREST and ALIVE studies were not large enough to demonstrate improvement in more pertinent end points, such as survival to hospital discharge, but nonetheless solidified the role of i.v. amiodarone as first-choice drug therapy for VT/VF in the year 2000 Advanced Cardiac Life Support (ACLS) guidelines.

Secondary Prevention Trials: Drugs versus Implantable Cardioverter Defibrillators

Three important randomized trials comparing ICDs with antiarrhythmic drugs for survivors of cardiac arrest or hemodynamically significant ventricular arrhythmias were completed in the 1990s: CASH, CIDS, and AVID (**Table 6.2**). Device technology was in a phase of rapid evolution, and concurrent with execution of the trials, perspectives on drug therapy were changing as well.

The CASH study, which began in 1987, randomized cardiac arrest survivors to amiodarone, metoprolol, ICD, or propafenone (42). The latter group was terminated early because of excess mortality compared with the ICD group. At long-term follow-up, a nonsignificant trend toward lower all-cause mortality favored the ICD group

TABLE 6.2. SURVIVAL TRIALS OF ICD THERAPY VERSUS CONVENTIONAL MEDICAL MANAGEMENT

	AVID (44)	CASH (42)	CIDS (43)	MADIT I (53)	MADIT II (55)
Pt population/entry criteria	Primary VF; or VT with syncope; or VT with EF ≤ 40% and significant symptoms	SCD survivors w/documented ventricular arrhythmias	VF; or cardiac arrest; sustained VT (poorly tolerated or EF ≤ 35%, or syncope with spontaneous or inducible VT)	Prior MI+EF ≤ 35%; NYHA class I–III + nonsustained VT	Prior MI, EF ≤ 30%, NYHA class I–III
Treatment	ICD vs. amiodarone or sotalol	ICD, amiodarone, metoprolol, or propafenone	ICD or amiodarone	ICD or conventional medical therapy	ICD or conventional medical therapy
Primary end point Results	All-cause mortality 39% lower mortality for ICD patients (at 3 yr 24.6% vs. 35.9%; $p < 0.02$)	All-cause mortality 38% lower mortality for ICD patients vs. amiodarone and metoprolol (36% vs. 44%; $p = 0.08$)	All-cause mortality 20% lower mortality for ICD patients (8.2%/yr vs. 10.2%/yr; $p = 0.14$)	All-cause mortality 54% lower mortality for ICD patients (17% vs. 39%; $p = 0.009$)	All-cause mortality 28% lower mortality for ICD patients (at 20 mo; 14.2% vs. 19.8%)

EF, ejection fraction; ICD, implantable cardiac defibrillator; VF, ventricular fibrillation; VT, ventricular tachycardia.
[a]Enrollment in the propafenone arm was stopped in 1992 because of a high mortality rate.

versus the combined amiodarone and metroprolol groups. CIDS was a "purer" and more recent comparison of ICDs versus amiodarone for survivors of cardiac arrest and documented unstable VT (43). As with CASH, a trend emerged in favor of ICDs for the end points of total and arrhythmic mortality, but again did not reach statistical significance. The AVID trial was the largest and most definitive of the three trials, randomizing more than 1,000 patients to ICD or antiarrhythmic drug (96% amiodarone) (44). AVID showed significantly better 2-year survival in the ICD group (75% vs. 64%; $p < 0.02$), leading many observers to conclude that CASH and CIDS were simply underpowered. Thus, in aggregate, the trials indicate that ICDs are superior to drug therapy. As a result, ICDs are now generally used as first-line treatment in the secondary-prevention population.

Primary Prevention Trials: Antiarrhythmic Drugs

In the 1970s and early 1980s, various investigators observed a high incidence of sudden death in survivors of acute MI, and identified methods of predicting increased risk for future arrhythmic events, including depressed ejection fraction, complex ventricular ectopy/nonsustained VT (NSVT) on ambulatory ECG monitoring, the presence of late potentials on signal-averaged ECG, and the induction of sustained tachycardias with invasive electrophysiologic study (EPS). These insights led to primary prevention trials in MI survivors, initially with antiarrhythmic drugs. Unfortunately, these trials demonstrated that with the exception of amiodarone, antiarrhythmic drugs actually appear to *increase* mortality in this patient population. In particular, Vaughan-Williams class I agents propafenone, encainide, flecainide (45), and moricizine (46) all demonstrated excess mortality compared with control groups in randomized studies of post-MI patients. In contrast, oral amiodarone appeared to reduce arrhythmic events and sudden death in several trials enrolling post-MI and CHF patients (48–51), although consistent improvements in all-cause mortality were not seen. A meta-analysis of amiodarone trials (52) suggested a small advantage in overall survival compared with placebo or alternative antiarrhythmic drugs. The recently approved class III antiarrhythmic drug dofetilide had a neutral effect on mortality in post-MI and CHF patients, but is currently approved for use only in AF (see AF section).

Primary Prevention Trials: Drugs versus Implantable Cardioverter Defibrillators

After the disappointing results of antiarrhythmic drug trials, primary prevention trials involving ICDs were completed. The ICD trials again focused on the post-MI population known to be at high risk for SCD, and the first two major trials—MADIT and MUSTT (53,54)—selected patients with low ejection fractions, NSVT, and inducible VT at EPS. As with the primary prevention trials, a clear advantage emerged in favor of ICDs compared with medical therapy with or without antiarrhythmic drugs.

More recently, the results of the MADIT II trial, which selected coronary patients on the basis of low ejection fraction alone (30% or less), were published, and demonstrated a statistically significant 31% relative reduction in mortality with prophylactic ICD implantation (55; see Table 6.2). Based on these results, the new ACC/AHA/NASPE Guidelines (59) now consider as a class IIa recommendation ICD therapy for patients with LVEF less than 30%, at least 1 month after MI and 3 months after coronary artery revascularization therapy.

Primary Prevention Trials: Noncoronary Cardiomyopathy Patients

In contrast to the progress in sudden death prevention in coronary disease patients outlined earlier, the question of whether antiarrhythmic drugs or ICDs provide additional mortality benefit for noncoronary cardiomyopathy patients beyond that provided by angiotensin-converting enzyme (ACE) inhibitors and β-blockers requires further study. Many cardiomyopathy patients were included in the amiodarone trials referenced earlier, suggesting a neutral to slightly beneficial effect on mortality.

Only one completed study, the Cardiomyopathy Trial (CAT), compared ICD with control in only nonischemic dilated cardiomyopathy (DCM) patients (57). The trial

was terminated before completion of full enrollment bec█
mortality in the control group; as a result, the study wa█
mortality difference between the two groups [26% (ICD) vs.█
ongoing trials, such as DEFINITE (see *Pacing Clin Electroph*█
SCD-HeFT (58) will provide additional data on ICD use in DCM█

CARDIAC PACING STUDIES

Traditionally, permanent pacemakers have been used for the treatme█
arrhythmias. Recently, however, evolving pacemaker technologies have sh█
in the management of tachyarrhythmias, CHF, and to a limited extent, ▐
syncope.

Pacemaker Mode Selection Trials

In clinical practice, most cardiologists implant dual-chamber pacemakers in patients
with bradyarrhythmias, except those with chronic AF. Despite the sound rationale
for physiologic dual-chamber pacing—including maintenance of AV synchrony, avoidance of retrograde ventriculoatrial (VA) conduction, and preservation of normal heart
rate response in patients with intact sinus node function—objective benefits of dual-
chamber pacing have proved difficult to quantify prospectively. Confirming prior retrospective data, several recent clinical trials have shown that atrial or dual-chamber
pacing, when compared with single-chamber ventricular (VVI) pacing, prevents pacemaker syndrome, and is associated with a lower incidence of new or permanent AF,
particularly among patients with sinus node dysfunction. However, improvements in
"harder" end points, such as stroke or death, were seen in one preliminary study (60)
but not confirmed in larger, later trials [CTOPP, MOST (62,63)]. Furthermore, in the
recent Dual Chamber and VVI Implantable Defibrillator (DAVID) Trial Investigators,
dual-chamber pacing was compared with ventricular backup pacing in 506 patients
with an implantable defibrillator and EF of 40% or less, and the backup pacing group
had a better 1-year survival free of death or hospitalization for CHF (83.9% vs. 73.3%;
relative hazard, 1.61; 95% CI, 1.06 to 2.44) (64), suggesting unnecessary pacing, which
might desynchronize the two ventricles, may be harmful.

Pacing for Vasovagal Syncope

Therapy for patients with frequent episodes of vasovagal syncope is generally unsatisfactory. Nonrandomized data previously suggested that a subset of vasovagal syncope
patients with pronounced cardio-inhibitory (bradycardia) physiology benefit from permanent pacing. To this end, pacemakers were developed that automatically pace at
high rates when triggered by prespecified decreases in intrinsic heart rate (rate-drop
response). In a randomized but unblinded trial of highly symptomatic patients with
bradycardia during tilt-table testing, implantation of pacemakers with rate-drop response resulted in a significant reduction in subsequent syncopal events (65). A fully
blinded follow-up study, however, resulted in less dramatic benefit (66). Pacemakers
thus remain a therapeutic option for selected vasovagal syncope patients with marked
tendency to bradycardia.

Pacing for Prevention of Atrial Fibrillation

Based on the observed benefits of standard right atrial pacing in preventing AF in sus-
ceptible patients (reviewed earlier), investigators have explored whether the development of specialized pacing software to provide automated atrial overdrive pacing or
the implantation of atrial leads at two separate sites can achieve even better suppression of AF than standard dual-chamber pacing. Overdrive right atrial pacing appears
to reduce the "burden" of AF somewhat (67), but the superiority of dual-site versus
single-site pacing has not been clearly established. Statistically significant findings
for particular end points and/or in specific subgroups have been reported with these

use of a lower than expected
underpowered to detect a
31.5%; p = NS). Several
ysiol 2000;23:338) and
populations.

nt of brady-
own utility
asovagal

e clinical relevance of the end points, and
ncertain (68–70).

leart Failure

ventricular dysfunction, 30% or more
ich block or intraventricular conduc-
:ions of the ventricular myocardium.
ietween ventricles appears to impair
:ributing to HF symptoms and possi-
rporate leads delivered through the
ion to the epicardial surface of the
ited latest in these patients. These
g, known as "resynchronization"

...mediate hemodynamic benefits from LV or BiV
.. .rials were performed with several different pacing sys-
...s Am Coll Cardiol 2002;39:194). Each of these studies had short- to
...uiate-term follow-up and documented improvements with LV or BiV pacing in
various subjective and objective measures of heart failure severity, including New York
Heart Association functional class; 6-minute walk test; peak oxygen consumption; and
QOL (71–74). In the MIRACLE study, 453 NYHA class III or IV patients with EF less
than 35% who underwent BiV pacing system placement were randomized to active
pacing (atrially synchronized BiV pacing) or no pacing for 6 months (74). The active-
pacing group had significant improvement in all measured parameters, including EF
and hospitalization for worsening HF.

These data resulted in a class IIa recommendation in the updated ACC/AHA/
NASPE Guidelines (59): "biventricular pacing in medically refractory, symptomatic
NYHA Class III or IV patients with idiopathic dilated or ischemic cardiomyopathy, pro-
longed QRS interval (130 milliseconds or more), LV end-diastolic diameter (LVEDD)
55 mm or more, and EF 35% or less." Such data also paved the way for Food and Drug
Administration (FDA) approval of dedicated BiV pacing systems (including ICDs with
BiV pacing capability).

The subsequently complete COMPANION trial enrolled 1,600 patients with class
III/IV CHF with QRS > 120 msec and found death and hospitalization was signifi-
cantly reduced with BiV pacing and BiV pacing plus ICD (CRT-D). In addition, the
CRT-D group had a highly significant 43% mortality reduction compared to optimal
drug therapy. It is important to note that these findings apply to only ~5% of the
U.S. heart failure population. However, given the high cost of these devices, criteria
for optimal patient selection is extremely important and subgroup analyses of the
COMPANION data will assist in this process.

REFERENCES

Atrial Fibrillation

Epidemiology

1. **Fuster V,** et al. ACC/AHA/ESC guidelines for the management of patients
   with atrial fibrillation: executive summary: a Report of the American College of
   Cardiology/American Heart Association Task Force on Practice Guidelines and the
   European Society of Cardiology Committee for Practice Guidelines and Policy Con-
   ferences (Committee to Develop Guidelines for the Management of Patients with
   Atrial Fibrillation), developed in Collaboration With the North American Society
   of Pacing and Electrophysiology. *J Am Coll Cardiol* 2001;38:1231–1266.

2. **Kopecky SL,** et al. The natural history of lone atrial fibrillation. *N Engl J Med*
   1987;317:669–674.

In this population-based study of Olmstead County, Minnesota, residents between
1950 and 1980, 3,623 persons were found to have AF, of whom 97 (2.7%) were younger

than 60 years (mean age, 44 years at diagnosis) and had no overt cardiovascular disease or precipitating illness. Among these lone AF patients, 21% had an isolated episode, 58% had recurrent AF, and 22% had chronic AF. At 15-year follow-up, only 1.3% of patients had had a stroke on a cumulative actuarial basis, and no difference was found in survival or stroke-free survival among patients with the three types of lone AF. Based on these findings, the authors suggest that routine anticoagulation may not be indicated in individuals with lone AF.

3. **Atrial Fibrillation Investigators.** Risk factors for stroke and efficacy of antithrombotic therapy in atrial fibrillation: an analysis of pooled data from 5 randomized controlled trials (AFASAK, SPAF, BAATAF, SPINAF, CAFA). *Arch Intern Med* 1994;154:1449–1457.

Pooled data from these five trials showed that warfarin use was associated with a 68% reduction in stroke risk (to 1.4%/yr) and 33% lower all-cause mortality. This significant benefit of warfarin also was present in patients with paroxysmal/intermittent AF [1.7%/yr (warfarin) vs. 5.7%/yr (placebo)]. Risk factors for thromboembolism were history of hypertension, prior stroke or TIA, diabetes, and age older than 65 years. A nonsignificant increase was seen in the frequency of major bleeding. Two of these five trials randomized patients to an aspirin group; the pooled risk reduction versus placebo was 36%.

4. **Benjamin EJ,** et al. Left atrial size and the risk of stroke and death: the Framingham Heart Study. *Circulation* 1995;92:835–841.

This analysis focused on 3,099 patients aged 50 years or older. For each 1-cm increase in left atrial size, the relative risk of stroke was 2.4 in men and 1.4 in women, and for death, 1.3 and 1.4 in men and women, respectively.

5. **Wood KA,** et al. Risk of thromboembolism in chronic atrial flutter. *Am J Cardiol* 1997;79:1043–1047.

Retrospective analysis of 86 patients referred for radiofrequency ablation. The annual risk of embolic events was 3% (1.6% after exclusion of patients with TIA and pulmonary embolism). In a logistic regression model, no significant independent predictors of increased thromboembolic risk were found.

6. **Benjamin EJ,** et al. Impact of atrial fibrillation on the risk of death. *Circulation* 1998;98:946–952.

Of 5,209 Framingham Study participants, in 296 men and 325 women, AF developed during 40 years of follow-up. AF patients were more likely (at baseline) to smoke and have hypertension, LV hypertrophy on ECG, history of MI, CHF, valvular disease, and stroke or TIA. AF was associated with an adjusted OR for death of 1.5 (95% CI, 1.2 to 1.8) in men and 1.9 (95% CI, 1.5 to 2.2) in women. The presence of AF increased the risk of dying at all ages. Most of the excess mortality was seen in the first 30 days after AF developed.

7. **Seidl K,** et al. Risk of thromboembolic events in patients with atrial flutter. *Am J Cardiol* 1998;82:580–583.

This retrospective analysis focused on 191 consecutive patients with atrial flutter. At an average follow-up of 26 months, embolic events had occurred in 11 (7%) patients. Acute (less than 48 hours) embolism occurred in four patients (three after DC cardioversion, one after catheter ablation). In multivariate analysis, the only independent predictor of embolic events was hypertension (OR, 6.5; 95% CI, 1.5 to 45).

Atrial Fibrillation Prevention after Surgery

8. **Andrews TC,** et al. Prevention of supraventricular arrhythmias after coronary artery bypass surgery: a meta-analysis of randomized controlled trials. *Circulation* 1991;84(suppl III):III-236.

This meta-analysis included 1,549 patients from 24 randomized, controlled studies. Patients were excluded if they had an LVEF less than 30%, insulin-dependent diabetes, AV block, sick sinus syndrome, and those undergoing noncardiac operations. The initiation of preoperative β-blockers was found to be more effective than postoperative initiation, and β-blocker therapy reduced post-CABG AF by 77%.

9. **Daoud EG,** et al. Preoperative amiodarone as prophylaxis against atrial fibrillation after heart surgery. *N Engl J Med* 1997;337:1785.

This prospective, randomized, double-blind study enrolled 124 patients scheduled to undergo elective cardiac surgery. Patients were randomized at least a week before surgery to oral amiodarone (600 mg per day for 7 days, and then 200 mg per day until hospital discharge), or placebo. Postoperative AF occurred significantly less in the amiodarone group (25% vs. 53%; $p = 0.003$). Amiodarone patients had a shorter and less costly hospital stay compared with placebo patients (6.5 vs. 7.9 days; $p = 0.04$; \$18,375 vs. \$26,491; $p = 0.03$). No significant differences were seen between the groups in nonfatal and fatal postoperative complications.

Rate versus Rhythm Control
10. **Wyse G,** for the Atrial Fibrillation Follow-up Investigation of Rhythm Management **(AFFIRM)** Investigators. Preliminary results presented at the American College of Cardiology Annual Scientific Session, Atlanta, GA, March 2002.

This prospective, randomized, multicenter study enrolled 4,060 patients with AF more than 6 hours but less than 6 months in duration. Eligible patients were aged 65 years or older or had one or more risk factors for stroke, could not have failed cardioversion, and had to be willing to accept randomization to rate versus rhythm control. Patients were randomized to rhythm control with electrical cardioversion and antiarrhythmic drugs (initially 39% amiodarone, 33% sotalol, and 15% IC agents) or to rate control with standard agents. Amiodarone was ultimately given to 60% of patients. Warfarin was continued indefinitely in the rate-control arm but could be discontinued at the local physicians' discretion in the rhythm-control arm if SR was maintained for 1 month. At follow-up (average, 3.5 years), no significant differences were found between the two groups in all-cause mortality (primary end point) and other major secondary end points including stroke [7.3% (rhythm control) vs. 5.7%; $p =$ NS].

11. **Crijns H,** Van Gelder IC, Rate Control vs. Electrical Cardioversion for persistent atrial fibrillation **(RACE).** Preliminary results presented at the American College of Cardiology Annual Scientific Session, Atlanta, GA, March 2002.

This smaller trial had a general structure similar to that of the AFFIRM, enrolling 256 patients in the rate-control group and 266 patients in the rhythm-control group. Discontinuation of warfarin after a period of SR was mandated by the study for the rhythm-control group. At 3 years, no statistically significant difference was seen between the groups in the primary composite end point of cardiovascular death, HF hospitalization, embolic events, severe bleeding, pacemaker implantation, or severe drug side effects [17.2% (rate control) vs. 22.0%]. Trends toward more embolic events, HF, and adverse drug events were seen in the rhythm-control arm. Event rates were higher in hypertensive patients.

Antiarrhythmic Drug Trials for Atrial Fibrillation
12. **Coplen SE,** et al. Efficacy and safety of quinidine therapy for maintenance of sinus rhythm after cardioversion: a meta-analysis of randomized controlled trials. *Circulation* 1990;82:1106–1116.

This analysis focused on six trials with 808 patients. Quinidine use was associated with less AF recurrence. At 3, 6, and 12 months, 69%, 58%, and 50% of quinidine-treated patients were in normal SR versus 45%, 33%, and 25% of controls. Despite the lower recurrence rates, the quinidine group had a higher all-cause mortality rate (2.9% vs. 0.8%; $p < 0.05$).

13. **Gosselink TM,** et al. Low-dose amiodarone for maintenance of sinus rhythm after cardioversion of atrial fibrillation or flutter. *JAMA* 1992;267:3289–3293.

This study was composed of 89 AF patients for whom previous therapy failed. A loading dose of amiodarone (600 mg over a 4-week period) was followed by an average daily dose of 204 mg/day. Fifteen (16%) patients converted to normal SR during loading; 90% were in SR after cardioversion, and 53% remained in normal SR at 3-year follow-up. No proarrhythmias were documented.

14. **Halinen MO,** et al. Comparison of sotalol with digoxin-quinidine for conversion of acute atrial fibrillation to sinus rhythm (the Sotalol-Digoxin-Quinidine trial). *Am J Cardiol* 1995;76:495–498.

This randomized trial was composed of 61 patients with paroxysmal AF randomized at less than 48 hours to sotalol, 80 to 320 mg (80-mg doses repeated if AF persisted; heart rate, 80 beats/min or more; BP, 120 mm Hg or more) or quinidine, 200 to 600 mg [digoxin given first (0.25 to 0.75 mg) if heart rate was greater than 100 beats/min]. The quinidine group had an increased conversion rate (86% vs. 52%). Sotalol was discontinued in 16 of 33 patients secondary to asymptomatic bradycardia or hypotension. Asymptomatic wide complex tachycardia occurred in 13% (sotalol, 27%).

15. **Galve E,** et al. Intravenous amiodarone in the treatment of recent-onset atrial fibrillation: results of a randomized, controlled trial. *J Am Coll Cardiol* 1996;27:1079–1082.

One hundred patients with AF less than 1 week in duration and not taking any antiarrhythmics were randomized to amiodarone, 5 mg/kg over a 30-minute period, and then 1,200 mg over a 24-hour period, or placebo. Both groups were given i.v. digoxin. At 24 hours, no differences occurred in the incidence of normal SR (68% vs. 60%; $p = 0.53$). Among nonconverters, the amiodarone group had a decreased average ventricular rate (82 vs. 91 beats/min). No differences were observed in the 15-day recurrence rate (12% vs. 10%).

16. **Stambler BS,** et al. Efficacy and safety for repeated intravenous doses of ibutilide for rapid conversion of atrial flutter or fibrillation. *Circulation* 1996;94:1613–1621.

This randomized trial was composed of 266 patients with sustained (3 hours to 45 days) AF or flutter. Patients received one or two 10-minute infusions of ibutilide, separated by 10 minutes (1.0 mg plus 0.5 mg or 1 mg plus 1 mg) or placebo. Ibutilide converted 47% of patients overall (vs. 2% with placebo), with better success in atrial flutter than in AF (63% vs. 31%). The average time to termination was 27 minutes. No significant differences were seen between dosing regimens. Polymorphic VT occurred in 8.3%, but was sustained in only 1.7%.

17. **Torp-Pedersen C,** et al., for the Danish Investigations of Arrhythmia and Mortality on Dofetilide **(DIAMOND-CHF)** Study Group. Dofetilide in patients with congestive heart failure and left ventricular dysfunction. *N Engl J Med* 1999;341:857–865 (see summary after reference 18).

18. **Kober L,** et al., for the Danish Investigations of Arrhythmia and Mortality on Dofetilide **(DIAMOND-MI)** Study Group. Effect of dofetilide in patients with recent myocardial infarction and left-ventricular dysfunction: a randomised trial. *Lancet* 2000;356:2052–2058.

The efficacy of dofetilide, an orally available class III antiarrhythmic drug, in the conversion of AF/flutter to normal SR was established in two unpublished, randomized, placebo-controlled trials: EMERALD (European and Australian Multicenter Evaluative Research on Atrial Fibrillation Dofetilide) and SAFIRE-D (Symptomatic Atrial Fibrillation Investigation and Randomized Evaluation of Dofetilide). Short-term conversion rates were approximately 10% for the 250-μg b.i.d. dose and approximately 30% for the 500-μg b.i.d. dose, compared with 1% for placebo (see *Physician's Desk Reference* package insert for details).

Given concerns over the use of antiarrhythmic drugs in patients with structural heart disease, additional safety studies were conducted. Dofetilide was compared with placebo in 1,518 subjects hospitalized with new or worsening CHF and LV dysfunction (DIAMOND-CHF) and 1,510 subjects with severe LV dysfunction after MI

(DIAMOND-MI). In patients with AF at baseline, dofetilide was much more effective than placebo at restoring SR (44% vs. 13% at 1 year; $p < 0.001$) and maintaining SR (hazard ratio, 0.35; $p < 0.001$). Furthermore, patients in SR at baseline were less likely to develop new AF with dofetilide than with placebo (2.0% vs. 6.6%; $p < 0.001$). No difference in total mortality was found in either trial. Torsades des pointes was seen in 3.3% of dofetilide patients in DIAMOND-CHF, but after adjustments in the dosing regimen, this was reduced to 0.9% in DIAMOND-MI. Dofetilide thus appears safe in the CHF/post-MI populations, but initiation of therapy must take place in hospital with careful dose calculation (based on creatinine clearance) and QT-interval monitoring.

19. **Roy D,** et al., for the Canadian Trial of Atrial Fibrillation **(CTAF)** Investigators. Amiodarone to prevent recurrence of atrial fibrillation. *N Engl J Med* 2000; 342:913–920.

Design: Prospective, randomized, multicenter trial. Mean follow-up of 16 months.
Purpose: To evaluate the efficacy of amiodarone in preventing recurrent AF.
Population: 403 patients with symptomatic AF.
Treatment: Amiodarone, sotalol, or propafenone (average daily doses at 1 year were 194 mg, 231 mg, and 554 mg, respectively).
Results: Only 35% of amiodarone patients had a documented recurrence of AF compared with 63% taking the other antiarrhythmics. Discontinuation of study drug due to adverse effects occurred in 18% of amiodarone patients and 11% of sotalol/propafenone patients ($p = 0.06$).
Comments: The superiority of amiodorone over sotalol was confirmed in the recently presented sotalol amiodorone (atrial) Fibrillation Efficacy Trial (SAFE-T); amiodarone prolonged time to new onset of AF four times longer than sotalol (NASPE 2003 Scientific Sessions, Washington, D.C.).

Electrical Cardioversion and Pericardioversion Anticoagulation

20. **Manning WJ,** et al. Cardioversion from atrial fibrillation without prolonged anticoagulation with the use of transesophageal echocardiography to exclude the presence of atrial thrombi. *N Engl J Med* 1993;328:750–755.

This study was composed of 94 patients with AF of more than 2 days' duration (average, 4.5 weeks). Eighty patients received heparin before cardioversion; 14 thrombi were seen by TEE versus only two of 14 seen on transthoracic echocardiography (two of these patients died suddenly, whereas the other 10 were cardioverted after prolonged oral anticoagulation). No embolic events occurred in the other patients [78 of 82 successfully cardioverted (47 by drugs)].

21. **Manning WJ,** et al. Transesophageal echocardiography facilitated early cardioversion from atrial fibrillation using short-term anticoagulation: final results of a prospective 4.5-year study. *J Am Coll Cardiol* 1995;25:1354–1361.

In this study of 230 patients (inclusion criteria were AF of more than 2 days' duration or of unknown duration), TEE identified 40 atrial thrombi in 34 patients, of whom 18 had successful cardioversion after prolonged anticoagulation. Among patients without thrombi, 95% had successful cardioversion without a thromboembolic event. Among patients without prolonged anticoagulation (i.e., warfarin for 1 month), none had thromboembolic events.

22. **Klein AL,** et al., for the Assessment of Cardioversion Using Transesophageal Echocardiography **(ACUTE)** Investigators. Use of transesophageal echocardiography to guide cardioversion in patients with atrial fibrillation. *N Engl J Med* 2001;344:1411–1420.

Design: Prospective, randomized, open, multicenter study. Primary end point: embolic events.
Purpose: To evaluate the safety and efficacy of TEE-guided cardioversion in patients with AF.
Population: 1,222 patients with AF of more than 48 hours' duration.

Exclusion Criteria: Included atrial flutter (and no history of AF), long-term warfarin therapy, hemodynamic instability, contraindications to TEE.
Treatment: Cardioversion after 3 or more weeks of warfarin or TEE-guided cardioversion. All received a minimum of 4 weeks of warfarin after cardioversion.
Results: No difference between the groups was found in the incidence of embolic events [0.5% (TEE-guided) vs. 0.8%]. The TEE approach was associated with lower rates of hemorrhage, mostly minor (2.9% vs. 5.5%; $p = 0.03$). The TEE group had a higher initial successful cardioversion rate (71.1% vs. 65.2%; $p = 0.03$); however, SR rates were similar at 8 weeks.

23. **Page RL,** et al. Biphasic versus monophasic shock waveform for conversion of atrial fibrillation: the results of an international randomized, double-blind multicenter trial. *J Am Coll Cardiol* 2002;39:1956–1963.

This prospective, randomized, double-blind, multicenter trial compared the effectiveness of monophasic versus biphasic shocks for the cardioversion of AF. The 203 patients were randomized to monophasic or biphasic shocking waveforms, and received successive shocks, as needed, at three shared energies (100, 150, and 200 joules), and then maximum output for the respective devices (200 J biphasic, 360 J monophasic) and, if necessary, a final crossover shock at maximum output of the alternate waveform. The success rate was higher for biphasic than for monophasic shocks at each of the three shared energy levels (100 J: 60% vs. 22%; 150 J: 77% vs. 44%; 200 J: 90% vs. 53%; $p < 0.0001$). On average, biphasic patients required fewer shocks (1.7 vs. 2.8; $p < 0.0001$) and lower total energy (217 J vs. 548 J, $p < 0.0001$) for successful conversion. The biphasic shock waveform also was associated with a lower frequency of dermal injury (17% vs. 41%; $p < 0.0001$).

24. Anticoagulation for Cardioversion Using Enoxaparin. Preliminary results presented at the Annual European Society of Cardiology meeting, Munich, September 2002.

This European study included 496 patients with nonvalvular AF scheduled to undergo elective cardioversion. Subjects were randomized to 72 hours of i.v. unfractionated heparin followed by phenprocoumon, or to enoxaparin, 1 mg/kg twice daily for 3 to 8 days followed by 40 or 60 mg b.i.d. Most (86%) of the cardioversions were TEE guided. The primary composite end point of all-cause mortality, neurologic events, embolic events, and major bleeding occurred in 4.8% of unfractionated heparin patients and 2.8% of enoxaparin patients ($p = NS$). Investigators concluded that enoxaparin was not inferior.

Long-term Anticoagulation Studies
25. **Albers GW.** Atrial fibrillation and stroke: 3 new studies, 3 new questions. *Arch Intern Med* 1994;154:1443–1448.

Analysis of the trials showed that anticoagulation therapy was associated with a reduction in stroke rates of approximately 50% compared with placebo, whereas aspirin reduced the risk by approximately 25%. No significant difference in stroke rates was noted between those with paroxysmal and chronic AF. Based on these data, the following recommendations were proposed: (a) in individuals younger than 60 years with no risk factors (history of previous stroke, TIA, diabetes, hypertension), no therapy is required (stroke risk is less than 0.5%/yr); (b) in patients aged 60 to 75 years with lone AF, aspirin only is adequate (risk is 2%/yr without therapy); and (c) patients older than 75 years or younger than 75 years with risk factors should be given anticoagulation with warfarin.

26. **Peterson,** et al. Atrial Fibrillation, Aspirin, Anticoagulation **(AFASAK)** study. Placebo-controlled, randomized trial of warfarin and aspirin for prevention of thromboembolic complications in chronic atrial fibrillation. *Lancet* 1989;333:175–178.

Design: Prospective, randomized, partially open (warfarin), partially blinded (aspirin vs. placebo) study. Follow-up period was 2 years. Primary end point was thromboembolic complications (TIA, minor stroke, nondisabling stroke, fatal stroke, or embolism to viscera or extremities).

Purpose: To assess the efficacy of low-dose warfarin in preventing strokes in patients with nonrheumatic AF.

Population: 1,007 patients aged 18 years with chronic AF.

Exclusion Criteria: Prior anticoagulation for 6 months, cerebrovascular events in the prior 1 month, blood pressure (BP) greater than 180/100 mm Hg.

Treatment: Low-dose warfarin [target prothrombin time (PT), 1.2 to 1.5 times control (approximate INR, 2.8 to 4.2)]; aspirin, 75 mg/day; or placebo.

Results: The warfarin group had significantly fewer thromboembolic complications [1.5% vs. 6.0% (aspirin) and 6.3% (placebo)]. Vascular death occurred in 0.9%, 3.6%, and 4.5% of the warfarin, aspirin, and placebo groups ($p < 0.02$). Warfarin patients had more frequent nonfatal bleeding (6.3% vs. 0.6% and none of aspirin and placebo patients).

27. Boston Area Anticoagulation Trial for Atrial Fibrillation **(BAATAF).** The effect of low-dose warfarin on the risk of stroke in patients with nonrheumatic atrial fibrillation. *N Engl J Med* 1990;323:1505–1511.

Design: Prospective, randomized, open, controlled, multicenter study. Mean follow-up period was 2.2 years. Primary end point was ischemic stroke.

Purpose: To assess the efficacy of low-dose warfarin in preventing strokes in patients with nonrheumatic AF.

Population: 420 patients (mean age, 63 years) with chronic or intermittent AF.

Exclusion Criteria: Prosthetic valves, severe HF, stroke in the prior 6 months, and contraindications to or requirement for aspirin or warfarin therapy.

Treatment: Warfarin [target PT, 1.2 to 1.5 times normal (achieved in 83%)]; aspirin was allowed in the control group.

Results: Trial was terminated early because of strong evidence in favor of warfarin. The warfarin group had 86% fewer strokes [0.41%/yr vs. 2.98%/yr (control group); $p = 0.002$] and a 62% lower death rate (2.25%/yr vs. 5.97%/yr; $p = 0.005$). The warfarin group had more minor hemorrhages (38 vs. 21 patients).

28. **SPAF** Investigators. Stroke Prevention in Atrial Fibrillation Study: final results. *Circulation* 1991;84:527–539.

Design: Prospective, randomized, partially open (warfarin), partially blind (aspirin vs. placebo), multicenter study. Primary events were ischemic stroke and systemic embolism. Mean follow-up was 1.3 years.

Purpose: To determine the efficacy and safety of warfarin and aspirin compared with placebo for the prevention of ischemic stroke and systemic embolism in patients with nonrheumatic AF.

Population: 1,330 patients with chronic or intermittent AF.

Exclusion Criteria: Prosthetic valves, mitral stenosis, MI in the prior 3 months, and stroke or TIA in the prior 2 years.

Treatment: Group 1 [627 patients (most 75 years or younger): warfarin (target PT, 1.3 to 1.8 times normal (approximate INR, 2.0 to 4.5)]; aspirin, 325 mg/day; or placebo. Group 2 (703 nonanticoagulation candidates): aspirin or placebo.

Results: Aspirin-treated patients had 67% fewer primary events than did placebo patients (3.6%/yr vs. 6.3%/yr; $p = 0.02$). In the warfarin-eligible patients, warfarin reduced the risk of primary events by 67% compared with placebo (2.3%/yr vs. 7.4%/yr; $p = 0.01$). Primary events or death were reduced 58% by warfarin ($p = 0.01$) and 32% by aspirin ($p = 0.02$). Disabling stroke or vascular death was reduced 54% by warfarin and a nonsignificant 22% by aspirin ($p = 0.33$). Significant bleeding rates were similar in all three groups (1.4% to 1.6%/yr). Significant risk factors for stroke were (a) prior cerebrovascular accident, (b) CHF within preceding 100 days, (c) hypertension, and among the echocardiographically assessed features, (d) left atrium more than 5 cm, and (e) LV dysfunction. If one clinical factor was present, the risk of stroke was 7%/yr; if two or all three factors were present, the risk was 18%/yr. The group without any risk factors (26%) had an event rate of only 1%/yr.

Comments: Placebo arm of group 1 was discontinued in late 1989 because of the strong evidence of superiority of both warfarin and aspirin over placebo.

29. **Connolly SJ,** et al. Canadian Atrial Fibrillation Anticoagulation study **(CAFA).** *J Am Coll Cardiol* 1991;18:349–355 (editorial, 301–302).

Design: Prospective, randomized, double-blind, placebo-controlled, multicenter study. Primary end point was nonlacunar ischemic stroke, other systemic embolism, and intracranial or fatal hemorrhage.
Purpose: To evaluate the effectiveness and safety of warfarin in AF patients.
Population: 378 patients with recurrent paroxysmal or chronic AF.
Exclusion Criteria: Clear indications or contraindications to anticoagulation, stroke, or TIA in the prior year, MI in the prior month, use of antiplatelet drug(s), and uncontrolled hypertension.
Treatment: Warfarin (target INR, 2 to 3) or placebo.
Results: Target INR was achieved with only 44% frequency (subtherapeutic values in 39.6%). The warfarin group had a nonsignificant 37% risk reduction in primary outcome events (3.5%/yr vs. 5.2%/yr; $p = 0.26$). Major/fatal and minor bleeding events were common with warfarin use (2.5%/yr vs. 0.5%/yr and 16%/yr vs. 9.4%/yr).
Comments: Trial was terminated early because of the AFASAK and SPAF results.

30. **Ezekowitz MD,** et al. VA Stroke Prevention in Nonrheumatic Atrial Fibrillation **(SPINAF).** Warfarin in the prevention of stroke associated with nonrheumatic atrial fibrillation. *N Engl J Med* 1992;327:1406–1412.

Design: Prospective, randomized, double-blind, placebo-controlled, multicenter study. Average follow-up period was 1.8 years. Primary end point was cerebral infarction.
Purpose: To evaluate whether low-intensity anticoagulation will decrease the risk of stroke in patients with nonrheumatic AF.
Population: 571 men, 46 with prior stroke, without echocardiographic evidence of rheumatic heart disease and AF on two ECG tracings 4 weeks apart.
Exclusion Criteria: Contraindications to or requirement for anticoagulation, BP greater than 180/105 mm Hg, and use of nonsteroidal antiinflammatory drugs.
Treatment: Warfarin (target INR, 1.4 to 2.8) or placebo.
Results: A 79% risk reduction was observed among patients without a history of stroke (0.9%/yr vs. 4.3%/yr; $p = 0.001$). Significant benefit also was seen in patients older than 70 years (0.9% vs. 4.8%/yr; $p = 0.02$) and with a history of prior stroke (6.1%/yr vs. 9.3%/yr). Major hemorrhage rates were similar [1.3%/yr (warfarin) vs. 0.9%/yr]. Cerebral infarction occurred more frequently among patients with a history of cerebral infarction [9.3%/yr (placebo group) and 6.1%/yr (warfarin group)].
Comments: An analysis of 516 evaluable admission computed tomography (CT) scans showed that 14.7% had one silent infarct. Strokes during the study were not predicted by infarct on admission CT scan, but rather by active angina [placebo group, 15% (angina) vs. 5%] (see *Circulation* 1995;92:2178).

31. European Atrial Fibrillation Trial **(EAFT).** Secondary prevention in nonrheumatic fibrillation after transient ischemic attack or minor stroke. *Lancet* 1993;342:1255–1262.

Design: Prospective, randomized, partially open (anticoagulant therapy), double-blind aspirin treatment, placebo-controlled, multicenter study. Primary end points were death from vascular disease, any stroke, MI, and systemic embolism. Mean follow-up period was 2.3 years.
Purpose: To evaluate and compare the effectiveness of oral anticoagulation and aspirin in AF patients with recent minor cerebrovascular events.
Population: 1,007 patients with nonrheumatic AF and minor stroke or TIA in the previous 3 months.
Exclusion Criteria: Use of nonsteroidal antiinflammatory or other antiplatelet drugs, MI in the prior 3 months, and scheduled coronary surgery or carotid endarterectomy within next 3 months.
Treatment: Group 1 (669 patients): warfarin (target INR, 2.5 to 4.0), or aspirin, 300 mg daily, or placebo. Group 2: Contraindications to anticoagulation; 338 patients.

Results: Anticoagulation was more effective than aspirin and placebo: 8% versus 15% and 17% annual rates of primary outcome events; risk of stroke was especially lower in warfarin-treated patients [4%/yr vs. 12%/yr (placebo)]. Overall, warfarin use was associated with 90 fewer vascular events per 1,000 patient years (vs. 40 with aspirin). Bleeding events were common in warfarin-treated patients [2.8%/yr vs. 0.9%/yr (aspirin patients)]. Analysis of group 2 patients showed that the optimal INR range was 2.0 to 3.9, with most bleeding complications occurring when the INR was greater than 5.0, and no significant treatment effect was seen if INR was less than 2.0 (see *N Engl J Med* 1995;333:5).

32. **SPAF II.** Warfarin versus aspirin for prevention of thromboembolism in atrial fibrillation. *Lancet* 1994;43:687–691.

Design: Prospective, randomized, open, parallel-group, multicenter study. Primary events were stroke and systemic embolism. Mean follow-up period was 2.3 years.
Purpose: To define the long-term benefits and risks associated with warfarin compared with aspirin, according to age and risk of thromboembolism.
Population: 1,100 patients, 715 patients aged 75 years or younger and 385 older than 75 years, with AF in the prior 12 months.
Exclusion Criteria: Lone AF if younger than 60 years, stroke or TIA in the prior 2 years.
Treatment: Warfarin (target INR, 2.0 to 4.5), or aspirin, 325 mg daily.
Results: No significant difference was observed between groups. However, 12 of 28 events in the warfarin group occurred while patients were not taking warfarin. Thus, a 50% difference in favor of warfarin is evident if these events are excluded. Event rates per year for patients aged 75 years or younger were 1.3% vs. 1.9% ($p = 0.24$); older than 75 years, 3.6% vs. 4.8% ($p = 0.39$). Low-risk younger patients (no hypertension, recent HF, or prior thromboembolism) had a low 0.5%/yr primary event rate. Among older patients, stroke rates were similar in the two treatment groups (aspirin, 4.3%/yr; warfarin, 4.6%/yr). Among warfarin-treated patients, the intracranial hemorrhage was significantly higher in older versus younger patients (1.6% vs. 4.2%; $p = 0.04$).
Comments: Randomization was performed separately for the two age groups.

33. **Hylek EM,** et al. An analysis of the lowest effective intensity of prophylactic anticoagulation for patients with nonrheumatic atrial fibrillation. *N Engl J Med* 1996;335:540–546.

This retrospective, case-control analysis focused on 74 consecutive patients with ischemic strokes taking warfarin (INR measured at admission) and 222 controls (INR measured closest to admission day of case patient). The risk of stroke increased significantly at INRs less than 2.0; the adjusted OR for stroke was 2.0 if the INR was 1.7 to 2.0, 3.3 if the INR was 1.5 to 2.0, and 6.0 if the INR was 1.3 to 2.0. Other independent risk factors were prior stroke (OR, 10.4), diabetes (OR, 2.9), hypertension (OR, 2.5), and smoking (OR, 5.7).

34. **SPAF III.** Adjusted-dose warfarin vs. low-intensity, fixed-dose warfarin and aspirin for high-risk patients with atrial fibrillation: SPAF III randomised clinical trial. *Lancet* 1996;348:633–638.

Design: Prospective, randomized, partially open, multicenter study. Primary events were ischemic stroke and systemic embolism. Mean follow-up period was 1.1 years.
Purpose: To compare the safety and effectiveness of a combination of low-intensity, fixed-dose warfarin plus aspirin with adjusted-dose warfarin in AF patients at high risk of stroke.
Population: 1,044 AF patients with one of the following: CHF or EF 25% or less, prior thromboembolism, systolic blood pressure (SBP) greater than 160 mm Hg, or woman older than 75 years.
Exclusion Criteria: Conditions requiring standard anticoagulation therapy and contraindications to aspirin or warfarin.
Treatment: Fixed-dose warfarin [initial INR, 1.2 to 1.5 (mean, 1.3)] and aspirin (325 mg/day) or adjusted-dose warfarin [INR, 2 to 3 (mean, 2.4)].

Results: Trial was terminated early. The low-INR group had 4 times more ischemic strokes and systemic emboli (7.9%/yr vs. 1/9%/yr; $p < 0.0001$). Rates of disabling stroke (5.6%/yr vs. 1.7%/yr; $p = 0.0007$) and of primary or vascular death (11.8%/yr vs. 6.4%/yr; $p = 0.002$) also were higher with combination therapy. Bleeding rates were similar. The greatest benefits of standard adjusted-dose warfarin were seen in patients with prior thromboembolism.

35. **Gullov AL,** et al., **AFASAK II.** Fixed minidose warfarin, aspirin alone and in combination, versus adjusted-dose warfarin for stroke prevention in atrial fibrillation. *Arch Intern Med* 1998;158:1513–1521 (editorial, 1487–1491).

Design: Prospective, randomized, controlled, single-center study. Primary end point was stroke and systemic thromboembolic events.
Purpose: To investigate the effects of minidose warfarin alone and in combination with aspirin in chronic AF patients.
Population: 677 patients (median age, 74 years) with chronic AF documented by ECG tracings at least 1 month apart.
Exclusion Criteria: Lone AF in patients 60 years or younger, SBP more than 180 mm Hg, diastolic BP more than 100 mm Hg, and stroke or TIA in the prior 6 months.
Treatment: Warfarin, 1.25 mg/day; warfarin, 1.25 mg/day; and aspirin, 300 mg/day; aspirin alone; or warfarin alone (target INR, 2 to 3).
Results: Trial was terminated early because of SPAF III results. One-year cumulative primary event rates were as follows: minidose warfarin, 5.8%; warfarin plus aspirin, 7.2%; aspirin alone, 3.6%; and adjusted-dose warfarin, 2.8% ($p = 0.67$). No significant differences were seen at 3 years. Major bleeding events were rare.

Investigational Anticoagulant

36. **SPORTIF III** (Third Stroke Prevention Using Oral Direct Thrombin Inhibitor Ximelagratan in Patients with Nonvalvular AF). Preliminary results presented at the 52nd ACC Scientific Session, Chicago IL, March 2003.

This open-label, randomized, multicenter trial enrolled 3,407 patients with nonvalvular AF and at least one other stroke factor. Patients received ximelagratan, 36 mg twice daily or warfarin (goal INR 2   3; mean 2.5). At mean follow-up of 21 months, the ximelagratan group had a 1.6% annualized rate of stroke or systemic embolic events. An on-treatment analysis found a significant 41% relative risk reduction with ximelagratan (1.3% / yr vs. 2.2% / yr, $p = 0.018$). Ximelagratan was also associated with a significantly reduced risk of major or minor bleeding complications (25.5% / vs. 29.5%, $p = 0.007$); but also an increased incidence of liver enzyme elevations (6.5% vs. 0.7%, $p = 0.001$). The later typically occured between 2 and 6 months, and enzyme normalized either spontanously or after cessation of treatment.

Ventricular Arrhythmias

Immediate Therapy: Automated External Defibrillators

37. **Weaver WD,** Hill D, Fahrenbruch CE, et al. Use of the automatic external defibrillator in the management of out-of-hospital cardiac arrest. *N Engl J Med* 1988;319:661–666.

This prospective study of 1,287 consecutive cardiac arrest victims compared outcomes of defibrillation performed by first-responder firefighters using automatic external defibrillators (AEDs) with paramedics, who on average arrive on scene slightly later. Among patients for whom defibrillation was attempted, survival to hospital discharge was better when administered by firefighters (30%) than when waiting slightly longer for paramedics (19%; $p < 0.001$).

38. **Valenzuela TD,** et al. Outcomes of rapid defibrillation by security officers after cardiac arrest in casinos. *N Engl J Med* 2000;343:1206–1209.

This study tracked outcomes of treating cardiac arrest victims at a number of casinos with AEDs operated by (minimally) trained security officers. Of 105 subjects whose initial rhythm was VF, 53% survived to hospital discharge. Survival was better for witnessed than for unwitnessed arrests, and when defibrillation was performed in less than versus more than 3 minutes (74% vs. 49%). These results suggest that use of AEDs by nonmedical personnel is feasible and effective.

39. **Page RL,** et al. Automated external defibrillator use aboard a domestic airline. *N Engl J Med* 2000;343:1210–1216.

In this pilot study, AEDs were furnished aboard aircraft of one domestic U.S. carrier. The 200 AED uses were reported, 99 of them for unconscious patients. Shocks were advised and delivered by the AEDs in 14 of 14 patients with VF, and in no patients with other rhythms (sensitivity and specificity of ECG diagnostics, both 100%). Survival to hospital discharge was 40% in the VF patients. Again, the use of AEDs by nonmedical personnel was supported.

Immediate Therapy: Intravenous Amiodarone
40. **Kudenchuk PJ,** et al. Amiodarone for resuscitation after out-of-hospital cardiac arrest due to ventricular fibrillation. *N Engl J Med* 1999;341:871–878.

Design: Prospective, randomized, placebo-controlled, double-blind single-center trial. Primary end point was survival to hospital admission. Patients were followed up to hospital discharge.
Purpose: To determine whether i.v. amiodarone, compared with placebo, improved survival to hospital admission in shock-refractory VT/VF.
Population: 504 adult subjects with nontraumatic out-of-hospital cardiac arrest with ongoing pulseless VT or VF after three defibrillations.
Treatment: Epinephrine,1 mg i.v., followed by amiodarone, 300 mg given as an i.v. push, or placebo, followed by standard advanced cardiac life support (ACLS)-guided resuscitative measures.
Results: Amiodarone group had a significantly higher survival to admission compared with the placebo group (44% vs. 33%; $p = 0.03$). Amiodarone was associated with higher frequency of hypotension (59% vs. 48%; $p = 0.04$) and bradycardia (41% vs. 25%; $p = 0.004$) compared with placebo

41. **Dorian P,** et al. Amiodarone as compared with lidocaine for shock-resistant ventricular fibrillation. *N Engl J Med* 2002;346:884–890. **(ALIVE)**

Design: Prospective, randomized, double-blind, controlled, single-center study. Primary end point was survival to hospital admission.
Purpose: To compare i.v. amiodarone with lidocaine for shock-refractory VT/VF.
Population: 347 adult subjects with nontraumatic out-of-hospital cardiac arrest with ongoing pulseless VF after three defibrillations, i.v. epinephrine and a fourth defibrillation, or recurrent VF after initially successful defibrillation.
Treatment: Amiodarone, 5-mg/kg i.v. push plus lidocaine placebo, or lidocaine, 1.5-mg/kg i.v. push plus amiodarone placebo, followed by standard ACLS-guided resuscitative measures. A second dose of the same study drug (2.5 mg/kg amiodarone or 1.5 mg/kg lidocaine) could be given if VF persisted.
Results: Survival to hospital admission was better with i.v. amiodarone than with lidocaine (22.8% vs. 12.0%; $p = 0.009$). Patients treated early (less than the median of 24 minutes from ambulance dispatch to study-drug administration) had better survival than those treated late, but within this subgroup, survival remained better with amiodarone (27.7% vs. 15.3%; $p = 0.05$).

Secondary Prevention Trials: Drugs versus Implantable Cardioverter Defibrillators
42. **Kuck KH,** et al. Randomized comparison of antiarrhythmic drug therapy with implantable defibrillators in patients resuscitated from cardiac arrest: the Cardiac Arrest Study Hamburg **(CASH).** *Circulation* 2000;102:748–754 (also see *Am Heart J* 1994;127:1139).

This prospective study, initiated in 1987, initially randomized survivors of SCD in 3:1 fashion to treatment with oral propafenone, amiodarone, or metoprolol or to

ICD implantation without concomitant antiarrhythmic drugs. The propafenone arm (56 patients) was terminated in 1992 after interim analysis revealed increased all-cause mortality and sudden death (12% vs. none; $p < 0.05$) with propafenone compared with ICD over an average follow-up of only 11 months. The remaining three arms of the study enrolled a total of 288 subjects: 99 ICD, 92 amiodarone, and 97 metoprolol. Final analysis at a mean follow-up of 57 months revealed a nonsignificant reduction in all-cause mortality favoring the ICD group over the combination of the amiodarone and metoprolol arms (36% vs. 44%; one-tailed p value, 0.08). The relative improvement in survival with ICD compared with amiodarone/metoprolol was greatest at 1 year (42%), and progressively declined as the duration of follow-up lengthened.

43. **Connolly SJ**, et al. Canadian implantable defibrillator study **(CIDS):** a randomized trial of the implantable cardioverter defibrillator against amiodarone. *Circulation* 2000;101:1297–1302.

This prospective, randomized study enrolled patients with documented VF or out-of-hospital cardiac arrest without a reversible cause, VT that was poorly tolerated or occurred in the presence of LVEF less than 35%, or syncope with spontaneous or inducible VT. Patients were randomized to oral amiodarone ($n = 331$; mean dose, 255 mg/day at 5 years) or ICD implantation ($n = 328$); 90% of ICD implants were transvenous. A moderate (21% to 28%) degree of crossover between groups occurred, and sotalol and β-blockers were more frequently used by ICD patients. Reductions in total mortality (8.2% vs. 10.2% per year; $p = 0.14$) and arrhythmic death (3.0% vs. 4.5% per year; $p = 0.09$) favored the ICD arm, but did not reach statistical significance. The trend toward improved survival with ICDs was viewed as consistent with the AVID trial, in which the survival benefit did reach statistical significance.

44. The Antiarrhythmics versus Implantable Defibrillators **(AVID)** Investigators. A comparison of antiarrhythmic-drug therapy with implantable defibrillators in patients resuscitated from near-fatal ventricular arrhythmias. *N Engl J Med* 1997;337:1576–1583.

Design: Prospective, randomized, open, multicenter study. Primary end point was all-cause mortality.

Purpose: To compare the efficacy of antiarrhythmic drugs (primarily amiodarone) with ICDs for secondary prevention of SCD.

Population: 1,016 subjects resuscitated from VF (45%) or hemodynamically unstable VT (55%) not due to a transient or correctable cause, with LVEF of 40% or less. Most (81%) had a clinical history of CAD.

Exclusion Criteria: Contraindication to amiodarone or ICD implantation.

Treatment: Patients were randomly assigned to antiarrhythmic drug treatment (96% amiodarone) or ICD implantation. Nearly all ICD implants were transvenous, with many pectoral. Crossover was approximately 10% in both groups. β-Blocker use was three- to fourfold higher among ICD versus amiodarone patients.

Results: Mortality was significantly lower in the ICD group than in the antiarrhythmic drug arm at 1 year (10.7% vs. 17.7%), 2 years (18.4% vs. 25.3%), and 3 years (24.6% vs. 35.9%; $p < 0.02$).

Comments: The study was criticized for the imbalance in β-blocker use, but the core conclusion of ICD superiority remains generally accepted.

Primary Prevention Trials: Antiarrhythmic Drugs

45. The Cardiac Arrhythmia Suppression Trial **(CAST)** Investigators. Preliminary report: effect of encainide and flecainide on mortality in a randomized trial of arrhythmia suppression after myocardial infarction. *N Engl J Med* 1989;321:406–412 (see also Chapter 4, ref. 165).

In 1,727 post-MI patients, encainide and flecainide led to a significantly higher mortality rate through 10 months of follow-up (7.7% vs. 3.0% for placebo; relative risk, 2.5; 95% CI, 1.6 to 4.5). Arrhythmic death also was higher with the I-C agents than with placebo (4.5% vs. 1.2%).

46. The Cardiac Arrhythmia Suppression Trial II (CAST II) Investigators. Effect of the antiarrhythmic agent moricizine on survival after myocardial infarction. *N Engl J Med* 1992;327:227–233 (see Chapter 4, ref. 165).

CAST-II enrolled 2,699 subjects 6 to 90 days after MI with an EF of 40% or less and six or more premature ventricular contractions (PVCs)/hour. Patients were randomized to placebo or the class I-C agent moricizine in the short-term (2 weeks; $n = 1,325$) and long-term (mean, 18 months; $n = 1,374$) protocols. The study was terminated early because of increased mortality associated with moricizine use in the 14-day protocol (2.6% vs. 0.5%; adjusted $p < 0.01$). Incidence of long-term deaths was similar (15% vs. 12%). The authors concluded that the use of moricizine after MI was not only ineffective but also harmful.

47. **Waldo AL,** et al. Survival with oral D-sotalol (SWORD) investigators. Effect of D-sotalol on mortality in patients with left ventricular dysfunction after recent and remote myocardial infarction. *Lancet* 1996;348:7–12 (see Chapter 4, ref. 165).

The 3,121 post-MI patients with an EF of 40% or less and NYHA class II to III HF were randomized to D-sotalol (100 to 200 mg, b.i.d.) or placebo. The D-sotalol arm exhibited higher all-cause mortality (5.0% vs. 3.1%), cardiac mortality (4.7% vs. 2.9%), and presumed arrhythmic deaths (3.6% vs. 2.0%) at a mean follow-up of 148 days (p values all <0.01).

48. **Doval HC,** et al., for the Grupo de Estudio de la Sobrevida en la Insuficiencia Cardiaca en Argentina (GESICA) investigators. Randomised trial of low-dose amiodarone in severe congestive heart failure. *Lancet* 1994;344:493–498.

This trial randomized 516 Argentinian patients with CHF to amiodarone, 300 mg/day, or placebo. A significant proportion of patients had Chagas disease or alcoholism as the etiologies of their LV dysfunction. The trial found a nonsignificant 27% reduction in sudden death ($p = 0.16$) and a significant reduction in total mortality (33.5% vs. 41.4%; $p = 0.02$) in favor of amiodarone.

49. **Singh SN,** et al., for the Survival Trial of Antiarrhythmic Therapy in Congestive Heart Failure (CHF-STAT) Investigators. Amiodarone in patients with congestive heart failure and asymptomatic ventricular arrhythmia. *N Engl J Med* 1995;333:377–382.

Entry criteria for CHF-STAT were symptomatic CHF, EF less than 40%, more than ten PVCs/hour, and cardiac enlargement. The majority (70%) of subjects had ischemic cardiomyopathy. The 674 subjects were randomized to amiodarone (maintenance dose, 300 mg/day) or placebo and followed up for a median of 45 months. Amiodarone showed no benefit in terms of overall mortality or SCD.

50. **Julian DG,** et al. Randomised trial of effect of amiodarone on mortality in patients with left ventricular dysfunction after recent myocardial infarction: EMIAT. *Lancet* 1997;349:667–674 (see Chapter 4, ref. xx).

In 1,486 post-MI patients with an EF of 40% or less, all-cause mortality was similar for amiodarone versus placebo, but a 35% risk reduction ($p = 0.05$) occurred in arrhythmic deaths. The authors concluded that the systematic prophylactic use of amiodarone after MI (with low EF) was not indicated, but the lack of proarrhythmia supports the use of amiodarone in patients for whom antiarrhythmic therapy is indicated for other reasons.

51. **Cairns JA,** et al. Randomised trial of outcome after myocardial infarction in patients with frequent or repetitive ventricular premature depolarisations CAMIAT. *Lancet* 1997;349:675–682 (also see Chapter 4, ref. xx).

CAMIAT randomized 1,202 postinfarct patients with frequent ventricular ectopy (more than ten premature ventricular depolarizations per hour) or NSVT to amiodarone or placebo. At a mean follow-up of 1.8 years, a reduction in combined resuscitated VF or arrhythmic death was found with amiodarone (4.5% vs. 6.9%; $p = 0.03$), but no significant difference was seen in all-cause mortality.

52. **Sim I,** et al. Quantitative overview of randomized trials of amiodarone to prevent sudden cardiac death. *Circulation* 1997;96:2823–2829.

This meta-analysis pooled the results of all trials randomizing subjects to amiodarone or alternative nondevice therapy (including placebo) for the prevention of sudden death, including a minority of subjects in secondary prevention studies. Across trials, amiodarone reduced total mortality by 19% when compared with active control or "usual care" but only 10% when compared with placebo. The treatment effect of amiodarone, when pooled, appeared to be independent of the clinical population studied (post-MI, CHF, or SCD survivors).

Primary Prevention Trials: Drugs versus Implantable Cardioverter Defibrillators
53. **Moss AJ,** et al., for the Multicenter Automated Defibrillator Implantation Trial **(MADIT)** Investigators. Improved survival with an implanted defibrillator in patients with coronary disease at high risk for ventricular arrhythmia. *N Engl J Med* 1996;335:1933–1940.

Design: Prospective, randomized, open, multicenter trial. The primary end point was all-cause mortality. Average follow-up was 27 months.
Purpose: To compare the efficacy of ICDs with standard medical therapy (generally including antiarrhythmic drugs) for primary prevention of SCD in coronary patients at high risk for SCD.
Population: 196 Adult patients with prior MI, documented NSVT, EF of 35% or less, and inducible VT or VF at EPS, not suppressible with i.v. procainamide.
Exclusion Criteria: Included previous cardiac arrest or VT with syncope; symptomatic hypotension; MI within 3 weeks; CABG surgery within 2 months; or PTCA within 3 months.
Treatment: Patients were randomly assigned to ICD implantation (50% transthoracic, 50% transvenous) or standard medical therapy. In the standard therapy group, 74% received amiodarone, 10% received type I antiarrhythmic drugs, and 7% received sotalol.
Results: Study enrollment was terminated prematurely when interim analysis passed prespecified stopping criteria. At follow-up, the mortality rate was 17% in the defibrillator group versus 39% in the conventional therapy group, a 54% reduction ($p = 0.009$).

54. **Buxton AE,** et al., for the Multicenter Unsustained Tachycardia Trial **(MUSTT)** Investigators. A randomized study of the prevention of sudden death in patients with coronary artery disease. *N Engl J Med* 1999;341:1882–1890.

Design: Prospective, randomized, open, multicenter trial. Primary end point was cardiac arrest or death from arrhythmia. Median follow-up duration was 39 months.
Purpose: To compare the efficacy of electrophysiologically guided therapy (antiarrhythmic drugs or ICDs if drugs failed) with standard medical therapy (not including antiarrhythmic drugs) for primary prevention of SCD in coronary patients at high risk for SCD.
Population: Adult patients with prior MI, documented NSVT, EF of 40% or less, and inducible VT or VF at EPS. Noninducible patients were followed up in a voluntary registry. The 704 inducible patients were randomized.
Exclusion Criteria: Syncope, sustained VT, or VF more than 48 hours after an acute MI; untreated exercise-induced ischemia.
Treatment: Standard medical therapy (not including antiarrhythmic drugs) or therapy based on serial EP testing, which consisted of an antiarrhythmic drug that suppressed VT inducibility, amiodarone (if two previous drug trials failed), or an ICD. Initially, ICDs were reserved for patients with three or more unsuccessful drug trials, but halfway through enrollment, this was relaxed to one or more. Ultimately, 46% of the EP-guided patients were discharged with ICDs, and 45% were treated with drugs: 26% class I, 10% amiodarone, 9% sotalol.
Results: Overall, the EP group showed a lower rate of cardiac arrest or arrhythmic death ($p = 0.04$) and lower total mortality (hazard ratio, 0.80; $p = 0.06$). However,

all the benefit was achieved among patients who had received an ICD (total mortality, 24% at 5 years), whereas patients treated with EP-guided antiarrhythmic drug therapy had a slightly higher mortality rate (55% at 5 years) compared with standard medical therapy without antiarrhythmic drugs (48%).

55. **Moss AJ,** et al., for The Multicenter Automatic Defibrillator Implantation Trial II **(MADIT II)** Investigators. Prophylactic implantation of a defibrillator in patients with myocardial infarction and reduced ejection fraction. *N Engl J Med* 2002;346:877–883.

Design: Prospective, randomized, open, multicenter trial. Primary end point was all-cause mortality. Average follow-up, 20 months.

Purpose: To compare the efficacy of ICDs with conventional medical therapy (primarily without antiarrhythmic drugs) for primary prevention of SCD in coronary patients at high risk for SCD.

Population: Adult patients with prior MI and EF of 30% or less.

Exclusion Criteria: FDA-approved indication for ICD implantation; NYHA class IV CHF; MI within 1 month; coronary revascularization procedure within 3 months; or other life-threatening condition.

Treatment: Patients were randomly assigned in 3:2 ratio to ICD implantation (all transvenous) or standard medical therapy. Amiodarone was used by 13% of ICD subjects and 10% of conventional therapy subjects at last study contact. Use of other cardiac medications, including β-blockers and ACE inhibitors, was well balanced between groups.

Results: Total mortality was 19.8% in the conventional therapy group and 14.2% in the ICD group (hazard ratio, 0.69; $p = 0.016$). Benefits were consistent across all subgroups. A trend toward an increased rate of hospitalization for CHF was seen in the ICD group (19.9% vs. 14.9%; $p = 0.09$); this finding may be related to ventricular pacing worsening CHF by creating dyssynchrony in the heart (also see DAVID results, ref. 63).

Comments: Based on these results, the updated ACC/AHA Guidelines include ICD implantation in post-MI patients with LVEF 30% or less as a class IIa recommendation.

Primary-prevention Trials: Noncoronary Cardiomyopathy Patients

56. **AMIOVERT.** Preliminary results presented at the Annual Scientific Session of American Heart Association, New Orleans, LA, November 2000.

This prospective study randomized 103 patients with nonischemic cardiomyopathy and asymptomatic NSVT to ICD implantation or oral amiodarone. An additional 75 patients who refused randomization were followed up in a registry. At 2 years, all-cause mortality was 11% in the ICD group and 12% in the amiodarone group ($p = $ NS). This was the first randomized comparison of amiodarone with ICDs in cardiomyopathy patients, but was probably underpowered to find a small difference in outcome.

57. **Bansch D,** et al., for the Cardiomyopathy Trial **(CAT)** Investigators. Primary prevention of sudden cardiac death in idiopathic dilated cardiomyopathy. *Circulation* 2002;105:1453–1458.

This prospective, randomized, multicenter trial enrolled 104 patients with recent onset of DCM (9 months or less), LVEF 30% or less, and in NYHA class II or III. CAD had to be excluded by angiography. Other exclusion criteria included history of MI, symptomatic bradycardia, VT, or VF. Patients were randomized to ICD or control. Trial was terminated early because 1-year mortality did not reach 30% in the control group. At mean follow-up of 5.5 years, no significant difference in mortality rates was found between the two groups (26.0% vs. 31.5%). The only predictor of mortality was impaired LVEF.

58. **Bardy GH,** et al., for the SCD-HeFT Pilot Investigators. Interim publication of results. *PACE Pacing Clin Electrophysiol* 1997;20(II):1148. (Sudden Cardiac Death in Heart Failure: **SCD-HeFT.**)

Entry criteria for SCD-HeFT include an EF of 35% of less and NYHA class II to III CHF. The cause of LV dysfunction could be either coronary or noncoronary; a significant proportion of both have been enrolled. This NHLBI-sponsored trial, which began in January 1997, has randomized an estimated 2,500 subjects to ICD or amiodarone versus placebo.

Cardiac Pacing Studies

Guidelines
59. **Gregoratos G,** et al., **ACC/AHA/NASPE 2002 Guideline** update for implantation of cardiac pacemakers and antiarrhythmia devices. Summary article: a report of the American College of Cardiology/American Heart Association Task Force on Practice Guidelines (ACC/AHA/NASPE Committee to Update the 1998 Pacemaker Guidelines). *Circulation* 2002;106:2145–2161.

Two notable changes to these updated guidelines are that the following are now considered class IIa recommendations: BiV pacing in selected patients with HF, and ICD therapy for patients with a LVEF of 30% or less at least 1 month after MI.

Mode-Selection Trials
60. **Andersen HR,** et al. Prospective randomized trial of atrial versus ventricular pacing in sick-sinus syndrome. *Lancet* 1994;344:1523–1528.

This Danish trial randomized 225 patients with sick-sinus syndrome to atrial or ventricular pacing. During the initially reported follow-up period (mean, 40 months), atrially paced patients had significantly less AF. This was associated with a reduction in stroke or peripheral arterial embolic events, which occurred in 20 patients in the ventricular group and in six patients in the atrial group ($p < 0.01$). At longer-term follow-up of 8 years, the benefits in AF and thromboembolic complications persisted (see *Lancet* 1997;350:2010). In addition, significant reductions were seen in total mortality (35% vs. 50%; $p = 0.045$) and HF severity.

61. **Lamas GA,** et al., for the Pacemaker Selection in the Elderly **(PASE)** Investigators. Quality of life and clinical outcomes in elderly patients treated with ventricular pacing as compared with dual-chamber pacing. *N Engl J Med* 1998;338:1097–1104.

This prospective, randomized, single-blinded, multicenter trial enrolled 407 patients older than 65 years who received dual-chamber pacemakers for bradycardia. Patients were then randomly assigned to a dual-chamber or ventricular-pacing mode. No significant differences between pacing modes were found for the primary end point of QOL or secondary end points of stroke or death. In patients with sinus node dysfunction, a trend toward less AF was seen with dual-chamber versus ventricular pacing (19% vs. 28%; $p = 0.06$). In addition, 26% of subjects assigned to ventricular pacing crossed over to dual-chamber pacing because of the symptoms of the pacemaker syndrome.

62. **Connolly SJ,** et al., for Canadian Trial of Physiologic Pacing **(CTOPP)** Investigators. Effects of physiologic pacing versus ventricular pacing on the risk of stroke and death due to cardiovascular causes. *N Engl J Med* 2000;342:1385–1391.

Design: Prospective, randomized, multicenter trial. Primary end point was stroke or cardiovascular death.

Purpose: To determine the benefits of physiologic (atrial or dual-chamber) pacing compared with ventricular pacing in patients with symptomatic bradycardia.

Population: 2,568 patients undergoing initial implantation of a permanent pacemaker for symptomatic bradycardia. Approximately 60% of patients had AV block, and 40% had sinus node dysfunction.

Exclusion Criteria: Chronic/persistent AF, prior AV junction ablation, limited life expectancy.

Treatment: Implantation of physiologic (atrial or dual-chamber) or ventricular pacing system.

Results: At 3 years, no significant difference was found in the primary end point of stroke or cardiovascular death between physiologic and ventricular pacing groups (4.9% vs. 5.5%). No significant differences in total mortality or CHF admission rates were seen. Physiologic pacing was associated with an 18% reduction in the incidence of AF (5.3%/year vs. 6.6%/year; $p = 0.05$).

63. **Lamas GA,** et al., for the Mode Selection Trial in Sinus-node Dysfunction **(MOST)** Investigators. Ventricular pacing or dual-chamber pacing for sinus-node dysfunction. *N Engl J Med* 2002;346:1854–1862.

Design: Prospective, randomized, multicenter study. Primary end point was death or nonfatal stroke.
Purpose: To determine the benefits of dual-chamber pacing compared with ventricular pacing in patients with sinus node dysfunction.
Population: 2,010 patients undergoing initial implantation of a dual-chamber pacemaker for sinus node dysfunction. Patients were required to be in SR at the time of randomization, but 45% had a history of AF.
Exclusion Criteria: Serious concurrent illness.
Treatment: All patients had dual-chamber pacemakers implanted, and then were randomized to dual-chamber (DDD) or ventricular (VVI) pacing modes.
Results: No difference was found between study groups in the incidence of death or nonfatal stroke. In adjusted analyses, small benefits favoring dual-chamber pacing were found for the secondary end points of hospitalization for HF (hazard ratio, 0.73; $p = 0.02$) and death, stroke, or hospitalization for HF (hazard ratio, 0.85; $p = 0.05$). Dual-chamber pacing was also associated with a lower incidence of any AF (hazard ratio, 0.79; $p = 0.008$) and progression to chronic AF (15% vs. 27% of those who had any AF; $p < 0.001$), and greater improvements in several QOL measures than with ventricular pacing. At the last follow-up, 31% of subjects originally assigned to ventricular pacing had crossed over to dual-chamber, about half of them for strictly defined pacemaker syndrome.
Comments: A subsequent secondary analysis revealed, as in MOST, a reduction not only in the incidence of AF with dual-chamber pacing, but also in the progression to chronic AF (2.8%/year vs. 3.8%/year with VVI pacing; $p = 0.016$) [see *J Am Coll Cardiol* 2001;38:167].

64. **Wilkoff BL,** et al., Dual Chamber and VVI Implantable Defibrillator **(DAVID)** Trial Investigators. Dual-chamber pacing or ventricular backup pacing in patients with an implantable defibrillator: the Dual Chamber and VVI Implantable Defibrillator (DAVID) Trial. *JAMA* 2002;288:3115–3123.

Design: Prospective, randomized, single-blind, parallel-group, multicenter trial. Primary end point was composite of death or first hospitalization for CHF.
Purpose: To determine the efficacy of dual-chamber pacing compared with backup ventricular pacing in patients with standard indications for ICD implantation but without indications for antibradycardia pacing.
Population: 506 patients with LVEF of 40% or less, no indication for antibradycardia pacemaker therapy, and no persistent atrial arrhythmias.
Treatment: All had an ICD with dual-chamber, rate-responsive pacing capability implanted. ICDs programmed to ventricular backup pacing at 40 per minute (VVI-40) or dual-chamber rate-responsive pacing at 70 per minute (DDDR-70).
Results: The VVI-40 group had a better 1-year survival free of composite end point [83.9% vs. 73.3% (for patients DDDR-70); relative hazard, 1.61; 95% CI, 1.06 to 2.44]. A trend toward lower mortality in the VVI-40 group was noted (6.5% vs. 10.1%; relative hazard, 1.61; 95% CI, 0.84 to 3.09).

Pacing for Vasovagal Syncope
65. **Connolly SJ,** et al., for the North American Vasovagal Pacemaker Study **(VPS)** Investigators. A randomized trial of permanent cardiac pacing for the prevention of vasovagal syncope. *J Am Coll Cardiol* 1999;33:16–20.

Design: Prospective, randomized, open, multicenter study. Primary end point was time to first recurrence of syncope.

Purpose: To determine whether permanent pacemakers with rate-drop algorithms can reduce the frequency of vasovagal syncope.

Population: 54 patients with six or more prior syncopal episodes and a positive head-up tilt-table test, with syncope or presyncope and "relative bradycardia" (definition differed depending on whether test was performed with isoproterenol).

Treatment: Pacemaker implantation or continuation of medical therapy (not standardized).

Results: Study was terminated prematurely at first interim data analysis when a large treatment effect favoring pacemaker implantation was observed. Syncope had occurred in 19 (70%) of 27 no-pacemaker patients and only six (22%) of 27 pacemaker patients ($p < 0.001$). Time to first recurrence was 54 days in the no-pacemaker group and 112 days in the pacemaker group. Additional reductions in the rate of presyncopal events were seen in the pacemaker group, but were not statistically significant.

66. **Connelly SJ,** et al., for the Second North American Vasovagal Pacemaker Study Investigators **(VPS-II).** Pacemaker therapy for prevention of syncope in patients with recurrent severe vasovagal syncope. *JAMA* 2003;289:2224–2229.

Design: Prospective, randomized, double-blind, multicenter study. Primary endpoint was time to first recurrence of syncope.

Purpose: To determine if pacing therapy reduces the risk of syncope in patients with vasovagal syncope.

Population: 100 patients with six or more prior syncopal episodes or ≥ 3 in prior two years and a positive tilt table test.

Treatment: Dual-chamber pacing (DDD) with rate drop response or (ODO).

Results: At 6 months, the cumulative risk of syncope was 40% for the ODO group and 31% for the DDD group. There was a nonsignificant 30% relative risk reduction in time to syncope with DDD pacing ($p = 0.14$). Lead dislodgement or repositioning occurred in 7 patients.

Pacing for Prevention of Atrial Fibrillation

67. **Carlson MD,** et al., Atrial Dynamic Overdrive Pacing Trial **(ADOPT).** Preliminary results presented at North American Society for Pacing and Electrophysiology (NASPE) Scientific Sessions, Boston, MA, 2001.

This study tested a specific pacing algorithm designed to pace the atrium above patients' intrinsic sinus rates to suppress AF, which is often triggered by atrial ectopic beats. Patients with sinus node dysfunction and two or more episodes of AF in the preceding month were randomized to dual-chamber pacing with or without this algorithm. Investigators reported an approximate 25% reduction in the "burden of AF."

68. **Fan K,** et al. Effects of biatrial pacing in prevention of postoperative atrial fibrillation after coronary artery bypass surgery. *Circulation* 2000;102:755–760.

In a cohort of 132 patients undergoing CABG surgery at a single center, patients were randomized to right atrial pacing (RA), left atrial pacing (LA), biatrial pacing (BA) or no pacing after surgery. Overdrive pacing at 90 beats/min or 10 beats/min above the intrinsic rate up to 120 beats/min was performed for 5 days in the active-pacing arms. Rates of AF lasting 10 or more minutes or requiring intervention were 12.5% in the BA group and 36%, 33%, and 42% in the LA, RA, and no-pacing groups, respectively ($p < 0.05$ for all comparisons). Total length of stay was reduced about 2 days in the BA-pacing group, compared with the no-pacing group.

69. **Greenberg MD,** et al. Atrial pacing for the prevention of atrial fibrillation after cardiovascular surgery. *J Am Coll Cardiol* 2000;35:1416–1422.

Another single-center study randomized 154 cardiac surgery (CABG and valve replacement) patients to RA, LA, BA, or no pacing for 72 hours after surgery at rates of 100 to 110 beats/min. β-Blocker use was strongly encouraged. AF lasting 1 hour or more and requiring urgent intervention occurred in 37.5% of subjects with no pacing, but in 8%, 20%, and 26% of subjects in the RA, LA, and BA groups, respectively. Thus all pacing patients combined were significantly less likely to have AF than were no-pacing patients (17% vs. 37.5%; $p < 0.005$), but in contrast to the previously mentioned study by Fan K, et al., biatrial pacing was no better than RA pacing.

70. **Saksena S,** et al. Improved suppression of recurrent atrial fibrillation with dual-site right atrial pacing and antiarrhythmic drug therapy (Dual-site Atrial Pacing for Prevention of Atrial Fibrillation, **DAPPAF**). *J Am Coll Cardiol* 2002;40:1140–1150.

This prospective, randomized, single blind, crossover study enrolled patients had dual-chamber pacemakers implanted, with two atrial leads: one in the traditional high RA position, and one in the low RA, outside the ostium of the coronary sinus. Patients were then assigned to one of three pacing modes: high RA overdrive, dual-site RA overdrive, or "support" (DDI or VDI at suggested rate of 50 beats/min) for 6 months, and then crossed over in random sequence to each of the other modes. Dislodgement of the "extra" low RA lead was infrequent (1.7%). As expected, the "support" mode of pacing did the worst in terms of tolerability and rate of recurrent AF. Patients in the dual-site RA group were somewhat less likely to cross over because of mode intolerance than were patients in the high-RA group (time to crossover, 5.8 vs. 4.7 months; $p < 0.01$) but had a similar proportion of mode-related adverse events. For the entire cohort, no significant difference was found between the dual-site and high-RA pacing groups for freedom from symptomatic AF or time to AF recurrence. *Post hoc* subgroup analysis did suggest the superiority of dual-site over high-RA pacing for AF suppression in patients with one or more AF episodes per week (hazard ratio, 0.62; $p = 0.006$), whereas a trend only was seen for patients taking antiarrhythmic drugs (hazard ratio, 0.67; $p = 0.06$).

Resynchronization Therapy for Congestive Heart Failure

71. **Auricchio A,** et al. Effect of pacing chamber and atrioventricular delay on acute systolic function of paced patients with congestive heart failure: the Pacing Therapies for Congestive Heart Failure (**PATH-CHF**) Study Group. *Circulation* 1999;99:2993–3001.

This single-blind study enrolled 42 patients with NYHA class III to IV CHF, EF less than 35%, and QRS durations greater than 120 milliseconds, mostly due to left bundle branch block. All patients received BiV systems with the LV lead placed via limited thoracotomy. After implantation, the immediate hemodynamic performances of three different pacing modes (RV, LV, and BiV) were compared: LV pacing alone appeared most favorable. Patients then entered a 3-month crossover phase to select the optimal mode for the long-term phase, followed by a 12-month period of active pacing. At 12 months, BiV and LV pacing, compared with baseline, were associated with statistically significant improvements in 6-minute walk (446 vs. 357 m; $p < 0.001$); peak oxygen consumption (1.19 vs. 0.97 L/min; $p = 0.019$); anaerobic threshold (0.91 vs. 0.76 L/min; $p = 0.018$); NYHA class (1.90 vs. 3.05; $p < 0.001$); and QOL (20 vs. 49; $p < 0.001$).

72. **Gras D,** et al. Cardiac resynchronization therapy in advanced heart failure: the multicenter InSync clinical study (**InSync**). *Eur J Heart Fail* 2002;4:311–320.

InSync was a nonrandomized study of BiV pacing, with all leads introduced transvenously. In the 103 subjects enrolled, on-treatment improvements (vs. baseline) were noted in NYHA class, QOL, and 6-minute walk. About half of the patients also had serial echocardiograms, and showed an increase in LVEF from 22% to 26% ($p = 0.006$). Only one procedure-related complication occurred.

73. **Cazeau S,** et al., for the Multisite Stimulation in Cardiomyopathies (**MUSTIC**) Study Investigators. Effects of multisite biventricular pacing in patients with heart failure and intraventricular conduction delay. *N Engl J Med* 2001;344:873–880.

Design: Prospective, randomized, single-blind, crossover, multicenter study. Primary end point was the 6-minute walk test.

Purpose: To assess the clinical benefits of BiV pacing (compared with no pacing) in HF patients with electrical conduction delays.

Population: 67 patients in SR with persistent NYHA class III symptoms despite optimal medical therapy; EF less than 35%; LVEDD, more than 60 mm; QRS duration of >150 milliseconds; and no other indication for pacemaker implantation. Nine patients withdrew before randomization, and 10 failed to complete both study phases.

Exclusion Criteria: Included hypertrophic or restrictive cardiomyopathy; treatable valve disease; acute myocarditis; recent acute coronary syndrome or revascularization procedure; approved indication for ICD implantation.

Treatment: All patients had fully transvenous BiV pacing systems implanted, with RA and RV endocardial leads and LV leads introduced via coronary sinus branches. Two weeks after implant, patients were randomized to consecutive 3-month periods of "inactive" pacing (VVI at 40 beats/min) or "active" pacing in a crossover design. Optimal AV delay for active pacing was determined by echocardiographic evaluation at the time of implant.

Results: Initial implantation success rate was 92%. Early lead dislodgement occurred in eight patients and was corrected in all but three. Active pacing, as compared with "inactive," resulted in significant improvement in the average distance walked in 6 minutes (399 vs. 325 m; $p < 0.001$). Active pacing also was associated with a 32% improvement in the QOL score ($p < 0.001$), and an 8% increase in maximal oxygen consumption ($p < 0.03$).

Comments: Similar benefits with BiV pacing were seen in 64 patients with chronic atrial fibrillation (see *Circulation* 2000;102:3349A).

74. **Abraham WT,** et al., for the Multicenter InSync Randomized Clinical Evaluation **(MIRACLE)** Study Group. Cardiac resynchronization in chronic heart failure. *N Engl J Med* 2002;346:1845–1853.

Design: Prospective, randomized, double-blind, controlled, multicenter trial. Primary end points were 6-minute walk, NYHA class, and QOL score.

Purpose: To assess the safety and efficacy of biventricular pacing, compared with no pacing, in CHF patients with intraventricular conduction delay.

Population: 453 NYHA class III to IV patients with EF of 35% or less, LVEDD, 55 mm or more; QRS duration of 130 milliseconds or more, and 6-minute walking distance of 450 m or less.

Treatment: All received transvenous BiV pacing systems and then were randomized to active pacing (atrially synchronized BiV pacing) or no pacing for 6 months.

Results: Initial implantation success rate was approximately 92%; 30 patients required subsequent repositioning or replacement of the LV pacing lead. Compared with the control group, patients successfully treated with BiV pacing had significantly greater improvements in 6-minute walking distance (+39 vs. +10 meters; $p = 0.005$); peak oxygen consumption (+1.1 vs. +0.2 mL/kg/min; $p = 0.009$); QOL (−18 vs. −9 points; $p = 0.001$); time on treadmill (+81 vs. +19 seconds; $p = 0.001$); and EF (+4.6% vs. −0.2%; $p < 0.001$). In addition, a significantly larger proportion of BiV patients improved one or more NYHA classes (68% vs. 38%; $p < 0.001$), and significantly fewer were hospitalized for worsening heart failure (hazard ratio, 0.50; $p = 0.02$).

75. **Young JB,** et al. Combined cardiac resynchronization and implantable cardioversion defibrillation in advanced chronic heart failure. The **MIRACLE ICD** trial. *JAMA* 2003;289:2685–2694.

Design: Prospective, randomized, double-blind, parallel-controlled, multicenter trial. Primary endpoints were changes between baseline and 6 months in quality of life (QOL), functional class, and 6 minute walk distance.

Purpose: To examine the efficacy and safety of combined CRT and ICD therapy in patients with NYHA Class III or IV CHF despite appropriate medical therapy.

Population: 369 patients with LVEF 35% or less, QRS duration of 130 msec, at high risk of life-insectening ventricular arrhythmeas, and in NYHA Class III or IV.

Treatment: All with ICD activated. Control group with cardiac resynchronization therapy (CRT) off.

Results: CRT group had a greater improvement in median QOL seuere ($p = 0.02$) and functional class ($p = 0.007$) compared to control group but there was no significant difference in change in 6 minute walk distance (55 m vs. 53 in, $p = 0.36$). CRT group did have a significant increse in peak oxygen consumption ($+ 1.1$ mL/kg/min vs. 0.1 [controls], $p = 0.04$).

76. **COMPANION** (Comparison of Medical Therapy, Pacing, and Defibrillation in Chronic Heart Failure. Preliminary results presented at 52nd ACC Scientific sessions, Chicago IL, March 2003.

This prospective, randomized, multicenter trial enrolled 1,600 patients with moderate or severe heart failure with QRS > 120 m sec and PR interval > 150 m sec. Patients were assigned in 1:2:2 fashion to optimal medical therapy, optimal drugs plus CRT, or optimal drugs plus CRT with ICD (CRT-D). At 1 year, the CRT and CRT-D groups had a significant 19% reduction in death or all cause hospitalization mortality was reduced by 43.4%. with CRT-D and a nonsignificant 23.9% with CRT alone. The CRT-D mortality benefit was similar in those with ischemic and nonishemic etiologies.

SUBJECT INDEX

A

Abciximab
  comparison with eptifibatide, 81
  as myocardial infarction treatment, 208–209
    comparison with stenting, 206
  in non–ST-elevation myocardial infarction, 164, 166
  as restenosis prophylaxis, 86
  as unstable angina treatment, 164, 166
  use in percutaneous coronary intervention patients, 77, 78, 80, 81
Abciximab before Direct Angiography and Stenting in MI Regarding Acute and Long-term Follow-up (ADMIRAL) trial, 208
Abdominojugular test, 290
Ablation
  atrioventricular junction, 327–328
  catheter-based, as atrial fibrillation treatment, 326
Abrupt closure, percutaneous coronary interventions-related, 84
N-Acetylcysteine (Mucomyst), renoprotective effects of, 85
ACME (Angioplasty Compared to Medicine) study, 81
ACS Multilink Coronary Stent Trial (ASCENT), 76
Acute coronary syndrome, plaque rupture associated with, 160
ACUTE II (Antithrombotic Combination Using Tirofiban and Enoxaparin) study, 165
Acute Infarction Ramipril Efficacy (AIRE) trial, 200, 293
Acute Myocardial Infarction Study of Adenosine (AMISTAD) trials, 210
Adenosine, as myocardial infarction treatment, 199t, 210
ADMIRAL (Abciximab before Direct Angiography and Stenting in MI Regarding Acute and Long-term Follow-up) trial, 208
Adrenergic agents, as congestive heart failure treatment, 292
AFASAK (Atrial Fibrillation, Aspirin, Anticoagulation) studies, 327t
AFCAPS/TexCAPS (Air Force/Texas Coronary Atherosclerosis Prevention study), 6, 15–16
AFFIRM (Atrial Fibrillation Follow-up Investigation of Rhythm Management) trial, 323
African American Study of Kidney Disease and Hypertension (ASSK) study, 11–12
AFTER (Aspirin/Anticoagulants Following Thrombolysis with Eminase in Recurrent Infarction) trial, 207
Aging, as cardiovascular disease risk factor, 13
AIRE (Acute Infarction Ramipril Efficacy) trial, 200, 293
Air Force/Texas Coronary Atherosclerosis Prevention (AFCAPS/TexCAPS) study, 6, 15–16
Alcohol intoxication, as atrial fibrillation cause, 321, 322
Alcohol use
  cardioprotective effects of, 13
  as hypertension cause, 10
Aldosterone antagonists, as congestive heart failure treatment, 296
ALIVE (Amiodarone as compared with lidocaine for shock-resistant ventricular fibrillation) trial, 328
Allergic reactions, to contrast agents, 74, 85
ALLHAT (Antihypertensive and Lipid-Lowering Treatment to Prevent Heart Attack Trial), 11
Alpha-Tocopherol Beta-Carotene Cancer Prevention (ATBC) trial, 2, 4
Alteplase, as myocardial infarction treatment, 202

American College of Cardiology, atrial fibrillation treatment guidelines of, 322
American College of Cardiology/American Heart Association
  antiplatelet and anticoagulant therapy guidelines of, 163, 164t
  exercise treadmill testing guidelines of, 169
American College of Cardiology/American Heart Association Classification, of stenosis morphology, 72
American Diabetes Association, 9
American Heart Association
  atrial fibrillation treatment guidelines of, 322
  omega-3 fatty acid supplementation recommendation of, 4
AMIGO (Atherectomy before Multilink Improves Lumen Gain and Clinical Outcomes) trial, 88
Amiodarone
  antiarrhythmic activity, in cardiac disease patients, 330
  as atrial fibrillation treatment, 323–324, 325
  as congestive heart failure treatment, 295, 296
  as immediate cardiac arrest treatment, 328
  implantable cardioverter defibrillator therapy versus, 328, 329t
  as myocardial infarction treatment, 199t
  as postoperative atrial fibrillation prophylaxis, 322–323
Amiodarone as compared with lidocaine for shock-resistant ventricular fibrillation (ALIVE) trial, 328
AMISTAD (Acute Myocardial Infarction Study of Adenosine) trials, 210
Amlodipine, as hypertension treatment, 11
AMRO (Amsterdam-Rotterdam) trial, 89
Analgesia, as myocardial infarction treatment, 210
Anemia, as congestive heart failure cause, 290
Aneurysm, coronary, stent-based exclusion of, 76
Angina
  stable, percutaneous transluminal coronary angioplasty treatment for, 81
  unstable
    clinical and laboratory findings in, 162–163
    epidemiology of, 160
    invasive treatment of, 167–168
    medical treatment of, 163–167
    noninvasive evaluation of, 168–169
    pathophysiology of, 160
    percutaneous coronary interventions in, 82
    prognosis, 169
    risk estimation in, 162–163, 163f
Angina with Extremely Serious Operative Mortality Evaluation (AWESOME) study, 91
Angiography, coronary
  indications for, 72
Angiography, coronary. See also Percutaneous transluminal coronary angiography
  in non–ST-elevation myocardial infarction, 167–168
  quantitative, 74
  in unstable angina, 167–168
Angioplasty Compared to Medicine (ACME) study, 81
Angioseal, 74
Angiotensin-converting enzyme inhibitors
  as congestive heart failure treatment, 292–293, 293t
  as hypertension treatment, 11
    in diabetes-associated hypertension, 9
  as myocardial infarction treatment, 199t, 200
  as restenosis prophylactic, 86
Angiotensin II-receptor antagonists
  as congestive heart failure treatment, 293–294
  as diabetes-associated hypertension treatment, 9
  as myocardial infarction treatment, 200

TRIAL ACRONYM INDEX